Encyclopedia of Diabetic Retinopathy

Encyclopedia of Diabetic Retinopathy

Edited by **Abigail Gipe**

FOSTER ACADEMICS

New Jersey

Published by Foster Academics,
61 Van Reypen Street,
Jersey City, NJ 07306, USA
www.fosteracademics.com

Encyclopedia of Diabetic Retinopathy
Edited by Abigail Gipe

International Standard Book Number: 978-1-63242-135-7 (Hardback)

Printed in China.

Contents

	Preface	**IX**
Part 1	**Pathophysiology/Basic Research**	**1**
Chapter 1	**Diabetic Retinopathy** Carlos César Lopes De Jesus	**3**
Chapter 2	**Gluco-Oxidation of Proteins in Etiology of Diabetic Retinopathy** Mohd Wajid Ali Khan, Kamalpreet Banga and Wahid Ali Khan	**17**
Chapter 3	**Cellular and Molecular Mechanism of Diabetic Retinopathy** Mohammad Shamsul Ola and Mohd Imtiaz Nawaz	**39**
Chapter 4	**Inner Blood-Retinal Barrier Transporters: Relevance to Diabetic Retinopathy** Yoshiyuki Kubo and Ken-ichi Hosoya	**67**
Chapter 5	**The Molecular Pathogenesis of Diabetic Retinopathy - A Spectrum of Pathology Caused by the Disruption of Inner Blood-Retinal Barrier** Byung Joo Lee, and Jeong Hun Kim	**85**
Chapter 6	**Fibrovascular Membranes Associated with PDR: Development of Molecular Targets by Global Gene Expression Profiling** Shigeo Yoshida, Keijiro Ishikawa, Mitsuru Arima, Ryo Asato, Yukio Sassa and Tatsuro Ishibashi	**109**
Part 2	**Inflammation and Angiogenesis**	**123**
Chapter 7	**Immunological Risk Factors for the Development and Progression of Diabetic Retinopathy** Katarzyna Zorena, Dorota Raczyńska, and Krystyna Raczyńska	**125**

Chapter 8 **Inflammation and Diabetic Retinopathy** **151**
Hongbin Lü

Chapter 9 **Inflammation and Angiogenesis in Diabetic Retinopathy** **163**
Ying Yang, Ying Zhang and Yiping Li

Part 3 Clinical Aspects of Diabetic Retinopathy and Retinal Functions **191**

Chapter 10 **Diabetic Macular Edema** **193**
Christina Antonopoulos and Manju Subramanian

Chapter 11 **Optical Coherence Tomography Findings in Diabetic Macular Edema** **207**
Desislava Koleva-Georgieva

Chapter 12 **The Effect of Diabetes Mellitus on Retinal Function** **231**
Zvia Burgansky-Eliash

Chapter 13 **Preventing Diabetic Retinopathy: Red Lesions Detection in Early Stages** **249**
C. Mariño, J. Novo, N. Barreira and M.G. Penedo

Part 4 Emerging Treatments and Concepts in Diabetic Retinopathy **271**

Chapter 14 **Prophylactic Medical Treatment of Diabetic Retinopathy** **273**
Akihiro Kakehashi, Ayumi Ota, Fumihiko Toyoda, Nozomi Kinoshita, Hiroko Yamagami, Hiroto Obata, Takafumi Matsumoto, Junichi Tsuji, Yoh Dobashi, Wilfred Y. Fujimoto, Masanobu Kawakami and Yasunori Kanazawa

Chapter 15 **Treatment of Diabetic Macular Edema - Latest Therapeutic Developments** **287**
Yeon Sung Moon and Na Rae Kim

Chapter 16 **Calcium Dobesilate in Prevention and Treatment of Diabetic Retinopathy** **305**
Oldřich Farsa

Chapter 17 **The Role of Sex Hormones in Diabetic Retinopathy** **331**
Jeffery G. Grigsby, Donald M. Allen, Richard B. Culbert,
Gerardo Escobedo, Kalpana Parvathaneni,
Brandi S. Betts and Andrew T.C. Tsin

Permissions

List of Contributors

Preface

Every book is a source of knowledge and this one is no exception. The idea that led to the conceptualization of this book was the fact that the world is advancing rapidly; which makes it crucial to document the progress in every field. I am aware that a lot of data is already available, yet, there is a lot more to learn. Hence, I accepted the responsibility of editing this book and contributing my knowledge to the community.

The purpose of this book is to present an elaborative analysis of latest concepts in pathogenesis, diagnosis and treatments of diabetic retinopathy. It encompasses a compilation of topics written by veteran authors, highlighting discussions on developments in comprehension of pathophysiology, growing concepts and immunological factors, considering clinical aspects and treatment techniques. The aim of this book is to serve as an efficient source of knowledge and enhance diagnosis and treatment options for those patients who face vision loss due to diabetic retinopathy.

While editing this book, I had multiple visions for it. Then I finally narrowed down to make every chapter a sole standing text explaining a particular topic, so that they can be used independently. However, the umbrella subject sinews them into a common theme. This makes the book a unique platform of knowledge.

I would like to give the major credit of this book to the experts from every corner of the world, who took the time to share their expertise with us. Also, I owe the completion of this book to the never-ending support of my family, who supported me throughout the project.

Editor

Part 1

Pathophysiology/Basic Research

1

Diabetic Retinopathy

Carlos César Lopes De Jesus
Federal University of Sao Paulo, Sao Paulo, Brazil

1. Introduction

Diabetes mellitus is a group of metabolic disorders characterized by chronic hyperglicemia resulting from peripheral resistance to insulin, reduction of pancreatic secretion of such substance and increase of glycosis hepatic production, causing, after a long time, a series of complications (1).

Clinical diabetes complications may affect the great and medium arteries - causing coronary artery disease and peripheral artery disease - or the little arteries, causing diabetic microangiopathy – retinopathy, nephropathy and neuropathy (2,3).

2. Pathophisiology

Elevated glycemia induces a series of bichemical and cellular abnormalities which may cause vascular alterations found in diabetic retinopathy (4,5,6). Mechanisms induced by hyperglycemia which can cause endothelial cells dysfunction include increase of polyol pathway flux, accelerated and non-enzimatic formation of advanced glycation end-products (AGES), increase in diacylglycerol formation (with consequent activation of protein kinase C – PKC), increase of hexosamine pathway flux and a disturbed oxi-reduction status (4,5,6,7). All these mechanisms may contribute to the known phisiological characteristics of diabetic complications through increase of cytokines and growing factors regulation, and through formation of oxygen and nitrogen derived free radicals (8).

2.1 Free radicals

A free radical can be defined as a chemical species that has a non-paired electron (9). It may be also considered as a fragment of a molecule (10). Thus, free radicals can be formed in three ways:

- By cliving a covalent link of a normal molecule, with each of the fragments retainning one of the paired electrons (10);
- When a normal molecule lose one electron (10) and
- When a normal molecule receives one electron (10).

The most relevant free radicals in biological systems are those derived from oxygen (9,10,11).

3. Oxidative stress

It is said that a cell suffers oxidative stress when formation of free radicals overcomes hability of cellular antioxidant system (12). That may happen when a lot of free radicals is formed, when endogenous antioxidant defenses are diminished or, more commonly, when both events occur (12). Excessive free radical production may damage any cellular structure, including membrane (lipid peroxidation), proteins (anomalous polimerization) and nucleus (desoxirribonucleic acid – DNA - lesion) (12).

In diabetes, free radical formation, together with antioxidant deficiency, increases with time and may have an important role in retinopathy development (13,14).

Retina is known as an important target of diabete mellitus (1). Because of its high oxygen requirement and due to its unsaturated lipid content, retina may be a selective site for free radical production and for lipid peroxidation (1).

In endothelial cells, intracellular hyperglycemia promotes an increase in superoxide radical production at mitochondrial level (10). It is thought that such increase of superoxide production is the activator process of all pathways enrolled in diabetic complications pathogenesis (10). It is also seen an increase in nitric oxide production (NO) that is particularly damaging because it reacts with oxygen and produces peroxynitrite, a powerful oxidant (10). Peroxynitrite is cytotoxic because it inhibits mitochondrial transportation of electrons, oxidizes sulphidril groups in proteins, begins lipid peroxidation without the necessity of transition metals and nitrates aminoacids (such as tyrosine), what affects many signal transduction pathways (10). Chronic hyperglycemia promotes non-enzimatic glycation of proteins and glycated proteins may increase oxidant generation by activating fagocytes or by releasing superoxide and hydrogen peroxyde directly (10). Besides, AGEs estimulate oxidant production through specific interactions with receptors that are present in vascular cells (10).

4. Alterations of blood flux regulation

Endothelins are the main endothelial vasoconstrictors (12). In endothelial cells of retinal vessels, main endothelin is the subtype ET-1, that is synthethized and released by the action of several factors (growth factors, cytokines and insulin, among others) and is negativelly controlled by prostaciclin, nitric oxide and heparin, among other substances (12). ET-1 interacts with specific membrane receptors that are present in vascular smooth muscle fibers (ETA and ETB) and it triggers a vasoconstrictor effect (12). In diabetic animals retina, synthesis and activity of ET-1 and ET-3 are increased and factors which inhibit such actions are decreased; thus, endothelins are considered one of the factors that contribute to a reduction of retinal blood flux and to endothelial capillary proliferation (12).

Among the vasodilating factors those which deserve a greater attention are prostaciclin and nitric oxide (12). Prostaciclin is formed from arachidonic acid through participation of cycloxigenase, to form ciclic endoperoxides, as it occurs in platelets (12). Main difference between prostaciclin synthesis in platelets and in endothelium is that the first involves thomboxane synthetase that produces thromboxane A2 (TxA2, a powerful vasoconstrictor and platelet agregant) while the last one involves prostaciclin synthetase (a powerful vasodilating and platelet disagregant) (12). Due to shared biochemical origin but opposed effects of both prostanoids, it is accepted that a proper balance between platelet thromboxane and vascular prostaciclin be fundamental to physiological interaction between platelets and vessel walls (12).

5. Vascular nitric oxide defficiency origin in diabete

In diabete, hyperglycemia may actvate PKC isoform bII in endothelial cells, what reduces calcium ingress in cells and, consequently, nitric oxide synthesis (15). Besides, PKC promotes superoxide generation in endothelial cells and it quenches in a reaction that produces the toxic radical peroxynitrite (15). This way, overactivation of PKC mediated by hyperglycemia may reduce the synthesis or accelerate the loss of nitric oxide (15).

Hyperglycemia also provides a substrate increase for endothelial aldose reductase (15). Such enzyme generates sorbitol from glucose in a reaction that oxidizes NADPH - and, this way, decreases disponibility of reducing co-factor for NO sintase (16).

Glycated tissue proteins (whose levels increase as a consequence of hyperglycemia) may generate superoxide in a non-enzymatic reaction that needs transition metal catalysis; such factor also contributes to NO deficiency associated to hyperglycemia (15). Besides, AGEs may also extinguish NO directly (15).

6. Pathogenic implications of NO deficiency

Vascular deficiency of NO may be critical for pathogenesis of micro and macrovascular complications of non-controlled diabetes mellitus (15). This may be appreciated in the light of physiological importance of basal activity of NO in maintaining an appropriate arteriolar vasodilation, stabilizing platelets and preventing excessive activation and circulating leucocyte adhesion (15). Loss of such activity may clearly promote ischaemia by inducing arteriolar vasoconstriction and microvascular occlusion by activated adhering leucocytes and thrombosis (15). Besides, NO increases sodium-potassium pump activity in arterial wall and in axons of peripheral nerve (15). Reduction of sodium-potassium pump activity in endothelial capillary cells exposed to hyperglycemia could, in the same way, be attributed to a lesser production of NO (15).

In diabetes, vasoconstrictor impact of NO deficiency is exacerbated by stimilus of PKC over endothelin production (15). There is also evidence that endothelial synthesis of PGI 1 (prostaciclin) tends to be subnormal in diabetics (15). Once prostaciclin, as well as protaglandin E1 (PGE1), present many physiological effects that are complementary to those of NO - including vasodilation - it is probable that an impairment in its production amplifies the pathogenic impact of NO deficiency (15).

In diabetes, NO deficiency and excessive activation of endothelial PKC cause an increased synthesis of Platelet Activating Factor (PAF) (15). Endothelial PAF, confined to luminal endothelial membrane, stimulates receptors in marginated leucocytes that circulate along post-capillary venules, inducing activation of these leucocytes and taking them to express β2-integrins (15). Such phenomenon possibilitates leucocytes to adhere tightly to endothelial surface (15). One of the main endothelial targets to which such endothelins adhere - ICAM-1 - is also estimulated by PKC activity (15).

Activated leucocytes also synthethize leucotrien B4 (LTB4), what also increases PKC activity more yet by estimulating phospholipase C-b (15).

Leucocytes are greater and more viscous than erithrocytes and the activation process increases their polymerization because of its action over actin (15). Thus, under conditions in which pressure gradient through capillaries is reduced - as in vascular beds supplied by estenotic arteries or in constricted arterioles - activated leucocytes become edged in capillaries, preventing vascular flux (15).

In diabetics, blood viscosity increases due to greater fibrinogen plasmatic levels and it may damage microcirculatory flux more yet (15). This way, these factors promote retinal hypoxia, which causes angiogenic factors release - more notably, vascular endothelial growth factors - which induce neovascularization (15).

7. Alterations of control mechanisms of growth factors

Among all growth factors, VEGF is the innermost factor related to retinal neovascularization because it takes part in formation of new vessels which appear after retinal ischaemia (12). VEGF is member of a great family of proteins with angiogenic and mitogenic capabilities (12). It is produced in retina in pigmented epitelium, in neurosensorial retina, in pericytes and in vascular smooth muscle layer (12). Even in the earliest stages of retinopathy (early or backgraund retinopathy) it is already observed an increased expression of (VEGF) messenger ribonucleic acid (mRNA) in retinal pigmented epitelium (12).

Studies about induction of permeability in retinal endothelial cells in culture showed that VEGF induces transitory and transcellular hyperpermeability, which involves nitric oxide synthase activation and nitric oxide formation (17). It is believed that such phase is followed by a sustained increase of paracellular permeability due to a reduction of ocludin protein of tight junctions and it involves urokinase receptor expression (uPAR), what may deflagrate plasmin formation and matrix metaproteinase activation (17).

VEGF, in turn, still promotes ICAM-1 expression by endothelial cell, what causes leucocyte activation and cytokine release leading to an amplification of inflammatory response (12,18).

8. Pigmented Epitelium Derived Factor (PEDF)

Besides causing vascular lesion, diabetes also presents an adverse and early impact over neural retina (2,12,18). Studies with diabetic patients showed early alterations in visual function, including damage of colored vision and contrast sensibility, and reduction of electroretinogram oscilatory potentials (2,12,18). Such alterations frequently precede microvascular lesions establishment and predict retinopathy worsening in a better way than clinical characteristics, suggesting that neurodegeneration, as well as vascular dysfunction, be an important characteristic of diabetic retinopathy (2,12,18). It was suggested that metabolic factors that cause such phenomenon include loss of trophic support mediated by insulin or a lesion due to excessive accumulation of hexosamine, α-Tumoral Necrosis Factor or glutamate (2,12,18). Data that show reduced levels of Pigmented Epitelium Derived Factor (PEDF) in ocular fluids and vitrectomy species of patients with diabetic retinopathy suggest that loss of PEDF contributes to neuroglial cells toxicity induced by diabetes (2,12,18).

PEDF occurs naturally in eye and it is expressed in multiple retinal cells, including retinal pigmented epithelial cells, glial cells, vascular endothelial cells and neurons (17). It was demonstrated that treatment with PEDF prevents retinal neovascularization in a model of ischaemic retinopathy (17). Recently it was verified that PEDF blocks the increase in vascular retinal permeability induced by ocular injections of VEGF (17). PEDF may also function as an antioxidant once it supresses reactive species generation mediated by NAD(P)H oxidase and blocks increase of expression of VEGF induced by oxidative stress (17). Studies of ocular fluids of patients with active neovascularization show an inverse correlation between VEGF levels (increased) and PEDF ones (decreased), suggesting that a change in balance between PEDF and VEGF levels may contribute to development of retinal neovascular disease (17).

Reductions of mRNA PEDF levels were related in endothelial cells in culture and in pericytes exposed to oxidative stress conditions, as well as in endothelial cells treated with TNF-α (17). Studies with cells in culture indicate that hypoxia and VEGF inhibit PEDF levels by increasing matrix metalloproteinases that degrade and inactivate PEDF (17).

9. Poly (ADP-ribose) polymerase and diabetic vascular disfunction

Poly(ADP-ribose)polymerase (PARP), also known as poly(ADP-ribose)synthase (PARS), is a nuclear enzyme abundant in eukaryotic cells that takes part in DNA repair in answer to genotoxic stress (19).

Compulsory trigger to PARP activation is DNA breakdown, which can be induced by a variety of environmental stimulations and free / oxidizing radicals, more notably hydroxil and peroxynitrite radicals (8,20).

When activated by DNA breakdown, PARP begins a cicle that consumes energy by transfering ADP ribose units from NAD+ to nuclear proteins (8,19). Such process results in a rapid depletion of intracellular supplies of NAD+ and ATP, reducing glycolisis tax (and mitochondrial respiration), as well as NADP levels (a co-factor for pentose way and of bio-reducing synthetic ways, involved in maintaning reduced glutatione pools), causing cellular dysfunction and death (8,19). It was showed that PARP activation occurs in a great variety of pathological states, including reperfusion lesion of colon, kidney, skeletal muscle and myocardium, inflammatory diseases such as colitis, diabetes and arthritis, septic and haemorragic shocks (8,19). It was demonstrated that PARP activation has also a central role in cardiovascular diseases, including encephalic vascular accident (EVA), atherosclerosis, cardiac ischaemic disease, doxorrubicin toxicity and diabetic cardiovascular disfunction (8).

PARP activation in answer to elevated glucose levels can be attenuated by SOD (8).

PARP activation may be relevant in endothelial cells dysfunction induced by hyperglycemia (8). Endothelial cells exposed to hyperglycemia during 1-2 days present an intense suppression of high energy phosphate cell levels, as well as NAD+ and NADPH levels (8). Since constitutive NO-sintetase (ec-NOS) is a NADPH-dependent enzyme, it is conceivable that NADPH cellular depletion in cells exposed to hyperglycemia be directly responsible for ec-NOS activity suppression and for reduction of endothelium dependent relaxing capacity of diabetic vessels (8). In diabetic patients, hyperglycemia effects over NADPH levels may be exacerbated by aldose redutase increased activity, which also depletes NADPH as well as generates reactive oxidants (8).

PARP activation in endothelial cells exposed to hyperglycemia may be a common factor among three of major hypotheses by which hyperglycemia causes diabetic complications: activation of PKC isoforms, increased flux of hesosamine pathway and AGEs increased formation (8,21). Each of these pathways may be activated by superoxide overproduction from mitochondrial electron transport chain and it is induced by hyperglycemia (8,21). Superoxide overproduction in endothelial cells exposed to hyperglycemia results from inhibition of activity of glyceraldeid-3-phosphate dehydrogense (GAPDH) enzyme, being PARP the mediator of such effect (8). Inhibition of GAPDH activity also activates pro-inflammatory transcription factor NF-κβ that is PKC-dependent in endothelial cells (8). Inhibition of GAPDH activity is a result of poly(ADP-ribosyl)ation of enzyme by PARP and can be reversed by inhibiting PARP (8). GAPDH is a multifunctional enzyme that presents effects as much in cytoplasm as in nucleus and it has been implicated not only in normal physiology (exportation of nuclear RNA, DNA replication, DNA repair, exocitotoxic membrane fusion, cytoskeletal organization and phosphotransferase activity), but also in pathological states, such as, neurodegenerative diseases (Parkinson's disease), cancer (prostate) and in viral pathogenesis, where it was demonstrated that GAPDH presents a role in apoptotic cellular death (8). It has been demonstrated that GAPDH is the link between PARP activation and endothelial cells diabetic dysfunction (8).

10. Vitamin C

10.1 Introduction

Vitamin C (ascorbic acid) is an essential micronutrient for normal body metabolism and it is present in fresh fruits, particularly in citrus ones, and in vegetables (15). Its deficiency causes scurvy (22).

Minimum necessary requirement of vitamin C is 60 mg/day for health and non-smoker people (22).

Vitamin C is a co-factor of several enzymes:

1. Pro-collagen-proline dehidrogenase (proline dehidrogenase) and procollagen lisine 5-dehidrogenase (lysine desidrogenase), involved in pro-collagen synthesis (22). Thus, vitamin C deficiency causes teeth losses, joint pains, bone and conective tissues disorders, and a deficient wound scar, all of which are characteristics of scurvy (22);
2. Deoxigenases, involved in carnitine biosynthesis, essential substance for long chain fat acids transportation to the interior of mitochondria (22). Thus, vitamin C deficiency results in fatigue and letargy, initial symptoms of scurvy (22);
3. Dopamine-monoxigenase, that catalyses conversion of dopamine into norepinephrine (22). Thus, norepinephrine deficiency must be related with depression, hipochondria and humor alterations that occur in scurvy (22).

Vitamin C was also implicated in cholesterol and biliary acids metabolism, through cholesterol 7α-monoxigense, and in adrenal steroid metabolism (22).

Other acitivties of vitamin C include thiol enzymes maintenance in a reduced state, and a saving effect of glutatione (an important intracellular antioxidant) and tetrahidrofolate (co-factor for cathecolamine synthesis) (22).

10.2 Antioxidant effect

According to the Panel on Dietary Antioxidants and Related Compounds of the Food and Nutrition Board, an antioxidant may be defined as a substance that reduces significantly the adverse effects of free radicals over normal physiological function (22).

Vitamin C (or L-ascorbic acid) is called electron donnor antioxidant due to its hability to prevent oxidation of other compounds by linking to their electrons (23). While ascorbic acid is oxidized in a stable and non-reactive form, free radicals are reduced to water and do not cause cellular lesion any longer (23).

Vitamin C scavenges superoxide and hydroperoxyl, watery peroxyl, oxygen singlet, ozone, peroxynitrite and nitrogen dioxide, nitroxide radicals and hypoclorous acid, protecting, this way, other substrates from oxidative lesion (16,22).

Besides, vitamin C regenerates α-tocopherol (vitamin E) from α-tocopheril radical (22). That is particularly important because α-tocopherol may act as a pro-oxidant in absence of co-oxidants like vitamin C (22).

10.3 Effects over coagulation, platelets and vessels

Studies showed an inverse association between vitamin C plasmatic concentrations and coagulation factors (22,24).

10.4 Effects over platelets

In vitro studies showed that physiological concentrations of vitamin C may increase PGE1 and PGI1 production, resulting in a reduction of platelet aggregation and thrombus formation (22). Besides, low concentrations of vitamin C are also associated to greater levels of Plasminogen Activating Inhibitor 1, a protein that inhibits fibrinolysis (22).

10.5 Vitamin C and nitric oxide

Other studies demonstrated that vitamin C restores endothelium depending vasodilation in diabetic type 1 patients and in acute hyperglycemia in health humans, while studies realized with type 2 diabetics showed varied results (24). Several mechanisms may be responsible for such effects and, probably, they are related to vitamin C antioxidant activity (22).

NO presents an important role in vasodilation and it also inhibits platelet aggregation and lecocyte adhesion (22). Studies showed that NO concentrations are reduced through its reaction with superoxide radicals and because of its release by oxidized LDL (22). This way, vitamin C may prevent NO breakdown by scavenging superoxide radicals or by preventing oxidized LDL formation (16,22,23).

10.6 Effects over capillary fragility

Vitamin C deficiency promotes the following alterations over vascular tissues: inner and basal membrane thickening, extra-cellular matrix accumulation due to a reduced sulfatation, endothelium tight junctions loss (with consequent increase of transcapilar escape tax - TET) and capillary fragility (24). Such findings are also met in diabetic microangiopathy (24).

10.7 Effects over diabetic complications

A recent report showed that all alterations induced by hyperglycemia - including aldose redutase, PKC and AGEs increases - are reversed by inhibiting free radicals production induced by glucose (25). Such fact gives the possibility that, by blocking glucose induced oxidative stress, it may also be possible to prevent lesions caused by other pathways (25).

Vitamin C presents a central role in antioxidant defense system and may help to mitigate oxidative stress associated to diabetic complications (22). In fact, there are reports that high dose vitamin C diets are associated to reversion of early signs of retinopathy and to normalization of capillary resistance in diabetes mellitus, confirming its antioxidant protector role in blood vessels lesion (9,26).

10.8 Intracellular transportantion of vitamin C

It is known the existence of two distict mechanisms of vitamin C transportation into the cells (25):

1. A sodium-dependent mechanism that is mediated by a pair of ascorbate carriers, which is predominant in hemato-encephalic barrier, osteoblasts, muscles, placenta, intestine walls, brush border kidney cells, liver, brain and in the majority of endocrine and neuroendocrine systems, and it is not affected by glucose plasmatic levels (25);
2. An extremely sensible mechanism to glucose blood levels and dependent of some members of glucose transporters family (GLUT) (25).

There are also some cellular types, as linfocytes and red blood cells, that use both ascorbate captation mechanisms (25).

Once dehidroascorbate (DHA) enters cells, it is converted into ascorbic acid and stored (25).

Glucose and DHA co-transportation by GLUT's in certain cellular types suggests a new causative mechanism of disease in these particular cellular types (25). Studies show an increase in free radicals production induced by hyperglycemia in target-organs affected by diabetes mellitus (25). Thus, it is suggested that free radicals production is the main causative pathway of diabetic complications (25).

Ascorbic acid functions as an important component of cellular defense against oxygen toxicity and lipid peroxidation caused by free radicals (13,26). Reduced ascorbic acid levels have been observed in diabetic patients, mainly in those with microangiopathy (13,26).

Ascorbic acid caption by cell is mediated by a process related to glucose transportation and it was demonstrated that a high glucose extracellular concentration in diabetics may damage such caption and accentuate problems related to deficiency of such vitamin (13,26).

That phenomenon would deprive cells of central antioidant and could cause accumulation of free radicals followed by activation of PKC and aldose redutase pathways and by AGEs production in diabetes (25).

Such effects are limited to certain specific cellular types that depend on glucose and DHA co-transportation by GLUT (25).

Since DHA and glucose compete for GLUT carriers, each of them can inhibit transportation of the other (25,26). Basal blood glucose in non-controlled diabetes is tipycally elevated and, during hiperglycemic episodes, it increases still more (25,26). Besides, ascorbate levels tend to be significantly reduced in non-controlled diabetes, even in diabetics who eat diets rich in such substance (25,26). It seems that ascorbate loss is due to its excretion (together with glucose) by the kidneys, to a blockade of its recaption due to a greater glucose concentration and to its reduced absorption by kidney tubules (due to osmotic diuresis and glucosuria) (25).

It is verified, in average, a reduction between 30 and 80% of normal taxes of entrance of DHA into cells (25). Thus, DHA transportation into nerves, retina, kidney and other tissues that are unique or mainly GLUT -dependent, will be intense and chronically reduced (25).

This way, it is probable that hyperglycemia results in a vitamin C deficiency in certain types of cells (such as peripheral neurons, pigmented cells and retinal vascular endothelial cells) which depend mainly or exclusively on GLUT carriers for vitamin C caption (25).

11. Preventing and treating diabetic complications

Thus, it is believed that ascorbic acid may prevent or even treat complications associated to diabetes by affecting proteic glycosilation (25,27), sensibility to insulin, retinal blood flux and oxidative stress (25,28).

11.1 Adverse effects of vitamin C

Adverse effects from excess of vitamin C are hemochromatosis or iron overload, an increase of uric acid and oxalate excretion (with consequent development of kidney stones), nausea, vomiting and diarrhea (29).

12. Superoxide dismutase

12.1 Physiopathology of diabetes chronic complications

According to what has already been said, diabetes chronic complications occur as a consequence of persistent hyperglycemia (7). Hyperglycemia, in turn, promotes glucose auto-oxidation, AGEs formation and its interaction with RAGEs, activation of several isoformes of PKC, induction of poliol pathway and an increase of flux of hexosamine pathway (7).

Recently, it was made a hypothesis according to which all these processes would be a consequence of an increase of superoxide production by respiratory mitochondrial chain during hyperglycemia (7,30).

Mitochondrial role in retinopathy pathogenesis is supported by reports which show that retinal mitochondria presents a dysfunction in diabetes (30,31). Eight-month diabetic rats (a duration in which capillary cell apoptosis is seen in retina) present an increase of citocrome c release in citosol and of Bax pro-apoptotic protein in mitochondria (30,31). Besides, incubation of retinal capillary cells in a hyperglycemic environment results in these precise abnormalities, which are accompanied by increased cellular apoptosis (30).

Retinal capillary cells apoptosis is an early event in diabetic retinopathy pathogenesis, and oxidative stress is linked to accelerated apoptosis of retinal capillary cells (30). Because it was demonstrated that retinal capillary cells are lost through apoptosis before other hystopathological alteration is detectable and because treatments that inhibit retinopathy development also inhibit apoptosis and caspase-3 activation, it is suggested that superoxide presents an important role in diabetic retinopathy pathogenesis (30).

This way, reduction in superoxide production by mitochondria or an increase in its tax of decomposition by antioxidants could block many of hyperglycemia pathological consequences (7).

13. SOD history

In 1938, Mann and Keilin described a blue-greened protein containing copper (hemocupprein), which they have isolated from ox blood (9,32). In 1953, a similar protein was isolated from horses' liver and it was called hepatocuprein (9).

In 1969, McCord and Fridovich related that an erithrocitic protein was capable of removing catalitically superoxide radical, that is, it functioned as a superoxide dismutase enzyme (SOD) (9,33). Posteriorly, it was demonstrated that SOD is identical to human erithrocuprein and to bovine hemocupprein described previously (31,33).

Soon, SODs were isolated from a variety of eucharyotes and prokaryotes (33). All eucharyotic SODs had copper and zinc (CuZnSOD), while procharyotic ones had manganese (MnSOD) (33). While he worked with chicken livers, Fridovich perceived that it contained two types of SOD, one localized in mitochondria and another one localized in cytosol (33). Surprisingly, mitochondrial SOD had manganese (33).

Similarity between mitochondrial and bacterial SODs suggests that mitochondria has evolved from an endocellular symbiotic relation with procharyotes (33).

Together with Fred Yost, Fridovich also isolated a SOD which contains iron (33).

Howard M. Steinman and cols. determined the complete sequence of aminoacids of CuZnSOD (33). Steinman and Robert L. Hill determined the sequence of the first 29 residues of ending amino of mitochondrial Mn dismutase, of bacterial Manganese dismutase and of bacterial Iron dismutase (33). Elevated degree of similarity of identity between bacterial and mitochondrial dismutases gave an additional support to endosymbiotic origin of mitochondria (33).

13.1 SOD actions

SOD constitutes primary defense against superoxide radicals and its reaction with such free radicals results in hydrogen peroxide formation (16).

Due to its mitochondrial localization, MnSOD is considered the first line of defense against oxidative stress (30).

It was demonstrated that there is less mitochondrial SOD activity in retina during capillary cells apoptosis and during the appearance of diabetic retinopathy hystopathological characteristics (30).

In vivo and in vitro studies suggest that MnSOD presents a protecting role against development of diabetic retinopathy because an increase in its expression in isolated retinal endothelial cells protects retinal capillary cells from oxidative stress induced by glucose and from capillary cells apoptosis (30).

13.2 Effect of MnSOD over "hiperglycemic memory"

A paradox in diabetes is called "hiperglycemic memory" and refers to a persistent progression of microvascular alterations induced by hyperglycemia during subsequent periods of normal glycemic homeostasis (34). That outstanding phenomenon occurred in eyes of diabetic dogs during a post-hyperglycemic period of euglycemia (34). Eyes were hystologically normal during 2,5 years before exposition to elevated and sustained glycemia (34). But, after a subsequent period of 2,5 years of normal glycemia, eyes developed severe retinopathy (34). Worsening of retinopathy, in spite of sustained normoglycemia, was also related in rats with streptozocin induced diabetes implicating that an isolated good glycemic control does not stop diabetic microangiopathy progression in its late stage (34).

Results from Epidemiology of Diabetes Interventions and Complications Study indicate that hiperglycemic memory also occurs in human patients (34). It was demonstrated that the effects of conventional and intensive treatments over occurrence and severity of post-study diabetic retinopathy and nephropathy persist until 4 years after Diabetes Control and Complications Trial, in spite of almost identical glycosilated hemoglobin values during the 4-year follow-up period (34). It is interesting that obtaining normoglycemia through pancreatic transplantation is not effective yet in reducing diabetic retinopathy progression (34). Other studies demonstrate that previous glycemic exposure and glycemic level at first visit also have influence over diabetic retinopathy development (34). The lesson from those studies is that achieving the best glycemic control when diabetes is diagnosed seems to be of outstanding importance once HbA1c levels already during the first year of disease are related to posterior development of diabetic retinopathy (34).

As it was suggested by Brownlee and cols., superoxide mitochondrial production induced by hyperglycemia (oxidative stress) may provide an explanation for development of complications during post-hyperglycemia normal glycemia periods (30,34).

Treatments that inhibit activation of apoptosis promoting enzyme and, consequently, diabetic retinopathy development, reduce oxidative stress in retina (30). Thus, it was observed that increases in MnSOD expression prevents oxidative stress induced by glucose in retinal endothelial cells (30). This way, MnSOD could be used in treatment of "hiperglycemic memory".

14. Adverse effects

Superoxide dismutase does not present known adverse effects (9).

15. Conclusion

There are evidences of a key-role of free radicals in diabetic retinopathy pathogenesis. Retina is rich in polyunsaturated fat acids and presents glucose oxidation and oxygen caption taxes greater than any other tissue, being, this way, extremely susceptible to increased oxidative stress. Alterations of enzyme activity of antioxidant system (such as superoxide dismutase) seem to be one of the possible sources of oxidative stress in diabetes. Recent evidences also point to a participation of oxygen reactive species in mithogenic cascade began by tyrosine kinase receptors of several growth factors, including Vascular Endothelial Growth Factor (VEGF). Antioxidants, at least, inhibit some metabolic abnormalities and pathological alterations induced by hyperglycemia. Therefore, it is reasonable to postulate that an antioxidant treatment may be useful to prevent diabetic retinopathy progression and that medication combinations could be necessary to prevent visual loss in diabetic patients. Ascorbic acid is present in great amounts in human eyes and its hability of scavenging oxygen reactive species may have importance in the treatment of diabetic retinopathy. Biological role of superoxide dimutase is scavenging superoxide, which is generated in vivo after exposition to oxygen. Retinal Pigmented Epithelium (RPE) has elevated levels of Manganese-Superoxide Dismutase and a reduction of its levels may be related to retinal lesion. Antioxidants, such as vitamin C and superoxide dismutase, may provide aditional beneficial effects to patients with diabetic retinopathy. Thus, vitamin C and superoxide dismutase present the potential of influencing positively ocular disease.

16. References

[1] Yildrim Z, Ucgun NI, Kilic N, Gursel E, Sepici-Dincel A, et al. Antioxidant enzymes and diabetic retinopathy. Annals of the New York Academy of Sciences 2007;1100:199-206.

[2] Siemianowicz K, Gminski J, Telega A, Wójcik A, Posielezna B, Grabowska-Bochenek R, Francuz T. Blood antioxidant parameters in patients with diabetic retinopathy. International Journal of Molecular Medicine 2004;14:433-437.

[3] Parikh A, Fantus IG. Screening and management of diabetic microvascular complications in older adults. Geriatrics and Aging 2004;7:22-30.

[4] Kurtul N, Bakan E, Aksoy H, Baykal O. Leucocyte lipid peroxidation, superoxide dismutase and catalase activities of type 2 diabetic patients with retinopathy. Acta Medica (Hradec Králowé) 2005;48(1):35-38.

[5] Bosco Adriana, Lerário Antonio Carlos, Soriano Danilo, Santos Rosa Ferreira dos, Massote Píndaro, Galvão Daniela et al . Retinopatia diabética. Arq Bras Endocrinol Metab [serial on the Internet]. 2005 Apr [cited 2008 Aug 22] ; 49(2): 217-227. Available from: http://www.scielo.br/scielo.php?script=sci_arttext&pid=S0004-27302005000200007&lng=en. doi: 10.1590/S0004-27302005000200007.

[6] Anderson JW. Metabolic abnormalities contributing to diabetic complications. I. Glucose metabolism in insulin-insensitive pathways. The American Journal of Clinical Nutrition 1975; 28:273-280.

[7] Green K, Brand MD, Murphy MP. Prevention of mitochondrial oxidative damage as a therapeutic strategy in diabetes. Diabetes 2004;53 Suppl 1:S110-S118.

[8] Mabley JG, Soriano FG. Role of nitrosative stress and poly(ADP-ribose) polymerase activation in diabetic vascular dysfunction. Current Vascular Pharmacology 2005;3:247-252.

[9] Halliwell B, Gutteridge JMC. Free Radicals in Biology and Medicine. Third Edition. Oxford: Oxford University Press, 1999:23;106 - 7.

[10] Palmieri B, Sblendorio V. Oxidative stress detection: what for? Part I. European Review for Medical & Pharmacological Sciences 2006;10:291-317.

[11] Campos EBP, Yoshida WB. O papel dos radicais livres na fisiopatologia da isquemia e reperfusão em retalhos cutâneos: modelos experimentais e estratégias de tratamento. Jornal Vascular Brasileiro 2004;3(4):357-366.

[12] De La Cruz JP, Gonzalez-Correa JA, Guerrero A, De la Cuesta FS, et al. Pharmacological approach to diabetic retinopathy. Diabetes/metabolism research and reviews 2004;20:91-113.

[13] Gupta MM, Chari S, Gupta MM, Chari S. Lipid peroxidation and antioxidant status in patients with diabetic retinopathy. Indian Journal of Physiology and Pharmacology 2005;49:187-92.

[14] Altomare E, Grattagliano I, Vendemaile G, Micelli-Ferrari T, Signorile A, Cardia L. Oxidative protein damage in human diabetic eye: evidence of a retinal participation. European Journal of Clinical Investigation 1997; 27:141-147.

[15] McCarty MF. Nitric oxide deficiency, leucocyte activation, and resultant ischemia are crucial to the pathogenesis of diebtic retinopathy/neuropathy - preventive potential of antioxidants, essential fatty acids, chromium, gikgkolides, and pentoxifylline. Medical Hypotheses 1998;50:435-449.

[16] Kowluru RA, Kennedy A. Therapeutic potential of anti-oxidants and diabetic retinopathy. Expert Opinion on Investigational Drugs 2001;10:1665-76.

[17] Caldwell RB, Bartoli M, Behzadian MA, El Remessy AE, Al Shabrawey M, Platt DH, et al. Vascular endothelial growth factor and diabetic retinopathy: role of oxidative stress. Current drug targets 2005;6:511-24.

[18] Mamputu JC, Renier G. Advanced glycation end-products increase monocyte adhesion to retinal endothelial cells through vascular endothelial growth factor-induced ICAM-1 expression: inhibitory effects of antioxidants. Journal of Leukocyte Biology 2004;75:1062-9.

[19] Pacher P, Liaudet L, Soriano FG, Mabley JG, Szabó É, Szabó C. The role of poly(ADP-ribose) polymerase activation in the development of myocardial and endothelial dysfunction in diabetes. Diabetes 2002;51:514-521.

[20] Szabó C, Mabley JG, Moeller SM, Shimanovich R, Pacher P, Virág L, et al. Part I: Pathogenetic role of peroxynitrite in he development of diabetes and diabetic vascular complications: studies with FP15, a novel potent peroxynitrite decomposition catalyst. Molecular Medicine 2002;8(10):571-580.

[21] Ceriello A. New insights on oxidative stress and diabetic complications may lead to a "causal" antioxidant therapy. Diabetes Care 2003;26(5):1589-1596.

[22] Carr AC, Frei B. Toward a new recommended dietary allowance for vitamin C based on antioxidant and health effects ih humans. Am. J. Clin. Nutr. 1999;69:1086-1107.

[23] Soro-Paavonen A, Forbes JM. Novel therapeutics for diabetic micro- and macrovascular complications. Current Medicinal Chemistry 2006;13:1777-88.

[24] Juhl B. Vitamin C treatment reduces transcapillary escape rate of albumin in type 1 diabetes. European Journal of Internal Medicine 2004;15:428-35.

[25] Root-Bernstein R, Busik JV, Henry DN. Are diabetic neuropathy, retinopathy and nephropathy caused by hyperglicemic exclusion of dehydroascorbate uptake by glucose transporters? J. Theor. Biol. 2002;216:345-359.

[26] Rema M, Mohan V, Bhaskar A, Shanmugasundaram KR. Does oxidant stress play a role in diabetic retinopathy? Indian J. Ophthalmol. 1995;43:17-21.

[27] Vinson J, Hsu C, Possanza C, Drack A, Pane D, Davis R, et al. Lipid peroxidation and diabetic complications: effect of antioxidant vitamins C and E. Advances in experimental medicine and biology 1944;366:430-2.

[28] Millen AE, Gruber M, Klein R, Klein BEK, Palta M, Mares JA. Relations of serum ascorbic acid and α-tocopherol to diabetic retinopathy in the Third National Health and Nutrition Examination Survey. American Journal of Epidemiology 2003;158:225-233.
[29] Campos S. Medicina Biomolecular e Radicais Livres. São Paulo, Francolor Artes Gráficas e Editora Ltda., 1996:Vol 1:137-143.
[30] Kowluru RA, Ho Y-S. Role of mitochondrial superoxide dismutase in the development of diabetic retinopathy. Investigative Ophthalmology and Visual Science 2006;47:1594-1599.
[31] Wikipedia The Free Encyclopedia [text on the Internet]. Los Angeles, The Wikimedia Foundation, Inc.; 2008 [cited 2009 Jan 12]. Disponível em: http://en.wikipedia.org/wiki/Bcl-2.
[32] McCord JM, Fridovich I. Superoxide dismutase. An enzymic function for erythrocuprein (hemocuprein). J. Biol. Chem. 1969;244(22):6049-6055.
[33] Kresge N, Simoni RD, Hill RL. Forty years of superoxide dismutase research: the work of Irwin Fridovich. J. Biol. Chem. 2006;281(22);issue of June 2:p.e17-e19.
[34] Balasubramanyam M, Rema M, Premanand C. Biochemical and molecular mechanisms of diabetic retinopathy. Current Science 2002;83:1506-14.

2

Gluco-Oxidation of Proteins in Etiology of Diabetic Retinopathy

Mohd Wajid Ali Khan[1,*], Kamalpreet Banga[2] and Wahid Ali Khan[3]
[1]I3-IRG, Department of Immunity, Infection and Biochemistry, Medical School of Cardiff, Cardiff University, Cardiff,
[2]School of Public Health, University of Saskatchewan, Health Sciences Building, Saskatoon,
[3]Department of Clinical Biochemistry, College of Medicine and Medical Science, King Khalid University, Abha,
[1]United Kingdom
[2]Canada
[3]Kingdom of Saudi Arabia

1. Introduction

Diabetes mellitus a chronic slow progressing catastrophe and is a major medical problem throughout the world. Diabetes causes an array of long-term systemic complications that have considerable impact on patient as well as society, as the disease typically affects individuals in their most productive years (Federman et al., 1994; Bhavsar et al., 2010). In addition, this increase appears to be greater among certain ethnic groups and in developing countries. Diabetic retinopathy is one of the main causes of diabetic complications. It causes visual impairment and finally blindness, a result of long-term accumulated damage to the small blood vessels in the retina. The proportion of blindness due to diabetic retinopathy ranges from close to 0% in most of Africa, to 3–7% in much of South-East Asia and the Western Pacific, to 15–17% in the wealthier regions of the Americas, Europe and the Western Pacific (Resnikoff et al. 2004; Zhang et al., 2010). According to the WHO fact sheet Aug. 2011, 346 million people worldwide have diabetes (World Health Organization [WHO], 2011). About 50% of persons with diabetes are unaware that they have the condition, although about 2 million deaths every year are attributable to complications of diabetes. After 15 years, about 2% of persons with diabetes become blind, and about 10% develop severe visual loss (WHO 2011). After 20 years, more than 75% of patients will have some form of diabetic retinopathy (Barcelo et al., 2003).

Post onset diabetes with increasing age, there is a higher risk of developing diabetic retinopathy and its complications, including diabetic macular oedema or proliferative diabetic retinopathy increases. The exact mechanism by which diabetes causes retinopathy remains unclear, but several theories have been postulated to explain the typical course and

*Corresponding Author

history of the disease (Crawford et al. 2009). Chronic hyperglycemia exerts protein gluco-oxidation, a process involving the non-enzymatic modification of tissue proteins by physiologic sugars in vivo, appears to play a central role in the pathogenesis of diabetic complications. One mechanism linking uncontrolled hyperglycaemia with tissue damage such as that in diabetic retinopathy is the formation and accumulation of advanced glycation end-products (AGE) (Hammes et al, 1996). *Ex vivo* and in vivo studies have indicated that AGE induce irreversible cross-links in long-living extracellular matrix (Brownlee et al., 1988; Fu et al., 1992; Sell et al., 1992; Sell et al., 1993) and, upon binding to specific cellular proteins, change the local concentrations of cytokines, growth factors and other bioactive molecules (Schleicher & Nerlich 1996; Vlassara et al, 1985). Accumulation of AGEs depends on both sugar concentration and the rate of protein turnover. Thus, some proteins that reach critical levels of AGE modification in sites where diabetic complications occur may turnover too quickly for normal levels of blood glucose to cause functional alterations, while proteins with a longer half-life would continue to be modified over a longer period of time (Brownlee 1995).

The relation between diabetes mellitus and oxidative stress is well known. With the onset of diabetes, persistent and chronic hyperglycemias causes increased production of free radicals through auto-oxidation of glucose, via nonenzymatic protein glycation and enhanced flux of glucose through the polyol pathway (Giugliano et al., 1996). The generation of reactive oxygen species and protein glycation are strictly interconnected (Palm et al, 2003). Levels of serum AGE are increased in diabetes mellitus before they have developed microvascular complications (Berg et al., 1997). These increased serum levels of AGE can predict changes in microvascular morphology in patients with diabetic retinopathy. Proteins containing AGE are highly immunogenic (Reddy et al., 1995) and anti-AGE antibodies were found in the sera of patients with diabetes (Shibayama et al, 1999; Baydanoff et al., 1996). Our research team has hypothesized that increase in the titre of anti-AGE antibodies has a direct role in the pathogenesis of diabetes microvascular complications especially diabetic retinopathy. Detection and characterization of antibodies against gluco-oxidative modified proteins could help in understanding the exact aetiology of gluco-oxidation of protein and diabetic retinopathy. Anti-gluco-oxidative modified proteins antibodies may potentially help in the prediction and /or prognosis of diabetes retinopathy. However the exact pathophysiology is yet to be ascertained.

2. Glycation

Reducing sugars such as glucose (or other reducing sugars as fructose, pentoses, galactose, mannose, ascorbate, xylulose) reacts nonenzymatically with free ε-amino groups in protein, lipids and nucleic acids through a series of reactions forming Schiff's bases and Amadori products to produce AGEs; and this process, also known as the Milliard reactions. In theory, every protein can be modified by glycation. Indeed, many protein-AGE adducts have been identified, *e.g.* glycated fibrinogen, collagen, albumin, herpes simplex glycoprotein B, hemoglobin, β2-microglobulin, and low density lipoprotein (Raj et al., 2000; Cribbs et al., 2000). Albumin is the most abundant protein in human serum, about 35-50 g/liter, and it is prone to glycation (Carter & Ho 1994). Non-enzymatic glycation of albumin occurs at multiple sites; glucose can attach to Lys199, Lys281, Lys439, and Lys525 as well as some other lysine and arginine residues and also at the N-terminal residues of polypeptides (Iberg & Fluckiger 1986). In fact, only a small number of factors are known to result in the variation of serum albumin. The alteration in the structure of albumin due to uncontrolled hyperglycemia causes vascular complications (Bourdon et al., 1999).

Glycation is a classical covalent reaction in which, by means of N-glycoside bonding, the sugar-protein complex is formed through a series of chemical reactions described for the first time by a chemist Louis Camille Maillard in 1912 (Sing et al., 2001). Maillard reactions are complex, multilayered, and can be analyzed in three steps. (i) The sugar-protein complex is formed first (Amadori rearrangement), an early product of non-enzymatic glycation leading to intermediary products which are precursors of all later compounds. (ii) Formation of numerous intermediary products, some of which are very reactive and continue the glycation reaction. (iii) Final phase consists of polymerization reaction of the complex products formed in the second step, whereby heterogeneous structures named advanced glycation end products (AGE) are formed (Fig. 1).

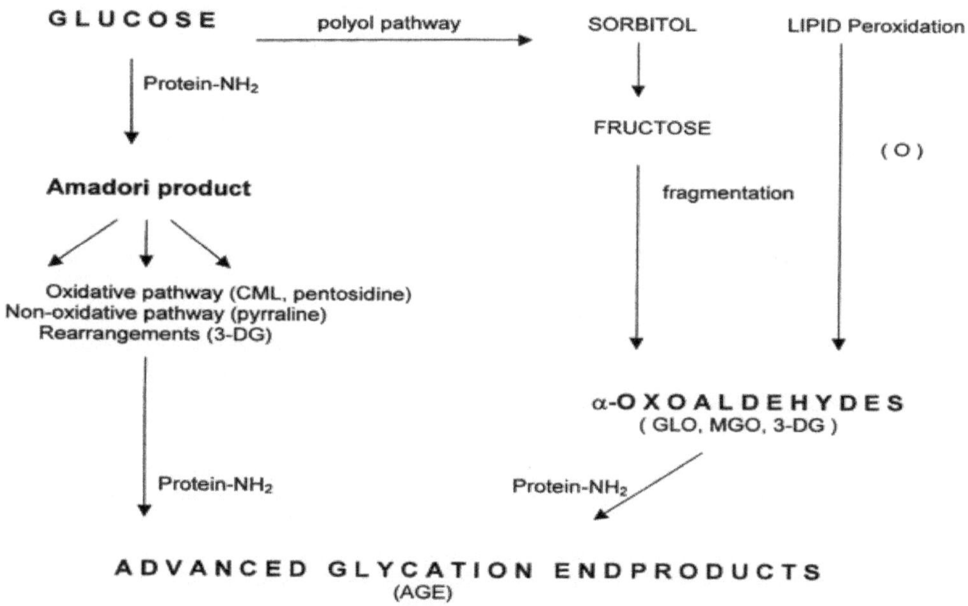

Fig. 1. Schematic presentation of potential pathway leading to AGE formation. The abbreviations given above are represented as, GLO=glyoxal; MG=methylglyoxal; 3-DG=3-deoxyglucosone; CML=carboxymethyl-lysine (Turk, 2001).

AGE constitute a heterogenous group of molecules (Peppa & Vlassara 2005) and its formation takes place continuously within the body during ageing, however it is extremely accelerated in diabetes (Vlassara & Palace 2002; Fu et al., 1996; Thorpe & Baynes 1996; Peppa et al., 2004). Some of the major AGEs are carboxymethyl lysine (CML) and pentosidine and also include many reactive intermediates or AGE-precursors such as 1- or 3-deoxyglucosone, methylglyoxal (MG) and their derivatives. AGE can cause tissue damage by two main pathways: they either form cross-links that disrupts the structure and function of short and long-lived proteins and lipids or they bind with specific and nonspecific cell surface receptors inducing deleterious consequences, leading to altered intracellular events that induce oxidative stress and inflammation (Vlassara & Palace 2002; Peppa et al., 2002; Peppa et al., 2004; Vlassara 2001). AGE induced pathogenesis of diabetic retinopathy occurs via alteration of small vessel wall integrity and structure, by inducing cytokines, growth factors and increased oxidative stress (Sheetz & King 2002; Vlassara & Palace 2002; Peppa et al., 2002; Peppa et al., 2004; Vlassara 2001; Stitt et al., 1997; Stitt 2001; Yamagishi et al., 2002). *Ex vivo*, retinal endothelial cells exposed to AGE overproduce vascular endothelial growth factor (VEGF) through oxidative stress induction, protein kinase-C pathway activation and abnormal endothelial nitric oxide synthase (eNOS) expression (Mamputu & Renier 2002; Chakravarthy et al., 1998). Retinal organ cultures show an increased glyoxal induced CML formation in association with increased apoptosis and cell death, restored by anti-AGE agents and antioxidants (Mamputu & Renier 2002). Increased AGE accumulation was found in the retinal pericytes of diabetic rats after 8 months of diabetes (Stitt et al., 1997). In addition, exogenous AGE-albumin administration in non-diabetic animals accumulated around and within the pericytes, colocalized with AGE receptors inducing retinal vessel wall thickening and loss of retinal pericytes (Xu et al., 2003; Clements et al., 1998). In humans, it has been found that with the increasing severity of retinopathy there is a proportional increase in AGE accumulation around retinal blood vessels (koya et al., 2002). Glycation of vitreous collagen was also observed in human donor eyeballs (Sulochana et al, 2003). In addition, studies using anti-AGE agents further support the role of AGE in diabetic retinopathy (Yamagishi et al., 2002; Chappey etal., 1997; Reber et al., 2003). AGE have also been linked to the changes associated with diabetic keratopathy through their effect in reducing corneal epithelial cell adhesion (Matsumoto et al., 1997). Furthermore, glycation of the vitreal collagen fibrils leading to dissociation from hyaluronan and resultant destabilization of the gel structure has been associated with vitreous liquefaction and posterior vitreous detachment in diabetes (Stevens 1998; Sebag et al., 1992; Stitt et al., 1998).

3. Pathophysiological mechanism of AGEs formation in diabetic retinopathy

The knowledge of gluco-oxidation of proteins and AGEs has considerably expanded over the years, and a large body of evidence has documented their implication in diabetes-related complications (Singh et al., 2001; Turk et al., 2001; Brownlee 2001; Monnier et al., 2005; Huebschmann et al., 2006). In the process of glycation, AGE peptides that are released as degradation products, which partly occur through proteolysis of the matrix component are commonly named as glycotoxins. Glycated proteins are toxic for neuronal cells, retinal capillary cells, leukocytes, pericytes, and endothelial cells (Takeuchi et al., 2000; Yamagishi et al., 2002; Lyons et al., 2000). Toxicity of glycated polypeptides may be due to the AGE modification or due to the aggregation state of the polypeptides. Glycotoxins are very reactive on entering blood circulation. Non elimination of these proteins through the kidneys leads to recirculating AGE peptides which can generate new AGE products that react with other plasma or tissue components. At this stage, glycation becomes an autonomic process, which significantly accelerates the progress of the complication (Turk 2001).

Immunoglobins are glycated differently according to their class. The glycation of immunoglobulin-M is twofold greater than that of immunoglobulin G, and can be related to the difference in amino acid composition. Albumin can be glycated at multiple sites. In diabetic patients, excessive glycation of fibrinogen and fibrin has been reported (Chappey et al., 1997). Hemoglobin is glycated at two sites: on the valine residue of the N-terminal β-chains at the ε-amino group of the α and β-chains, and at the N-termini of the α-chains (McDonald et al., 1978). Other intracellular and membrane proteins of red blood cells (RBC) are also glycated, for example Spectrin, a major RBC membrane protein, band 3 transmembrane protein, and band 4-1 (Retnaikes et al., 1987; Bryszewska & Szosland 1988). Hence glycation results in RBC deformability and an increased adherence to endothelium. Membrane proteins of platelets can also be glycated. Increased binding of fibrinogen and platelet aggregation observed in diabetic patients can be related to the glycation of adenosine diphosfate receptors. Lipids can also contribute to the modifications of platelet functions in diabetes (Chappey et al., 1997). Hyperglycemia can also induce protein aggregation which is associated with diabetes and its complications. Gluco-oxidation of proteins induces refolding of globular proteins, accompanied by the formation of cross β-structure (Bouma et al., 2003).

Gluco-oxidation of proteins forms complex and irreversible molecules, which accumulate in the retinal vasculature of patients with diabetes and streptozotocin-induced diabetic rats (Hammes et al., 1999; Stitt et al., 1997) and have been implicated in the development of diabetic retinopathy (Boehm et al., 2004 Genuth et al., 2005). Chronic exposure of the endothelium to AGEs has been shown to increase retinal vascular permeability in vivo (Stitt et al., 2000) and *ex vivo* (Leto et al., 2001). AGEs, however, have also been shown to increase capillary permeability acutely (Sampietro et al., 1987). Activation of AGE recepter (RAGE) and production of oxygen free radicals have been shown to mediate cellular responses to AGEs; however, the signalling pathways involved in the early permeability response are unknown (Kislinger et al., 1999; Bonnardel-Phu et al., 1999).

It has been suggested that, in diabetes, oxidative stress plays a key role in the pathogenesis of vascular complications, both microvascular and macrovascular, and an early marker of such damage is the development of an endothelial dysfunction (Giugliano et al., 1996; Cai & Harrison 2000). Evidence implicates hyperglycemia-derived oxygen free radicals as mediators of diabetic complications. Recently recognized relationship between α-oxoaldehydes and biologically important macromolecules highlights the intermediate step of advanced glycation cascade (Beisswenger et al., 2003a; Beisswenger et al., 2003b; Thornalley 2005). Diabetic individuals may exhibit elevated levels of iron and free copper ions (Cutler 1978; Mateo et al., 1978), which in the presence of glycated proteins *ex vitro* have been shown to generate free radicals (Hunt 1994). The accumulation of glycated material in tissues that contain free copper ion contribute to the generation of free radical mediated damage. These highly reactive species are capable of causing oxidative degradation of protein *ex vivo* (Hunt 1994). The formation of α-dicarbonyl compounds is known to be an essential step for the cross-linking of proteins and subsequent free radical generation (Rahbar & Figarola 2003). Methylglyoxal is increased 5-6 fold; in adult onset, non-insulin dependent diabetes mellitus as compared to healthy individuals. In the presence of oxidative stress, glycation of proteins by methylglyoxal is enhanced. This may underlie the link of glycation and oxidative stress with diabetic complications, and may also contribute to pathological processes of ageing.

Structural and functional modification of host-protein is a common feature of all AGEs irrespective of their generating precursors. Through their effects on the functional properties of extracellular matrix, intracellular signal transduction and protein function, AGEs may contribute to the pathogenesis of diabetic retinopathy (Poukupec et al., 2003). A mechanism by which AGE-modified proteins may exert their effect is binding to RAGE identified on a variety of cells including endothelial and smooth muscle cells, and by internalization and degradation *via* monocyte/macrophage AGE-receptors. Using radiolabeled AGE proteins it has been shown that several cells, such as human and mouse monocyte, macro-phage and lymphocyte, bind these types of glycated compounds in a relatively selective way (Gilcrease & Hoover 1990; Imani et al., 1993). Gluco-oxidative modified proteins bind to these cells in a saturable manner with a dissociation constant in the range of 50–200 mmol/l^{-1}. The putative receptors for AGE have been isolated from cell membranes and purified, and were reported to have different molecular weights: 30–50 KD for renal tissue, 36–83 KD for a macrophage cell line, 60–90 KD for liver cells (Yang et al., 1991; Skolnik et al., 1991). A carbohydrate-binding protein of 35 KD named Galectin 3 is present on lymphocytes, macrophages, endothelial, mesangial, smooth muscle cells, and fibroblasts, and binds AGE with a higher affinity than other carbohydrates (Vlassara et al., 1995).

Increased hyperglycemia caused protein gluco-oxidation and/or glucose auto-oxidation enhanced formation of AGEs, stimulate the expression of RAGE and hence NADPH oxidase activation. Activation of NADPH oxidase increased the production of free reactive oxygen radicals can up-regulate vascular endothelial growth factor (VEGF) in retinal cells via nuclear transcription factors (eg. NF-kappaB) potentially promoting retinal neovascularisation and increasing permeability to proteins across the retinal barrier. Increased RAGE expression has been found on endothelial cells, vascular smooth muscle cells and cardiac myocytes of diabetic patients (Schmidt et al., 1999). It has been reported that ligation of AGE with RAGE causes activation of intracellular signaling, gene expression, and production of proinflammatory cytokines and free radicals, thus playing an important role in the development and progression of diabetic micro- and macroangiopathy (Kim et al., 2005).

4. Oxidative stress and diabetic retinopathy

Diabetic retinopathy pathogenesis is multifactorial, and the precise mechanisms are unclear. Several mechanisms have been proposed, including enhanced free radical production ROS (Brownlee et al., 1998; Koya & King 1998). Oxidative stress is increased in the retina in diabetes, and it is considered to play an important role in the development of retinopathy (Manikanth et al., 2010; Armstrong et al., 1998). It has been already proved that oxidative stress and hyperglycemia are central to chronic pathogenesis of diabetic retinopathy (Turk 2010). Increased levels of free radicals have a direct effect on *in vivo* protein. Oxidative stress induced modification of proteins is initiated mainly by reactions with hydroxyl radical; however, the course of the oxidation process is determined by the availability of oxygen and superoxide radical or its protonated form ($HO_2^{\cdot}$). Collectively, these ROS can lead to oxidation of amino acid residue side chains, cross-linking of soluble and/or membrane-bound proteins, oxidation of the protein backbone resulting in protein damage and yielding larger aggregates fragmentation. In the meantime, it has been shown that other forms of ROS may yield similar products and that transition metal ions can substitute for hydroxyl and superoxide radicals in some of the reactions (Berlett & Stadtman 1997). Even peptide bonds are subject to oxidative modification by ROS (Adams et al., 1999; Dhalla et al., 2000; Schoonover 2001).

Animal studies have demonstrated that oxidative stress contributes not only to the development of diabetic retinopathy but also to the resistance of retinopathy to reverse after good glycemic control is reinstituted—the metabolic memory phenomenon (Berg et al., 1997). Various mechanisms have been suggested to contribute to the formation of these reactive oxygen-free radicals. Glucose auto-oxidation is one of the major sources of ROS that is generated by oxidative pathways of glycation. Glucose exists in equilibrium with its enediol, which can undergo auto-oxidation to form an enediol radical. This radical reduces molecular oxygen to generate the superoxide radical and becomes oxidized itself to a dicarbonyl ketoaldehyde that reacts with protein amino groups forming a ketoamine, **Fig. 2** (Wolff and Dean 1987a). Ketoamine are similar to, although more reactive, than Amadori products and participate in AGE formation (Ahmed et al., 2005). The superoxide anion radicals undergo dismutation to hydrogen peroxide, which if not degraded by catalase or glutathione peroxidase, and in the presence of transition metals, can lead to production of extremely reactive hydroxyl radicals (Wolff and Dean 1987; Jiang et al., 1990).

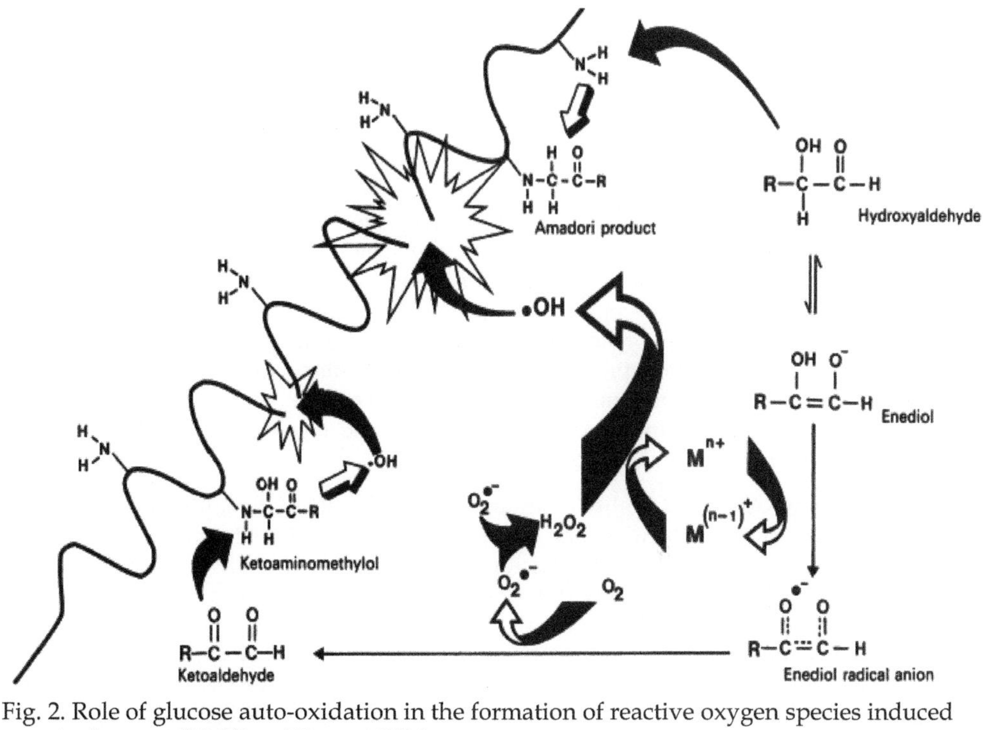

Fig. 2. Role of glucose auto-oxidation in the formation of reactive oxygen species induced protein damage (Wolff and Dean 1987a).

In hyperglycemic conditions, most of the carbonyl compounds generated by glycation need oxidative steps in their formation. The protein dicarbonyl compounds can participate in AGE formation and are referred to as glyco-oxidative products (Liggins & Furth 1997). Studies in diabetic rats showed elevated levels of superoxide in retinal cells with high glucose levels (Du et al., 2003; Cui et al., 2006), as well as increased levels of hydrogen peroxide (Ellis et al., 2000). Normally retinal blood vessels have tight junctions that protect them from leaking. Prolonged hyperglycemia damages the tight junctions by oxidative stress and the vessels become leaky allowing fluid or blood to seep into the retina, thus resulting in the swelling of the retina (Harhaj & Antonetti 2004). Recently the etiology behind the production of superoxide in endothelial cells in diabetic complications has been elucidated (Brownlee 2001). There are four pathways suggested to be involved in the pathogenesis of diabetic complications due to increased production of free radical (increased polyol pathway flux, increased advanced glycosylation end product formation, activation of protein kinase C, and increased hexosamine pathway flux (Nishikawa et al., 2000; Du et al., 2002). In diabetes, the activities of antioxidant defense enzymes responsible for scavenging free radicals and maintaining redox homeostasis such as SOD, glutathione reductase, glutathione peroxidase, and catalase are diminished in the retina (Kowluru et al., 2001; Haskins et al., 2003). The intracellular antioxidant GSH is probably the most important antioxidant in the cell and acts as an ROS scavenger and modulates intracellular redox state (Meister 1988). The levels of this intracellular antioxidant are decreased in the retina in diabetes (Kern et al., 1994), and enzymes responsible for its metabolism are compromised (Lou 2003). Some nonenzymic antioxidants such as vitamin C, vitamin E, and β-carotene are also depressed during hyperglycemia induced oxidative stress (Ford et al., 2003).

5. Autoantibodies in diabetes complications

The lack of an immune response to self when responses to environmental antigens are retained is due to immunological tolerance. The role of tolerance, or lack of tolerance, is important to the understanding of autoimmune diseases and transplantation immunobiology (Mackay 2000). A loss of natural tolerance (to self) underlies all autoimmune diseases. Many more individuals develop autoimmune phenomena than autoimmune disease. Immune-mediated (Type I) diabetes results from an organ-specific autoimmune-mediated loss of insulin-secreting β cells. This chronic destruction process involves both cellular and hormonal components detectable in the peripheral blood, months or even years, before the onset of clinical diabetes (Kukreja & Maclaren 1999). In order to elicit an immune response, a molecule must be recognized as non-self by the biological system.

Proteins containing AGE are highly immunogenic and anti-AGE antibodies have been found in the sera of patients with diabetes (Reddy et al., 1995; Shibayama et al, 1999; Baydanoff et al., 1996). Several AGE structures have been identified including pyrraline, pentosidine (Sell & Monnier 1989), (carboxymethyl)lysine (Ahmed et al., 1986), and crosslines (Nakamura et al., 1992). Immunological studies using antibodies specific for these compounds have confirmed their presence in vivo (Ienaga et al., 1995). However, it is still not known whether one of these compounds contributes, as a major AGE structure, to the pathogenesis of these diseases, or whether other structures may involve in this process. Immunological approaches have been attempted to determine the major AGE structures expressed in vivo. Using AGE-BSA as an antigen, researchers prepared a monoclonal anti-AGE antibody (6D12) in mice as well as a polyclonal anti-AGE antibody in rabbits (Hoeiuchi et al., 1986). Immunoreactivity studies of these antibodies have demonstrated an interesting observation: both antibodies react with AGE samples obtained from proteins, peptides, lysine derivatives, and monoaminocarboxylic acids, suggesting the presence of a common AGE structures in these AGE preparations. Immunologic studies using 6D12 monoclonal antibodies have disclosed the presence of AGE in several tissues and their potential involvement in disease processes. Anti-AGE antibodies use as a potential biomarker of AGE depositions during diabetes and its associated secondary complications.

There is increasing evidence of the presence of anti-AGE antibodies in diabetes and its complications. The role of these antibodies and specifically which particular anti-AGE antibodies are involved in the aetiology of diabetic micro- and macrovascular complications is, however, yet to be established. The possibility of effective therapeutic intervention stresses the importance of detecting anti-AGE antibodies, and advancements in measuring anti-AGE antibodies using reliable methods will help determine the role they have in the pathogenesis of many diseases, especially diabetes and its complications.

Antibodies against AGE structures led to the discovery that only a minor proportion of AGE are detectable by autoflourescence and they form to a greater extent in intracellularly than extracellularly because several glucose fragmentation products which occur during the metabolism of glucose in the cell are more reactive than glucose itself (Giardino et al., 1994). It was also found that the non-flourescent CML is the major epitope against which AGE-antibodies are directed (Reddy et al., 1996). Some AGE-antibodies used so far have not been characterized at all. To circumvent this problem researchers applied antibodies directed against the proteins that are abundantly available in blood and more exposed to blood glucose levels in diabetes mellitus as representative markers for the gluco-oxidative pathway. Anti-HSA antibodies have been observed in diabetes (Eilat *et al.*, 1981), a fivefold greater occurrence than in nondiabetic persons (Gregor *et al.*, 1986). Proteins containing AGEs are highly immunogenic and CML is one of the major epitopes recognised by anti-AGE antibodies (Reddy *et al.*, 1995; Ikeda *et al.*, 1996). The presence of AGE-antibodies in the serum of streptozotocin-diabetic rats as well as in a small number of diabetic patients have been reported (Shibayama *et al.*, 1999) AGE can exert their immunogenicity, demonstrate that presence of AGEs-immune complexes (AGE-IC) in the diabetic patients that may play a role in the artherogenesis (Turk *et al.*, 2001). Interactions of AGE autoantibodies with AGEs as a continuously produced antigen result in the formation of AGE-ICs that may play role in diabetic complications (Jakus and Rietbrock, 2004). The analysis of the frequency distribution profile shows that 14% of the diabetic subjects display significant antibody binding to AGE-HSA than the control subjects (Vay *et al.*, 2000).

6. Autoantibodies against gluco-oxidative modified proteins in diabetic retinopathy

The autoantibodies have always been important for clinical interest due to their potential role in screening, diagnosis, monitoring treatment of effectiveness and prognosis. Non-enzymatic glycation of proteins can lead to the formation of reactive AGEs, which are thought to be implicated in the formation of micro- and macrovascular complications in diabetes mellitus. Proteins such as serum albumin, collagen, elastin, lens crystalline, are particularly susceptible to glucose modification (Festa et al., 1998). Elevated serum levels of these glycated proteins were detected in diabetic subjects moreover, higher levels of glycated form of proteins or AGEs were found in diabetic patients with secondary complications such as retinopathy, nephropathy and artherosclerosis (Nicoloff et al., 2000; Nicoloff 2001; Ahmed 2005). Previous studies showed reactive AGE can directly alter the physical and structural properties of the extracellular matrix, for instance, by inducing collagen cross-linking, basement membrane thickening, and covalent trapping of plasma proteins such as LDL and IgG (Bouma et al., 2003). *Ex vivo* HSA was incubated with glucose at the concentration of 50 mM for 5 weeks at 37°C under aerobic conditions (Khan et al., 2007). Biochemical, spectral, electrophoretic, circular dichroism spectropolarimetric, and thermodynamic analyses confirmed that the structure and stability of HSA is significantly affected by glucose induced modification. Recently we showed that gluco-oxidation of proteins alter the structural complexity of the molecule and make them highly immunogenic (Khan et al., 2010). Ex vivo designed gluco-oxidative modified human serum albumin (RG-HSA) were used as an antigen and the titres of antibodies against (RG-HSA-Abs) it were screened in both types of diabetic patients, as well as screening was also done in diabetic patients with complications like retinopathy, nephropathy and artherosclerosis (Table 1). Interestingly, diabetic patients with associated complications (retinopathy, nephropathy and atherosclerosis) generated higher autoantibodies against gluco-oxidative modified HSA than controls and diabetic subjects without secondary complications. This above contention supports that gluco-oxidative proteins are toxic and highly immunogenic. From overall cohort of diabetic patients, the highest recognition of RG-HSA as an antigen by circulatory autoantibodies from diabetic retinopathy as compared to diabetic nephropathy and atherosclerosis (Table 1).

Groups	Sera positive for RG-HSA[1]	Sera positive for N-HSA[2]	Sera positive for both antigens	Carbonyl content (nmol/mg protein)
Type 1 diabetes (n = 30)	21 (52 ± 5.5)	-	1 (43 ± 4.7[1]; 51 ± 5.2[2])	2.9 ± 0.35
Type 2 diabetes (n = 30)	16 (48 ± 4.7)	-	2 (47 ± 4.7[1]; 43 ± 5.2[2], 45 ± 3.3[1]; 41 ± 4.7[2])	2.8 ± 0.4
Diabetes retinopathy (n = 12)	8 (76 ± 4.5)	-	-	3.9 ± 0.5
Diabetes nephropathy (n = 12)	7 (69 ± 3.1)	1 (41 ± 4.7)	-	3.5 ± 0.35
Diabetes atherosclerosis (n = 14)	9 (67 ± 4.0)	-	1 (55 ± 4.1[1]; 55 ± 2.8[2])	3.3 ± 0.55
Controls NH (n = 60)	-	-	-	2.3 ± 0.42

Table 1. Detection of N-HSA-Abs and RG-HSA-Abs and the estimation of carbonyl contents as oxidative stress in the sera of various diabetic groups and control. ELISA plate coated with the respective antigen (20 μg/ml). Sera positive means serum samples which gave inhibition greater than 30%, as less than that may be due to non specific bindings. n denotes the number of sera tested. Values in parentheses are mean ± SD of maximum percent inhibition of positive serum samples at 20 μg/ml of competitor. [1]ROS-glycated and [2]native HSA were used as inhibitor.

Diabetic retinopathic patients also exhibited maximum amount of carbonyl content, which showed a significant correlation between high oxidative stress and presence of anti-RG-HSA antibodies. Clinical and Laboratory examination was also done for 96 diabetic patients (66 males and 30 females) and 60 normal human (41 males and 19 females) serve as controls. According to the data given in Table 2, oxidative stress with chronic hyperglycemia and advanced age has been considered a potential risk factor in the development of autoantibodies in retinopathy and other diabetic complications as well. AGEs are products of oxidative modifications of glycated proteins, which damage blood proteins. High oxidative stress and toxic blood glucose levels are found to be the common factors behind the generation of high autoantibodies and the progression of disease complications.

Subjects	Number of subjects	Age Years	Duration of disease Years	Fasting blood glucose (mg/dL)	HbA_{1C} (%)
Type 1 diabetic	30	36 ± 14	9 ± 3	254 ± 32	7.4 ± 0.6
Type 2 diabetic	30	44 ± 11	7 ± 3.6	263 ± 28	7.1 ± 0.4
Diabetic retinopathy	12	68 ± 2.9	21 ± 5	434 ± 11	9.0 ± 0.4
Diabetic nephropathy	12	62 ± 4.3	18 ± 3.3	394 ± 13	9.2 ±0.6
Diabetic atherosclerosis	12	59 ± 3.6	17 ± 3.6	390 ± 15	8.8 ± 0.3
Control NH	60	32 ± 9.5	–	88 ± 9.8	5.8 ± 0.4

Table 2. Clinical characterization of the patients and normal control subjects. For the blood glucose estimations, blood was collected in oxalated fluoride containers and the assays were performed immediately. Values are in mean ± SD. NH represents normal human subjects.

Gluco-oxidative modified HSA was immunized in the white New-Zealand rabbit that exhibited high titre of anti-glycated albumin antibodies in the serum of experimental animals (Khan et al., 2010). High titre showed immunogenicity of the gluco-oxidative modified proteins. These antibodies were proven to be a potential probe for the detection of protein lesion in blood proteins during diabetes mellitus. ELISA experiments of these antibodies with the isolated blood proteins such as albumin, IgG and RBC membrane from the diabetic patients showed high recognition. It means that during hyperglycemia there is damage of blood proteins that modifies the normal conformation of and hence generate new-epitopes that share binding specificity with the ex vivo designed gluco-oxidative modified albumin. Moreover, anti-gluco-oxidative modified HSA antibodies showed cross reaction with proteins such as BSA, poly L-lysine, immunoglobulins that were incubated ex vivo with 25 μM of glucose or fructose for 20 days. These findings suggests that paratopes of anti-gluco-oxidative albumin antibodies recognise common epitopes that are present in most gluco-oxidative modified proteins.

During diabetes, persistent hyperglycemia causes increased production of free radicals, especially ROS in all tissues by glucose auto-oxidation, protein glycation and due to decreased destruction by nonenzymic and enzymic catalase , glutathione peroxidase, and superoxide dismutase activity (Kowluru et al., 2001; Baynes & Thorpe 1999; Haskins et al., 2003). The level of these antioxidant enzymes critically influences the susceptibility of various tissues to oxidative stress and is associated with the development of complications in diabetes. Also this is particularly relevant and dangerous for the beta islet, which is among those tissues that have the lowest levels of intrinsic antioxidant defences (West 2000; Robertson 2004). In diabetes mellitus, alterations in the endogenous free radical scavenging defence mechanisms may lead to ineffective scavenging of reactive oxygen species, resulting in oxidative damage and tissue injury.

Antibodies against glutamic acid decarboxylase-65 (GAD65Abs) are often considered to be an epiphenomenon resulting from the autoimmune destruction of the pancreatic beta cells in type 1 diabetes. Previous studies suggest that they are involved in antigen processing and presentation and thus modulate the immune response (Banga et al., 2004). Because of the high diagnostic sensitivity for autoimmune diabetes, the presence of GAD65Ab is currently used to identify subjects at high risk for the disease. GAD65Abs are detected in about 60% of new-onset cases of type 1 diabetes, and high levels of these autoantibodies were also reported in diabetic patients with secondary complications (such as retinopathy and nephropathy), the leading cause of blindness and renal failure (Falorini et al., 1998; Bonifecio et al., 1995; Jakuc & Reitbrock 2004). The exact aetiology behind these complications is not completely clear. In our recent study; ROS modified GAD65 was found to be more immunogenic in T1D than its native form (Khan et al., 2009). GAD65Abs in T1D are predominantly directed at conformational epitopes located in the middle region of the molecule, whereas they also recognize linear epitopes and epitopes located in the middle, COOH- and NH2-terminuses (Hampe et al., 2000). Shifts in GAD65 epitopes were detected in a subgroup of newly diagnosed children within the first 12 months after disease onset (Hampe et al., 1999). Moreover, epitope spreading has gained credence as a major driver underlying autoimmunity (Cheung & Wong 2007). Growing evidence suggests that ROS plays an important role in the initiation and progression of diabetes and its associated complications. These increased levels of free radicals pose a direct toxic effect on GAD65 and increase its immunogenicity. Specificity of autoantibodies for epitopes on GAD65 and their levels may be a better indicator of impending or actual destruction of islet beta-cells and increasing complications associated with diabetes.

In our 2009 study (Khan et al., 2009), while searching for a potential epitopes, high titre autoantibodies were detected in type 1 diabetes patients. GAD65 was considered a potential marker for type 1 diabetes. GAD65 was exposed to hydroxyl radical (ROS-GAD65), induced structural and conformational alterations were observed and investigated. Presence of autoantibodies against them were found in diabetes patients. Higher titres of autoantibodies were detected against ROS modified GAD65 (ROS-GAD65-Abs) in type 1 diabetic patients as compared to unmodified native GAD65. Increased levels of ROS in type 1 diabetes by molecular pathways or over produced metal catalyzed reactions modified GAD65 and induced biophysical structural alterations that would probably alter immunogenicity leading to induction and elevated levels of autoantibodies in type 1 diabetes. The data demonstrates possible role of ROS in presenting neo-epitopes that may be one of the factors in antigen-driven autoimmune response. Specificity of autoantibodies for epitopes on GAD65 and their levels may be a better indicator of impending or actual destruction of islet beta-cells and increasing complications associated with diabetes. The etiology of ROS-GAD65 in the pathogenesis of diabetic complications was further investigated in patients' diabetic complications in our new study (Khan et al., 2011). In this finding, significantly high levels of circulating ROS-GAD65Abs were detected in complicated diabetic patients especially in retinopathy as compared to uncomplicated type1 diabetic patients (Table 3).

Subjects	Age years	Gender (M:F)	Smoking duration Years	Duration of disease Years	Fasting blood glucose (mg/dl)	HbA_{1C} (%)	ROS-GAD65-Abs (MMPI)	Hyper-tension 140/90 (%)	Carbonyl Content (nmol/mg protein)
Uncomplicated T1D (n=60)	30 ± 09	37:23	*8(5±3.4)	09 ± 5.6	238 ± 27	7.9 ± 0.7	50.6 ± 7.2*	36(60)	3.0 ± 0.22
Complicated T1D Nephropathy (n=20)	37 ± 11	12:8	*14(6±3.8)	14 ± 4.9	311 ± 21	8.8 ± 0.6	70.3 ± 8.2	17(85)	3.4 ± 0.28
Complicated T1D Retinopathy (n=20)	42 ± 14	11:9	*17(8 ± 3.6)	17 ± 4.3	335 ± 17	9.3 ± 0.7	74.5 ± 6.5	16(80)	3.9 ± 0.31
Control (n=50)	32 ± 8	28:22	–	–	96 ± 11.2	5.8 ± 0.4	7.2 ± 3.7	4(8)	2.1 ± 0.17

Table 3. Clinical and laboratory data from complicated and uncomplicated T1D patients; normal human subjects serve as controls. Data are means ± SD. The sign "* "represents number of smokers from given total respective subjects. For blood glucose estimations, blood was collected in oxalated fluoride containers and the assays were performed immediately. Hypertension is defined as sitting systolic blood pressure ≥140mmHg and/or diastolic blood pressure ≥90 mmHg or the use of antihypertensive medication. Signs * represents 20 number of sera from different patients in the respective group. R-GAD65-Abs (Antibodies against ROS modified GAD65).

This risk of the disease may be enhanced due to acceleration in the formation of free radicals with gradual increase in duration of disease. Smoking and hypertension were also associated with increased antibody production in diabetic retinopathy. Gluco-oxidative stress leads to conformational alterations in native GAD65 protein which could increase or expose cryptic epitopes. Dynamic changes in the GAD65Abs binding pattern suggest subsequent epitopes spreading with disease progression. Concomitantly, these two studies on GAD65 provide us the evidences that hyperglycemia, age, oxidative stress, smoking, and as well as extent of blood protein glycation (HbA1C) participate in etiology of increased GAD65Ab immunogenicity implicated in diabetic retinopathy.

The exact mechanism for the formation of these autoantibodies and progression of diabetic retinopathy is still not well explained. We hypothesized that anti-gluco-oxidative protein autoantibodies bind to soluble glycated proteins and form an intermediary immune complex in the bloodstream that can bind to the basement membranes of the retinal blood vessels. At these sites they can activate complement cascade, resulting in damage to the walls of microvascular cappillaries associated with diabetic retinopathy. This phenomenon results in local necrosis of the vessels. If there is no continuous source of antigen, under conditions of controlled hyperglycemia then gluco-oxidative modified proteins are cleared and the disease can be controlled. However, if there is chronic hyperglycemia that enhances a continuing modification of blood protein, formation of increased immune complexes cause chronic autoimmune pathogenesis of diabetic retinopathy.

Gluco-oxidation associated damage of proteins due to hyperglycemia can be enhanced due to multiple factors such as duration of disease, age, smoking and hypertension and hence can accelerate production of autoantibodies. This suggests that it is perhaps the rate of accumulation rather than the absolute concentration of gluco-oxidative proteins that is important. The exact mechanism behind the production of these autoantibodies is yet to be elucidated. However it stands to reason that the measurement of serum levels of gluco-oxidative proteins or anti-gluco-oxidative modified protein antibodies is important for estimation of an increased risk for development of diabetic retinopathy.

7. Conclusion

Gluco-oxidation is considered to be an important pathophysiological mechanism in the development of diabetic retinopathy. Gluco-oxidation leads to toxicity of blood proteins in diabetic retinopathic patients. Considerable amounts of AGEs are formed from blood proteins that subsequently develop into immune complexes with anti-AGE antibodies in retinopathic subjects. The ROS and gluco-oxidative modified protein autoantibodies were detectable in high titers in patients suffering from diabetic retinopathy. Chronic hyperglycemia and increased age, that are often seen in such cases, have proven to cause abnormally high production of free radicals with decreased antioxidant defence system. Proteins are damaged by the concomitant effect of glycation and oxidative stress leading to conformational alterations in native structure which could induce neo-epitopes or may increase exposed cryptic epitopes. Dynamic changes in the autoantibody binding patterns suggest subsequent epitope spreading with disease progression. Immune complexes of gluco-oxidative proteins and antibodies against them possibly activate complement cascade system and hence destroy capillaries within the retina. Measurement of these autoantibodies could be useful in assisting the prediction of the development of disease even before non-proliferative diabetic retinopathy. Reduction in the levels of glycation and ROS may lead to decrease in *in vivo* protein modifications, thus delaying the progression of diabetic retinopahy.

8. References

Adams AK, Wermuth EO, McBride PE. (1999) Antioxidant vitamins and the prevention of coronary heart disease. *Am Fam Physc,* 60, 895-904.

Ahmed MU, Thorpe SR, Baynes JW. (1986) Identification of Ne-(carboxymethyl)lysine as a degradation product of fructose lysine in glycated protein. *J Biol Chem,* 261, 4889-4894.

Ahmed N, Babaei-Jadidi R, Howell KS, Beisswenger JP, Thornalley JP. (2005) Degradation products of proteins damaged by glycation, oxidation and nitration in clinical type 1 diabetes. *Diabetologia,* 48, 1590-1603.

Ahmed N. (2005) Advanced glycation endproducts--role in pathology of diabetic complications. *Diabetes Res Clin Pract,* 67, 3-21.

Armstrong D, Ueda T, Ueda T, et al. (1998) Lipid hydroperoxide stimulates retinal neovascularization in rabbit retina through expression of tumor necrosis factor-alpha, vascular endothelial growth factor and platelet-derived growth factor. *Angiogenesis* 2, 93–104.

Banga JP, Moore JK, Duhindan N, Madec AM, Vanendert PM, Orgiazzi J, Endl J. (2004) Modulation of antigen presentation by autoreactive B cell clonesspecific for GAD65 from a type I diabetic patient. *Clin Exp Immunol,*135, 74-84.

Barcelo A, Aedo C, Rajpathak S, Robles S. (2003) The cost of diabetes in Latin America and the Caribbean. *Bulletin of the World Health Organization,* 81:19–27.

Baydanoff S, Konova E, Ivanova N. (1996). Determination of anti-AGE antibodies in human serum. *Glucoconjugate J*, 13, 335– 339.

Baynes JW, Thorpe SR. (1999) Role of oxidative stress in diabetic complications: a new perspective on an old paradigm. *Diabetes*, 48(1), 1–9.

Beisswenger PJ, Howell SK, Nelson RG, Mauer M, Szergold BS (2003a) alpha-Oxoaldehyde metabolism and diabetic complications. *Biochem Soc Trans*, 31, 1358-1363.

Beisswenger PJ, Howell SK, Smith K, Szwergold BS. (2003b) Glyceraldehyde-3-phosphate dehydrogenase activity as an independent modifier of methylglyoxal levels in diabetes. *Biochim Biophys Acta*, 1637: 98-106.

Berg TJ, Bangstad HJ, Torjesen PA, Osterby R, Bucala R, Hanssen KF. (1997a). Advanced glycation end products in serum predict changes in the kidney morphology of patients with insulin-dependent diabetes mellitus. *Metabolism* 46, 661– 665.

Berlett BS, Stadtman ER. (1997) Protein oxidation in aging, disease, and oxidative Stress. *J Biol Chem*, 272, 20313–20316.

Bhavsar AR, Emerson GG, Emerson MV, Browning DJ. (2010) Diabetic Retinopathy. In: Browning DJ. *Epidemiology of Diabetic Retinopathy*. Springer, New York.

Boehm BO, Schilling S, Rosinger S, Land GE, Land GK, Kienthsch-Engel R, Stahl P. (2004) Elevated serum levels of N(epsilon)-carboxymethyl-lysine, an advanced glycation end product, are associated with proliferative diabetic retinopathy and macular oedema. *Diabetologia* 47, 1376–1379.

Bonifacio E, Genovese S, Braghi S. (1995) Islet autoantibody markers in IDDM: Risk assessment strategies yielding high sensitivity. *Diabetol*, 38, 816-822.

Bonnardel-Phu E, Wautier JL, Schmidt AM, Avila C, Vicaut E. (1999) Acute modulation of albumin microvascular leakage by advanced glycation end products in microcirculation of diabetic rats in vivo. *Diabetes*,48, 2052–2058.

Boulanger E, Puisieux F, Gaxatte C, Wautier JL. (2007) Aging: role and control of glycation. *Rev Med Interne* 28(12), 832-840.

Boulanger E, Wautier JL, Dequiedt P, Schmidt AM. (2006) Glycation, glycoxidation and diabetes mellitus. *Nephrol Ther*, 2(1), S8-16.

Bouma B, Kroon-Batenbury JML, Wu PY, Brunjes B, Posthuma G, Kranenburg O, DeGroot GP, Voest EE, Gebbink GBFM. (2003) Glycation induces formation of amyloid cross-beta structure in albumin. *J Biol Chem*, 278, 41810-41819.

Bourdon E, Lorea N, Blache D. (1999) Glucose and free radicals impair the antioxidant properties of serum albumin. *FASEB J*, 13, 233-244.

Brownlee M, Cerami A, Vlassara H. (1998) Advanced glycosylation end products in tissue and the biochemical basis of diabetic complication. *N Engl J Med* 318, 1315–21.

Brownlee M. (1995) Advanced protein glycosylation in diabetes and aging. *Annu Rev Med*, 46, 223-234.

Brownlee M. (1996) Advanced glycation end products in diabetic complications. *Curr Opin Endocrinol Diabetes*, 3, 291–97.

Brownlee M. (2001) Biochemistry and molecular cell biology of diabetic complications. *Nature*, 414, 813-820.

Brownlee M. (2005) The pathobiology of diabetic complications – a unifying mechanism. *Diabetes*, 54, 1615-1625.

Bryszewska M, Szosland K. (1988)Association between glycation of erythrocyte membrane fluidity. *Ann Clin Res*, 21, 49–51.

Cai H, Harrison DG. (2000) Endothelial dysfunction in cardiovascular disease: the role of oxidant stress. *Circ Res*, 87, 840–844.

Carter CD, Ho XJ. (1994) Structure of serum albumin. *Adv Prot Chem*, 45, 153-203.

Chakravarthy U, Hayes RG, Stitt AW, McAuley E, Archer DB. (1998) Constitutive nitric oxide synthase expression in retinal vascular endothelial cells is suppressed by high glucose and advanced glycation end products. *Diabetes* 47, 945-952.

Chappey O, Dosquet C, Wautier MP, Wautier JL. (1997) Advanced glycation end products, oxidant stress and vascular lesions. *Eur J Clin Invest* 27, 97–108.

Cheung N, Wong TY. (2007) Obesity and Eye Diseases. *Survey of Ophthalmology*, 52, 180–95.

Clements RS Jr, Robison WG Jr, Cohen MP. (1998) Anti-glycated albumin therapy ameliorates early retinal microvascular pathology in db/db mice. *J Diab Comp* 12, 28-33.

Crawford TN, Alfaro DV 3rd, Kerrison JB, Jablon EP. (2009) Diabetic retinopathy and angiogenesis. *Curr Diabetes Rev*, 5(1), 8-13.

Cribbs DH, Azizeh BY, Cotman CW, LaFerla FM. (2000) Fibril formation and neurotoxicity by a herpes simplex virus glycoprotein B fragment with homology to the Alzheimer's A beta peptide. *Biochemistry*, 39, 5988–5994.

Cui Y, Xu X, Bi H, Zhu Q, Wu J, Xia X, Qiushi R, Ho PC. (2006) Expression modification of uncoupling proteins and MnSOD in retinal endothelial cells and pericytes induced by high glucose: the role of reactive oxygen species in diabetic retinopathy. *Experimental Eye Research*, 83, 807–816.

Cutler P. (1989) Deferoxamine therapy in high-ferritin diabetes. *Diabetes*, 38, 1207-1210.

Dhalla NS, Temsah RM, Netticadan T. (2000) Role of oxidative stress in cardiovascular diseases. *J Hypertens*, 18, 655-673

Du XL, Edelstein D, Rossetti L, Fantus IG, Goldberg H, Ziyadeh F, Wu J, Brownlee M. (2002) Hyperglycemia-induced mitochondrial superoxide overproduction activates the exosamine pathway and induces plasminogen activator inhibitor-1 expression by increasing Sp1 glycosylation. *Proc NatlAcad Sci USA*, 97, 12222–12226.

Du Y, Miller CM, Kern TS. (2003) "Hyperglycemia increases mitochondrial superoxide in retina and retinal cells," *Free Radical Biology and Medicine*, 35(11), 1491–1499.

Eilat D, Fischel R, Zlotnick A. (1981) Albumin-immunoglobulin complexes in human serum: classification and immunochemical analysis. *Scand J Imminol*, 14, 77-83.

Ellis EA, Guberski DL, Somogyi-Mann M, and Grant MB. (2000) Increased H2O2, vascular endothelial growth factor and receptors in the retina of the BBZ/WOR diabetic rat. *Free Radical Biology and Medicine*, 28(1), 91–101.

Falorni A, Kassi G, Murdolo G, Calcinaro F. (1998) Controversies on humoral immune markers of insulin-dependent diabetes mellitus. *J Ped Endocrinol Metab*, 11, 307-317.

Federman JL, Gouras P, Schubert H. (1994) Systemic diseases. In: Podos SM, Yanoff M, eds., (pp, 7-24) Vol9, *Retina and Vitreous: Textbook of Ophthalmology.*

Festa A, Schmolzer B, Schernthaner G, Menzel EJ. (1998) Differential expression of receptors for advanced glycation end products on monocytes in patients with IDDM. *Diabetologia*, 41, 674– 680.

Ford ES, Mokdad AH, Giles WH, and Brown DW. (2003)The metabolic syndrome and antioxidant concentrations:findings from the Third National Health and Nutrition Examination Survey. *Diabetes*, 52(9), 2346–2352.

Fu MX, Knecht KJ, Thorpe SR, Baynes JW (1992) The role of oxygen in cross-linking and chemical modifications of collagen by glucose. *Diabetes*, 41, 42-48.

Fu MX, Requena JR, Jenkins AJ, Lyons TJ, Baynes JW, Thorpe SR. (1996) The advanced glycation end product, Nepsilon-(carboxymethyl)lysine, is a product of both lipid peroxidation and glycoxidation reactions. *J Biol Chem* 271, 9982-9986.

Genuth S, Sun W, Cleary P, Sell DR, Dahms W, Malone J, Sivitz W, Monnier VM. (2005) Glycation and carboxymethyllysine levels in skin collagen predict the risk of future 10-year progression of diabetic retinopathy and nephropathy in the diabetes control and complications trial and epidemiology of diabetes interventions and complications participants with type 1 diabetes. *Diabetes,* 54, 3103–3111.

Giardino I, Edelstein D, Brownlee M (1994) Nonenzymatic glycosylation in vitro and in bovine endothelial cells alters basic fibroblast growth factor activity. *J Clin Invest,* 94, 110-117

Gilcrease MZ, Hoover RL. (1990) Activated human monocytes exhibit receptor-mediated adhesion to a non-enzymatically glycosylated proteinsubstrate, *Diabetologia,* 33, 329–33.

Giugliano D, Ceriello A, Paolisso G. (1996) Oxidative stress and diabetic vascular complications. *Diabetes Care,* 19, 257–267.

Gregor I, Iberg N, Berger W, Fluckiger R. (1986) Albumin directed antibodies in diabetes; demonstration of human serum albumin-directed IgM autoantibodies. *Diabetologia,* 29, 481-484.

Hammes HP, Alt A, Niwa T, Clausen JT, Bretzel RG, Brownlee M, Schleicher ED. (1999) Differential accumulation of advanced glycation end products in the course of diabetic retinopathy. *Diabetologia,* 42, 728–736.

Hammes HP, Weiss A, Hess S, Araki N, Horiuchi S, Brownlee M, Preissner KT. (1996) Modification of vitronectin by advanced glycation alters functional properties in-vitro and the diabetic retina. *Lab Invest,* 75, 325-338.

Hampe CS, Hammerle LP, Bekris L, Ortqvist E, Kockum I, Rolandsson O,Landin-Olsson M, Torn C, Persson B, Lernmark A. (2000) Recognition of glutamicacid decarboxylase (GAD) by autoantibodies from different GADantibody-positive phenotypes. *J Clin Endocrinol Metab,* 85, 4671-4679.

Hampe CS, Ortqvist E, Persson B, Schranz DB, Lernmark A. (1999) Glutamate decarboxylase (GAD) autoantibody epitope shift during the first year of type 1 diabetes. *Horm Metab Res,* 31, 553-557.

Harhaj NS and Antonetti DA. (2004) Regulation of tight junctions and loss of barrier function in pathophysiology. *Int J of Biochem Cell Biol,* 36(7), 1206–1237.

Haskins K, Bradley B, Powers K, Fadok V, Flores S, Ling X, Pugazhenthi S, Reusch J, Kench J. (2003) Oxidative stress in type 1 diabetes, *Ann NY Acad Sci,* 1005,43–54.

Horiuchi S, Murakami M, Takata K, Morino Y. (1986) Scavenger receptor for aldehyde-modified proteins. *J Biol Chem,* 261, 4962-4966.

Huebschmann G, Regensteiner JG, Vlassara H, Reusch JE. (2006) Diabetes and advanced glycoxidation end products. *Diabetes Care,* 29, 1420-1432.

Hunt JV. (1994) In "Free Radicals in the Environment, Medicine and Toxicology", Nohl H, Esterbauer H, Rice-Evans C. eds., (pp, 137-162), Richeliu Press, London.

Iberg N, Fluckiger R. (1986) Nonenzymatic glycosylation of albumin in vivo. Identification of multiple glycosylated sites. *J Biol Chem,* 261, 13542-13545.

Ienaga K, Nakamura K, Hochi T, Nakazawa Y, Fukunaga Y, Kakita H, Nakano K. (1995) Crosslines, fluorophores in the AGE-related cross-linked proteins. *Contrib Nephrol, 112*, 42-51.

Ikeda K, Higashi T, Sano H, Jinnouchi Y, Yoshida M, Araki T, Ueda S, Horiuchi S. (1996) *N*-(Carboxymethyl)lysine protein adduct is a major immunological epitope in proteins modified with advanced glycation end products of the Maillard reaction. *Biochemistry* , 35, 8075-8083.

Imani F, Horii Y, Suthanthiran M, Skolnik EY, Makita Z, Sharma V, Sehaipal P, Vlassara H. (1993) Advanced glycosylation end product-specific receptors on human and rat T-lymphocytes mediates synthesis of interferon gamma: role in tissue remodeling. *J Exp Med,* 178, 2165–72.

Jakus V, Rietbrock N. (2004) Advance glycation end-products and the progress of diabetic vascular complications. *Physiol Res,* 53, 131-142.

Jiang ZY, Woollard AC, Wolff SP. (1990) Hydrogen peroxide production during experimental protein glycation. *FEBS Lett,* 268(1), 69–71.

John WG, Lamb EJ. (1993) the Millard or browning reaction in diabetes. *Eye,* 7, 230-237.

Kameda Y, Makita Z. (2000) Neurotoxicity of advanced glycation end-products for cultured cortical neurons. *J Neuropathol Exp Neurol,* 59, 1094–1105.

Khan MWA, Rasheed Z, Khan WA, Ali R. (2007) Biochemical, biophysical and thermodynamical analysis of *in vitro* glycated human serum albumin, *Biochemistry (Mosc)*, 72, 146-152.

Khan MWA, Sherwani S, Khan WA, Moinuddin , Ali R. (2009) Characterization ofhydroxyl radical modified GAD65: a potential autoantigen in type 1 diabetes. *Autoimmunity,* 42, 150-158.

Khan MWA., Banga K., Mashal SN., Khan WA. (2011) Detection of autoantibodies against reactive oxygen species modified glutamic acid decarboxylase-65 in type 1 diabetes associated complications. *BMC Immunol,* 12:19-26.

Khan MWA., Qadrie ZL., Khan WA. (2010) Antibodies against gluco-oxidative modified HSA-detected in diabetes associated complications, *Int Arch Allergy Immunol,* 153, 207-214.

Kim W, Hudson BI, Moser B, Guo J, Rong LL, Lu Y, Qu W , Lalla E, Lerner S, Chen Y, Shi Du Yan S, D'Agati V, Naka YU, Ramasamy R, Herold K, Yan SF, Schmidt AM. (2005) Receptor for advanced glycation end products and its ligands: a journey from the complications of diabetes to its pathogenesis. *Ann N Y Acad Sci,* 1043, 553-561.

Kislinger T, Fu C, Huber B, Qu W, Taquchi A, Du Yan S, Hoffmann M, Yan SF, Pischetsrieder M, Stern D, Schmidt AM. (1999) N(epsilon)-(carboxymethyl)lysine adducts of proteins are ligands for receptor for advanced glycation end products that activate cell signaling pathways and modulate gene expression. *J Biol Chem,* 274, 31740–31749.

Koenig RJ, Blobstein SH, Cerami A. (1977) Structure of carbohydrate of hemoglobin Aic. *J Biol Chem,* 252, 2992-2997.

Koga K, Yamagishi S, Okamoto T, Inagaki Y, Amano D, Akeuchi M, Makita Z. (2002) Serum levels of glucose-derived advanced glycation end products are associated with the severity of diabetic retinopathy in type 2 diabetic patients without renal dysfunction. *Int J Clin Pharmacol Res* 22, 13-17.

Kowluru RA, Tang J, and Kern TS. (2001) Abnormalities of retinal metabolism in diabetes and experimental galactosemia. VII. Effect of long-term administration of antioxidants on the development of retinopathy. *Diabetes*, 50(8), 1938–1942.

Koya D, King GL. (1998) Protein kinase C activation and the development of diabetic complications. *Diabetes* 47, 859–66.

Kukreja A, Maclaren KN. (1999) Autoimmunity and diabetes. *J Clin Endocrin Metabol*, 84: 4371-4382.

Leto G, Pricci F, Amadio L, Iacobini C. (2001) Increased retinal endothelial cell monolayer permeability induced by the diabetic milieu: role of advanced non-enzymatic glycation and polyol pathway activation. *Diabetes Metab Res Rev*,17, 448–458.

Liggins J, Furth JA. (1997) Role of protein-bound carbonyl groups in the formation of advanced glycation endproducts. *Biochim Biophys Acta*, 1361: 123-129.

Lou MF (2003) Redox regulation in the lens. Prog Retin Eye Res 22(5), 657-682.

Lyons TJ, Li W, Wojciechowski B, Wells-Knecht MC, Wells-KnechtK. J., and Jenkins, A. J. (2000) Aminoguanidine and the effects of modified LDL on cultured retinal capillary cells. *Invest Ophthalmol Vis Sci*, 41, 1176–1180

Mackay IR. (2000) Tolerance and autoimmunity. *BMJ* 321, 93-96.

Mamputu JC, Renier G. (2002) Advanced glycation end products increase, through a protein kinase C-dependent pathway, vascular endothelial growth factor expression in retinal endothelial cells. Inhibitory effect of gliclazide. *J Diab Comp* 16, 284-293.

ManiKanth SB,Kalishwaralal K, Sriram M, Pandian SBRK, Youn H, Eom S, Gurunathan S. (2010) Anti-oxidant effect of gold nanoparticles restrains hyperglycemic conditions in diabetic mice. *J Nanobiotechnology* 8, 16-24.

Mateo MCM, Bustamante JB, Cantalapiedra MAG. (1978) Selinium, zinc, copper and insulin in diabetes millitus. *Biomed*, 29, 56-58.

Matsumoto K, Ikeda K, Horiuchi S, Zhao H, Abraham EC. (1997) Immunochemical evidence for increased formation of advanced glycation end products and inhibition by aminoguanidine in diabetic rat lenses. *Biochem Biophys Res Commun* 241, 352-354.

McDonald MJ, Shapiro R, Bleichman M, Solway J, Bunn HF. (1978) Glycosylated minor components of human adult hemoglobin. *J Biol Chem*, 253, 2327–32.

Meister A. (1988) Glutathione metabolism and its selective modification. *J Biol Chem*, 263(33), 17205–17208.

Monnier VM, Sell DR, Genuth S. (2005) Glycation products as markers and predictors of the progression of diabetic complications. *Ann NY Acad Sci*, 1043, 567-581.

Nakamura, K., Hasegawa, T., Fukunaga, Y., & Ienaga, K. (1992) Crosslines A and B as candidates for the fluorophores in ageand diabetes-related cross-linked proteins, and their diacetates produced by Millard reaction of a-N-acetyl-L-lysine with D glucose. *J Chem Soc Chem Commun*, 14, 992-994.

Nicoloff G, Baydanoff S, Stanimirova N, Petrova CH, Christova P. (2000) Relationship between elastin-derived peptides and the development of diabetic microvascular complications—a longitudinal study in children with Type 1 (insulin-dependent) diabetes mellitus. *Gen Pharmacol*, 35, 59- 64.

Nicoloff G, Baydanoff S, Stanimirova N, Petrova CH, Christova P. (2001) Detection of serum collagen type IV in children with Type 1 (insulin-dependent) diabetes mellitus—a longitudinal study. *Pediatr Diabetes*, 2, 184–190.

Nishikawa T, Edelstein D, Du X-L, Yamagishi S, Matsumura T, Kaneda Y, Yorek M, Beebe D, Oates P, Hammes HP, GiardinoI, Brownlee M. (2000) Normalizing mitochondrial superoxide production blocks three pathways of hyperglycaemic damage. *Nature,* 404, 787–790.

Palm F, Cederberg J, Hansell P, Liss P, Carlsson OO. (2003) Reactive oxygen species cause diabetes-induced decrease in renal oxygen tension. *Diabetologia,* 46, 1153–1160.

Peppa M, Uribarri J, Vlassara H. (2002) Advanced glycoxidation: A new risk factor for cardiovascular disease? *Cardiovasc Toxicol* 2, 275-287.

Peppa M, Uribarri J, Vlassara H. (2004) The role of advanced glycation end products in the development of atherosclerosis. *Curr Diab Rep* 4, 31-36.

Peppa M, Vlassara H. (2005) Advanced glycation end products and diabetic complications: A General overview. Hormones 4(1), 28-37.

Poukupec R, Kalauz M, Turk N, Turk Z. (2003) Advanced glycation endproducts in human diabetic and non-diabetic cataractous lenses. *Graefes Arch Clin Exp Ophthalmol,* 241, 378-384.

Prevention of blindness from diabetes mellitus. (2005) Report of a WHO consultation in Geneva, Switzerland 9–11 November 2005.

Rahbar S, Figarola LJ. (2003) Novel inhibitors of advanced glycation endproducts *Arch Biochem Biophys* 419(1), 63-79.

Raj DS, Choudhury D, Welbourne TC, Levi M. (2000) Advanced glycation end products: a Nephrologist's perspective. *Am J Kidney Dis,* 35, 365–380.

Ratnaikes S, Blake D, Shevenan P. (1987) Enzymatic glycation may decrease activity of erythrocyte *S*-aminolevulinate dehydratase in diabetes mellitus. *Clin Chem,* 33, 1807–1810.

Reber F, Geffarth R, Kasper M, Reichenbach A, Schleicher ED, Siegner A, Funk RH. (2003) Graded sensitiveness of the various retinal neuron populations on the glyoxal-mediated formation of advanced glycation end products and ways of protection. *Graefes Arch Clin Exp Ophthalmol* 241, 213-225.

Reddy S, Bichler J, Wells-Knecht KJ, Thorpe SR, Baynes JW. (1995) Nε-(carboxymethyl)lysine is a dominant advanced glycation end product (AGE) antigen in tissue proteins. *Biochemistry,* 34, 10872– 10878.

Resnikoff S, Pascolini D, Etyaale D, Kocur I, Pararajasegaram R, Pokharel GP, Mariotti SP. (2004) Global data on visual impairment in the year 2002. *Bulletin of the World Health Organization,* 82, 844–851.

Robertson, R.P. (2004) Chronic oxidative stress as a central mechanism for glucose toxicity in pancreatic islet beta cells in diabetes. *J Biol Chem,* 279(41), 42351–42354.

Schleicher E, Nerlich A (1996) The role of hyperglycaemia in the development of diabetic complications. *Horm Metab Res,* 28, 367-373.

Schmidt AM, Yan SD, Wautier JL, Stern D. (1999) Activation of receptor for advanced glycation end products – a mechanism for chronic vascular dysfunction in diabetic vasculopathy and atherosclerosis. *Circ Res,* 84, 489- 497.

Schoonover LL. (2001) Oxidative stress and the role of antioxidants in cardiovascular risk reduction. *Prog Cardiovasc Nurs,* 16(1), 30-32.

Sebag J, Buckingham B, Charles MA, Reiser K. (1992) Biochemical abnormalities in vitreous of humans with proliferative diabetic retinopathy. *Arch Ophthalmol* 110, 1472-1476.

Sell DR, Monnier VM. (1989) Structure elucidation of a senescence cross-link from human extracellular matrix. Implication of pentoses in the aging process. *J Biol Chem,* 264, 21597-21602

Sell DR, Carlson EC, Monnier VM (1993) Differential effects of type 2 (noninsulin-dependent) diabetes mellitus on pentosidine formation in skin and glomerular basement membrane. *Diabetes,* 40, 190-196.

Sell DR, Lapolla A, Odetti P, Fogarty J, Monnier VM (1992) Pentosidine formation in skin correlates with severity of complication in individuals with long-standing IDDM. *Diabetes* 41, 1286-1292.

Sheetz MJ, King GL. (2002) Molecular understanding of hyperglycemia.s adverse effects for diabetic complications. *JAMA* 288, 2579-2588.

Shibayama R, Araki N, Nagai R, Horiuchi S. (1999) Autoantibody against Ne-(carboxymethyl) lysine an advanced glycation end product of the Maillard reaction. *Diabetes,* 48, 1842– 1849.

Singh R, Barden A, Mori T, Beilin L. (2001) Advanced glycation end-products: a review. *Diabetologia,* 44, 129-146.

Skolnik EY, Yang Z, Makita Z, Radoff S, Kirstein M, Vlassara H. (1991) Human and rat mesangial cell receptors for glucose-modified proteins:potential role in kidney tissue remodeling and diabetic nephropathy. *J Exp Med,* 174, 931–39.

Stevens A. (1998) The contribution of glycation to cataract formation in diabetes. *J Am Optom Assoc* 69, 519-530.

Stitt AW, Bhaduri T, McMullen CB, Gardiner TA, Archer DB. (2000) Advanced glycation end products induce blood-retinal barrier dysfunction in normoglycemic rats. *Mol Cell Biol Res Comm,* 3, 380 –388.

Stitt AW, Li YM, Gardiner TA, Bucala R, Archer DB, Vlassara H. (1997) Advanced glycation end products (AGEs) co-localise with AGE receptors in the retinal vasculature of diabetic and of AGE-infused rats. *Am J Pathol,*150, 523–531.

Stitt AW, Moore JE, Sharkey JA, Murphy G, Simpson DA, Bucala R, Vlassara H, Archer DB. (1998) Advanced glycation end products in vitreous: Structural and functional implications for diabetic vitreopathy. *Invest Ophthalmol Vis Sci* 39, 2517-2523.

Stitt AW. (2001) Advanced glycation, an important pathological event in diabetic and age related ocular disease. *Br J Opthalmol* 85, 746-753.

Sulochana KN, Ramprasad S, Coral K, Lakshmi S, Punitham R, Angayarkanni N, Ramakrishnan S. (2003) Glycation and glycoxidation studies in vitro on isolated human vitreous collagen. *Med Sci Monit* 9(6), 219-224.

Swallow AJ. (1960) In *Radiation Chemistry of Organic Compounds,* Swallow AJ, eds., (pp. 211–224), Pergamon Press, New York.

Takeuchi M, Bucala R, Suzuki T, Ohkubo T, Yamazaki M, Koike T, Kameda Y, Makita Z. (2000) Neurotoxicity of advanced glycation end-products for cultured cortical neurons. *J Neuropathol Exp Neurol,* 59(12), 1094-1105.

Thornalley PJ. (2005) Dicarbonyl intermediates in the Maillard reaction. *Ann NY Acad Sci,* 1043, 111-117.

Thorpe SR, Baynes JW. (1996) Role of the Maillard reaction in diabetes mellitus and diseases of aging. *Drugs Aging* 9, 69-77.

Traverso N, Menini S, Cottalasso D, Odetti P, Marinari MU, Pronzata AM. (1997) Mutual interaction between glycation and oxidation during non-enzymatic protein modification. *Biochim Biophys Acta*, 1336, 409-418.

Turk Z, Ljubik S, Turk N, Benko B. (2001) Detection of autoantibodies against advanced glycation end products and AGE-immune complexes in serum of patients with diabetes mellitus. *Clin Chim Acta*, 303, 105–115.

Turk Z. (2001) Glycation and compications of diabetes. *Diabetol Croat*, 30, 49-54.

Turk Z. (2010) Glycotoxines, Carbonyl Stress and Relevance to Diabetes and Its Complications. *Physiol Res*, 59, 147-156.

Vay D, Vidali M, Allochis G, Cusaro C, Rolla R, Mottaram E, Bellomo G, Albano E. (2000) Antibodies against advanced glycation end product Nepsilon-(carboxymethyl)lysine in healthy controls and diabetic patients. *Diabetologia*, 43, 1385-1388.

Vlassara H, Brownlee M, Cerami A (1985) High-affinityreceptor-mediated uptake and degradation of glucosemodified proteins: a potential mechanism for the removal of senescent macromolecules. *Procl Natl Acad Sci USA*, 82, 5588-5592.

Vlassara H, Li YM, Imani F, Wojciechowicz D, Yang Z, Liu FT, Cerami A. (1995) Identification of Galectin-3 as a high affinity binding protein for advanced glycation end products (AGE): a new member of the AGE receptor complex. *Mol Med*, 1, 634–46.

Vlassara H, Palace MR. (2002) Diabetes and advanced glycation endproducts. *J Intern Med* 251: 87-101.

Vlassara H. (2001) The AGE-receptor in the pathogenesis of diabetic complications. *Diabetes Metab Res Rev* 17, 436-443.

Wautier JL, Guillausseau PJ. (1988) Diabetes, advanced glycation endproducts and vascular disease. *Vasc Med*, 3, 131-137.

West IC. (2000) Radicals and oxidative stress in diabetes. *Diabetic Med*, 17, 171–180.

Wolff SP, Dean RT (1987) Glucose autooxidation and protein modification. The potential role of ìautooxidative glycosylation in diabetes. *Biochem J*, 245, 243-250.

World Health Organization (2011) Diabetes fact sheet N°312.

Xu X, Li Z, Luo D. (2003) Exogenous advanced glycosylation end products induce diabetes-like vascular dysfunction in normal rats: a factor in diabetic retinopathy. *Graefes Arch Clin Exp Ophthalmol* 241, 56-62.

Yamagishi S, Inagaki Y, Amano S, Okamoto T, Takeuchi M, Makita Z. (2002) Pigment epithelium-derived factor protects cultured retinal pericytes from advanced glycation end product-induced injury through its antioxidative properties. *Biochem Biophys Res Commun* 296, 877-882.

Yamagishi S, Inagaki Y, Okamoto T, Amano S, Koga K, Takeuchi M, Makita Z. (2002) Advanced glycation end product-induced apoptosis and overexpression of vascular endothelial growth factor and monocyte chemoattractant protein-1 in human-cultured mesangial cells. *J Biol Chem*, 277, 20309–20315

Yang Z, Makita Z, Horii Y, Brunelle S, Cerami A, Sehaipal P, Suthanthiran M, Vlassara H. (1991) Two novel rat liver membrane proteins, that bind advanced glycosylation end products, relationship to macrophage receptor glucose-modified proteins. *J Exp Med*, 174, 515–24.

Zhang X, Saaddine JB, Chou CF, Cotch MF, Cheng YJ, Geiss LS, Gregg EW, Albright AL, Klein BE, Klein R. (2010) Prevalence of diabetic retinopathy in the United States, 2005-2008. *JAMA*, 304(6), 649-656.

3

Cellular and Molecular Mechanism of Diabetic Retinopathy

Mohammad Shamsul Ola and Mohd Imtiaz Nawaz
Department of Ophthalmology, College of Medicine, King Saud University, Riyadh, KSA

1. Introduction

Diabetic retinopathy (DR) is one of the most common complications of diabetes affecting millions of working adults worldwide, in which the retina, a part of the eye becomes progressively damaged, leading to vision loss and blindness. Tremendous efforts have been made to identify biochemical mechanisms which led to the recognition of hyperglycemia, hypertension and dyslipidemia as major risk factors in DR. Consequently, tight glycemic control, blood pressure control and lipid-lowering therapy have all shown proven benefits in reducing the incidence and progression of DR. However, despite tight glycemic control, blood pressure control and lipid-lowering therapy, the number of DR patients keeps growing and therapeutic approaches are limited [Ismail-Beigi F, 2010; Patel A, 2008]. For last several decades, laser photocoagulation and vitrectomy remain as the two conventional approaches for treating sight-threatening conditions such as macular edema and proliferative DR (PDR).

The increased levels of metabolites in diabetic patients and in various animal models of the disease have been shown to induce several unrelated and interrelated biochemical pathways implicated in the progression of the DR. Disturbed level of several metabolites in addition to hyperglycemia and hormonal factors systemically and within diabetic retina change the production pattern of a number of mediators including growth factors, neurotrophic factors, cytokines/chemokines, vasoactive agents, inflammatory molecules, and adhesion molecules resulting in increased blood flow, increased capillary permeability, altered cell turnover (apoptosis) and finally in angiogenesis. In this chapter a major emphasis is given on diabetic induced metabolic changes in the retina which induces a range of molecules and pathways involved early in the pathophysiology of DR which are briefly discussed and those major cascades of events are shown in the schematic diagram as depicted in Fig.1.

2. Hyperglycemia

2.1 Advanced Glycation end products (AGEs)

AGE's are formed via non-enzymatic condensation reaction between reducing glucoses and amine residues of proteins, lipids or nucleic acids that undergo a series of complex reaction to give irreversible cross linked complex group of compounds termed as AGEs. Some of the best chemically characterized AGEs in human are carboxymethyllysine (CML), carboxyethyllysine (CEL), and pentosidine which act a markers for formation and accumulation of AGE in hyperglycemia. CML and other AGEs have been localized to retinal blood vessels of diabetes patients and were found to correlate with the degree of retinopathy suggesting the pathophysiological role of AGE's in diabetes [Stitt AW, 2001]. Increased AGEs formation and accumulation has been found in retinal vessels of diabetic animals, in human serum with type 2 diabetes and in vitreous cavity of people with diabetic retinopathy [Goh SY, 2008; Goldin A, 2006].

Retinal pericytes have been shown to accumulate AGEs during diabetes, implicating pericytes loss which can induce blood-retinal barrier dysfunction [Stitt AW, 2000]. In addition, AGE induces leukocyte adherence that leads to breakdown of blood-retinal barrier via increased leukocyte adhesion to cultured retinal microvascular endothelial cells (ECs) by inducing intracellular cell adhesion molecule-1 (ICAM-1) expression [Moore TC, 2003]. Also retinal vascular endothelial growth factor (VEGF) has been found to induce ICAM-1 expression, thus leading to leukostasis and breakdown of blood-retinal barrier, suggesting AGE-elicited pro-inflammation, may be modulated by the blockage of VEGF [Joussen AM, 2002; Ishida S, 2003]. AGEs increases monocyte chemoattractant protein-1 (MCP-1) and ICAM-1 expression in microvascular ECs through intracellular reactive oxygen species (ROS) generation, thereby inducing T-cell adhesion to ECs [Yamagishi S, 2007; Inagaki Y, 2003].

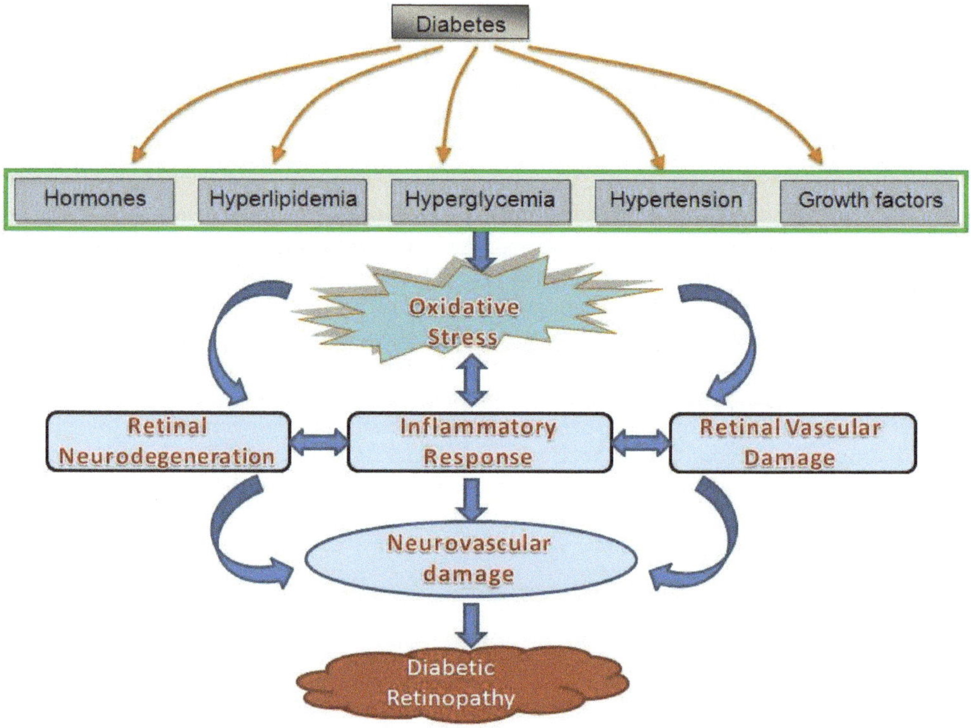

Fig. 1. General features for diabetes induced neurovascular damage in diabetic retinopathy

AGEs disturb retinal microvascular homeostasis by overproduction of VEGF through the interaction with receptor of advanced glycation end products (RAGE) [Yamagishi S, 2002] and the AGE-RAGE axis could be involved in the development and progression of DR by eliciting pericyte apoptosis and dysfunction [Yamagishi S, 2009]. AGEs induces the activation of nuclear factor-B (NF-κB), with simultaneous increase in the ratio of Bcl-2/Bax, and activity of caspase-3, a key enzyme in the execution of apoptosis of pericytes [Yamagishi S, 2002; Denis U, 2002].

Recently, potential therapeutic role of pigment epithelial growth factor (PEDF) as angiostatic, neurotrophic, neuroprotective, antioxidative, and anti-inflammatory properties are widely being discussed and its potential therapeutic property could be exploited as a new option for the treatment of vascular complications in diabetic patients [Yamagishi S, 2008]. Since PEDF levels are decreased in aqueous or vitreous humor in patients with PDR than control, suggesting that loss of PEDF in the eye may contribute to the pathogenesis of PDR [Tombran-Tink J, 2003; Yamagishi S, 2008]. PEDF inhibits the AGE-induced ROS generation and subsequently prevents apoptotic cell death [Yamagishi S, 2008] and also inhibits AGE-induced retinal vascular hyperpermeability in endothelial cells by suppressing nicotinamide adenine dinucleotide phosphate (NADPH)-oxidase mediated ROS generation and subsequently VEGF expression [Sheikpranbabu S, 2010 (a), 2010 (b)]. The work by Yamagishi and his group have shown that injection of AGEs to normal rats increase RAGE and ICAM-1 expression that induced retinal leukostasis and hyperpermeability, however the process was blocked by simultaneous treatment with PEDF that completely inhibited superoxide generation and NF-κB activation in AGE-exposed endothelial cells [Yamagishi S, 2006, 2007]. There is also a significant correlation between the vitreous AGE and VEGF levels and furthermore, both AGEs and VEGF levels (inversely) and PEDF (positively) are associated with the total anti-oxidant status in the vitreous fluid [Yokoi M, 2005, 2007]. All these observations support the concept that PEDF is a potential anti-oxidative agent and anti-inflammatory, that could block the AGE-VEGF axis, thereby may ameliorate the progression of PDR [Yamagishi S, 2009]. Many therapeutic drugs are also being used such as aminoguanidine, pyridoxamine and LR-90 that inhibit glycation reactions and or conversion of early products to AGEs [Abu El-Asrar AM, 2009]. However many such AGE formation inhibitors are still early in clinical trials.

2.2 Protein Kinase C (PKC)

Protein Kinase (PKCs) is a family of about 13 isoforms that are widely distributed in various mammalian tissues. In hyperglycemic state, some of the PKC isoforms are produced primarily from enhanced *de novo* synthesis of diacylglycerol (DAG) from glucose to glycerol 3-phosphate, which act an upstream activator for various isoforms of PKCs, a family of serine/threonine kinases that mediates unique function [Inoguchi T, 1994]. The activities of the classic isoforms (PKC-α, -β1/2, and PKC-δ) are greatly enhanced by DAG and have been linked to vascular dysfunctions and pathogenesis of DR [Geraldes P, 2010]. Hyperglycemia primarily activates the β and δ isoforms of PKC in cultured vascular cells [Koya D, 1997]. Excessive PKC activation underlies microvascular ischaemia, leakage, and angiogenesis in DR. Some of the changes due to PKCs activation include: increase in blood flow, basement membrane thickening, extracellular matrix expansion, vascular permeability, angiogenesis, apoptosis, leukocyte adhesion, and cytokine activation [Aiello LP, 2006; Avignon A, 2006; Das Evcimen N, 2007; Geraldes P, 2010].

In the diabetic retina, hyperglycemia not only activates protein kinase C but also mitogen-activated protein kinase (MAPK) to increase the expression of a unknown targets of PKC signaling, like SHP-1 (Src homology-2 domain–containing phosphatase-1), a protein tyrosine phosphatase. This signaling cascade leads to platelet-derived growth factor (PDGF) receptor-β dephosphorylation and a reduction in downstream signaling from this receptor, resulting in pericyte apoptosis.[Geraldes P, 2009].

PKC isoform selective inhibitors are likely new therapeutics, which can delay the onset or stop the progression of diabetic vascular disease. The highly selective PKCβ activation and its inhibition by ruboxistaurin mesylate have been most extensively studied [Davis MD, 2009]. Clinical studies have shown that ruboxistaurin prevented loss of visual acuity in diabetic patients [Gálvez MI, 2009]. Thus, PKC activation involving several isoforms is likely to be responsible for some of the pathologies in diabetic retinopathy.

2.3 Polyol pathway

In diabetes, hyperglycemia activates polyol pathway, where a part of excess glucose are metabolized to sorbitol which is then converted to fructose [Lorenzi M, 2007]. Aldose reductase (AR) is the key and rate limiting enzyme in polyol pathway, and both galactose and glucose are substrates to this enzyme and compete with each other while being reduced to galactitol and sorbitol, respectively. Under physiological conditions glucose is poorly reduced by AR to sorbitol. By contrast, under diabetic condition the intracellular glucose levels are elevated, the polyol pathway of glucose metabolism becomes active and sorbitol is produced [Lorenzi M, 2007; Gabbay KH, 1973; Barba I, 2010]. AR, reduces glucose to sorbitol using NADPH as a cofactor, thereby reducing the NADPH level [B. Lass` egue, 2003] which results in less glutathione and increase in oxidative stress, a major factor in retinal damage [Chung SS, 2003; Brownlee M, 2002]. Retinas from diabetic patients with retinopathy showed high expression of AR protein in nerve fibers, ganglion cells and Müller cells than from nondiabetic individuals [Dagher Z, 2004]. Similarly excess accumulation of sorbitol has been found in various tissues including retina of diabetic animals and also in human retinas from nondiabetic eye donors exposed to high glucose similar to the level in nondiabetic rats retina incubated under identical conditions [Lorenzi M, 2007; Chung SS, 2005]. We also measured rate of polyols formation in *ex vivo* rat retinas that gave evidence of increased flux through the polyol pathway with increase in the duration of diabetes and with hyperglycemia [Ola MS, 2006]. The use of inhibitor of aldose reductase in many animal models has prevented the early activation of complement in the wall of retinal vessels, apoptosis of vascular pericytes and endothelial cells and the development of acellular capillaries [Dagher Z, 2004].

Accumulated sorbitol within retina may cause osmotic stress and also the byproducts of polyol pathway, fructose-3-phosphtae and 3-deoxyglucosone are powerful glycosylating agents that enter in the formation of AGEs, which are an important factor for the pathogenecity of diabetic retinopathy. Biochemical consequences of polyol pathway activation as studied in the retina of experimentally diabetic rats show an increased nitrotyrosine [Obrosova IG, 2005], lipid peroxidation products and depletion of antioxidant enzymes [Obrosova IG, 2003].Thus, activation of the polyol pathway initiate and multiply several mechanisms of cellular damage by activation and interaction of aldose reductase and other pathogenetic factors such as formation of AGE, activation of oxidative-nitrosative stress, PKC pathway and poly(ADP-ribose) polymerase that may further lead to initiation of inflammation and growth factor imbalances [Obrosova IG, 2011]. The use of fidarestat, an inhibitor of aldose reductase counteracts diabetes-associated retinal oxidative-nitrosative stress and poly (ADP-ribose) polymerase formation [Obrosova IG, 2005] supporting an important role for aldose reductase in diabetes and rationale for the development of aldose reductase inhibitors for counteraction of polyol pathway [Drel VR, 2008].

2.4 Hexosamine pathway

The hexosamine biosynthesis pathway is another hyperglycemic induced pathway which has been implicated in diabetic pathogenesis [Giacco F, 2010]. Increased expression of an enzyme called GFAT (glutamine: fructose-6 phosphate amidotransferase) causes the diversion of some of glycolytic metabolites such as fructose-6 phosphate to the hexosamine pathway producing UDP (uridine diphosphate)-N-acetylglucosamine which is a substrate used for the post-translational modification of intracellular factors including transcription factors [Nerlich AG, 1998; Brownlee M, 2005]. Du and coworkers have shown the role of hyperglycemia in activation of hexosamine pathway that increases the expression of plasminogen activator inhibitor-1 (PAI-1) and transforming growth factor-β1 (TGF-β1), which are deleterious for diabetic blood vessels and may contribute to the pathogenesis of diabetic complications [Du XL, 2000]. Hyperglycaemia results in increased glucosamines may cause insulin resistance in skeletal muscle and adipocytes and heamoglobin-A1c (HbA1c) which significantly correlates with basal GFAT activity in Type 2 diabetes [Yki-Järvinen H, 1996; Buse MG, 2006]. Few studies suggest that hexosamine biosynthetic pathway may cause retinal neurodegeneration via either affecting the neuroprotective effect of insulin or through the induction of apoptosis possibly by altered glycosylation of proteins [Nakamura M, 2001].

The ability of benfotiamine, a lipid soluble thiamine, to inhibit simultaneously the hexosamine pathway along with AGE formation and PKC pathways might be clinically useful in preventing the development and progression of diabetic pathogenesis arising due to hyperglycemia induced vascular damage [Hammes HP, 2003].

2.5.1 Poly (ADP-ribose) Polymerase (PARP)

Poly (ADP-ribose) Polymerase (PARP) is a nuclear enzyme residing as an inactive form which gets activated after the cell receives the DNA damaging signals. Increased intracellular glucose generates increased ROS in the mitochondria, which induces DNA strand breaks, thereby activating PARP. Once activated, PARP depletes its substrate, NAD^+ molecule, by breaking into nicotinic acid and ADP-ribose, slowing the rate of glycolysis and mitochondrial function. By inhibiting mitochondrial superoxide or ROS production with either MnSOD or UCP-1, prevented both modification of glyceraldehyde 3-phosphate dehydrogenase (GAPDH) by ADP-ribose and reduction of its activity by hyperglycemia [Du X, 2003]. PARP was found to decrease the GAPDH activity, activate the polyol and PKC pathways, increases intracellular AGE formation and activates hexosamine pathway flux which trigger the production of reactive oxygen and nitrogen species, playing a role in the pathogenesis of endothelial dysfunction and diabetic complications. PARP also potentiates NF-κB activation resulting in increase of the expression of NF-κB dependent genes such as ICAM-1, MCP-1 and TNF-α with increase in leukostasis and producing greater oxidative stress. PARP inhibition suppresses NF-κB activation and expression of adhesion molecule in cultured endothelial cells under high glucose [Zheng L, 2004]. More recently, Drel et al., demonstrated an increase in PARP activity in streptozotocin induced diabetic rats and PARP inhibitors reduced retinal oxidative-nitrosative stress, glial activation, and cell death in palmitate exposed pericytes and endothelial cells [Drel VR, 2009].

2.5.2 Peroxisome Proliferator Activator Receptor-γ (PPAR- γ)

PPAR-γ is a member of ligand-activated nuclear receptor superfamily, which plays an important role in carbohydrate metabolism, angiogenesis and inflammation [Malchiodi-Albedi F, 2008; Yanagi Y, 2008]. PPAR-γ is highly expressed in retinal cells, macropahges and other cell types that influence inflammation such as microglial cells, a resident macrophage present both in brain and retina, indicating that PPAR-γ might modulate diabetes induced activation of these cells involved in inflammation and neurodegeneration [Bernardo A, 2006]. The recent work by Tawfik and group has shown the down regulation of PPAR-γ expression in oxygen induced retinopathy in an experimental model of diabetes [Tawfik A, 2009]. In streptozotocin induced diabetic mice deficient in PPAR-γ expression had increased leukostasis and leakage compared to wild type control mice, indicating that endogeneous PPAR-γ and its activation by specific ligands is critical for inhibiting leukostasis and leakage in diabetic mice [Muranaka K, 2006]. PPAR-γ also acts as agonist by inhibiting the VEGF-stimulated proliferation, migration and tube formation in PPAR-γ expressing retinal endothelial cells [Murata T, 2000]. In diabetic patients, PPAR-γ agonists have been shown to reduce several markers of inflammation such as serum levels of c-reactive protein, interleukin-6 (IL-6), monocyte chemoattractant protein (MCP-1) and matrix metallo ptoteinase 9 (MMP-9) [Agarwal R, 2006]. *In-vitro* studies showed that PPAR-γ agonists suppress activated NF-κB and decrease ROS generation in blood mononuclear cells [Aljada A, 2001]. Many such studies suggest the use of PPAR-γ agonists in the treatment of diabetic retinopathy.

2.6 Oxidative stress

The retina is highly metabolic active tissue, making it susceptible to increased oxidative stress. Diabetes disturbs the cellular homeostasis in the normal retina by metabolic dysregulation of glucose, lipids, amino acids and other metabolites which causes oxidative stress, implicating in the in the pathogenesis of diabetic retinopathy.

Oxidative stress is believed to play a pivotal role in the development of diabetic retinopathy by damaging retinal cells [Sato H, 2005]. However, the potential sources of ROS, is still unclear although a number of studies showed that high glucose and the diabetic state stimulate flux through the glycolytic pathway, increases cytosolic NADH, tissue lactate-to-pyruvate ratios, and tricarboxylic acid cycle flux thereby producing excess level of ROS [Madsen-Bouterse SA, 2008; Ido Y, 1997; Obrosova IG, 2001]. ROS can be produced by activation of AGE, aldose reductase, hexosamine and PKC pathways induced by hyperglycemia, altered lipoprotein metabolism, excess level of excitatory amino acids and altered growth factor or cytokines/chemokines activities [Ola MS, 2006; Kanwar M, 2009]. Oxidative stress creates a vicious cycle of damage to macromolecules by amplifying the production of more ROS and activates other metabolic pathways that are detrimental to the development of diabetic retinopathy. However, it is still unclear whether oxidative stress has a primary role in the pathogenesis of diabetic complication, occurs at an early stage in diabetes or it is a consequence of the tissue damage. Other sources of oxidative stress are the activation of NADPH oxidase which may increase superoxide, induction of xanthine oxidase, decreased tissue concentration of endogenous antioxidants such as glutathione and impaired activities of antioxidant defense enzymes such as superoxide dismutase (SOD) and catalase [Sonta T, 2004; Al-Shabrawey M, 2008; Madsen-Bouterse SA, 2008].

To develop novel therapeutic strategies that specifically target ROS is actually desired for patients with PDR. The use of PEDF as a therapeutic option which has a anti-oxidative, anti-angiogenic, neuroprotective and anti-inflammatory properties could be used to block pathways that leads the production of ROS [Yamagishi S, 2011]. Vitamin E has a protective role against lipid peroxidation, whereas its effects on protein and DNA oxidation are less pronounced [Pazdro R, 2010].

3. Hyperlipidaemia

Increased level of plasma lipid has been found to be involved in the pathogenesis of microvascular disease [Ansquer JC, 2009]. High content of lipid in diabetic patients increases the risk of diabetic retinopathy and particularly diabetic macular edema [van Leiden HA, 2002]. Still it is unclear how altered lipids level affect the onset and progression of diabetic retinopathy, may be through alterations in metabolic processes that alters concentration of serum compounds such as ketone bodies, acylcarnitine and oxidized fatty acids [Adibhatla RM, 2007]. There is a growing body of evidence suggest that serum lipid/fatty acid composition, concentration and tissue distribution contribute to the development and severity of this disease [Berry EM, 1997; Kowluru RA, 2007; Nagao K, 2008]. The contribution of lipids/fatty acid may be particularly important in the context of type I diabetes, where hypoglycemia and hyperglycemia co-exist.

The major sources of fatty acids/lipids are from the modern diets (Western in particular) that have a high fat content [Hu FB, 2001]. Not only these diets have high caloric content, but also have high levels of saturated and trans-fatty acids (SFA), rather than the generally beneficial cis-monounsaturated or polyunsaturated fatty acids. Thus understanding the details of metabolic response of diabetic mice to Western diets may aid in understanding, how dietary lipid/fatty acids contribute to the complication of diabetes. The sensitivity of retina to fatty acid is well documented and thus understanding how diet affects the levels of these key metabolites will provide important new information about their role in DR [Giovanni JP, 2005; Adibhatla RM, 2007]. Very long chain unsaturated fatty acids such as docosahexaenoic acids (DHA) are essential for retinal development and function, and free fatty acids in this class have been shown to be protective against age related macular degeneration in a mouse model [Connor KM, 2007]. Diet high in SFA and deficient in the precursors of important retinal fatty acids may adversely affect retinal function or increase the pathology. In the context of type I diabetes, a high fat diet may also increase oxidative stress [Kowluru RA, 2007] and contributes to the inflammatory response [Fox TE, 2006] as well as alter metabolism and metabolite pools in the retina [Antonetti DA, 2006].

ETDR (early treatment of diabetic retinopathy) study demonstrated that elevated serum lipid levels are associated with an increased risk of retinal hard exudates, accompanying diabetic macular edema with an increased risk of visual impairment. The presence of hard exudates in diabetic retinopathy patients has been shown to be associated with increased serum cholesterol levels [Li J, 2009; Rodriguez-Fontal M, 2009]. The therapeutic use of lipid lowering drugs such as fibrates and cholesterol lowering drug, statins, may have great potential in the treatment of diabetic retinopathy.

4. Renin Angiotensin System (RAS)

Hypertension has been identified as a major risk factor of microvascular complications leading to small vessel dysfunction, manifesting the state of diabetic retinopathy. In patients with diabetic retinopathy, tight control of blood pressure delays the progression of the disease and growing evidence suggests that RAS plays an important role in the regulation of blood pressure. The RAS is an enzymatic cascade in which angiotensinogen is the precursor of the angiotensin peptides. The cascade begins with the conversion of the inactive form of renin, prorenin, to active renin [Satofuka S, 2009]. Renin converts angiotensinogen to angiotensin-1 (Ang I) which is further cleaved by angiotensin converting enzyme (ACE) to angiotensin-II (Ang II). Ang II is the main effector peptide of the RAS, acting primarily on two receptors, the angiotensin type I (AT-1) and angiotensin type 2 (AT22). Ang II is known to cause systemic and, local blood pressure via its constrictor effect by upregulation of angiotensin II type 1 receptor.

A number of investigators studied components of retinal RAS (Ang I, Ang II, renin, ACE, AT-1, AT-2) in the retina and increased levels of prorenin, rennin and angiotensin II have been reported in the vitreous of patients with PDR and diabetic macular edema (DME) suggesting the involvement of RAS in pathogenesis of diabetic retinopathy [Noma H, 2009; Nagai N, 2005]. Ang II is also a growth factor, promoting differentiation, apoptosis and the deposition of extracellular matrix [Otani A, 2001; Suzuki Y, 2003]. Ang II potentiates deleterious effect of AGEs by inducing RAGE expression in hypertensive eye and can be blocked by telmisartan, an inhibitor of ACE, indicating a link between AGE-RAGE and the RAS which may be involved in the pathogenesis of diabetic retinopathy.

Angiotensin induce cell growth, proliferation and the deposition of extracellular matrix proteins via stimulation of growth factors such as transforming growth factor (TGF-β), platelet-derived growth factor (PDGF), vascular endothelial growth factor (VEGF), and connective tissue growth factor (CTGF) [Ruperez M, 2003]. There is evidence that the AT-2 receptor also influences pathological angiogenesis in rats with oxygen induced retinopathy and blockade of the AT-2 receptor was shown to reduce retinal angiogenesis and expression of VEGF, VEGFR-2 and angiopoietin-2. In diabetic rats both AT-1 and AT-2 receptor blockade attenuate the rise in retinal VEGF expression [Zhang X, 2004]. Blockade of the RAS at the level of ACE inhibition or angiotensin reduces the rise in retinal VEGF and VEGFR-2 that occurs in diabetic rats and transgenic rats with OIR and attenuates vascular pathology including vascular leakage, proliferation of endothelial cells, angiogenesis [Kim JH, 2009], leukostasis [Chen P, 2006] and inflammation [Egami K, 2003]. Recently, Nagai et al. studied the involvement of RAS and NF-kB pathway in diabetic induced retinal inflammation by upregulation of ICAM-1, MCP-1 and VEGF which are attenuated by AT-1 receptor blocker [Nagai N, 2007]. Therefore, RAS plays an important role in the pathogenesis of diabetic retinopathy and this has led a major interest in RAS inhibitors to prevent retinopathy.

5. Hormones

Several hormones such as insulin, aldosterone, adrenomesdulin, growth hormone (GH) and endothelin have been found to be implicated in diabetic retinopathy [Wilkinson-Berka JL, 2008]. Insulin stimulates anabolic functions and prevents the breakdown of skeletal muscle tissue. In diabetes, the loss of insulin signaling profoundly alters carbohydrate, lipids, amino acids and protein metabolism in a range of tissues including retina, altering nutrients pool and resulting in metabolic dysregulation that ultimately induces tissue damage. Also, the loss of insulin action in diabetic patients causes muscle loss [Serrarbassa PD, 2008]. Numerous studies towards understanding whether the role of insulin concise to its effect on blood level only or extend its role in maintaining retinal homoeostasis reveals the neurotrophic action of insulin [Meyer-Franke A, 1995] pointing to the possibilities that exogenous insulin have a role in the treatment of DR via its neurotrophic actions [Reiter CE, 2006]. Few studies also describe the role of insulin in inflammatory processes [Fort PE, 2009]. Data and research from the Diabetes Control and Complications Trial (DCCT, Diabetes, 1995), as a study by Barber et al. demonsonstrated that administration of exogenous insulin reduces the risk and progression of retinopathy [Barber AJ, 1998]. Use of several implantable hydrogels with degradable and thermoresponsive properties are widely being tested for slow and sustained local release of insulin to the retina [Misra GP, 2009; Kang Derwent JJ, 2008]. However further investigations of both efficiency and potency of such locally administered insulin needs a more indepth studies and research.

Growth factors (GH) have been recently found in vitreous fluid of human, in which they regulate retinal function and provide markers of ocular dysfunction. The presence of GH in the human vitreous suggests that vitreous GH may be involved in the pathogenesis of various forms of ocular diseases including PDR [Harvey S, 2009; Malhotra C, 2010]. It has been shown that the low GH concentrations in the vitreous of diabetic patients may correlate with retinal neurodegeneration making it a marker to follow progression of diabetes [Ziaei M, 2009]. Systemic inhibition of GH or insulin like growth factor (IGF-1) or both, may have therapeutic potential in preventing some forms of retinopathy [Smith LE, 1997]. Thus growth hormone may play a major role in the progression of diabetic retinopathy in combination with IGF-I and VEGF.

6. Inflammation and diabetic retinopathy

Many of the molecular and functional changes that are characteristic of inflammation have been detected in retinas from diabetic animals or humans, and in retinal cells under diabetic conditions which support the potential role of proinflammatory cytokines, chemokines and other inflammatory markers in DR [Adamis AP, 2008]. Joussen et al, have shown that CD18-/- and ICAM-1-/- mice have significantly fewer adherent leukocytes which is associated with fewer damaged endothelial cells and lesser vascular leakage [Joussen AM, 2004]. Leukostasis is a condition that is characterized by abnormal intravascular leukocyte aggregation and clumping which play a major role in inflammatory process in patient with DR [Tamura H, 2005; Tadayoni R, 2003]. Leukostatsis has been shown to be increased in retinas of diabetic animals and contributes to the capillary nonperfusion and also suggests that increased leukocyte-endothelial cell adhesion and retinal leukostasis as an early event associated with areas of vascular non-perfusion that leads to the development of diabetic retinopathy [Chibber R, 2007; Kern TS, 2007; Joussen AM, 2004; Ishida S, 2003].

The role of proinflammatory transcription factors that are responsible for inflammatory process includes the production of proinflammatory mediators such as NF-κB, specificity protein 1 (Sp1), activator protein 1 (AP-1), PPARs and other members of the nuclear receptor superfamily [Rahman I, 2002; Yang SR, 2006]. A variety of diabetes induced metabolic factors including AGEs, PKC, polyols and oxidative stress may activate NF-κB and thereby release proinflammatory cytokines, chemokines and other inflammatory mediator proteins [Gao X, 2008 (a)].

Proinflammatory cytokines such as Interleukin-1β (IL-1β), Tumor necrosis Factor-α (TNF-α) and IL-6 were found to be significantly higher in vitreous of PDR than in control patient and their role in retinal pathogenesis leading to PDR have been characterized. Increased levels of IL-1β, is detected in vitreous fluid of the patients with PDR [Demircan N, 2006; Sato T, 2009] and in the retina from diabetic rats [Vincent JA, 2007] suggesting that IL-1β might have an important role in the pathogenesis of diabetic retinopathy. Using the IL-1 receptor antagonist (IL-1Ra) which causes a blockade of IL-1 activity reduces tissue inflammation in the type 2 diabetic rat [Ehses JA, 2009]. TNF-α is a potent proinflammatory cytokine that is involved in various immunologic and pathologic reactions including upregulation of proliferation, differentiation and cell death [Gao X, 2007, 2008 (b)]. The data provides the evidence of the activation of the local synthesis of TNF-α along with other cytokines such as Endothelin-1 (ET-1) and IL-6 in PDR [Adamiec-Mroczek J, 2010]. Furthermore, the role of several cell adhesion molecules such as soluble vascular cell adhesion protein-1 (sVCAM) and soluble ICAM have been shown to correlate with the vitreous VCAM-1 and TNF-α concentration [Adamiec-Mroczek J, 2009; Adamiec-Mroczek J, 2008]. In addition, increased level of TNF-α in diabetic plasma has been shown to induce leukocyte cell adhesion [Ben-Mahmud BM, 2004]. The role TNFα is critical for the later complications and progression of blood retinal barrier (BRB) breakdown. In diabetes induced TNF-α knockout mice the BRB breakdown was completely suppressed showing that TNFα is essential for progression BRB breakdown and would be a good therapeutic target to prevent BRB breakdown, retinal leukostasis, and apoptosis associated with DR [Huang H, 2011]. Increased level of IL-6 is detected in vitreous fluid of the patients with PDR and DME [Noma H, 2009; Murugeswari P, 2008]. Serum level of IL-6 in patients with both type 1 and type 2 diabetes were also found to be increased [Myśliwiec M, 2008; Bertoni AG, 2010]. Levels of soluble IL-6 receptor in the vitreous and serum of patients with PDR was found to be significantly higher than control [Kawashima M, 2007]. Increased level of IL-6 was found to be related to retinal vascular permeability and the severity of DME [Noma H, 2009; Noma H, 2010]. Up-regulation of IL-6 increase leukocyte-endothelial interaction which contributes to breakdown of BRB in diabetes [Adamis AP, 2008].

Chemokines such as MCP-1, IP-10, IL-8 and stromal derived factor-1 (SDF-1) have been also found to play a potential role in pathogenesis of diabetic retinopathy [Murugeswari P, 2008; Yoshimura T, 2009]. MCP-1 which is a strong activator of macrophages and monocytes, have been shown to be involved in the pathogenesis of DR where vitreous MCP-1 levels are increased in PDR compared with those in controls [Maier R, 2008; Hernández C, 2005]. The angiogenic effect of MCP-1 was completely inhibited by a VEGF inhibitor, suggesting that MCP-1 induced angiogenesis is mediated through pathways involving VEGF [Hong KH, 2004].The increased MCP-1 expression contributes to the development of neovascularization and fibrosis in proliferative vitreoretinal disorders [Yoshida S, 2003]. Abu El-Asrar and others have found increased levels of IP-10 in the vitreous humor samples from eyes with PVR and PDR patients [Abu El-Asrar AM, 2006;Maier R, 2008] and IP-10 expression under both *in vitro* and *in vivo* conditions has been shown to be induced by VEGF, indicating a potent angiogenesis factor in PDR [Maier R, 2008]. VEGF induced augmentation of IP-10 expression is a major mechanism underlying its proinflammatory function. In age-related macular degeneration, IP-10 is also marked as early biomarkers to understand the regulation and neovascular response [Mo FM, 2010]. The work by Liu shows that diabetic tears exhibited elevated levels of pro-angiogenic cytokines such as IP-10 and MCP-1 than anti-angiogenic cytokines [Liu J, 2010]. IL-8 is angiogenic and inflammatory mediator which is elevated in vitreous of patients with PDR in comparison to control subjects [Murugeswari P, 2008; Petrovic MG, 2007]. It has been shown that IL-8 is produced by endothelial and glial cells in the retina with ischemic angiogenesis [Yoshida A, 1998] where it could act as a marker of ischaemic inflammatory reaction, and play a role in deteriorating visual acuity by DR progression [Petrovič MG, 2010].

In humans, vitreous SDF-1 concentration increases as proliferative diabetic retinopathy progresses [Butler JM, 2005; Sonmez K, 2008]. Abu El-Asrar and coworkers have shown that expression of SDF-1 and its receoptor CXCR4 in PDR epiretinal membranes [Abu El-Asrar AM, 2006; Abu El-Asrar AM, 2011]. SDF-1 is upregulated in ischemic tissue establishing an SDF-1 gradient favoring recruitment of EPCs from peripheral blood to sites of ischemia, thereby accelerating neovascularization. The intravitreal injection of bevacizumab and triamcinolone in patient with PDR potentially diminishes the level of SDF-1 that in turn eliminate diffuse macular edema, and cause regression of active aberrant neovascularization (NV) suggesting the possible role of SDF-1 in the pathogenesis of the adverse visual consequences of DR [Arimura N, 2009; Brooks HL Jr, 2004].

The role of various growth factors such as epidermal growth factor (EGF), VEGF, basic FGF, granulocyte colony-stimulating factor (G-CSF) and granulocyte-macrophage colony-stimulating factor (GM-CSF) in the retinal pathogenesis have been evaluated. Schallenberg and his group have shown that the hematopoietic cytokine, GM-CSF and its receptor are expressed within rat and human retina where GM-CSF reduced apoptosis and protected injured retinal ganglion cells by activating the ERK1/2 pathway [Schallenberg M, 2009].

7. Neuronal damage in diabetic retinopathy

7.1 Neurodegeneration

A pathogenic mechanism of nerve damage in diabetic retinopathy begins shortly after the onset of diabetes. Several clinical tools such as multifocal electroretinography (ERG), flash ERG, contrast sensitivity, color vision, and short-wavelength automated perimetry, all detect neuronal dysfunction at early stages of diabetes [Han Y, 2004; Bearse MA, 2004; Fletcher EL, 2007]. Occurrence of many functional changes in the retina can be identified before the development of vascular pathology, suggesting that they result from a direct effect of diabetes on the neural retina [Lieth E, 2004]. Diabetic mice develop capillary lesion that are characteristic of the early stages of DR and cause pathologic progression resulting due to neuronal loss or upregulation of glial fibrillary acidic protein (GFAP) in retinal glial cells [Feit-Leichman RA, 2005]. Van Dijk and his group has shown the gradual and selective thinning of mean ganglion cell/inner plexiform retinal layer in type 1 diabetic patients [van Dijk HW, 2009] which further supports the concept that early DR includes a neurodegenerative sign [van Dijk HW, 2010; Peng PH, 2009]. Retinal glial cells that play important roles in maintaining the normal function of the retina, after the onset of diabetes the normal function of these cells are altered and compromised. They are known to become gliotic displaying altered potassium siphoning, GABA uptake, glutamate excitoxicity and are also known to express several modulators of angiogenic factors. In addition to metabolic stress, there are many growth factors involved in process of neuronal death in DR suggesting further investigation into the mechanism of neurodegenaration [Whitmire W, 2011].

7.2 Apoptosis

Even before the emergence of the concept of programmed cell death (PCD)/apoptosis in diabetes, studies have identified a pyknotic bodies in histological sections of the retina of people with diabetes [Bloodworth JM Jr, 1962; Wolter JR, 1962]. Diabetes causes chronic loss of inner retinal neurons by increasing the frequency of apoptosis as studied in streptozotocin-induced diabetic mice [Martin PM, 2004]. Many findings suggest that the visual loss associated with DR could be associated not only to an early phase of photoreceptor loss but also to later microangiopathy [Park SH, 2003], so both retinal neurodegeneration and retinal microangiopathy should be considered as sign and onset of DR [Ning X, 2004]. Caspases, the enzymes involved in apoptosis are also elevated in retinas of diabetic rats thus making them as markers for apoptosis [Mohr S, 2002]. The role of pro-inflammatory cytokine (IL-1β) and caspase-1 in diabetes-induced mice have shown that caspase-1/IL-1β signaling pathways play an important role in degeneration of retinal capillaries [Vincent JA, 2007] and its inhibition might represent a new strategy to inhibit capillary degeneration in diabetic retinopathy [Mohr S, 2008]. The increased expression of apoptotic mediators, Bcl-2 in the vascular endothelium inhibits the diabetes-induced degeneration of retinal capillaries and superoxide generation [Kern TS, 2010; Susnow N, 2009].

Several studies also demonstrate that the expression of Bax (Bcl-2 associate X protein), pro-apoptotic protein is associated with degenerative diseases and are increased in retinas of diabetic rats, confirming the increase in apoptosis within the inner retina as a component of DR [Podesta F, 2000]. Involvement of TNF-α and AGE, in retinal pericyte apoptosis through activation of the pro-apoptotic transcription factor Forkhead box O1 (FOXO1) establishes the possible mechanism of apoptosis in DR [Alikhani M, 2010].

7.3 Glutamate excitotoxicity

Glutamate is the excitatory neurotransmitter in the retina, but it is neurotoxic when present in excessive amounts. Crucial role in the disruption of glutamate homeostasis in diabetic retina is due to decrease in the ability of Müller cells to remove the excess amount of glutamate from the extracellular space causing excitotoxicity leading to neurodegeneration [Li Q, 2002; Diederen RM, 2006]. Extracellular glutamate is transported into Müller cells by glutamate transporters (GLAST) and amidated by glutamine synthetase (GS) to the non-toxic amino acid, glutamine. Yu XH and coworkers have shown a linear correlation between time-dependent reduction in GS expression and the time course of diabetic retinopathy, making GS as a possible biomarker for evaluating the severity of diabetic retinopathy [Yu XH, 2009]. At postsynaptic neurons, two major classes of receptors referred to as amino-3-hydroxy-5-methyl-4-isoxazolepropionic acid (AMPA) receptors and N-methyl-D-aspartate (NMDA) are activated by excess glutamate. The major causes for cell death following activation of NMDA receptors are the influx of calcium and sodium into cells, the generation of free radicals linked to the formation of AGEs and/or advanced lipoxidation endproducts (ALEs) as well as defects in the mitochondrial respiratory chain. Thus, glutamate may play an important role in the progression of disease and treatment by glutamate inhibitors may decrease neurotoxicity [Ola MS, 2011].

7.4 Role of neurotrophic factors

Neurotrophic factors play important roles in regulating growth, maintenance and survival of neurons [Mattson MP, 2004]. The role of brain derived neurotrophic factors (BDNF) in metabolism is supported by studies on BDNF-deficient mice which develop obesity and hyperphagia in early adulthood [Kernie SG, 2000] whereas, when it administered to normal mice or rats, it has no effect on blood glucose levels, indicating that BDNF exerts its effects by enhancing insulin sensitivity [Ono M, 1997] and activates several signaling pathways including phosphatidylinositol-3 kinase/Akt [Cotman CW, 2005]. Plasma levels of BDNF were decreased in humans with type 2 diabetes accompany impaired glucose metabolism [Krabbe KS, 2007] and act like a biomarkers of insulin resistance [Fujinami A, 2008]. Recently to understand the mechanism of action of BDNF under normal and hypoxic condition in Müller cells, BDNF treated cells increased glutamate uptake and also up regulated glutamine synthetase (GS) during hypoxia which may underlie neuroprotective effects of BDNF [Min D, 2011]. The therapeutic merit of BDNF was also evaluated by injecting it in diabetic mice, which not only ameliorated glucose metabolism [Yamanaka M, 2008 (a)] but also prevented the development of diabetes in pre-diabetic mice [Yamanaka M, 2008 (b)]. Treatment with ciliary neurotrophic factor (CNTF) in combination with brain derived neurotrophic factor (BDNF) is shown to rescue photoreceptors in retinal explants, conveying its neuroprotective effects [Azadi S, 2007].

Several studies have shown an elevated level of Nerve Growth Factor (NGF), another potent neurotrophic factor, which contributes to neurogenic inflammation [Barhwal K, 2008]. NGF level was significantly elevated in the PDR samples as compared to controls, indicating that NGF might be a potent angiogenic factor in the pathogenesis of PDR [Chalam KV, 2003].

Another neurotrophic includes Basic Fibroblast Growth Factor (bFGF), which is important for survival and maturation of both glial cells and neurons and play an important role in regeneration after neural injury [Bikfalvi A, 1997; Molteni R, 2001]. Study found an increase in bFGF concentration in vitreous samples from patients with PDR [Sivalingam A, 1990] revealing that bFGF is a potent angiogenic factor playing an important role in the pathogenesis of neovascularization in DR [Wong CG, 2001]. Studies also suggest that bFGF have a therapeutic value for diabetic neuropathy when injected with cross-linked gelatin hydrogel in streptozotocin-induced diabetic rats [Nakae M, 2006].

Glial cell line-derived neurotrophic factor (GDNF) is a member of the transforming growth factor-β (TGF-β)-related neurotrophic factor family. GDNF promotes photoreceptor survival during retinal degeneration mediated by interaction of the neurotrophic factors via receptors in Müller glial cells that in turn release secondary factors that act directly to rescue photoreceptors [Harada C, 2003].

8. Conclusions

As described in this chapter, extensive research progress has been made in investigating the pathophysiology of the disease, however, due to non availability of human retinal samples and also due to lack of proper animal model of DR, the exact molecular mechanism has not been elucidated, making therapeutic a difficult task. Therefore, research using large diabetic animal models which develop clinical signs of retinopathy are needed which may provide a correlation of the systemic metabolic profiles and retinal pathology with human studies to better understand the exact molecules and pathway(s) involved in DR. In addition, neurodegeneration and loss of neuronal functions as early signs of DR have been detected which may implicate later in vascular pathology. Precise molecular studies are required towards understanding the neurovascular damage in DR. These insights would be helpful in better understanding of the biochemical and molecular changes especially early in the diabetic retina for effective therapies towards prevention and amelioration of DR.

9. Acknowledgements

Authors acknowledge funding from Dr Nasser Al-Rashid Research Chair in Ophthalmology, King Saud University, KACST (ARP 30-23) and Deanship of Scientific Research (RGP-VPP-052) for the research support.

10. References

[1] Abu El-Asrar AM, Struyf S, Kangave D, Geboes K, Van Damme J. Chemokines in proliferative diabetic retinopathy and proliferative vitreoretinopathy. *Eur Cytokine Netw.* 2006 Sep;17(3):155-65.

[2] Abu El-Asrar AM, Struyf S, Verbeke H, Van Damme J, Geboes K. Circulating bone-marrow-derived endothelial precursor cells contribute to neovascularization in diabetic epiretinal membranes. *Acta Ophthalmol.* 2011 May;89(3):222-8.

[3] Abu El-Asrar AM, Al-Mezaine HS, Ola MS. Pathophysiology and management of diabetic retinopathy. *Expert Review of Ophthalmology*, 2009, 4, 627-647.

[4] Adamiec-Mroczek J, Oficjalska-Młyńczak J, Misiuk-Hojło M. Proliferative diabetic retinopathy-The influence of diabetes control on the activation of the intraocular molecule system. *Diabetes Res Clin Pract.* 2009 Apr;84(1):46-50.

[5] Adamiec-Mroczek J, Oficjalska-Młyńczak J, Misiuk-Hojło M. Roles of endothelin-1 and selected proinflammatory cytokines in the pathogenesis of proliferative diabetic retinopathy: Analysis of vitreous samples. *Cytokine*. 2010 Mar;49(3):269-74.

[6] Adamiec-Mroczek J, Oficjalska-Młyńczak J. Assessment of selected adhesion molecule and proinflammatory cytokine levels in the vitreous body of patients with type 2 diabetes--role of the inflammatory-immune process in the pathogenesis of proliferative diabetic retinopathy. *Graefes Arch Clin Exp Ophthalmol*. 2008 Dec;246(12):1665-70.

[7] Adamis AP, Berman AJ. Immunological mechanisms in the pathogenesis of diabetic retinopathy. *Semin Immunopathol*. 2008 Apr; 30(2):65-84.

[8] Adibhatla RM, Hatcher JF. Role of Lipids in Brain Injury and Diseases. *Future Lipidol*. 2007 Aug;2(4):403-422.

[9] Agarwal R. Anti-inflammatory effects of short-term pioglitazone therapy in men with advanced diabetic nephropathy. *Am J Physiol Renal Physiol*. 2006 Mar;290(3):F600-5.

[10] Aiello LP, Davis MD, Girach A, Kles KA, Milton RC, Sheetz MJ, Vignati L, Zhi XE, PKC-DRS2 Group. Effect of ruboxistaurin on visual loss in patients with diabetic retinopathy. *Ophthalmology*. 2006 Dec;113(12):2221-30.

[11] Alikhani M, Roy S, Graves DT. FOXO1 plays an essential role in apoptosis of retinal pericytes. *Mol Vis*. 2010 Mar 10;16:408-15.

[12] Aljada A, Garg R, Ghanim H, Mohanty P, Hamouda W, Assian E, Dandona P. Nuclear factor-kappaB suppressive and inhibitor-kappaB stimulatory effects of troglitazone in obese patients with type 2 diabetes: evidence of an antiinflammatory action?. *J Clin Endocrinol Metab*. 2001 Jul;86(7):3250-6.

[13] Al-Shabrawey M, Rojas M, Sanders T, Behzadian A, El-Remessy A, Bartoli M, Parpia AK, Liou G, Caldwell RB. Role of NADPH oxidase in retinal vascular inflammation. *Invest Ophthalmol Vis Sci*. 2008 Jul;49(7):3239-44.

[14] Ansquer JC, Foucher C, Aubonnet P, Le Malicot K. Fibrates and microvascular complications in diabetes--insight from the FIELD study. *Curr Pharm Des*. 2009;15(5):537-52.

[15] Antonetti DA, Barber AJ, Bronson SK, Freeman WM, Gardner TW, Jefferson LS, Kester M, Kimball SR, Krady JK, LaNoue KF, Norbury CC, Quinn PG, Sandirasegarane L, Simpson IA; JDRF Diabetic Retinopathy Center Group. Diabetic retinopathy: seeing beyond glucose-induced microvascular disease. *Diabetes*. 2006 Sep;55(9):2401-11.

[16] Arimura N, Otsuka H, Yamakiri K, Sonoda Y, Nakao S, Noda Y, Hashiguchi T, Maruyama I, Sakamoto T. Vitreous mediators after intravitreal bevacizumab or triamcinolone acetonide in eyes with proliferative diabetic retinopathy. *Ophthalmology*. 2009 May;116(5):921-6.

[17] Avignon A, Sultan A. PKC-B inhibition: a new therapeutic approach for diabetic complications?. *Diabetes Metab*. 2006 Jun;32(3):205-13.

[18] Azadi S, Johnson LE, Paquet-Durand F, Perez MT, Zhang Y, Ekström PA, van Veen T. CNTF+BDNF treatment and neuroprotective pathways in the rd1 mouse retina. *Brain Res*. 2007 Jan 19;1129(1):116-29.

[19] Barba I, Garcia-Ramírez M, Hernández C, Alonso MA, Masmiquel L, García-Dorado D, Simó R. Metabolic fingerprints of proliferative diabetic retinopathy: an 1H-NMR-based metabonomic approach using vitreous humor. *Invest Ophthalmol Vis Sci*. 2010 Sep;51(9):4416-21.

[20] Barber AJ, Lieth E, Khin SA, Antonetti DA, Buchanan AG, Gardner TW. Neural apoptosis in the retina during experimental and human diabetes. Early onset and effect of insulin. *J Clin Invest.* 1998;102(4):783-91.

[21] Barhwal K, Hota SK, Prasad D, Singh SB, Ilavazhagan G. Hypoxia-induced deactivation of NGF-mediated ERK1/2 signaling in hippocampal cells: neuroprotection by acetyl-L-carnitine. *J Neurosci Res.* 2008 Sep;86(12):2705-21.

[22] Bearse MA Jr, Han Y, Schneck ME, Barez S, Jacobsen C, Adams AJ. Local multifocal oscillatory potential abnormalities in diabetes and early diabetic retinopathy. *Invest Ophthalmol Vis Sci.* 2004;45(9):3259-65.

[23] Ben-Mahmud BM, Mann GE, Datti A, Orlacchio A, Kohner EM, Chibber R. Tumor necrosis factor-alpha in diabetic plasma increases the activity of core 2 GlcNAc-T and adherence of human leukocytes to retinal endothelial cells: significance of core 2 GlcNAc-T in diabetic retinopathy. *Diabetes.* 2004 Nov;53(11):2968-76.

[24] Bernardo A, Minghetti L. PPAR-gamma agonists as regulators of microglial activation and brain inflammation. *Curr Pharm Des.* 2006;12(1):93-109.

[25] Berry EM. Dietary fatty acids in the management of diabetes mellitus. *Am J Clin Nutr.* 1997 Oct;66(4 Suppl):991S-997S.

[26] Bertoni AG, Burke GL, Owusu JA, Carnethon MR, Vaidya D, Barr RG, Jenny NS, Ouyang P, Rotter JI. Inflammation and the incidence of type 2 diabetes: the Multi-Ethnic Study of Atherosclerosis (MESA). *Diabetes Care.* 2010 Apr;33(4):804-10.

[27] Bikfalvi A, Klein S, Pintucci G, Rifkin DB. Biological roles of fibroblast growth factor-2. *Endocr Rev,* 1997; 18: 26-45.

[28] Bloodworth JM Jr. Diabetic retinopathy. *Diabetes.* 1962;11:1-22.

[29] Brooks HL Jr, Caballero S Jr, Newell CK, Steinmetz RL, Watson D, Segal MS, Harrison JK, Scott EW, Grant MB. Vitreous levels of vascular endothelial growth factor and stromal-derived factor 1 in patients with diabetic retinopathy and cystoid macular edema before and after intraocular injection of triamcinolone. *Arch Ophthalmol.* 2004 Dec;122(12):1801-7.

[30] Brownlee M. Biochemistry and molecular cell biology of diabetic complications. *Nature.* 2001 Dec 13;414(6865):813-20.

[31] Brownlee M. The pathobiology of diabetic complications: a unifying mechanism. *Diabetes.* 2005 Jun;54(6):1615-25.

[32] Buse MG. Hexosamines, insulin resistance, and the complications of diabetes: current status. *Am J Physiol Endocrinol Metab.* 2006 Jan;290(1):E1-E8.

[33] Butler JM, Guthrie SM, Koc M, et al. SDF-1 is both necessary and sufficient to promote proliferative retinopathy. *J Clin Invest.* 2005 Jan;115(1):86-93.

[34] Chalam KV, Agarwal N, Agarwal R, Wordinger R, Vinjamaram S. Evaluation And Comparision Of Vitreal Ngf Levels In Human Proliferative Diabetic Retinopathy And Proliferative Vitreoretinopathy *Invest Ophthalmol Vis Sci* 2002;43: E-Abstract 1310.

[35] Chen P, Scicli GM, Guo M, Fenstermacher JD, Dahl D, Edwards PA, Scicli AG. Role of angiotensin II in retinal leukostasis in the diabetic rat. *Exp Eye Res.* 2006 Nov;83(5):1041-51.

[36] Chibber R, Ben-Mahmud BM, Chibber S, Kohner EM. Leukocytes in diabetic retinopathy. *Curr Diabetes Rev.* 2007 Feb;3(1):3-14.

[37] Chung SS, Chung SK. Aldose reductase in diabetic microvascular complications. *Curr Drug Targets*. 2005 Jun;6(4):475-86.

[38] Chung SS, Ho EC, Lam KS, Chung SK. Contribution of polyol pathway to diabetes-induced oxidative stress. *J Am Soc Nephrol*. 2003 Aug;14(8 Suppl 3):S233-6.

[39] Connor KM, SanGiovanni JP, Lofqvist C, Aderman CM, Chen J, Higuchi A, Hong S, Pravda EA, Majchrzak S, Carper D, Hellstrom A, Kang JX, Chew EY, Salem N Jr, Serhan CN, Smith LE. Increased dietary intake of omega-3-polyunsaturated fatty acids reduces pathological retinal angiogenesis. *Nat Med*. 2007 Jul;13(7):868-73.

[40] Cotman CW. The role of neurotrophins in brain aging: aperspective in honor of Regino Perez-Polo. *Neurochem Res*, 2005, 30:877–881.

[41] Dagher Z, Park YS, Asnaghi V, Hoehn T, Gerhardinger C, Lorenzi M. Studies of rat and human retinas predict a role for the polyol pathway in human diabetic retinopathy. *Diabetes*. 2004 Sep;53(9):2404-11.

[42] Das Evcimen N, King GL The role of protein kinase C activation and the vascular complications of diabetes. *Pharmacol Res*. 2007 Jun;55(6):498-510.

[43] Davis MD, Sheetz MJ, Aiello LP, Milton RC, Danis RP, Zhi X, Girach A, Jimenez MC, Vignati L; PKC-DRS2 Study Group. Effect of ruboxistaurin on the visual acuity decline associated with long-standing diabetic macular edema. *Invest Ophthalmol Vis Sci*. 2009 Jan;50(1):1-4.

[44] Demircan N, Safran BG, Soylu M, Ozcan AA, Sizmaz S.Determination of vitreous interleukin-1 (IL-1) and tumour necrosis factor (TNF) levels in proliferative diabetic retinopathy. *Eye*. 2006 Dec;20(12):1366-9.

[45] Denis, U.; Lecomte, M.; Paget, C.; Ruggiero, D.; Wiernsperger, N. Lagarde, M. Advanced glycation end-products induce apoptosis of bovine retinal pericytes in culture: involvement of diacylglycerol/ceramide production and oxidative stress induction. *Free Radic. Biol. Med*, 2002, 33(2), 236-247.

[46] Derubertis FR, Craven PA. Activation of protein kinase C in glomerular cells in diabetes: mechanism and potential links to the pathogenesis of diabetic glomerulopathy. *Diabetes*. 1994;43:1–8.

[47] Diederen, R.M., La Heij, E.C., Deutz, N.E., 2006. Increased glutamate levels in the vitreous of patients with retinal detachment. *Exp. Eye Res*. 83, 45–50.

[48] Drel VR, Pacher P, Ali TK, Shin J, Julius U, El-Remessy AB, Obrosova IG. Aldose reductase inhibitor fidarestat counteracts diabetes-associated cataract formation, retinal oxidative-nitrosative stress, glial activation, and apoptosis. *Int J Mol Med*. 2008 Jun;21(6):667-76.

[49] Drel VR, Xu W, Zhang J, Kador PF, Ali TK, Shin J, Julius U, Slusher B, El-Remessy AB, Obrosova IG. Poly(ADP-ribose)polymerase inhibition counteracts cataract formation and early retinal changes in streptozotocin-diabetic rats. *Invest Ophthalmol Vis Sci*. 2009 Apr;50(4):1778-90.

[50] Du X, Matsumura T, Edelstein D, Rossetti L, Zsengeller Z, Szabo C, Brownlee M: Inhibition of GAPDH activity by poly(ADP-ribose) polymerase activates three major pathways of hyperglycemic damage in endothelial cells. *J Clin Invest* 112:1049–1057, 2003.

[51] Du XL, Edelstein D, Rossetti L, Fantus IG, Goldberg H, Ziyadeh F, Wu J, Brownlee M. Hyperglycemia-induced mitochondrial superoxide overproduction activates the

hexosamine pathway and induces plasminogen activator inhibitor-1 expression by increasing Sp1 glycosylation. *Proc Natl Acad Sci U S A*. 2000 Oct 24;97(22):12222-6.

[52] Egami K, Murohara T, Shimada T, Sasaki K, Shintani S, Sugaya T, Ishii M, Akagi T, Ikeda H, Matsuishi T, Imaizumi T. Role of host angiotensin II type 1 receptor in tumor angiogenesis and growth. *J Clin Invest*. 2003 Jul;112(1):67-75.

[53] Ehses JA, Lacraz G, Giroix MH, Schmidlin F, Coulaud J, Kassis N, Irminger JC, Kergoat M, Portha B, Homo-Delarche F, Donath MY. IL-1 antagonism reduces hyperglycemia and tissue inflammation in the type 2 diabetic GK rat. *Proc Natl Acad Sci U S A*. 2009 Aug 18;106(33):13998-4003.

[54] Feit-Leichman RA, Kinouchi R, Takeda M, Fan Z, Mohr S, Kern TS, Chen DF. Vascular damage in a mouse model of diabetic retinopathy: relation to neuronal and glial changes. *Invest Ophthalmol Vis Sci*. 2005 Nov;46(11):4281-7.

[55] Fletcher EL, Phipps JA, Ward MM, Puthussery T, Wilkinson-Berka JL. Neuronal and glial cell abnormality as predictors of progression of diabetic retinopathy. *Curr Pharm Des*. 2007;13(26):2699-712.

[56] Fort PE, Freeman WM, Losiewicz MK, Singh RS, Gardner TW. The retinal proteome in experimental diabetic retinopathy: up-regulation of crystallins and reversal by systemic and periocular insulin. *Mol Cell Proteomics*. 2009 Apr;8(4):767-79.

[57] Fox TE, Han X, Kelly S, Merrill AH 2nd, Martin RE, Anderson RE, Gardner TW, Kester M. Diabetes alters sphingolipid metabolism in the retina: a potential mechanism of cell death in diabetic retinopathy. *Diabetes*. 2006 Dec;55(12):3573-80.

[58] Fujinami A, Ohta K, Obayashi H, Fukui M, Hasegawa G, Nakamura N, Kozai H, Imai S, Ohta M Serum brain-derived neurotrophic factor in patients with type 2 diabetes mellitus: Relationship to glucose metabolism and biomarkers of insulin resistance. *Clin Biochem*. 2008 Jul;41(10-11):812-7.

[59] Gabbay KH. The sorbitol pathway and the complications of diabetes. *N Engl J Med*. 1973;288:831–836.

[60] Gálvez MI. Rubosixtaurin and other PKC inhibitors in diabetic retinopathy and macular edema. *Curr Diabetes Rev*. 2009 Feb;5(1):14-7.

[61] Gao X, Belmadani S, Picchi A, Xu X, Potter BJ, Tewari-Singh N, Capobianco S, Chilian WM, Zhang C. Tumor necrosis factor-alpha induces endothelial dysfunction in Lepr(db) mice. *Circulation*. 2007 Jan 16;115(2):245-54.

[62] Gao X, Zhang H, Belmadani S, Wu J, Xu X, Elford H, Potter BJ, Zhang C. Role of TNF-alpha-induced reactive oxygen species in endothelial dysfunction during reperfusion injury. *Am J Physiol Heart Circ Physiol*. 2008 (a) Dec;295(6):H2242-9.

[63] Gao X, Zhang H, Schmidt AM, Zhang C. AGE/RAGE produces endothelial dysfunction in coronary arterioles in type 2 diabetic mice. *Am J Physiol Heart Circ Physiol*. 2008 (b) Aug;295(2):H491-8.

[64] Geraldes P, Hiraoka-Yamamoto J, Matsumoto M, Clermont A, Leitges M, Marette A, Aiello LP, Kern TS, King GL. Activation of PKC-delta and SHP-1 by hyperglycemia causes vascular cell apoptosis and diabetic retinopathy. *Nat Med*. 2009;15:1298–1306.

[65] Geraldes P, King GL. Activation of protein kinase C isoforms and its impact on diabetic complications. Circ Res. 2010;106:1319–1331.

[66] Giacco F, Brownlee M. Oxidative stress and diabetic complications. *Circ Res*. 2010 Oct 29;107(9):1058-70.

[67] Giovanni JP, Chew EY. The role of omega-3 long-chain polyunsaturated fatty acids in health and disease of the retina. *Prog Retin Eye Res.* 2005 Jan;24(1):87-138.

[68] Goh SY, Cooper ME. Clinical review: The role of advanced glycation end products in progression and complications of diabetes. *J Clin Endocrinol Metab.* 2008 Apr;93(4):1143-52.

[69] Goldin A, Beckman JA, Schmidt AM, Creager MA. Advanced glycation end products: sparking the development of diabetic vascular injury.*Circulation.* 2006 Aug 8;114(6):597-605.

[70] J, Bierhaus A, Nawroth P, Hannak D, Neumaier M, Bergfeld R, Giardino I, Brownlee M. Benfotiamine blocks three major pathways of hyperglycemic damage and prevents experimental diabetic retinopathy. *Nat Med.* 2003 Mar;9(3):294-9.

[71] Han Y, Adams AJ, Bearse MA Jr, Schneck ME. Multifocal electroretinogram and short-wavelength automated perimetry measures in diabetic eyes with little or no retinopathy. Arch *Ophthalmol.* 2004;122(12):1809-15.

[72] Harada C, Harada T, Quah HM, Maekawa F, Yoshida K, Ohno S, Wada K, Parada LF, Tanaka K. Potential role of glial cell line-derived neurotrophic factor receptors in Müller glial cells during light-induced retinal degeneration. *Neuroscience.* 2003;122(1):229-35.

[73] Harada T, Harada C, Mitamura Y, Akazawa C, Ohtsuka K, Ohno S, Takeuchi S, Wada K. Neurotrophic factor receptors in epiretinal membranes after human diabetic retinopathy. *Diabetes Care.* 2002 Jun;25(6):1060-5.

[74] Harvey S, Parker E, Macdonald I, Sanders EJ. Growth hormone is present in the human retina and vitreous fluid. *Neurosci Lett.* 2009 May 22;455(3):199-202.

[75] Hernández C, Segura RM, Fonollosa A, Carrasco E, Francisco G, Simó R. Interleukin-8, monocyte chemoattractant protein-1 and IL-10 in the vitreous fluid of patients with proliferative diabetic retinopathy. *Diabet Med.* 2005 Jun;22(6):719-22.

[76] Hong KH, Ryu J, Han KH. Monocyte chemoattractant protein-1-induced angiogenesis is mediated by vascular endothelial growth factor-A. *Blood.* 2005 Feb 15;105(4):1405-7.

[77] Hu FB, van Dam RM, Liu S. Diet and risk of Type II diabetes: the role of types of fat and carbohydrate. *Diabetologia.* 2001 Jul;44(7):805-17.

[78] Huang H, Gandhi JK, Zhong X, Wei Y, Gong J, Duh EJ, Vinores SA. TNF{alpha} Is Required for Late BRB Breakdown in Diabetic Retinopathy, and Its Inhibition Prevents Leukostasis and Protects Vessels and Neurons from Apoptosis. *Invest Ophthalmol Vis Sci.* 2011 Mar 10;52(3):1336-44.

[79] Hueber A, Wiedemann P, Esser P, Heimann K. Basic fibroblast growth factor mRNA, bFGF peptide and FGF receptor in epiretinal membranes of intraocular proliferative disorders (PVR and PDR). *Int Ophthalmol* 1996-97; 20: 345-50.

[80] Ido Y, Kilo C, Williamson JR. Cytosolic NADH/NAD+, free radicals, and vascular dysfunction in early diabetes mellitus. *Diabetologia.* 1997 Jul;40 Suppl 2:S115-7.

[81] Inagaki, Y.; Yamagishi, S.; Okamoto, T.; Takeuchi, M. ; Amano, S. Pigment epithelium-derived factor prevents advanced glycation end products-induced monocyte chemoattractant protein-1 production in microvascular endothelial cells by suppressing intracellular reactive oxygen species generation. *Diabetologia,* 2003, 46(2), 284-287.

[82] Inoguchi T, Xia P, Kunisaki M, Higashi S, Feener EP, King GL. Insulin's effect on protein kinase C and diacylglycerol induced by diabetes and glucose in vascular tissues. *Am J Physiol* 1994;267:E369–79.

[83] Ishida S, Yamashiro K, Usui T, Kaji Y, Ogura Y, Hida T, Honda Y, Oguchi Y, Adamis AP. Leukocytes mediate retinal vascular remodeling during development and vaso-obliteration in disease. *Nat Med.* 2003 Jun;9(6):781-8.

[84] Ishida, S. ; Usui, T. ; Yamashiro, K.; Kaji, Y.; Ahmed, E.; Carrasquillo, K. G.; Amano, S.; Hida, T.; Oguchi, Y.; Adamis, A. P. VEGF164 is proinflammatory in the diabetic retina. *Invest. Ophthalmol. Vis. Sci.*, 2003, 44(5), 2155-2162.

[85] Ismail-Beigi F, Craven T, Banerji MA, Basile J, Calles J, Cohen RM, Cuddihy R, Cushman WC, Genuth S, Grimm RH Jr, Hamilton BP, Hoogwerf B, Karl D, Katz L, Krikorian A, O'Connor P, Pop-Busui R, Schubart U, Simmons D, Taylor H, Thomas A, Weiss D, Hramiak I; ACCORD trial group. Effect of intensive treatment of hyperglycaemia on microvascular outcomes in type 2 diabetes: an analysis of the ACCORD randomised trial. *Lancet.* 2010 Aug 7;376(9739):419-30.

[86] Joussen AM, Poulaki V, Le ML, Koizumi K, Esser C, Janicki H, Schraermeyer U, Kociok N, Fauser S, Kirchhof B, Kern TS, Adamis AP. A central role for inflammation in the pathogenesis of diabetic retinopathy. *FASEB J.* 2004 Sep;18(12):1450-2.

[87] Joussen AM, Poulaki V, Qin W, Kirchhof B, Mitsiades N, Wiegand SJ, Rudge J, Yancopoulos GD, Adamis AP. Retinal vascular endothelial growth factor induces intercellular adhesion molecule-1 and endothelial nitric oxide synthase expression and initiates early diabetic retinal leukocyte adhesion in vivo. *Am J Pathol.* 2002 Feb;160(2):501-9.

[88] Kador PF, Randazzo J, Blessing K, Makita J, Zhang P, Yu K, Hosoya K, Terasaki T. Polyol formation in cell lines of rat retinal capillary pericytes and endothelial cells (TR-rPCT and TR-iBRB). *J Ocul Pharmacol Ther.* 2009 Aug;25(4):299-308.

[89] Kang Derwent JJ, Mieler WF. Thermoresponsive hydrogels as a new ocular drug delivery platform to the posterior segment of the eye. *Trans Am Ophthalmol Soc.* 2008;106:206-13; discussion 213-4.

[90] Kanwar M, Kowluru RA. Role of glyceraldehyde 3-phosphate dehydrogenase in the development and progression of diabetic retinopathy. *Diabetes.* 2009 Jan;58(1):227-34.

[91] Kawashima M, Shoji J, Nakajima M, Kamura Y, Sato Y. Soluble IL-6 receptor in vitreous fluid of patients with proliferative diabetic retinopathy. *Jpn J Ophthalmol.* 2007 Mar-Apr;51(2):100-4.

[92] Kern TS, Du Y, Miller CM, Hatala DA, Levin LA (2010) Overexpression of Bcl-2 in vascular endothelium inhibits the microvascular lesions of diabetic retinopathy. *Am J Pathol* 176:2550–2558.

[93] Kern TS, Miller CM, Du Y, Zheng L, Mohr S, Ball SL, Kim M, Jamison JA, Bingaman DP. Topical administration of nepafenac inhibits diabetes-induced retinal microvascular disease and underlying abnormalities of retinal metabolism and physiology. *Diabetes.* 2007 Feb;56(2):373-9.

[94] Kernie SG, Liebl DJ, Parada LF (2000) BDNF regulates eating behavior and locomotor activity in mice. *EMBO J* 19:1290–1300.

[95] Kim JH, Kim JH, Lee YM, Ahn EM, Kim KW, Yu YS. Decursin inhibits VEGF-mediated inner blood-retinal barrier breakdown by suppression of VEGFR-2 activation. *J Cereb Blood Flow Metab.* 2009 Sep;29(9):1559-67.
[96] Kowluru RA, Chan PS. Oxidative stress and diabetic retinopathy. *Exp Diabetes Res.* 2007;2007:43603.
[97] Koya D, Jirousek MR, Lin YW, Ishii H, Kuboki K, King GL. Characterization of protein kinase C beta isoform activation on the gene expression of transforming growth factor-beta, extracellular matrix components, and prostanoids in the glomeruli of diabetic rats. *J Clin Invest.*1997;100:115–126.
[98] Krabbe KS, Nielsen AR, Krogh-Madsen R, Plomgaard P, Rasmussen P, Erikstrup C, Fischer CP, Lindegaard B, Petersen AM, Taudorf S, Secher NH, Pilegaard H, Bruunsgaard H, Pedersen BK. Brain-derived neurotrophic factor (BDNF) and type 2 diabetes. *Diabetologia.* 2007 Feb;50(2):431-8. Epub 2006 Dec 7.
[99] Lassègue B, Clempus RE. Vascular NAD(P)H oxidases: specific features, expression, and regulation. *Am J Physiol Regul Integr Comp Physiol.* 2003 Aug;285(2):R277-97.
[100] Li J, Wang JJ, Chen D, Mott R, Yu Q, Ma JX, Zhang SX. Systemic administration of HMG-CoA reductase inhibitor protects the blood-retinal barrier and ameliorates retinal inflammation in type 2 diabetes. *Exp Eye Res.* 2009 Jun 15;89(1):71-8.
[101] Li Q, Puro DG. Diabetes-induced dysfunction of the glutamate transporter in retinal Müller cells. *Invest Ophthalmol Vis Sci.* 2002 Sep;43(9):3109-3116.
[102] Lieth E, Gardner TW, Barber AJ, Antonetti DA; Penn State Retina Research Group. Retinal neurodegeneration: early pathology in diabetes. *Clin Experiment Ophthalmol.* 2000;28(1):3-8.
[103] Liu J, Shi B, He S, Yao X, Willcox MD, Zhao Z. Changes to tear cytokines of type 2 diabetic patients with or without retinopathy. *Mol Vis.* 2010 Dec 31;16:2931-8.
[104] Lorenzi M. The polyol pathway as a mechanism for diabetic retinopathy: attractive, elusive and resilient. *Exp Diabetes Res.* 2007:61038.
[105] Madsen-Bouterse SA, Kowluru RA. Oxidative stress and diabetic retinopathy: pathophysiological mechanisms and treatment perspectives. *Rev Endocr Metab Disord.* 2008 Dec;9(4):315-27.
[106] Maier R, Weger M, Haller-Schober EM, El-Shabrawi Y, Wedrich A, Theisl A, Aigner R, Barth A, Haas A. Multiplex bead analysis of vitreous and serum concentrations of inflammatory and proangiogenic factors in diabetic patients. *Mol Vis.* 2008 Mar 27;14:637-43.
[107] Malchiodi-Albedi F, Matteucci A, Bernardo A, Minghetti L. PPAR-gamma, Microglial Cells, and Ocular Inflammation: New Venues for Potential Therapeutic Approaches. *PPAR Res.* 2008;2008:295784.
[108] Malhotra C. Proliferative diabetic retinopathy in acromegaly. *Oman J Ophthalmol.* 2010 May;3(2):96-7.
[109] Martin PM, Roon P, Van Ells TK, Ganapathy V, Smith SB. Death of retinal neurons in streptozotocin-induced diabetic mice. *Invest Ophthalmol Vis Sci.* 2004 Sep;45(9):3330-6.
[110] Mattson MP, Maudsley S, Martin B (2004) BDNF and 5-HT: adynamic duo in age-related neuronal plasticity and neurodegen- erative disorders. *Trends Neurosci* 27:589–594.

[111] Meyer-Franke A, Kaplan MR, Pfrieger FW, Barres BA. Characterization of the signaling interactions that promote the survival and growth of developing retinal ganglion cells in culture. *Neuron*. 1995 Oct;15(4):805-19.

[112] Min D, Xiao-Bo X, Si-Qi X. BDNF regulates GLAST and glutamine synthetase in mouse retinal Müller cells. *J Cell Physiol*. 2011 Mar 29. doi: 10.1002/jcp.22762. [Epub ahead of print]

[113] Misra GP, Singh RS, Aleman TS, Jacobson SG, Gardner TW, Lowe TL. Subconjunctivally implantable hydrogels with degradable and thermoresponsive properties for sustained release of insulin to the retina. *Biomaterials*. 2009 Nov;30(33):6541-7.

[114] Mo FM, Proia AD, Johnson WH, Cyr D, Lashkari K. Interferon gamma-inducible protein-10 (IP-10) and eotaxin as biomarkers in age-related macular degeneration. *Invest Ophthalmol Vis Sci*. 2010 Aug;51(8):4226-36.

[115] Mohr S, Xi X, Tang J, Kern TS. Caspase activation in retinas of diabetic and galactosemic mice and diabetic patients. *Diabetes*. 2002 Apr;51(4):1172-9.

[116] Mohr, S., Caspase-1/interleukin-1beta signaling in diabetic retinopathy. *Acta Ophthalmologica*. 2008, 86, S243.

[117] Molteni R, Fumagalli F, Magnaghi V, Roceri M, Gennarelli M, Racagni G, Melcangi RC, Riva MA. Modulation of fibroblast growth factor-2 by stress and corticosteroids: from developmental events to adult brain plasticity. *Brain Res Brain Res Rev*. 2001 Nov;37(1-3):249-58.

[118] Moore TC, Moore JE, Kaji Y, Frizzell N, Usui T, Poulaki V, Campbell IL, Stitt AW, Gardiner TA, Archer DB, Adamis AP. The role of advanced glycation end products in retinal microvascular leukostasis. *Invest Ophthalmol Vis Sci*. 2003 Oct;44(10):4457-64.

[119] Muranaka K, Yanagi Y, Tamaki Y, Usui T, Kubota N, Iriyama A, Terauchi Y, Kadowaki T, Araie M. Effects of peroxisome proliferator-activated receptor gamma and its ligand on blood-retinal barrier in a streptozotocin-induced diabetic model. *Invest Ophthalmol Vis Sci*. 2006 Oct;47(10):4547-52.

[120] Murata T, He S, Hangai M, Ishibashi T, Xi XP, Kim S, Hsueh WA, Ryan SJ, Law RE, Hinton DR. Peroxisome proliferator-activated receptor-gamma ligands inhibit choroidal neovascularization. *Invest Ophthalmol Vis Sci*. 2000 Jul;41(8):2309-17.

[121] Murugeswari P, Shukla D, Rajendran A, Kim R, Namperumalsamy P, Muthukkaruppan V. Proinflammatory cytokines and angiogenic and anti-angiogenic factors in vitreous of patients with proliferative diabetic retinopathy and eales' disease. *Retina*. 2008 Jun;28(6):817-24.

[122] Myśliwiec M, Myśliwska J, Zorena K, Balcerska A, Malinowska E, Wiśniewski P.Interleukin 6 -174(G>C) gene polymorphism is related to celiac disease and autoimmune thyroiditis coincidence in diabetes type 1 children. *Diabetes Res Clin Pract*. 2008 Oct;82(1):108-12.

[123] Nagai N, Izumi-Nagai K, Oike Y, Koto T, Satofuka S, Ozawa Y, Yamashiro K, Inoue M, Tsubota K, Umezawa K, Ishida S. Suppression of diabetes-induced retinal inflammation by blocking the angiotensin II type 1 receptor or its downstream nuclear factor-kappaB pathway. *Invest Ophthalmol Vis Sci*. 2007 Sep;48(9):4342-50.

[124] Nagai N, Noda K, Urano T, Kubota Y, Shinoda H, Koto T, Shinoda K, Inoue M, Shiomi T, Ikeda E, Tsubota K, Suda T, Oike Y, Ishida S. Selective suppression of pathologic,

but not physiologic, retinal neovascularization by blocking the angiotensin II type 1 receptor. *Invest Ophthalmol Vis Sci.* 2005 Mar;46(3):1078-84.
[125] Nagao K, Yanagita T. Bioactive lipids in metabolic syndrome. *Prog Lipid Res.* 2008 Mar;47(2):127-46.
[126] Nakae M, Kamiya H, Naruse K, Horio N, Ito Y, Mizubayashi R, Hamada Y, Nakashima E, Akiyama N, Kobayashi Y, Watarai A, Kimura N, Horiguchi M, Tabata Y, Oiso Y, Nakamura J. Effects of basic fibroblast growth factor on experimental diabetic neuropathy in rats. *Diabetes.* 2006 May;55(5):1470-7.
[127] Nakamura M, Barber AJ, Antonetti DA, LaNoue KF, Robinson KA, Buse MG, Gardner TW. Excessive hexosamines block the neuroprotective effect of insulin and induce apoptosis in retinal neurons. *J Biol Chem.* 2001 Nov 23;276(47):43748-55.
[128] Nerlich AG, Sauer U, Kolm-Litty V, Wagner E, Koch M, Schleicher ED. Expression of glutamine:fructose-6-phosphate amidotransferase in human tissues: evidence for high variability and distinct regulation in diabetes. *Diabetes.* 1998 Feb;47(2):170-8.
[129] Ning X, Baoyu Q, Yuzhen L, Shuli S, Reed E, Li QQ. Neuro-optic cell apoptosis and microangiopathy in KKAY mouse retina. *Int J Mol Med.* 2004 Jan;13(1):87-92.
[130] Noma H, Funatsu H, Mimura T, Harino S, Hori S. Aqueous humor levels of vasoactive molecules correlate with vitreous levels and macular edema in central retinal vein occlusion. *Eur J Ophthalmol.* 2010 Mar-Apr;20(2):402-9.
[131] Noma H, Funatsu H, Mimura T, Harino S, Hori S. Vitreous levels of interleukin-6 and vascular endothelial growth factor in macular edema with central retinal vein occlusion. *Ophthalmology.* 2009 Jan;116(1):87-93.
[132] Obrosova IG, Kador PF. Aldose reductase/polyol inhibitors for diabetic retinopathy. *Curr Pharm Biotechnol.* 2011 Mar 1;12 (3):373-85.
[133] Obrosova IG, Minchenko AG, Vasupuram R, White L, Abatan OI, Kumagai AK, Frank RN, Stevens MJ. Aldose reductase inhibitor fidarestat prevents retinal oxidative stress and vascular endothelial growth factor overexpression in streptozotocin-diabetic rats. *Diabetes.* 2003 Mar;52(3):864-71.
[134] Obrosova IG, Pacher P, Szabó C, Zsengeller Z, Hirooka H, Stevens MJ, Yorek MA. Aldose reductase inhibition counteracts oxidative-nitrosative stress and poly(ADP-ribose) polymerase activation in tissue sites for diabetes complications. *Diabetes.* 2005 Jan;54(1):234-42.
[135] Obrosova IG, Stevens MJ, Lang HJ. Diabetes-induced changes in retinal NAD-redox status: pharmacological modulation and implications for pathogenesis of diabetic retinopathy. *Pharmacology.* 2001;62(3):172-80.
[136] Ola MS, Berkich DA, Xu Y, King MT, Gardner TW, Simpson I, LaNoue KF. Analysis of glucose metabolism in diabetic rat retinas. *Am J Physiol Endocrinol Metab.* 2006 Jun;290(6):E1057-67.
[137] Ola MS, Hosoya KI, Lanoue KF. Regulation of glutamate metabolism by hydrocortisone and branched chain keto acids in cultured rat retinal Müller cells (TR-MUL). *Neurochem Int.* 2011 Jul 3. [Epub ahead of print]
[138] Ono M, Ichihara J, Nonomura T et al (1997) Brain-derived neurrophic factor reduces blood glucose level in obese diabetic mice but not in normal mice. *Biochem Biophys Res Commun* 238:633–637.

[139] Otani A, Takagi H, Oh H, Koyama S, Honda Y. Angiotensin II induces expression of the Tie2 receptor ligand, angiopoietin-2, in bovine retinal endothelial cells. *Diabetes.* 2001 Apr;50(4):867-75.
[140] Park SH, Park JW, Park SJ, Kim KY, Chung JW, Chun MH, Oh SJ. Apoptotic death of photoreceptors in the streptozotocin-induced diabetic rat retina. *Diabetologia.* 2003 Sep;46(9):1260-8.
[141] Patel A, MacMahon S, Chalmers J, Neal B, Billot L, Woodward M, Marre M, Cooper M, Glasziou P, Grobbee D, Hamet P, Harrap S, Heller S, Liu L, Mancia G, Mogensen CE, Pan C, Poulter N, Rodgers A, Williams B, Bompoint S, de Galan BE, Joshi R, Travert F & ADVANCE Collaborative Group. Intensive blood glucose control and vascular outcomes in patients with type 2 diabetes. *N Engl J Med.* 2008 Jun 12;358(24):2560-2572.
[142] Pazdro R, Burgess JR. The role of vitamin E and oxidative stress in diabetes complications. *Mech Ageing Dev.* 2010 Apr;131(4):276-86.
[143] Peng PH, Lin HS, Lin S. Nerve fibre layer thinning in patients with preclinical retinopathy. *Can J Ophthalmol.* 2009 Aug;44(4):417-22.
[144] Petrovič MG, Korošec P, Košnik M, Hawlina M. Association of preoperative vitreous IL-8 and VEGF levels with visual acuity after vitrectomy in proliferative diabetic retinopathy. *Acta Ophthalmol.* 2010 Dec;88(8):e311-6.
[145] Petrovic MG, Korosec P, Kosnik M, Hawlina M. Vitreous levels of interleukin-8 in patients with proliferative diabetic retinopathy. *Am J Ophthalmol.* 2007 Jan;143(1):175-6.
[146] Podestà F, Romeo G, Liu WH, Krajewski S, Reed JC, Gerhardinger C, Lorenzi M. Bax is increased in the retina of diabetic subjects and is associated with pericyte apoptosis in vivo and in vitro. *Am J Pathol.* 2000 Mar;156(3):1025-32.
[147] Rahman I. Oxidative stress, transcription factors and chromatin remodelling in lung inflammation. *Biochem Pharmacol.* 2002 Sep;64(5-6):935-42.
[148] Reiter CE, Wu X, Sandirasegarane L, Nakamura M, Gilbert KA, Singh RS, Fort PE, Antonetti DA, Gardner TW. Diabetes reduces basal retinal insulin receptor signaling: reversal with systemic and local insulin. *Diabetes* 2006; 55:1148-56.
[149] Rodriguez-Fontal M, Kerrison JB, Alfaro DV, Jablon EP.Metabolic control and diabetic retinopathy. *Curr Diabetes Rev.* 2009 Feb;5(1):3-7.
[150] Ruperez M, Lorenzo O, Blanco-Colio LM, Esteban V, Egido J, Ruiz-Ortega M. Connective tissue growth factor is a mediator of angiotensin II-induced fibrosis. *Circulation,* 2003108, 1499–1505.
[151] Sato H, Sato S, Kawasaki AR, Yamamoto AT, Yamashita, BT Yamashita H. A Retinal Cell Damage Due to Oxidative Stress in Diabetic Retinopathy. *Invest Ophthalmol Vis Sci* 2005;46: E-Abstract 443.
[152] Sato T, Kusaka S, Shimojo H, Fujikado T. Simultaneous analyses of vitreous levels of 27 cytokines in eyes with retinopathy of prematurity. *Ophthalmology.* 2009 Nov;116(11):2165-9.
[153] Satofuka S, Ichihara A, Nagai N, Noda K, Ozawa Y, Fukamizu A, Tsubota K, Itoh H, Oike Y, Ishida S. (Pro)renin receptor-mediated signal transduction and tissue renin-angiotensin system contribute to diabetes-induced retinal inflammation. *Diabetes.* 2009 Jul;58(7):1625-33.

[154] Schallenberg M, Charalambous P, Thanos S. GM-CSF regulates the ERK1/2 pathways and protects injured retinal ganglion cells from induced death. *Exp Eye Res.* 2009 Nov; 89(5):665-77.

[155] Serrarbassa PD, Dias AF, Vieira MF. New concepts on diabetic retinopathy: neural versus vascular damage. *Arq Bras Oftalmol.* 2008 May-Jun;71(3):459-63.

[156] Sheikpranbabu S, Haribalaganesh R, Lee KJ, Gurunathan S. Pigment epithelium-derived factor inhibits advanced glycation end products-induced retinal vascular permeability. *Biochimie.* 2010 (a), 92(8):1040-51.

[157] Sheikpranbabu S, Ravinarayanan H, Elayappan B, Jongsun P, Gurunathan S. Pigment epithelium-derived factor inhibits vascular endothelial growth factor-and interleukin-1beta-induced vascular permeability and angiogenesis in retinal endothelial cells. *Vascul Pharmacol.* 2010 (b), 52(1-2):84-94.

[158] Sivalingam A, Kenney J, Brown GC, Benson WE, Donoso L. Basic fibroblast growth factor levels in the vitreous of patients with proliferative diabetic retinopathy. *Arch Ophthalmol* 1990; 108:869-72.

[159] Smith LE, Kopchick JJ, Chen W, Knapp J, Kinose F, Daley D, Foley E, Smith RG, Schaeffer JM. Essential role of growth hormone in ischemia-induced retinal neovascularization. *Science.* 1997 Jun 13;276(5319):1706-9.

[160] Sonmez K, Drenser KA, Capone A Jr, Trese MT. Vitreous levels of stromal cell-derived factor 1 and vascular endothelial growth factor in patients with retinopathy of prematurity. *Ophthalmology.* 2008 Jun;115(6):1065-1070.

[161] Sonta T, Inoguchi T, Tsubouchi H, Sekiguchi N, Kobayashi K, Matsumoto S, Utsumi H, and Nawata H. Evidence for contribution of vascular NAD(P)H oxidase to increased oxidative stress in animal models of diabetes and obesity. *Free Radic Biol Med* 37: 115–123, 2004.

[162] Stitt AW 2001 Advanced glycation: an important pathological event in diabetic and age related ocular disease. *Br J Ophthalmol* 85:746–753.

[163] Stitt AW, Bhaduri T, McMullen CB, Gardiner TA, Archer DB. Advanced glycation end products induce blood-retinal barrier dysfunction in normoglycemic rats. *Mol Cell Biol Res Commun.* 2000 Jun;3(6):380-8.

[164] Susnow N, Zeng L, Margineantu D, Hockenbery DM (2009) Bcl-2 family proteins as regulators of oxidative stress. *Semin Cancer Biol* 9:42–49.

[165] Suzuki, Y., Ruiz-Ortega, M., Lorenzo, O., Ruperez, M., Esteban, V., & Egido, J. (2003). Inflammation and angiotensin II. *Int. J. Biochem. Cell Biol.*, 35, 881–900.

[166] Tadayoni R, Paques M, Gaudric A, Vicaut E. Erythrocyte and leukocyte dynamics in the retinal capillaries of diabetic mice. *Exp Eye Res.* 2003 Oct;77(4):497-504.

[167] Tamura H, Miyamoto K, Kiryu J, Miyahara S, Katsuta H, Hirose F, Musashi K, Yoshimura N. Intravitreal injection of corticosteroid attenuates leukostasis and vascular leakage in experimental diabetic retina. *Invest Ophthalmol Vis Sci.* 2005 Apr;46(4):1440-4.

[168] Tawfik A, Sanders T, Kahook K, Akeel S, Elmarakby A, Al-Shabrawey M. Suppression of retinal peroxisome proliferator-activated receptor gamma in experimental diabetes and oxygen-induced retinopathy: role of NADPH oxidase. *Invest Ophthalmol Vis Sci.* 2009 Feb;50(2):878-84.

[169] The Diabetes Control and Complications Trial/Epidemiology of Diabetes Interventions and Complications ResearchGroup. Retinopathy and nephropathy in

patients with type 1 diabetes four years after a trial of intensive therapy. *N Engl J Med* 2000; 342:381-9.

[170] The relationship of glycemic exposure (HbA1c) to the risk of development and progression of retinopathy in the diabetes control and complications trial. Diabetes 1995; 44:968-83.

[171] Tombran-Tink J, Barnstable CJ. PEDF: a multifaceted neurotrophic factor. *Nat Rev Neurosci* 2003;4:628–36.

[172] van Dijk HW, Kok PH, Garvin M, Sonka M, Devries JH, Michels RP, van Velthoven ME, Schlingemann RO, Verbraak FD, Abràmoff MD. Selective loss of inner retinal layer thickness in type 1 diabetic patients with minimal diabetic retinopathy. *Invest Ophthalmol Vis Sci.* 2009 Jul;50(7):3404-9.

[173] van Dijk HW, Verbraak FD, Kok PH, Garvin MK, Sonka M, Lee K, Devries JH, Michels RP, van Velthoven ME, Schlingemann RO, Abràmoff MD. Decreased retinal ganglion cell layer thickness in patients with type 1 diabetes. *Invest Ophthalmol Vis Sci.* 2010 Jul;51(7):3660-5.

[174] van Leiden HA, Dekker JM, Moll AC, Nijpels G, Heine RJ, Bouter LM, Stehouwer CD, Polak BC. Blood pressure, lipids, and obesity are associated with retinopathy: the hoorn study. *Diabetes Care.* 2002 Aug;25(8):1320-5.

[175] Vincent JA, Mohr S. Inhibition of caspase-1/interleukin-1beta signaling prevents degeneration of retinal capillaries in diabetes and galactosemia. *Diabetes.* 2007 Jan;56(1):224-30.

[176] Whitmire W, Al-Gayyar MM, Abdelsaid M, Yousufzai BK, El-Remessy AB. Alteration of growth factors and neuronal death in diabetic retinopathy: what we have learned so far. *Mol Vis.* 2011 Jan 28;17:300-8.

[177] Wilkinson-Berka JL, Miller AG. Update on the treatment of diabetic retinopathy. *ScientificWorldJournal.* 2008 Feb 6;8:98-120.

[178] Wolter JR. Diabetic retinopathy. *Am J Ophthalmol.* 1961;51:1123-41.

[179] Wong CG, Rich KA, Liaw LH, Hsu HT, Berns MW. Intravitreal VEGF and bFGF produce florid retinal neovascularization and hemorrhage in the rabbit. *Curr Eye Res* 2001; 22: 140-7.

[180] Yamagishi S, Amano S, Inagaki Y, Okamoto T, Koga K, Sasaki N, Yamamoto H, Takeuchi M, Makita Z. Advanced glycation end products-induced apoptosis and overexpression of vascular endothelial growth factor in bovine retinal pericytes. *Biochem Biophys Res Commun.* 2002 Jan 25;290(3):973-8.

[181] Yamagishi S, Matsui T, Nakamura K, Takeuchi M, Imaizumi T. Pigment epithelium-derived factor (PEDF) prevents diabetes- or advanced glycation end products (AGE)-elicited retinal leukostasis. *Microvasc Res.* 2006 Jul-Sep;72(1-2):86-90.

[182] Yamagishi S, Matsui T, Nakamura K, Ueda S, Noda Y, Imaizumi T. Pigment epithelium derived factor (PEDF): its potential therapeutic implication in diabetic vascular complications. *Curr Drug Targets* 2008;9:1025–9.

[183] Yamagishi S, Matsui T, Nakamura K, Yoshida T, Takeuchi M, Inoue H, Yoshida Y, Imaizumi T. Pigment-epithelium-derived factor suppresses expression of receptor for advanced glycation end products in the eye of diabetic rats. *Ophthalmic Res.* 2007;39(2):92-7.

[184] Yamagishi S, Matsui T. Advanced glycation end products (AGEs), oxidative stress and diabetic retinopathy. *Curr Pharm Biotechnol.* 2011 Mar 1;12(3):362-8.

[185] Yamagishi S. Advanced glycation end products and receptor-oxidative stress system in diabetic vascular complications. *Ther Apher Dial*. 2009 Dec;13(6):534-9.
[186] Yamagishi, S.; Matsui, T.; Nakamura, K.; Inoue, H.; Takeuchi, M.; Ueda, S.; Okuda, S. ; Imaizumi, T. Olmesartan blocks inflammatory reactions in endothelial cells evoked by advanced glycation end products by suppressing generation of reactive oxygen species. *Ophthalmic. Res.*, 2007, 40(1), 10-15.
[187] Yamanaka M, Itakura Y, Ono-Kishino M, Tsuchida A, Nakagawa T, Taiji M. Intermittent administration of brain-derived neurotrophic factor (BDNF) ameliorates glucose metabolism and prevents pancreatic exhaustion in diabetic mice. *J Biosci Bioeng*. 2008 (a) Apr;105(4):395-402.
[188] Yamanaka M, Itakura Y, Tsuchida A, Nakagawa T, Taiji M.Brain-derived neurotrophic factor (BDNF) prevents the development of diabetes in prediabetic mice. *Biomed Res*. 2008 (b) Jun;29(3):147-53.
[189] Yanagi Y. Role of Peoxisome Proliferator Activator Receptor gamma on Blood Retinal Barrier Breakdown. *PPAR Res*. 2008;2008:679237.
[190] Yang SR, Chida AS, Bauter MR, Shafiq N, Seweryniak K, Maggirwar SB, Kilty I, Rahman I. Cigarette smoke induces proinflammatory cytokine release by activation of NF-kappaB and posttranslational modifications of histone deacetylase in macrophages. *Am J Physiol Lung Cell Mol Physiol*. 2006 Jul; 291(1):L46-57.
[191] Yki-Järvinen H, Daniels MC, Virkamäki A, Mäkimattila S, DeFronzo RA, McClain D. Increased glutamine:fructose-6-phosphate amidotransferase activity in skeletal muscle of patients with NIDDM. *Diabetes*. 1996 Mar;45(3):302-7.
[192] Yokoi M, Yamagishi S, Sato A et al. Positive association of pigment epithelium-derived factor (PEDF) with total anti-oxidant capacity in the vitreous fluid of patients with proliferative diabetic retinopathy. *Br J Ophthalmol* 2007;91:885–7.
[193] Yokoi M, Yamagishi SI, Takeuchi M, Ohgami K, Okamoto T, Saito W, Muramatsu M, Imaizumi T, Ohno S. Elevations of AGE and vascular endothelial growth factor with decreased total antioxidant status in the vitreous fluid of diabetic patients with retinopathy. *Br J Ophthalmol*. 2005 Jun;89(6):673-5.
[194] Yoshida A, Yoshida S, Khalil AK, Ishibashi T, Inomata H. Role of NF-kappaB-mediated interleukin-8 expression in intraocular neovascularization. Invest Ophthalmol *Vis Sci*. 1998 Jun;39(7):1097-106.
[195] Yoshida S, Yoshida A, Ishibashi T, Elner SG, Elner VM. Role of MCP-1 and MIP-1alpha in retinal neovascularization during postischemic inflammation in a mouse model of retinal neovascularization. *J Leukoc Biol*. 2003 Jan;73(1):137-44.
[196] Yoshimura T, Sonoda KH, Sugahara M, Mochizuki Y, Enaida H, Oshima Y, Ueno A, Hata Y, Yoshida H, Ishibashi T.Comprehensive analysis of inflammatory immune mediators in vitreoretinal diseases. *PLoS One*. 2009 Dec 4;4(12):e8158.
[197] Yu XH, Zhang H, Wang YH, Liu LJ, Teng Y, Liu P. Time-dependent reduction of glutamine synthetase in retina of diabetic rats. *Exp Eye Res*. 2009 Dec;89(6):967-71.
[198] Zhang X, Lassila M, Cooper ME, Cao Z. Retinal expression of vascular endothelial growth factor is mediated by angiotensin type 1 and type 2 receptors. *Hypertension*. 2004 Feb;43(2):276-81.
[199] Zheng L, Szabó C, Kern TS. Poly(ADP-ribose) polymerase is involved in the development of diabetic retinopathy via regulation of nuclear factor-kappaB. *Diabetes*. 2004 Nov;53(11):2960-7.

[200] Ziaei M, Tennant M, Sanders EJ, Harvey S. Vitreous growth hormone and visual dysfunction. *Neurosci Lett.* 2009 Aug 21;460(1):87-91.

4

Inner Blood-Retinal Barrier Transporters: Relevance to Diabetic Retinopathy

Yoshiyuki Kubo and Ken-ichi Hosoya
University of Toyama
Japan

1. Introduction

Diabetic retinopathy is a frequent complication of diabetes, and leads to acquired blindness. A variety of gene and molecules have been studied to clarify its pathophysiological mechanism. The retina is involved in the vision process and contains neuronal cells that are the most sensitive to changes in the retinal environment, and the physiological barrier structure is important for maintaining optimal retinal homeostasis. The blood-retinal barrier (BRB) is composed of two cellular barriers, the tight junction of the retinal capillary endothelial cells (inner BRB) and the retinal pigment epithelial cells (outer BRB), restricting nonspecific material transport between the circulating blood and the retina. However, the specific transport of low molecular weight compounds, that is the supply of nutrients and elimination of undesired toxic compounds, is carried out by membrane transporter molecules at the BRB, suggesting that they are closely related to diabetic retinopathy. Since it is also known that two thirds of the human retina is nourished by the inner BRB (Cunha-Vaz, 2004; Hosoya & Tomi, 2005), in this chapter, we will describe the relationship between diabetic retinopathy and the membrane transporter molecules expressed at the inner BRB.

2. Structure and function of the inner BRB

In 1913, Schnaudigel was the first to propose the concept of the BRB. In his experiment, the retina showed similarity to the blood-brain barrier (BBB), that is, the retina was not stained with dye injected intravenously although peripheral tissues were stained (Schnaudigel, 1913). The tight junctions of retinal pigment epithelial (RPE) cells form the outer BRB, and the choriocapillaries are fenestrated while the inner BRB consists of multiple cells, retinal endothelial cells, pericytes and glial cells, and Müller cells are representative retinal glial cells. The inner BRB is formed by tight junctions of the retinal endothelial cells that are covered by pericytes and glial cells (Figure 1). Since the endothelial barrier is formed by a network complex including neurons, Müller cells/astrocytes and endothelial cells which control the function of retinal capillaries, the inner BRB can be thought of as a 'glio-vascular unit' (Kim et al., 2006).

2.1 Cellular interaction

The functional properties of the inner BRB are inducible by paracrine interactions with pericytes and glial cells. For example, in the endothelial cells, several barrier properties and host-derived angiogenesis are induced by injection of type I astrocytes into the anterior eye chamber of rats (Janzer & Raff, 1987; Janzer, 1997), and the barrier properties of bovine-derived retinal endothelial cells are increased by co-culture with rat brain-derived astrocytes (Gardner et al., 1997). These pieces of evidence suggest that retinal glial cells (Müller cells and astrocytes) acts in a similar manner to astrocytes in the brain, and imply that the barrier function of the inner BRB is modified by several factors secreted from astrocytes. It is known that Müller cells produce several factors to enhance the barrier function of blood vessels in the retina (Tout et al., 1993). In experiments with TR-MUL cells, conditionally immortalized rat Müller cells, TR-MUL cells produce transforming growth factor-beta (TGF-β) to increase the activity of barrier marker proteins expressed in the TR-iBRB cells, conditionally immortalized rat retinal capillary endothelial cells, suggesting that Müller cells contribute to the regulation of barrier function (Abukawa et al., 2009). In addition, it has been reported that there is involvement of glia cell-derived neurotropic growth factors in the TGF-β family, interleukin-6, and basic fibroblast growth factor (bFGF), in barrier regulation (Abbott, 2002). Pericytes produce angiopoietin-1 to modify the barrier function of endothelial cells (Hori et al., 2004). The gap junction-mediated interaction between pericytes, endothelial cells and contractile cells is involved in the regulation of blood flow (Bandopadhyay et al., 2001). It is also known that pericytes exhibit contraction in the presence of endothelin-1, angiotensin II, ATP and hypoxia, and relaxation in the presence of CO_2, NO, and adenosine (Matsugi et al,. 1997a; Matsugi et al., 1997b; Chen & Anderson, 1997).

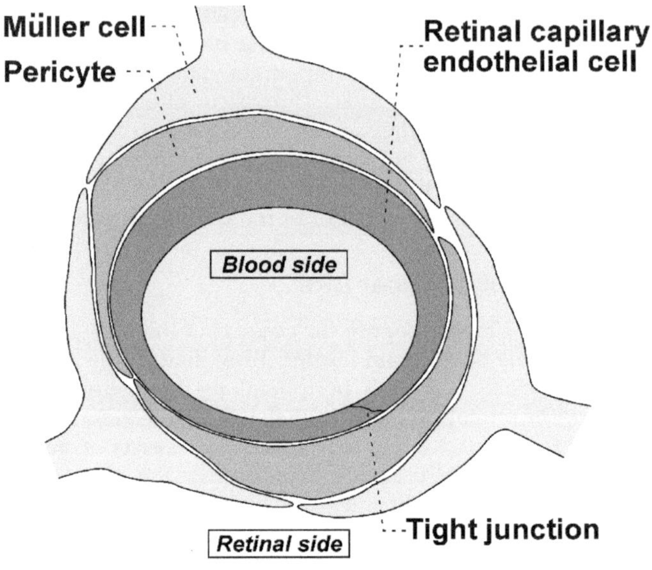

Fig. 1. Structure of inner Blood-Retinal Barrier (BRB)

2.2 Molecular aspects of the barrier structure

At the inner BRB, the retinal endothelial cells form a tightly sealed monolayer, separating the abluminal (retina side) and luminal (blood side) domains of the retinal endothelium, and prevent paracellular transport of materials across endothelial cells between the retina and circulating blood (Wolburg et al., 2009). In particular, D-mannitol, a representative non-permeable paracellular marker, exhibits very low blood-to-retina influx permeability while D-glucose and amino acids, the substrates of membrane transporter molecules, exhibit over a 300-fold higher permeability than that of D-mannitol (Puchowicz et al., 2004; Hosoya & Tachikawa, 2009). These pieces of evidence strongly suggest that the inner BRB is a selective barrier for the retina. In order to maintain the tightly sealed monolayer, it is important for the retinal endothelial cells to be connected via a junctional complex including adherens junctions and tight junctions. Tight junctions are formed by signaling, scaffolding and transmembrane proteins, and it is known that the junctional adhesion molecules (JAM), occuludin and claudin play a role in the tight junctions (Hirase et al., 1997; Furuse et al., 1998; Bazzoni et al, 2005). The quantitative transcript analysis of rodent retinal endothelial cells shows markedly higher expressions of claudin-5, occludin, and JAM-1 than non-retinal endothelial cells (Tomi & Hosoya, 2004; Tachikawa et al., 2008). ZO-1, ZO-2 and ZO-3, accessory proteins, belong to the zonula occludens family, and are involved in linking the actin cytoskeleton and the cytoplasmic tails of the occludin and claudin complex (Anderson et al., 1995; Haskins et al., 1998). In addition, the seal between the retinal endothelial cells is enhanced by catenins and vascular endothelial cadherin (VE-cadherin) (Bazzoni & Dejana, 2004). An anti-sense nucleotide study has suggested that occludin plays an important role in the functional regulation of the inner BRB since the barrier permeability is increased by a reduction in occludin expression (Kevil et al., 1998). In addition, the expression of occludin is reduced in experimentally conditioned-diabetes, suggesting a change in retinal barrier function in patients with diabetic retinopathy (Antonetti et al., 1998). Other reports have suggested that vascular endothelial growth factor (VEGF) and nitric oxide (NO) have an effect on the increase in retinal barrier permeability. In the presence of vascular endothelial growth factor (VEGF), the cultured endothelial cells exhibit reduced occludin expression and increased barrier permeability across the endothelial cell monolayers (Yaccino et al., 1997), and the NO synthesis or release has been reported to increase the vascular permeability (Mark et al., 2004). Thus, it is thought that VEGF and NO are closely involved in retinal barrier function in diabetic retinopathy since the retina exhibits enhanced production of these factors in hypoxia (Kaur et al., 2006). In addition, hypoxia-ischemia leads to the production of reactive oxygen species (ROS) that cause oxidative stress and affect neovascularization in the diabetic eyes and retinopathy of prematurity (ROP) (Augustin et al., 1993; Saugstad & Rognum, 1988). Therefore, the physiological and pathological roles of VEGF, NO and ROS are important in retinal barrier function, and the suppression of their production or function will help in the clinical treatment of diabetic retinopathy, retinal hypoxia, ischemic central retinal vein occlusion, and other conditions (Kaur et al., 2008).

2.3 Transport system across the barrier

The paracellular impermeability of hydrophilic molecules is governed by the tight junctions in the retinal capillary endothelium. However, it is essential that retinal neural cells, such as photoreceptor cells, are able to take up sources of energy and eliminate undesired materials. Thus, transcellular transport by retinal capillary endothelial cells is needed for a variety of low molecular weight compounds, such as D-glucose, amino acids and their metabolites (Niemeyer, 1997; Tachikawa et al., 2007). Regarding the mechanisms of transcellualr transport, there are three transport systems at the inner BRB, namely, passive diffusion, receptor-mediated transport and carrier-mediated transport (Figure 2). In particular, carrier-mediated transport is the most important for the uptake of essential nutrients and elimination of discarded metabolites, and this can be subdivided into facilitated transport, primary active efflux transport and secondary active influx and efflux transport (Hosoya & Tachikawa, 2009). In general, the membrane transporter is the 12 membrane-spanning membrane protein widely found in a variety of species ranging from bacteria to humans (Kubo et al., 2000; Kubo et al., 2005), and it is protein responsible for carrier-mediated transport. ATP-binding cassette (ABC) transporter and Solute carrier (SLC) transporter are involved in primary active efflux transport and secondary influx and efflux transport, respectively (Figure 3). It has been shown that a variety of influx membrane transporters, such as GLUT1 for D-glucose, are expressed in retinal capillary endothelial cells (Table 1), and they contribute to the retinal uptake of essential nutrients. It is also important to eliminate unwanted metabolites and toxic compounds from the retina. While facilitative and secondary active influx transport systems mediated by influx membrane transporters contribute to the influx of nutrients at the inner BRB, the elimination involves primary active and secondary active efflux transport systems. The efflux transport systems are mediated by ABC transporters, such as MDR1 (P-gp), and SLC transporters, such as OAT3 (Table 1). Research of membrane transporters uses a variety of analytical methods (Kubo et al., 2007). In particular, in the study of the inner BRB, integration plot and retinal uptake index analyses are available to study the *in vivo* blood-to-retina transport (Hosoya & Tomi, 2008), and TR-iBRB cells, the model cell line of retinal capillary endothelial cells, are useful for studying *in vitro* transport mechanisms (Hosoya & Tomi, 2005; Hosoya et al., 2001a).

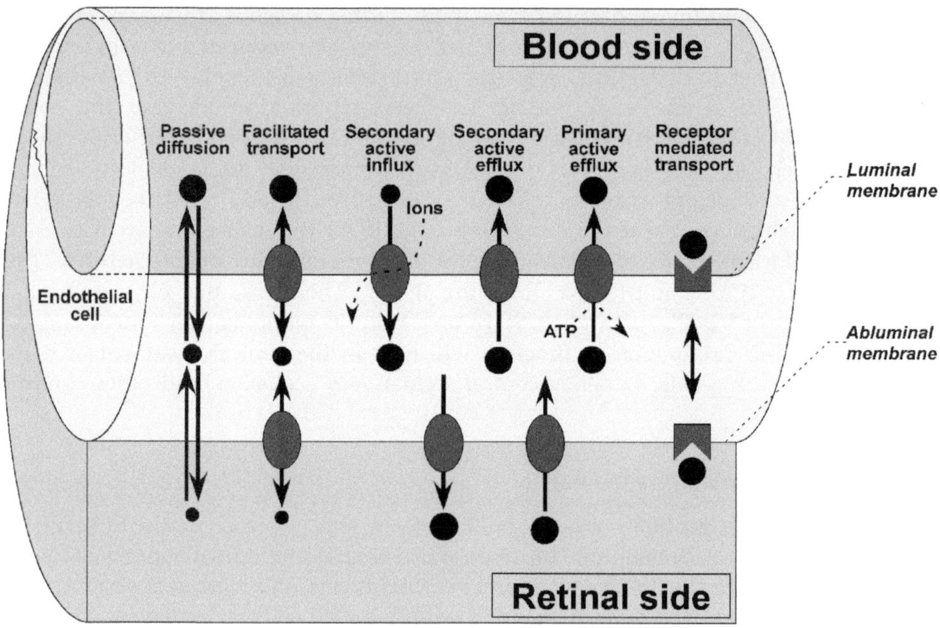

Fig. 2. Transport Systems in the inner BRB

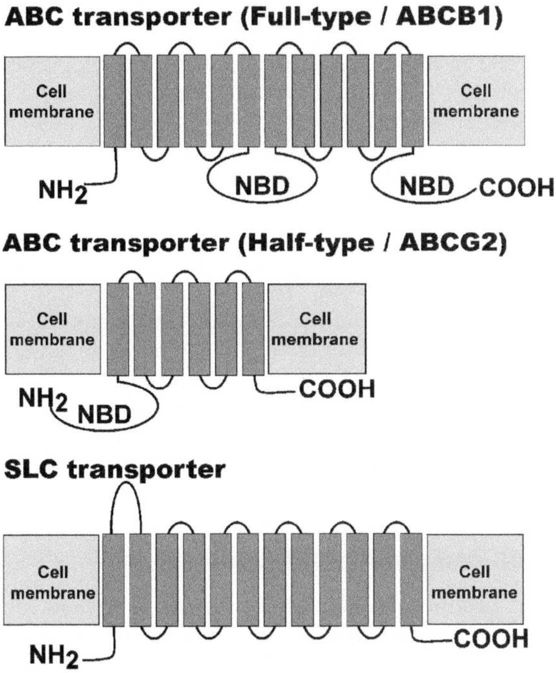

Fig. 3. Structure of Membrane Transporter

3. Hyperglycemia and glucose transporter (GLUT1)

Hyperglycemia (an increased blood D-glucose concentration) is the most important symptom exhibited by diabetic patients, and this has severe effects on the development of diabetic retinopathy (Cai & Boulton, 2002). At the inner BRB, the retinal endothelial cells express facilitative glucose transporter, GLUT1 that recognizes hexoses and dehydroascorbic acid (DHA) as substrates (Vera et al., 1993). GLUT1 mainly mediates the influx transport of D-glucose across the inner BRB. GLUT1 exhibits an asymmetrical localization at the inner BRB, and the abluminal expression of GLUT1 protein is 2- and 3-times higher than that on the luminal membrane (Takata K et al., 1992; Fernandes et al., 2003), suggesting that GLUT1 suppresses glucose accumulation in the retinal interstinal fluid. Regarding the influx permeability rate, the blood-to-retina transport is 544 and 2440 microL/(min· g retina) for D-glucose and DHA, respectively (Puchowicz et al., 2004; Hosoya et al., 2004). DHA is the oxidized form of ascorbic acid (vitamin C), one of the representative antioxidants, and rapidly undergoes cellular reduction to ascorbic acid, resulting in the higher permeability rate of DHA (Hosoya et al., 2008b). According to the K_m values of GLUT1 for D-glucose (5 mM) and DHA (93 microM) and the physiological plasma concentration of D-glucose (~5 mM) and DHA (~10 microM) (Hosoya et al., 2004; Ennis et al., 1982), GLUT1-mediated DHA influx transport across the inner BRB is not inhibited completely under normal and healthy conditions. However, under diabetic conditions, the elevated plasma concentration of D-glucose (>20 mM, hyperglycemia) causes a reduction in GLUT1-mediated DHA transport from the blood to the retina (Minamizono et al., 2006), showing that the retina of diabetic patients is subject to increased oxidative stress.

4. Hyperosmolality mediated by GLUT1

For all cells in the body, it is important to maintain a physiologically optimal osmolality. Sorbitol, a popular sweetener, works as a common organic osmolyte in cells. In the retinal cells, it is known that the cellular polyol pathway is responsible for sorbitol production from D-glucose (Vinores et al., 1993). The rate-limiting enzyme involved in sorbitol production is aldose reductase encoded by the *AR2* gene located on 7q35 which is thought to be a possible susceptible region for diabetic retinopathy (Patel et al., 1996). Under diabetic conditions, hyperglycemia enhances the intracellular accumulation of sorbitol because of the increased GLUT1-mediated facilitative D-glucose transport to the retina and stimulated cellular aldose reductase activity (Iannello et al., 1999). The elevated concentration of sorbitol causes hyperosmolality which stimulates lactate production and intracellular water and reduces the uptake of O_2 (Stevens et al., 1993; Lim et al., 2001). Therefore, GLUT1 is closely involved in the dysfunction and loss of retinal cells, including the capillary endothelial cells in diabetes. Although the change in GLUT1 expression also needs to be considered for a better understanding of the pathological and therapeutic aspects of diabetic retinopathy, both up- and down-regulation of GLUT1 have been reported in the retina with diabetes (Kumagai et al., 1996; Badr et al., 2000), and this remains controversial.

5. Advanced glycation end products (AGEs)

Advanced glycation end products (AGEs) are the result of a chemical chain reaction (non-enzymatic reaction). During normal aging and metabolism, glucose binds to the amino groups of proteins, through the Maillard reaction, Schiff base, and Amadori rearrangement, to produce Amadori products such as glycolhemoglobin (HbA1c) and glycolalbumin that are used to diagnose diabetes. The Amadori products undergo dehydration, hydrolysis and cleavage to form alpha-dicarbonyl compounds, such as glyoxal, methylglyoxal and 3-deoxyglucosone, that have a much greater ability than glucose to accelerate protein glycation. After further reactions, such as oxidation and degradation, irreversible AGEs are produced finally (Brownlee et al., 1988; Takeuchi & Makita Z, 2001).

5.1 AGE effects on the inner BRB

AGEs is the generic term that includes a number of compounds such as pentosidine, pyrraline, crossline, and N (epsilon)-(carboxymethyl) lysine. Interestingly, there are reports of the expression of receptors for AGEs, such as RAGE, on the cellular surface (Schmidt at al. 1992; Neeper et al., 1992). Under diabetic conditions, hyperglycemia promotes the production and accumulation of AGEs, and it is suggested that AGEs are closely related to the pericytes loss in diabetic retinopathy (Brownlee et al., 1988). As described previously, the retinal capillary is composed of endothelial cells, pericytes and glial cells, and it has been reported that the pericytes interacts with the endothelial cells to suppress the undesirable proliferation and prostacyclin production of endothelial cells and to protect these endothelial cells from harmful events (Yamagishi et al., 1993a; Yamagishi et al., 1993b). Therefore, the loss of pericytes, observed during the early stage of diabetic retinopathy, can be an exacerbating factor leading to the induction of neoangiogenesis via VEGF production, thrombus and hypoxia via prostacylin suppression in the retinal capillary endothelial cells. According to a recent report, the loss of pericytes is caused by AGEs and their receptors that inhibit the proliferation of pericytes and induce their apoptosis (Yamagishi et al., 1995; Yamagishi et al., 2002).

5.2 Taurine homeostasis and TAUT

It has been reported that the reactivity of AGEs can be blocked by the administration of taurine (Nandhini et al., 2004). Taurine is a non-essential amino acid which is thought to have a neuroprotective role as an osmolyte and antioxidant in the retina. In the body, taurine is synthesized from L-cysteine, and cysteine sulfinic acid decarboxylase is the rate-limiting enzyme involved in taurine biosynthesis. Interestingly, it is known that the retina is rich in taurine although the activity of cysteine sulfinic acid decarboxylase is low (Lin et al., 1985). This suggests the physiological importance of blood-to-retina taurine transport across the inner BRB for the maintenance of retina homeostasis. The taurine transport system is mediated by TAUT, which accepts taurine (K_m = 22.2 microM) for Na^+- and Cl^--dependent transport (Tomi et al., 2007). The expression of TAUT has been demonstrated in human primary retinal endothelial cells and TR-iBRB cells. Regarding the influx permeability rate, the blood-to-retinal transport is 259 microL/(min · g retina) for taurine (Tomi et al., 2007), and it has been confirmed that the substrates of TAUT have inhibitory effects on retinal taurine uptake (Törnquist et al., 1986). In a study with knockout mice, *taut*$^{-/-}$ mice exhibited an 80 to 90% reduction in taurine levels in the retina when compared with wild-type mice, showing that TAUT is responsible for the retinal homeostasis of taurine (Warskulat et al., 2007). Diabetic patients exhibit taurine deficiency, and a recent report shows that a reduced level of taurine in the retina causes the loss of cone photoreceptor and retinal ganglion cells, suggesting that retinal taurine deficiency is one of the exacerbating factors for diabetic retinopathy (Franconi et al., 1995; Jammoul et al., 2010). Reports have been published describing that taurine administration reduces the severity of the symptoms of diabetes (Barber, 2003; Moloney et al., 2010; Nakamura et al., 1999).

6. Oxidative stress

Oxidative stress is one of the exacerbating factors of diabetic retinopathy. Under normal conditions, it is important to protect the retina from light-induced oxidative stress, and the cellular uptake and synthesis of antioxidants can contribute to prevent the development of diabetic retinopathy. Catalase, superoxide dismutase (SOD) and glutathione peroxidase are representative cellular enzymatic systems that combat oxidative stress (Roginsky et al., 2001; Sozmen et al., 2001; Mates et al., 1999). Under diabetic conditions, down-regulation of SOD and glutathione peroxidase have been reported (Agardh et al., 1998; Agardh et al., 2000; Kern et al., 1994; Kowluru et al., 1997), and ROS are supposed to be generated by the production of AGE signaling via receptors for AGEs, the polyol pathway and enhanced metabolism of eicosannoid (Nourooz-Zadeh & Pereira 2000). Recently, TR-iBRB cells have been reported to show ROS-induced down-regulation of GLUT1 protein expression at the cellular plasma membrane, and proteasome and protein kinase B have been shown to be involved in this mechanism, suggesting that ROS disrupt glucose homeostasis in the retina (Fernandes et al, 2011). Regarding the enzymatic availability of NADPH, glutathione reductase, reducing the oxidized glutathione (GSSG) to glutathione (GSH), competes with aldose reductase in the polyol pathway, suggesting inhibitory effects on the retinal enzymes (Sato et al., 1999; Bravi et al., 1997). In glutathione synthesis, xCT, the membrane transporter expressed in retinal capillary endothelial cells, plays an important role in transporting L-cystine across the inner BRB from the circulating blood. xCT is the representative molecule for the system X_c^- and forms a heterodimer with 4F2hc to transport L-cystine and L-glutamate. TR-iBRB cells exhibits Na^+-independent L-cystine uptake (Km=9.2 microM), which is inhibited by substrates of xCT. xCT is one of the important molecules involved in the biosynthesis of GSH which is a potent endogenous antioxidant. The expression and activity of xCT has been reported to be up-regulated in response to oxidative conditions (Tomi et al., 2002), and it is expected that the expressional and functional alterations of xCT will have an effect on the development of the diabetic retinopathy, regulating the retinal GSH level.

Transporter	Alias	Substrates	Transport Direction	References
SLC2A1	GLUT1	D-Glucose	Influx	Puchowicz et al., 2004
		DHA	Influx	Hosoya et al., 2004
SLC5A6	SMVT	Biotin	Influx	Ohkura et al., 2010
SLC6A6	TAUT	Taurine	Influx	Törnquist et al, 1986
		GABA	Influx	Tomi et al., 2007
SLC6A8	CRT	Creatine	Influx	Nakashima et al., 2004
SLC6A9	GlyT	Glycine	Influx	Okamoto et al., 2009
SLC7A1	CAT1	L-Arginine	Influx	Tomi et al., 2009
SLC7A5	LAT1	L-Leucine	Influx	Törnquist et al, 1986 Tomi et al., 2005
SLC7A11	xCT	L-Cystine	Influx	Tomi et al., 2002
		L-Glutamate	Influx	Hosoya et al., 2001b
SLC16A1	MCT1	L-Lactate	Influx	Gerhart et al., 1999 Alm et al., 1985 Hosoya et al., 2001c
SLC19A1	RFC1	MTF	Influx	Hosoya K et al., 2008a
SLC22A5	OCTN2	L-Carnitine	Influx	Tachikawa et al., 2010
SLC22A8	OAT3	Organic anions	Efflux	Kikuchi et al., 2003 Somervaille et al., 2003 Hosoya et al., 2009
SLC29A2	ENT2	Nucleosides	Influx	Nagase et al., 2006 Baldwin et al., 2004,
SLC38A2	ATA2 SNAT2	L-Proline L-Alanine	Efflux Efflux	Yoneyama et al., 2010 LaNoue et al., 2001 Levkovitch-Verbin et al., 2002
SLCO1A4	OATP1A4 oatp2	Organic anions	Efflux	Nakakariya et al., 2008 Katayama et al., 2006 Noé et al., 1994 Gao et al., 2002 Sugiyama et al., 2001
ABCB1	MDR1 P-gp	Lipophilic drugs Organic cations	Efflux	Hosoya et al., 2001a Maines et al., 2005 Shen et al., 2003 BenEzra et al., 1990a BenEzra et al., 1990b
ABCC4	MRP4	Organic anions	Efflux	Tagami et al., 2009 Smeets et al., 2004 Uchida et al., 2007
ABCG2	BCRP MTX	Organic anions	Efflux	Asashima et al., 2006 Boulton et al., 2001

DHA dehydroascorbic acid; GABA gamma-aminobutyric acid; MTF methyltetrahydrofolate

Table 1. Membrane Transporters Identified at the inner BRB

7. Conclusion

In this chapter, we have described membrane transporters, such as GLUT1 for D-glucose and DHA, TAUT for taurine, and xCT for L-cystine and L-glutamate, which are mainly involved in the uptake of nutrients across the inner BRB under normal physiological conditions. However, under diabetic conditions, these membrane transporters have accelerating or decelerating roles in retinal capillary endothelial cells, and precise quantification of their expressional alteration in diabetes will provide information about the detailed pathological features of diabetic retinopathy. To date, although it has been shown that a variety of membrane transporters are expressed in retinal capillary endothelial cells (Table 1), there is still insufficient information about them to allow us to have a complete picture of retinal homeostasis, and further studies are needed. Therefore, there is still the possibility that several known membrane transporters play roles in diabetic retinopathy. Regarding the drug treatment of diabetic retinopathy, the membrane transporters are expected to be used in pharmacokinetic predictions and retina-specific drug delivery systems. At the inner BRB, OCTN2 and MCT1 are thought to accept drugs as their substrates (Ohashi et al., 1999; Tamai et al., 1999), and novel drug transport systems have also been suggested (Hosoya et al., 2010). Therefore, retina-specific delivery is a potential for aldose reductase inhibitors, such as sorbinil, ranirestat and epalrestat, that can suppress the cell death of the retinal capillary endothelium (Goldfarb et al., 1991; Narayanan et al., 1993). Furthermore, over 400 identified gene/protein molecules belong to the membrane transporter family, and over 100 molecules are 'orphan transporters' and their expression, localization, function, substrates and roles need to be fully identified. In addition, it is thought that there are also a number of unidentified membrane transporter genes, and new research reports on novel membrane transporters can be seen even now (Kawahara et al., 2009). Therefore, new discoveries and findings will be made as a result of the study of the membrane transporters expressed at the inner BRB, and advances in this field will contribute to our understanding of the pathological and therapeutic aspects of diabetic retinopathy.

8. References

Abbott, N.J. (2002). Astrocyte-endothelial interactions and blood-brain barrier permeability. *Journal of Anatomy*, Vol.200, pp. 629-638

Abukawa, H.; Tomi, M.; Kiyokawa, J.; Hori, S.; Kondo, T.; Terasaki, T. & Hosoya, K. (2009). Modulation of retinal capillary endothelial cells by Müller glial cell-derived factors. *Molecular Vision*, Vol.15, pp. 451-457

Agardh, C.D.; Agardh, E.; Hultberg, B.; Qian, Y. & Ostenson, C.G. (1998). The glutathione levels are reduced in Goto-Kakizaki rat retina, but are not influenced by aminoguanidine treatment. *Current Eye Research*, Vol.17, pp. 251–256

Agardh, E.; Hultberg, B. & Agardh, C. (2000). Effects of inhibition of glycation and oxidative stress on the development of cataract and retinal vessel abnormalities in diabetic rats. *Current Eye Research*, Vol.21, pp. 543–549

Alm, A. & Törnquist, P. (1985). Lactate transport through the blood-retinal and the blood-brain barrier in rats. *Ophthalmic Research*, Vol.17, pp. 181-184

Anderson, J.M.; Fanning, A.S.; Lapierre, L. & Van Itallie C.M. (1995). Zonula occludens (ZO)-1 and ZO-2: membrane-associated guanylate kinase homologues (MAGuKs) of the tight junction. *Biochemical Society Transactions,* Vol.23, pp. 470-475

Antonetti, D.A.; Barber, A.J.; Khin, S.; Lieth, E.; Tarbell, J.M. & Gardner, T.W. (1998). Vascular permeability in experimental diabetes is associated with reduced endothelial occludin content: vascular endothelial growth factor decreases occludin in retinal endothelial cells. *Diabetes,* Vol.47, pp. 1953-1959

Asashima, T.; Hori, S.; Ohtsuki, S.; Tachikawa, M.; Watanabe, M.; Mukai, C.; Kitagaki, S.; Miyakoshi, N. & Terasaki, T. (2006). ATP-binding cassette transporter G2 mediates the efflux of phototoxins on the luminal membrane of retinal capillary endothelial cells. *Pharmaceutical Research,* Vol.23, pp. 1235-1242

Augustin, A.J.; Breipohl, W.; Böker, T.; Lutz, J. & Spitznas, M. (1993). Increased lipid peroxide levels and myeloperoxidase activity in the vitreous of patients suffering from proliferative diabetic retinopathy. *Graefe's Archive for Clinical and Experimental Ophthalmology,* Vol.231, pp. 647-650

Badr, G.A.; Tang, J.; Ismail-Beigi, F. & Kern, T.S. (2000). Diabetes downregulates GLUT1 expression in the retina and its microvessels but not in the cerebral cortex or its microvessels. *Diabetes,* Vol.49, pp. 1016-1021

Baldwin, S.A.; Beal, P.R.; Yao, S.Y.; King, A.E.; Cass, C.E. & Young, J.D. (2004). The equilibrative nucleoside transporter family, SLC29. *Pflügers Archiv,* Vol.447, pp. 735-743

Bandopadhyay, R. ; Orte, C. ; Lawrenson, J.G. ; Reid, A.R. ; De Silva, S. & Allt, G. (2001). Contractile proteins in pericytes at the blood-brain and blood-retinal barriers. *Journal of Neurocytology,* Vol.30, pp. 35-44

Barber, A. J. (2003). A new view of diabetic retinopathy: a neurodegenerative disease of the eye. *Progress in Neuro-Psychopharmacology and Biological Psychiatry,* Vol.27, pp. 283-290

Bazzoni, G. & Dejana, E. (2004). Endothelial cell-to-cell junctions: molecular organization and role in vascular homeostasis. *Physiological Reviews,* Vol.84, pp. 869-901

Bazzoni, G.; Tonetti, P.; Manzi, L.; Cera, M.R.; Balconi, G. & Dejana, E. (2005). Expression of junctional adhesion molecule-A prevents spontaneous and random motility. *Journal of Cell Science,* Vol.118, pp. 623-632

BenEzra, D. & Maftzir, G. (1990a). Ocular penetration of cyclosporin A. The rabbit eye. *Investigative Ophthalmology and Vision Science,* Vol.31, pp. 1362-1366

BenEzra, D. & Maftzir, G. (1990b). Ocular penetration of cyclosporine A in the rat eye. *Archives of Ophthalmology,* Vol.108, pp. 584-587

Boulton, M; Rozanowska, M. & Rozanowski, B. (2001). Retinal photodamage. *Journal of Photochemistry and Photobiology B,* Vol.64, pp. 144-161

Bravi, M.C.; Pietrangeli, P.; Laurenti, O.; Basili, S.; Cassone-Faldetta, M.; Ferri, C. & De Mattia, G. (1997). Polyol pathway activation and glutathione redox status in non-insulin- dependent diabetic patients. *Metabolism,* Vol.46, pp. 1194–1198

Brownlee, M.; Cerami, A. & Vlassara, H. (1988). Advanced glycosylation end products in tissue and the biochemical basis of diabetic complications. *New England Journal of Medicine,* Vol.318, pp. 1315-1321

Cai, J. & Boulton, M. (2002). The pathogenesis of diabetic retinopathy: old concepts and new questions. *Eye,* Vol.16, pp. 242-260

Chen, Q. & Anderson, D.R. (1997). Effect of CO_2 on intracellular pH and contraction of retinal capillary pericytes. *Investigative Ophthalmology and Vision Science*, Vol.38, pp. 643-651

Cunha-Vaz, J.G. (2004). The blood-retinal barriers system. Basic concepts and clinical evaluation. *Experimental Eye Research*, Vol.78, pp. 715-721

Ennis, S.R.; Johnson, J.E. & Pautler, E.L. (1982). In situ kinetics of glucose transport across the blood-retinal barrier in normal rats and rats with streptozocin-induced diabetes. *Investigative Ophthalmology and Vision Science*, Vol.23, pp. 447-456

Fernandes, R.; Suzuki, K. & Kumagai, A.K. (2003). Inner blood-retinal barrier GLUT1 in long-term diabetic rats: an immunogold electron microscopic study. *Investigative Ophthalmology and Vision Science*, Vol.44, pp. 3150-3154

Fernandes, R.; Hosoya, K. & Pereira, P. (2011). Reactive oxygen species downregulate glucose transport system in retinal endothelial cells. *American Journal of Physiology-Cell Physiology*, Vol.300, pp. 927-936

Franconi, F.; Bennardini, F.; Mattana, A.; Miceli, M.; Ciuti, M.; Mian, M.; Gironi, A.; Anichini, R. & Seghieri, G. (1995). Plasma and platelet taurine are reduced in subjects with insulindependent diabetes mellitus: effects of taurine supplementation. *American Journal of Clinical Nutrition*, Vol.61, pp. 1115-1119

Furuse, M.; Fujita, K.; Hiiragi, T.; Fujimoto, K. & Tsukita, S. (1998). Claudin-1 and -2: novel integral membrane proteins localizing at tight junctions with no sequence similarity to occludin. *Journal of Cell Biology*, Vol.141, pp. 1539-1550

Gao, B.; Wenzel, A.; Grimm, C.; Vavricka, S.R.; Benke, D.; Meier, P.J. & Remè, C.E. (2002). Localization of organic anion transport protein 2 in the apical region of rat retinal pigment epithelium. *Investigative Ophthalmology and Vision Science*, Vol.43, pp. 510-514

Gerhart, D.Z.; Leino, R.L. & Drewes, L.R. (1999). Distribution of monocarboxylate transporters MCT1 and MCT2 in rat retina. *Neuroscience*, Vol.92, pp. 367-375

Gardner, T.W.; Lieth, E.; Khin, S.A.; Barber, A.J.; Bonsall, D.J.; Lesher, T.; Rice, K. & Brennan, W.A. Jr. (1997). Astrocytes increase barrier properties and ZO-1 expression in retinal vascular endothelial cells. *Investigative Ophthalmology and Visual Science*, Vol.38, pp. 2423-2427

Goldfarb, S.; Ziyadeh, F.N.; Kern, E.F. & Simmons, D.A. (1991). Effects of polyol-pathway inhibition and dietary myo-inositol on glomerular hemodynamic function in experimental diabetes mellitus in rats. *Diabetes*, Vol.40, pp. 465–471

Haskins, J.; Gu, L.; Wittchen, E.S.; Hibbard, J. & Stevenson, B.R. (1998). ZO-3, a novel member of the MAGUK protein family found at the tight junction, interacts with ZO-1 and occludin. *Journal of Cell Biolology*, Vol.141, pp. 199-208

Hirase, T.; Staddon, J.M.; Saitou, M.; Ando-Akatsuka, Y.; Itoh, M.; Furuse, M.; Fujimoto, K.; Tsukita, S. & Rubin, L.L. (1997). Occludin as a possible determinant of tight junction permeability in endothelial cells. *Journal of Cell Science*, Vol.110, pp. 1603-1613

Hori, S.; Ohtsuki, S.; Hosoya, K.; Nakashima, E. & Terasaki, T. (2004). A pericyte-derived angiopoietin-1 multimeric complex induces occludin gene expression in brain capillary endothelial cells through Tie-2 activation in vitro. *Journal of Neurochemistry*, Vol.89, pp. 503-513

Hosoya, K.; Tomi, M.; Ohtsuki, S.; Takanaga, H.; Ueda, M.; Yanai, N.; Obinata, M. & Terasaki, T. (2001a). Conditionally immortalized retinal capillary endothelial cell lines (TR-iBRB) expressing differentiated endothelial cell functions derived from a transgenic rat. *Experimental Eye Research*, Vol.72, pp. 163-172

Hosoya, K.; Saeki, S. & Terasaki, T. (2001b). Activation of carrier-mediated transport of L-cystine at the blood-brain and blood-retinal barriers in vivo. *Microvascular Research*, Vol.62, pp. 136-142

Hosoya, K.; Kondo, T.; Tomi, M.; Takanaga, H.; Ohtsuki, S. & Terasaki, T. (2001c). MCT1-mediated transport of L-lactic acid at the inner blood-retinal barrier: a possible route for delivery of monocarboxylic acid drugs to the retina. *Pharmaceutical Research*, Vol.18, pp. 1669-1676

Hosoya, K.; Minamizono, A.; Katayama, K.; Terasaki, T. & Tomi, M. (2004). Vitamin C transport in oxidized form across the rat blood-retinal barrier. *Investigative Ophthalmology and Vision Science*, Vol.45, pp. 1232-1239

Hosoya, K. & Tomi, M. (2005). Advances in the cell biology of transport via the inner blood-retinal barrier: establishment of cell lines and transport functions. *Biological Pharaceutical Bulletin*, Vol.28, pp. 1-8

Hosoya, K. & Tomi, M. (2008). Inner blood-retinal barrier: transport biology and methodology. In: *Drug Absorption Studies-In Situ, In Vitro and In Silico Models*, Ehrhardt, C. & Kim, K.J. 321-338, AAPS Press-Springer, ISBN978-0-387-74900-6, New York

Hosoya, K.; Fujita, K. & Tachikawa, M. (2008a). Involvement of reduced folate carrier 1 in the inner blood-retinal barrier transport of methyltetrahydrofolate. *Drug Metabolism and Pharmacokinetics*, Vol.23, pp. 285-292

Hosoya, K.; Nakamura, G.; Akanuma, S.; Tomi, M. & Tachikawa, M. (2008b). Dehydroascorbic acid uptake and intracellular ascorbic acid accumulation in cultured Müller glial cells (TR-MUL). *Neurochemistry International*, Vol.52, pp. 1351-1357

Hosoya, K.; Makihara, A.; Tsujikawa, Y.; Yoneyama, D.; Mori, S.; Terasaki, T.; Akanuma, S.; Tomi, M. & Tachikawa, M. (2009). Roles of inner blood-retinal barrier organic anion transporter 3 in the vitreous/retina-to-blood efflux transport of p-aminohippuric acid, benzylpenicillin, and 6-mercaptopurine. *Journal of Pharmacology and Experimental Therapeutics*, Vol.329, pp. 87-93

Hosoya, K. & Tachikawa, M. (2009). Inner blood-retinal barrier transporters: role of retinal drug delivery. *Pharmaceutical Research*, Vol.26, pp. 2055-2065

Hosoya, K.; Yamamoto, A.; Akanuma, S. & Tachikawa, M. (2010). Lipophilicity and transporter Influence on blood-retinal barrier permeability: a comparison with blood-brain barrier permeability. *Pharmaceutical Research*, Vol.27, pp. 2715-2724

Iannello, S.; Cavaleri, A.; Camuto, M. & Belfiore, F. (1999). In vitro inhibition of glucose phosphorylation by an aldosereductase inhibitor (Tolrestat) in some non-insulin sensitive rabbit tissues. *Journal of Diabetes Complications*, Vol.13, pp. 68–73

Jammoul, F.; Dégardin, J.; Pain, D.; Gondouin, P.; Simonutti, M.; Dubus, E.; Caplette, R.; Fouquet, S.; Craft, C.M.; Sahel, J.A. & Picaud, S. (2010). Taurine deficiency damages photoreceptors and retinal ganglion cells in vigabatrin-treated neonatal rats. *Molecular and Cellular Neuroscience*, Vol.43, pp. 414-421

Janzer, R.C. & Raff, M.C. (1987). Astrocytes induce blood-brain barrier properties in endothelial cells. *Nature*, Vol.325, pp. 253-257

Janzer, R.C. (1997). The blood-brain barrier: cellular basis. *Journal of Inherited Metabolic Disease*, Vol.16, pp. 639-647

Katayama, K.; Ohshima, Y.; Tomi, M. & Hosoya, K. (2006). Application of microdialysis to evaluate the efflux transport of estradiol 17-beta glucuronide across the rat blood-retinal barrier. *Journal of Neuroscience Methods*, Vol.156, pp. 249-256

Kaur, C.; Sivakumar, V. & Foulds, W.S. (2006). Early response of neurons and glial cells to hypoxia in the retina. *Investigative Ophthalmology and Vision Science*, Vol47, pp. 1126-1141

Kaur, C.; Foulds, W.S. & Ling, E.A. (2008). Blood-retinal barrier in hypoxic ischaemic conditions: basic concepts, clinical features and management. *Progress in Retinal and Eye Research*, Vol.27, pp. 622-647

Kawahara, A.; Nishi, T.; Hisano, Y.; Fukui, H.; Yamaguchi, A. & Mochizuki, N. (2009). The sphingolipid transporter spns2 functions in migration of zebrafish myocardial precursors. *Science*, Vol.323, pp. 524-527

Kern, T.S.; Kowluru, R.A & Engerman, R.L. (1994). Abnormalities of retinal metabolism in diabetes or galactosemia: ATPases and glutathione. *Investigative Ophthalmology and Visual Science*, Vol.35, pp. 2962–2967

Kevil, C.G.; Okayama, N.; Trocha, S.D.; Kalogeris, T.J.; Coe, L.L.; Specian, R.D.; Davis, C.P. & Alexander J.S. (1998). Expression of zonula occludens and adherens junctional proteins in human venous and arterial endothelial cells: role of occludin in endothelial solute barriers. *Microcirculation*, Vol.5, pp. 197-210

Kikuchi, R.; Kusuhara, H.; Sugiyama, D. & Sugiyama, Y. (2003). Contribution of organic anion transporter 3 (Slc22a8) to the elimination of *p*-aminohippuric acid and benzylpenicillin across the blood-brain barrier. *Journal of Pharmacology and Experimental Therapeutics*, Vol.306, pp. 51-58

Kim, J.H.; Kim, J.H.; Park, J.A.; Lee, S.W.; Kim, W.J.; Yu, Y.S. & Kim, K.W. (2006). Blood-neural barrier: intercellular communication at glio-vascular interface. *Journal of Biochemstry and Molecular Biology*, Vol.39, pp. 339-345

Kowluru, R.N.; Keern, T.S. & Engerman, R.L. (1997). Abnormalities of retinal metabolism in diabetes or experimental galactosemia. IV. Antioxidant defense system. *Free Radical Biology and Medicine*, Vol.22, pp. 587–592

Kubo, Y.; Konishi, S.; Kawabe, T; Nada, S. & Yamaguchi, A. (2000). Proximity of periplasmic loops in the metal-Tetracycline/H(+) antiporter of *Escherichia coli* observed on site-directed chemical cross-linking. *Journal of Biological Chemistry*, Vol.275, pp. 5270-5274

Kubo, Y.; Sekiya, S.; Ohigashi, M.; Takenaka, C.; Tamura, K.; Nada, S.; Nishi, T.; Yamamoto, A. & Yamaguchi, A. (2005). ABCA5 resides in lysosomes, and ABCA5 knockout mice develop lysosomal disease-like symptoms. *Molecular Cellular Biology*, Vol.25, pp. 4138-4149

Kubo, Y.; Kato, Y. & Tsuji, A. (2007). Experimental Approaches to Study Drug Transporters. In: *Drug Transporters: Molecular Characterization and Role in Drug Disposition (Wiley Series in Drug Discovery and Development*, You, G. & Morris, M.E. 533-556, Wiley, ISBN 978-0-471-78491-3, New Jersey

Kumagai, A.K.; Vinores, S.A. & Pardridge, W.M. (1996). Pathological upregulation of inner blood-retinal barrier Glut1 glucose transporter expression in diabetes mellitus. *Brain Research*, Vol.706, pp. 313-317

LaNoue, K.F.; Berkich, D.A.; Conway, M., Barber, A.J.; Hu, L.Y.; Taylor, C. & Hutson, S. (2001). Role of specific aminotransferases in de novo glutamate synthesis and redox shuttling in the retina. *Journal of Neuroscience Research*, Vol.66, pp. 914-922

Levkovitch-Verbin, H.; Martin, K.R.; Quigley, H.A.; Baumrind, L.A.; Pease, M.E. & Valenta, D. (2002). Measurement of amino acid levels in the vitreous humor of rats after chronic intraocular pressure elevation or optic nerve transection. *Journal of Glaucoma*, Vol.11, pp. 396-405

Lim, S.S.; Jung, S.H.; Ji, J.; Shin, K.H. & Keum, S.R. (2001). Synthesis of flavenoids and their effects on aldose reductase and sorbitol accumulation in streptozotocin-induced diabetic rat tissues. *Journal of Pharmacy and Pharmacology*, Vol.53, pp. 653–668

Lin, C.T.; Song, G.X. & Wu, J.Y. (1985). Ultrastructural demonstration of L-glutamate decarboxylase and cysteinesulfinic acid decarboxylase in rat retina by immunocytochemistry. *Brain Research*, Vol.331, pp. 71-80

Maines, L.W.; Antonetti, D.A.; Wolpert, E.B. & Smith, C.D. (2005). Evaluation of the role of P-glycoprotein in the uptake of paroxetine, clozapine, phenytoin and carbamazapine by bovine retinal endothelial cells. *Neuropharmacology*, Vol.49, pp. 610-617

Mark, K.S.; Burroughs, A.R.; Brown, R.C.; Huber, J.D. & Davis, T.P. (2004). Nitric oxide mediates hypoxia-induced changes in paracellular permeability of cerebral microvasculature. *American Journal of Physiology Heart and Circulatory Physiology*, Vol.286, pp. 174-180

Mates, J.M.; Perez-Gomez, C. & Nunez de Castro, I. (1999). Antioxidant enzymes and human diseases. *Clinical Biochemistry*, Vol.32, pp. 595–603

Matsugi, T.; Chen, Q. & Anderson, D.R. (1997a). Contractile responses of cultured bovine retinal pericytes to angiotensin II. *Archives of Ophthalmology*, Vol.115, pp. 1281-1285

Matsugi, T.; Chen, Q. & Anderson, D.R. (1997b).Adenosine-induced relaxation of cultured bovine retinal pericytes. *Investigative Ophthalmology and Vision Science*, Vol.38, pp. 2695-2701

Minamizono, A.; Tomi, M. & Hosoya, K. (2006). Inhibition of dehydroascorbic acid transport across the rat blood-retinal and -brain barriers in experimental diabetes. *Biological Pharmaceutical Bulletin*, Vol.29, pp. 2148-2150

Moloney, M.A.; Casey, R.G.; O'Donnell, D.H.; Fitzgerald, P.; Thompson, C. & Bouchier-Hayes, D.J. (2010). Two weeks taurine supplementation reverses endothelial dysfunction in young male type 1 diabetics. *Diabetes and Vascular Disease Research*, Vol.7, pp. 300-301

Nagase, K.; Tomi, M.; Tachikawa, M. & Hosoya, K. (2006). Functional and molecular characterization of adenosine transport at the rat inner blood-retinal barrier. *Biochimica et Biophysica Acta*, Vol.1758, pp. 13-19

Nakakariya, M.; Shimada, T.; Irokawa, M.; Koibuchi, H.; Iwanaga, T.; Yabuuchi, H.; Maeda, T. & Tamai, I. (2008). Predominant contribution of rat organic anion transporting polypeptide-2 (Oatp2) to hepatic uptake of beta-lactam antibiotics. *Pharmaceutical Research*, Vol.25, pp. 578-585

Nakamura, T.; Ushiyama, C.; Suzuki, S.; Shimada, N.; Ohmuro, H.; Ebihara, I. & Koide, H. (1999). Effects of taurine and vitamin E on microalbuminuria, plasma metalloproteinase-9, and serum type IV collagen concentrations in patients with diabetic nephropathy. *Nephron*, Vol.83, pp. 361-362

Nakashima, T.; Tomi, M.; Katayama, K.; Tachikawa, M.; Watanabe, M.; Terasaki, T. & Hosoya, K. (2004). Blood-to-retina transport of creatine via creatine transporter (CRT) at the rat inner blood-retinal barrier. *Journal of Neurochemistry*, Vol.89, pp. 1454-1461

Nandhini, A.T.; Thirunavukkarasu, V. & Anuradha, C.V. (2004). Stimulation of glucose utilization and inhibition of protein glycation and AGE products by taurine. *Acta Physiologica Scandinavica*, Vol.181, pp. 297-303.

Narayanan, S. (1993). Aldose reductase and its inhibition in the control of diabetic complications. *Annals of Clinical and Laboratory Science*, Vol.23, pp. 148–158

Neeper, M.; Schmidt, A.M.; Brett, J.; Yan, S.D.; Wang, F.; Pan, Y.C.; Elliston, K.; Stern, D. & Shaw, A. (1992). Cloning and expression of a cell surface receptor for advanced glycosylation end products of proteins. *Journal of Biological Chemistry*, Vol.267, pp. 14998-15004

Niemeyer, G. (1997). Glucose concentration and retinal function. *Clinical Neuriscience*, Vol.4, pp. 327-335

Noé, B.; Hagenbuch, B.; Stieger, B. & Meier, P.J. (1994). Isolation of a multispecific organic anion and cardiac glycoside transporter from rat brain. *PNAS*, Vol.94, pp. 10346-10350.

Nourooz-Zadeh, J. & Pereira, P. F. (2000). isoprostanes, potential specific markers of oxidative damage in human retina. *Ophthalmic Research*, Vol.32, pp. 133–137

Ohashi, R.; Tamai, I.; Yabuuchi, H.; Nezu. J.I.; Oku, A.; Sai, Y.; Shimane, M. & Tsuji, A. (1999). Na(+)-dependent carnitine transport by organic cation transporter (OCTN2): its pharmacological and toxicological relevance. *Journal of Pharmacology and Experimental Therapeutics*, Vol.291, pp. 778-784

Ohkura, Y.; Akanuma, S.I.; Tachikawa, M. & Hosoya, K. (2010). Blood-to-retina transport of biotin via Na(+)-dependent multivitamin transporter (SMVT) at the inner blood-retinal barrier. *Experimental Eye Research*, Vol.91, pp. 387-392

Okamoto, M.; Akanuma, S.; Tachikawa, M. & Hosoya, K. (2009). Characteristics of glycine transport across the inner blood-retinal barrier. *Neurochemistry International*, Vol.55, pp. 789-795

Patel, A.; Hibberd, M.L.; Millward, B.A. & Demaine, A.G. (1996). Chromosome 7q35 and susceptibility to diabetic micro-vascular complications. *Journal of Diabetes Complications*, Vol.10, pp. 62–67

Puchowicz, M.A.; Xu, K.; Magness, D.; Miller, C.; Lust, W.D.; Kern, T.S. & LaManna, J.C. (2004).Comparison of glucose influx and blood flow in retina and brain of diabetic rats. *Journal of Cerebral Blood Flow and Metabolism*, Vol.24, pp. 449-457

Roginsky, V. & Barsukova, T. (2001). Superoxide dismutase inhibits lipid peroxidation in micelles. *Chemistry and Physics of Lipids*, Vol.111, pp. 87–91

Sato, S.; Secchi, E.F.; Lizak, M.J.; Fukase, S.; Ohta, N.; Murata, M.; Tsai, J.Y. & Kador, P.F. (1999). Polyol formation and NADPH-dependent reductases in dog retinal capillary pericytes and endothelial cells. *Investigative Ophthalmology and Visual Science*, Vol.40, pp. 697–704

Saugstad, O.D. & Rognum, T.O. (1988). High postmortem levels of hypoxanthine in the vitreous humor of premature babies with respiratory distress syndrome. *Pediatrics*, Vol.81, pp. 395-398.

Schmidt, A.M.; Vianna, M.; Gerlach, M.; Brett, J.; Ryan, J.; Kao, J.; Esposito, C.; Hegarty, H.; Hurley, W.; Clauss, M. et al. (1992). Isolation and characterization of two binding proteins for advanced glycosylation end products from bovine lung which are present on the endothelial cell surface. *Journal of Biological Chemistry*, Vol.267, pp. 14987-14997

Schnaudigel O. (1913). Die vitale farbung mit trypanblau an auge. *Graefe's Archive for Clinical and Experimental Ophthalmology*, Vol.86, pp. 93-105

Shen, J.; Cross, S.T.; Tang-Liu, D.D. & Welty, D.F. (2003). Evaluation of an immortalized retinal endothelial cell line as an in vitro model for drug transport studies across the blood-retinal barrier. *Pharmaceutical Research*, Vol.20, pp. 1357-1363

Smeets, P.H.; van Aubel, R.A.; Wouterse, A.C.; van den Heuvel, J.J. & Russel, F.G. (2004). Contribution of multidrug resistance protein 2 (MRP2/ABCC2) to the renal excretion of p-aminohippurate (PAH) and identification of MRP4 (ABCC4) as a novel PAH transporter. *Journal of the American Society of Nephrology*, Vol.15, pp. 2828-2835

Somervaille, T.C.; Hann, I.M.; Harrison, G.; Eden, T.O.; Gibson, B.E.; Hill, F.G.; Mitchell, C.; Kinsey, S.E.; Vora, A.J. & Lilleyman, J.S. (MRC Childhood Leukaemia Working Party). (2003). Intraocular relapse of childhood acute lymphoblastic leukaemia. *British Journal of Haematology*, Vol.121, pp. 280-288

Sozmen, E.Y.; Sozmen, B.; Delen, Y. & Onat, T. (2001). Catalase/superoxide dismutase (sod) and catalase/paraoxonase (pon) ratios may implicate poor glycemic control. *Archives of Medical Research*, Vol.32, pp. 283–287

Stevens, M.J.; Henry, D.N.; Thomas, T.P.; Killen, P.D. & Greene, D.A. (1993). Aldose reductase gene expression and osmotic dysregulation in cultured human retinal pigment epithelial cells. *American Journal of Physiology*, Vol.265, pp. E428–E438

Sugiyama, D.; Kusuhara, H.; Shitara, Y.; Abe, T.; Meier, P.J.; Sekine, T.; Endou, H.; Suzuki, H. & Sugiyama Y. (2001). Characterization of the efflux transport of 17beta-estradiol-D-17beta-glucuronide from the brain across the blood-brain barrier. *Journal of Pharmacology and Experimental Therapeutics*, Vol.298, pp. 316-322

Tachikawa, M.; Hosoya, K.; Ohtsuki, S. & Terasaki, T. (2007). A novel relationship between creatine transport at the blood-brain and blood-retinal barriers, creatine biosynthesis, and its use for brain and retinal energy homeostasis. *Subcellular Biochemistry*, Vol.46, pp. 83-98

Tachikawa, M.; Toki, H.; Tomi, M. & Hosoya, K. (2008). Gene expression profiles of ATP-binding cassette transporter A and C subfamilies in mouse retinal vascular endothelial cells. *Microvascular Research*, Vol.75, pp. 68-72

Tachikawa, M.; Takeda, Y.; Tomi, M. & Hosoya, K. (2010). Involvement of OCTN2 in the transport of acetyl-L-carnitine across the inner blood-retinal barrier. *Investigative Ophthalmology and Vision Science*, Vol.51, pp. 430-436

Tagami, M.; Kusuhara, S.; Honda, S.; Tsukahara, Y. & Negi, A. (2009). Expression of ATP-binding cassette transporters at the inner blood-retinal barrier in a neonatal mouse model of oxygen-induced retinopathy. *Brain Research*, Vol.1283, pp. 186-193

Takata, K.; Kasahara, T.; Kasahara, M.; Ezaki, O. & Hirano, H. (1992). Ultracytochemical localization of the erythrocyte/HepG2-type glucose transporter (GLUT1) in cells of the blood-retinal barrier in the rat. *Investigative Ophthalmology and Vision Science*, Vol.33, pp. 377-383

Takeuchi, M. & Makita, Z. (2001). Alternative routes for the formation of immunochemically distinct advanced glycation end-products in vivo. *Current Molecular Medicine*, Vol.1, pp. 305-315

Tamai, I.; Sai, Y.; Ono, A.; Kido, Y.; Yabuuchi, H.; Takanaga, H.; Satoh, E.; Ogihara, T.; Amano, O.; Izeki, S. & Tsuji, A. (1999). Immunohistochemical and functional characterization of pH-dependent intestinal absorption of weak organic acids by the monocarboxylic acid transporter MCT1. *Journal of Pharmacy and Pharmacology*, Vol51, pp. 1113-1121

Tomi, M.; Hosoya, K.; Takanaga, H.; Ohtsuki, S. & Terasaki, T. (2002). Induction of xCT gene expression and L-cystine transport activity by diethyl maleate at the inner blood-retinal barrier. *Investigative Ophthalmology and Vision Science*, Vol.43, pp. 774-779

Tomi, M. & Hosoya, K. (2004). Application of magnetically isolated rat retinal vascular endothelial cells for the determination of transporter gene expression levels at the inner blood-retinal barrier. *Journal of Neurochemistry*, Vol. 91, pp. 1244-1248

Tomi, M.; Mori, M.; Tachikawa, M.; Katayama, K.; Terasaki, T. & Hosoya, K. (2005). L-type amino acid transporter 1-mediated L-leucine transport at the inner blood-retinal barrier. *Investigative Ophthalmology and Vision Science*, Vol.46, pp. 2522-2530

Tomi, M.; Terayama, T.; Isobe, T.; Egami, F.; Morito, A.; Kurachi, M.; Ohtsuki, S.; Kang, Y.S.; Terasaki, T. & Hosoya, K. (2007). Function and regulation of taurine transport at the inner blood-retinal barrier. *Microvascular Research*, Vol.73, pp. 100-106

Tomi, M.; Kitade, N.; Hirose, S.; Yokota, N.; Akanuma, S.; Tachikawa, M. & Hosoya K. (2009). Cationic amino acid transporter 1-mediated L-arginine transport at the inner blood-retinal barrier. *Journal of Neurochemistry*, Vol.111, pp. 716-725

Törnquist, P. & Alm, A. (1986). Carrier-mediated transport of amino acids through the blood-retinal and the blood-brain barriers. *Graefe's Archive for Clinical and Experimental Ophthalmology*, Vol.224, pp. 21-25

Tout, S.; Chan-Ling, T.; Holländer, H. & Stone, J. (1993). The role of Müller cells in the formation of the blood-retinal barrier. *Neuroscience*, Vol.55, pp. 291-301.

Uchida, Y.; Kamiie, J.; Ohtsuki, S. & Terasaki, T. (2007). Multichannel liquid chromatography-tandem mass spectrometry cocktail method for comprehensive substrate characterization of multidrug resistance-associated protein 4 transporter. *Pharmaceutical Research*, Vol.24, pp. 2281-2296

Vera, J.C.; Rivas, C.I.; Fischbarg, J. & Golde, D.W. (1993). Mammalian facilitative hexose transporters mediate the transport of dehydroascorbic acid. *Nature*, Vol.364, pp. 79-82

Vinores, S.A.; Van Niel, E.; Swerdloff, J.L. & Campochiaro, P.A. (1993). Electron microscopic immunocytochemical demonstration of blood–retinal barrier breakdown in human diabetics and its association with aldose reductase in retinal vascular endothelium and retinal pigment epithelium. *Histochemical Journal*, Vol.25, pp. 648–663

Warskulat, U.; Heller-Stilb, B.; Oermann, E.; Zilles, K.; Haas, H.; Lang, F. & Häussinger, D. (2007). Phenotype of the taurine transporter knockout mouse. *Methods in Enzymology*, Vol.428, pp. 439-458

Wolburg, H.; Noell, S.; Mack, A.; Wolburg-Buchholz, K. & Fallier-Becker, P. (2009). Brain endothelial cells and the glio-vascular complex. *Cell and Tissue Research*, Vol.335, pp. 75-96

Yaccino, J.A.; Chang, Y.S.; Hollis, T.M.; Gardner, T.W. & Tarbell J.M. (1997). Physiological transport properties of cultured retinal microvascular endothelial cell monolayers. *Current Eye Research*, Vol.16, pp. 761-768

Yamagishi, S.; Kobayashi, K. & Yamamoto, H. (1993a). Vascular pericytes not only regulate growth, but also preserve prostacyclin-producing ability and protect against lipid peroxide-induced injury of co-cultured endothelial cells. *Biochemical and Biophysical Research Communications*, Vol.190, pp. 418-425

Yamagishi, S.; Hsu, C.C.; Kobayashi, K. & Yamamoto, H. (1993b). Endothelin 1 mediates endothelial cell-dependent proliferation of vascular pericytes. *Biochemical and Biophysical Research Communications*, Vol.191, pp. 840-846

Yamagishi, S.; Hsu, C.C.; Taniguchi, M.; Harada, S.; Yamamoto, Y.; Ohsawa, K.; Kobayashi, K. & Yamamoto, H. (1995). Receptor-mediated toxicity to pericytes of advanced glycosylation end products: a possible mechanism of pericyte loss in diabetic microangiopathy. *Biochemical and Biophysical Research Communications*, Vol.213, pp. 681-687

Yamagishi, S.; Amano, S.; Inagaki, Y.; Okamoto, T.; Koga, K.; Sasaki, N.; Yamamoto, H.; Takeuchi, M. & Makita, Z. (2002). Advanced glycation end products-induced apoptosis and overexpression of vascular endothelial growth factor in bovine retinal pericytes. *Biochemical and Biophysical Research Communications*, Vol.290, pp. 973-978

Yoneyama, D.; Shinozaki, Y.; Lu, W.L.; Tomi, M.; Tachikawa, M. & Hosoya, K. (2010). Involvement of system A in the retina-to-blood transport of L-proline across the inner blood-retinal barrier. *Experimental Eye Research*, Vol.90, pp. 507-513

5

The Molecular Pathogenesis of Diabetic Retinopathy - A Spectrum of Pathology Caused by the Disruption of Inner Blood-Retinal Barrier

Byung Joo Lee[1,2] and Jeong Hun Kim[1,2]
[1]*Fight against Angiogenesis-Related Blindness (FARB) Laboratory, Seoul Artificial Eye Center Clinical Research Institute, Seoul National University Hospital*
[2]*Department of Ophthalmology, College of Medicine, Seoul National University Republic of Korea*

1. Introduction

1.1 Epidemiology of diabetic retinopathy

Among diverse microvascular complications of diabetes, diabetic retinopathy is a leading cause of adulthood blindness in the United States. According to the report of Eye Diseases Prevalence Research Group, the estimated incidence of diabetic retinopathy reaches up to 3.4% in US general population (Kempen et al., 2004). The incidence of retinopathy is increasing according to the duration of diabetes. In type I diabetes patients with duration of 20 years or more, the prevalence of any diabetic retinopathy reaches 100% (Klein et al., 1984b). Diverse classification criteria was introduced in diabetic retinopathy, but the presence of retinal new vessel (definition: any new vessels arising from retina or optic disc, extending to the inner surface of retina or into the vitreous cavity) is the most frequently used criterion because of its clinical significance. Panretinal photocoagulation is indicated in proliferative diabetic retinopathy (PDR) with high risk characteristics, where there is a dramatically increased risk of severe visual loss within 2 years (26.2%) compared to that of PDR without high risk characteristics (7%) (The Diabetic Retinopathy Study Research Group [ETDRS], 1987).

1.2 Anatomical and functional changes involved in diabetic retinopathy

The earliest clinical finding in diabetic retinopathy is the presence of microaneurysms and/or retinal dot hemorrhages. Pathologically, thickening of capillary basement membrane, loss of pericytes are early signs of diabetic retinopathy (Cunha-Vaz, 1978; Garner, 1993). Along with perivascular extracellular matrix, pericytes contribute to the stability of retinal microvessels. Pericytes share their basement membrane with retinal endothelial cells and postulated to mechanically stabilize retinal vasculature through N-cadherin-mediated adherence junctions located in peg–socket contacts (Gerhardt & Betsholtz, 2003). Moreover, pericytes communicate with endothelial cell through several mediators to regulate recruitment and proliferation of pericytes, proliferation of endothelial cells and the functional integrity of blood-retinal barrier. Loss of pericytes is putative cause of microaneurysm formation in diabetic retinopathy. In a more advanced stage, acellular capillaries and vitreo-retinal neovascularization are the characteristic histo-pathologic findings. Loss of retinal capillary cellular components involves both endothelial cells and pericytes. The mechanism of cell loss is to be elucidated, but throughout the diabetic retinal vasculature, increased apoptosis was observed in both animal models and human specimens (Mizutani et al., 1996).

1.3 General patho-physiology of diabetic retinopathy

In non-proliferative diabetic retinopathy, increased vascular permeability and retinal ischemia secondary to retinal capillary drop-out are two major patho-physiologic processes. Proliferation of new vessels and/or fibrous tissue is the hallmark of proliferative diabetic retinopathy. Unlike to normal retinal vessels, newly formed vessels in proliferative diabetic retinopathy are leaky due to the presence of endothelial fenestrae and incompetency of junctions (Wallow & Geldner, 1980; Williams et al., 1988) and usually accompany fibrous proliferation. These features of new vessels are responsible for the aggravation of retinal edema and development of retinal and/or vitreous hemorrhage in PDR patients. Moreover, a contraction of posterior vitreous surface which are adherent to the fibrovascular membrane usually results in the traction retinal detachment. In this chapter, we further discuss about the pathogenesis of diabetic retinopathy in an aspect of blood-retinal barrier dysfunction.

2. Blood-retinal barrier: In health and disease (diabetic retinopathy)

In the mammalian brain, molecular exchange between blood vessel and neuron is tightly regulated by the structure named blood-brain barrier (BBB). Ions, neurotransmitters, macromolecules like plasma proteins, toxins, metabolites and nutrients are regulated for neuronal homeostasis. Several mechanisms are involved in the selective exchange of molecule through BBB. There are two distinctive routes for circulating blood component to reach the central nervous system (CNS): transcellular and paracellular pathway (Pardridge, 1999). Microvasculature of central nervous system is consisted with non-fenestrated endothelium sealed by intercellular adherent junction and tight junction. Under normal functioning BBB, paracellular pathway is restricted by these structures.

As a part of CNS, retina also has functional barrier called blood-retinal barrier (BRB). Neural retina receives dual blood supply from retinal vessels and choroidal vessels. Retinal vessels and choroidal vessels are separated from neural retina by inner and outer BRB, respectively. In a narrow definition, inner BRB is a tight junction between retinal vascular endothelium (resembles the BBB proper of brain) and outer BRB means a tight junction between retinal pigment epithelium (resembles the blood-CSF barrier of brain). Among the two kinds of BRB, inner BRB is responsible for the pathogenesis of diabetic retinopathy.

Inner blood-retinal barrier is composed of diverse cellular component including endothelial cells, pericytes and Müller cells. Pericytes ensheathe the retinal microvascular endothelium and share their basement membrane with endothelial cells. Pericytes are connected to endothelial cells through the N-cadherin mediated adherent junction. Müller cells have spatial proximity with endothelium and communicate with endothelium through their foot-processes. Each endothelial cell is interconnected with adjacent endothelial cell through tight junctions and adherent junctions to provide barrier function. Non-selective diffusion of molecules through the paracellular pathway is thightly regulated by those structures and limited exchange of molecules happens through the transcellular pathways (carrier mediated transport, transcytosis and lipophilic diffusion).

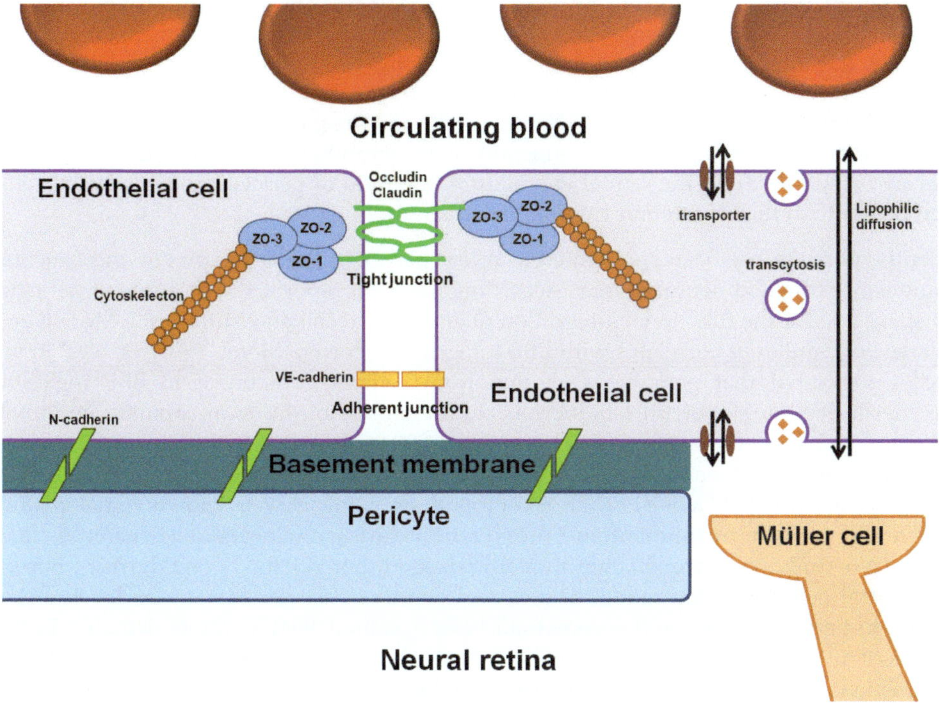

Fig. 1. A schematic view of the inner blood-retinal barrier

2.1 Molecular components of tight junction

Tight junction is constituted by various kinds of proteins. Transmembrane proteins like occludin and claudin interconnect endothelial cell with adjacent endothelium and exert a barrier function (Furuse et al., 1998; Russ et al., 1998). Cytoplasmic accessory proteins like zonular occludens (ZO) 1-3, cingulin, 7H6 antigen and cadherin-5 connect transmembrane proteins to cytoskelecton (Gumbiner et al., 1991; Persidsky et al., 2006). Tight junction proteins not only function as a barrier regulating paracellular diffusion, but also work as signaling complex (Gonzalez-Mariscal et al., 2008).

2.2 Molecular pathways across the BRB

Molecular exchange across the inner BRB is allowed through paracellular pathway and transcellular pathway (Pardridge, 1999). Paracellular pathway is restricted by tight junction and limited exchange of substances occurs according to a concentration gradient.

Transcellular pathway involves diffusion of lipophilic molecule, carrier mediated transport and transcytosis (Abbott et al., 2006).

2.3 Cellular components involved in the inner BRB

2.3.1 Pericyte

Retinal capillaries are covered by pericytes and pericytes exist in proximity to the endothelial cell (sharing basement membrane with endothelial cell). The spatial relationship facilitates the interaction of these two cells. Pericytes communicate with endothelial cells through diverse mediators like angiopoietins, transforming growth factor-β (TGF-β), platelet-derived growth factor-B (PDGF-B) and sphingosine-1-phosphate (S1P). Pericytes also form a heterocytic adherent junction with endothelial cells through N-cadherin (Navarro et al., 1998). In the retinal vasculature, the ratio of pericytes to endothelial cells is even higher than that of cerebral vasculature, reaching as high as 1:1.

Recently, pericyte has been spotlighted as a key player in the development and functional maintenance of blood-neural barrier. According to recent reports, the presence of pericyte is indispensable for the functional integration of endothelial cell and Müller cell. Moreover, its coverage of capillaries correlates with BBB integrity (Shepro & Morel, 1993). Several in vitro studies suggested that pericyte is an important cellular component in BBB regulation. Pericyte derived angiopoietin-1 induces occludin expression in brain capillary endothelial cell via Tie-2 receptor activation (Hori et al., 2004). TGF-β1/TGF-β receptor signaling between pericyte and endothelial cell plays an important role in enhancing BBB function (Dohgu et al., 2005). PDGF-B/PDGF receptor- β signaling is well known signal pathway involved in pericyte recruitment and proliferation during angiogenesis (Enge et al., 2002). For in vivo study, pericyte ablation model is needed, but Pdgfb -/- or Pdgfrb-/- mice, an ideal mural cell deficiency model, shows wide spread vascular leakage and hemorrhage leading to perinatal lethality (Leveen et al., 1994; Soriano, 1994). Perinatal lethality in these knock-out mice model made it difficult to analyze the role of pericyte in postnatal BBB dysfunction. More recently, studies using viable animal models of pericyte depletion provided an insight into the role of pericyte in BBB formation and regulation (Akagi et al., 1983; Thanabalasundaram et al., 2010).

The loss of pericyte is one of the earliest pathologic changes of diabetic retinopathy. The mechanism of pericyte loss in diabetic retinopathy is still unclear. Apoptosis triggered by hyperglycemia is presumed mechanism of pericyte loss in diabetic patients. Increased formation of advanced glycation end product (AGE) (Stitt et al., 1997) and aldose reductase expression in pericyte (Akagi et al., 1983) were suggested as the cause of pericyte loss under hyperglycemic condition. However, selective loss of pericyte is still to be elucidated because these mechanisms are common in various cell types. Pericyte loss not only results in the dysfunction of inner BRB, but also provides an important predisposing condition for the pathologic angiogenesis (Hammes et al., 2002). Under physiologic condition, pericytes inhibit the proliferation of endothelial cell. At the beginning of angiogenesis, the precedent denudation of pericytes from the pre-existing forefront of blood vessel is required for the mobilization of endothelial cells (Bergers & Benjamin, 2003; Yancopoulos et al., 2000). Endothelial hyperplasia which predispose for angiogenic sprouting can occur in the absence of pericytes.

2.3.2 Müller cells

In the development of primate retina, glial cells enter into the retina from the optic nerve and invade to the peripheral retina. Glial cells are involved in diverse process of retinal vascular development. First, glial cells secrete VEGF in response to hypoxic condition, resulting in retinal vascularization (Kim et al., 2010b). Second, a growing body of evidences showed that Müller cell, a predorminant constituent of the retinal glial cell, forms 'neurovascular unit' with endothelial cell and neuron to regulate blood flow of neural tissue and blood-neural barrier function. In vitro studies using retinal vascular endothelial cell co-cultured with glial cell or cultured with conditioned medium from glial cell demonstrated that glial cell is important in barrier properties including the expression of tight junction proteins (Gardner, 1995; Gardner et al., 1997). Several glial cell derived growth factors like angiopoietin-1, basic fibroblast growth factor (bFGF), glial derived growth factor (GDGF) and TGF-β are reported to induce the blood-neural barrier phenotype in vitro (Abbott et al., 2006). The src-suppressed C kinase substrate (SSeCKS) expressed in glial cell regulates the barrier integrity by the regulation of VEGF (potent mediator of vascular permeability) and angiopoietin-1 (involved in vascular maturation and barriergenesis) level (Lee et al., 2003).

Glial cell has a spatial proximity with endothelial cell and interconnected with basal laminar of endothelium via the end-foot processes. In the BBB, perivascular end-foot of glial cells contains abundant orthogonal arrays of particles (OAPs) in a polarized manner which is constituted with aquaporin 4 (AQP4) and the polarity of AQP4 localization in glial endfeet is disrupted under pathologic condition involving BBB impairment (Wolburg-Buchholz et al., 2009). In the perivascular endfeet of Müller cells, the expression of AQP4 also had been identified (Nagelhus et al., 1998). Agrin, an extracellular heparansulfate proteoglycan, is a factor that is known to affect this polarity of perivascular glial endfeet (Fallier-Becker et al., 2011; Wolburg et al., 2009) and suggested to be participated in the BBB development (Barber & Lieth, 1997).

Under diabetic condition both hypoxia and hyperglycemia can affect Müller cells leading to the breakdown of BRB. In the animal model of hypoxic retinopathy, hypoxia induced apoptotic loss of Müller cell leads to the subsequent BRB failure (Chan-Ling & Stone, 1992), pathologic angiogenesis and vitreous hemorrhage (Zhang & Stone, 1997). Moreover, in hypoxic retinopathy, Müller cell derived VEGF is essential pathogenic molecule resulting BRB disruption and pathologic neovascularization (Weidemann et al., 2010). Pathologic changes of retinal glia were also noted in the hyperglycemic condition. According to a study using streptozocin induced diabetic rat, Müller cell showed generalized regression throughout the retina from the early stage of diabetes before the BRB dysfunction (Rungger-Brandle et al., 2000). Furthermore, in diabetic rat, the alteration of perivascular Müller glial aquaporins was noted especially in the superficial retinal vessels which might affect the barrier function (Iandiev et al., 2007).

2.3.3 Endothelial cell

Retinal capillaries are consisted by non-fenestrated endothelium and the basement membrane of retinal vascular endothelium is continuous. Tight junction between retinal micro-vascular endothelial cells is the anatomical basis of the inner BRB. Retinal vascular endothelium forms a homocytic interconnection with adjacent cell via tight junction and adherent junction. Beside tight junction, adherent junction stabilizes the BRB providing mechanical force. VE-cadherin is major molecule involved in endothelial-endothelial adherent junctional complex (Navarro et al., 1998). The luminal side of retinal vascular endothelium has negative charge due to the glycocalyx coat which contributes to the barrier function toward negatively charged molecules and the loss of this surface charge causes dysfunction of BRB (Lin, 1988).

Endothelial cell of retinal capillary expresses diverse transporters for selective molecular exchange between neural retina and circulation. Enzymatic activity vascular endothelial also contribute to barrier property through regulating the metabolism of substances from circulating blood to retina and vice versa.

2.3.4 Neuron

Retinal blood flow is tightly regulated according to the activity of retinal neurons. Metabolic need of ganglion cells is supposed to be an important factor in vascular development of retina. Intercellular communications between endothelial cells, Müller cells and neurons are expected to play a pivotal role in the formation and functioning of BRB. Diabetic retinopathy is a kind of progressive neuropathy. Retinal neuropathy in diabetes could be a consequence of preceding diabetic vascuopathy. However, there are some evidences that diabetes itself could be the cause of retinal neuropathy. In streptozocin induced early diabetic rats, increased apoptosis of neuron was documented especially in retinal ganglion cells and Müller cells (Hammes et al., 1995). Moreover, post-mortem human specimen from diabetic patients showed that apoptosis of neuronal cell could occur prior to clinically significant diabetic vasculopathy and the location of neuronal death had nothing to do with the presence of focal vascular lesions (Barber et al., 1998). These results suggest retinal neuronal apoptosis may not be the result of diabetic vasculopathy.

3. Disruption of inner blood-retinal barrier in diabetic retina

3.1 Protein Kinase C (PKC)

In the diabetic retina, cellular accumulation of diacylglycerol which activates PKC to translocate into plasma membrane and to acquire phosphorylation activities has been documented (Dempsey et al., 2000; Newton, 1997; Xia et al., 1994). Hyperglycemia induced the activation of PKC is associated with the pathologic changes of diabetic retinopathy. The exact mechanism of PKC induced vascular leakage in diabetic retinopathy still remains unclear, but PKC, especillay β-isoform is considered as a key mediator of VEGF induced BRB disruption and retinal neovascularization (Aiello et al., 1997; Xia et al., 1996). Recently, it is reported that PKCδ is also associated with the pathogenesis of diabetic retina through inducing the decrement of endothelial tight junction protein (ZO-1, 2) expression and subsequent vascular hyperpermeability in diabetic retina (Kim et al., 2010a). In addition, PKC mediated occludin phosphorylation is reported to participate in the VEGF stimulated vascular leakage (Harhaj et al., 2006). Some investigators also suggested nitric oxide (NO) pathway as a potential downstream target of PKC induced vascular permeability. In an experiment using coronary venule, PKC regulated vascular leakage partially relies on the endothelial NO synthesis (Huang & Yuan, 1997).

3.2 Advanced Glycation Endproducts (AGEs)

Long-term exposure to hyperglycemic environment results in a non-enzymatic glycation of protein, lipid and nucleic acid to form a heterogenous group of irreversible adducts called

AGEs. The clinical implication of AGEs is well documented in patients with diabetes. Among type 1 diabetic patients, skin levels of glycated collagen (Amadori product) and carboxymethyllysine (a kind of AGEs) showed correlation with the progression of diabetic retinopathy (Genuth et al., 2005). Vitreous level of hydroimidazolone, one of the most prominent AGEs, is reported to be increased in patients with type 2 diabetes (Fosmark et al., 2007).

AGEs and its receptor RAGE (receptor of AGEs) are known to exert a pivotal role in diabetic vascular complication such as retinopathy and nephropathy. Dysfunction of BRB in diabetic retinopathy is also caused by AGEs associated mechanism. First, dysfunction and apoptosis of pericyte, a key cellular component in the formation and maintenance of BRB are suggested as a mechanism of AGEs related BRB breakdown in diabetes. In streptozocin induced diabetic rats, significant deposition of AGEs and expression of RAGE were noted in pericytes of the capillary beds (Stitt et al., 1997). AGEs showed toxicity to pericyte in vitro and this toxic effect is mediated by AGE-RAGE interaction (Yamagishi et al., 1995). ROS generation through AGE-RAGE interaction results in oxidation of DNA, membrane lipid peroxidation and subsequent apoptotic pericyte death (Yamagishi et al., 2002b). In addition, AGEs regulate the expression of growth factors from pericyte which participate in the BRB function (Shimizu et al., 2011; Yamagishi et al., 2002a). Second, AGEs are involved in inflammatory reactions which cause the disturbance of BRB function. In diabetes, AGEs are accumulated in the vascular wall to stimulate proinflammatory reaction (Yan et al., 2003). These adducts not only activate leukocytes (Chibber et al., 2000) but also involved in the regulation of endothelial adhesion molecules. According to experimental study, blocking the interaction between AGEs and RAGE could effectively ameliorate retinal ICAM-1 expression, leukostasis and subsequent BRB breakdown in diabetic animal (Kaji et al., 2007).

Because diverse mechanisms are involved in the pathogensis of BRB breakdown in diabetic retinopathy, the evaluation on the effect of AGEs in non-diabetic indivisual is required for elucidating the role of AGEs in barrier dysfunction. In vivo studies using normo-glycemic animal showed that infusion of AGEs could induce vasculopathy resembling that of diabetes (Vlassara et al., 1992) and BRB breakdown associated with overexpression of VEGF (Stitt et al., 2000).

3.3 Sorbitol

Under hyperglycemia, glucose is converted to intracellular sorbitol by aldose reductase. Intracellular accumulation of sorbitol results in an osmotic damage to retinal vascular endothelium and pericytes. In a postmortem electron microscopic study of diabetic eye, BRB disruption and increased aldose reductase expression in the vascular cells participates in BRB formation (retinal vascular endothelial cells and Müller cells) were found which suggest that aldose reductase induced intracellular accumulation of sorbitol in vascular cell might contribute to the BRB breakdown in diabetes (Vinores et al., 1993). However, a randomized clinical trial of sorbinil, an aldose reductase inhibitor, in patients with diabetic retinopathy ended with little success in preventing retinopathy progression (Sorbinil Retinopathy Trial Research Group, 1990).

3.4 Vascular Endothelial Growth Factor (VEGF)

VEGF is not only a potent angiogenic growth factor, but also a strong vascular permeability enhancer. There are four different isoform of VEGF produced by alternative splicing of the same gene: $VEGF_{121}$, $VEGF_{165}$, $VEGF_{189}$ and $VEGF_{206}$. Among these isoforms, $VEGF_{165}$ is the predominant isoform with optimal characteristics of bioavailability and bioactivity (Ferrara et al., 2003). The expression of VEGF is regulated mainly by oxygen tension. Under hypoxic condition, hypoxia-inducible factor (HIF)-1 binds to hypoxia response element (HRE) of the VEGF gene and activates genes participate in cellular response to hypoxia (Carmeliet et al., 1998; Jiang et al., 1996). VEGF expression is also controlled by diverse growth factors and inflammatory cytokines. In patients with proliferative diabetic retinopathy, vitreous level of VEGF is elevated and effectively reduced after panretinal laser photocoagulation (Aiello et al., 1994) because of a decreased metabolic need of neural retina which leads to amelioration of tissue hypoxia. Oxidative stress and pro-inflammatory cytokine is also suggested to be implicated in VEGF upregulation of diabetic retina (Frey & Antonetti, 2011; Giacco & Brownlee, 2010). VEGF exerts biological activity through specific receptor tyrosine kinases: VEGFR-1 and VEGFR-2. VEGFR-1 is considered as 'decoy' receptor which prevents VEGF from binding to VEGFR-2. Pro-angiogenic and vasopermeable effect of VEGF is mainly mediated by VEGF-2.

VEGF induces retinal vascular hyperpermeability through both transcellular pathway and paracellular pathway. VEGF induces pinocytotic vesicular transport by upregulation of the vesiculo-vacuolar organelle (VVO) formation (Feng et al., 1999). In paracellular pathway, VEGF affects both of tight junction and adherent junction. The expression and assembly of tight junction protein ZO-1 and occludin are reduced by the VEGF (Antonetti et al., 1998; Wang et al., 2001). Post-translational regulation of tight junction protein by phosphorylation is also responsible for the VEGF mediated vascular hyperpermeability (Antonetti et al., 1999; Harhaj et al., 2006). Phosphorylation and disorganization of VE-cadherin, a major component of adherent junction between microvascular endothelial cells are another pathogenic change associated with VEGF induced vascular leakage (Esser et al., 1998; Kevil et al., 1998). Moreover, in patients with diabetic retinopathy, over-expressed VEGF upregulates adhesion molecules (ICAM-1, VCAM-1 and E-selectin) and enhances leukocyte adhesion (Kim et al., 2001). During the process of angiogenesis, local concentration of VEGF also perturbs pericyte coverage and maturation of blood vessels (Greenberg et al., 2008). In the animal model of diabetes, the VEGF mediated BRB breakdown and the restoration of BRB by an inhibition of VEGF action are well documented from the early stage of diabetic retinopathy (Murata et al., 1995; Qaum et al., 2001). Now a days anti-VEGF agents are widely used in the treatment of diabetic macular edema.

3.5 Carbonic Anhydrase (CA)

CA is a ubiquitous enzyme that catalyzes the interconversion of carbon dioxide and bicarbonate to regulate pH of tissue and to help transport of carbon dioxide. Presence of CA in the posterior segment of human eye has been proven (Wistrand et al., 1986), but the significance of CA in the pathogenesis of diabetic retinopathy was underestimated until recently. According to comparative proteomic analysis of vitreous from non-diabetic, diabetic without retinopathy versus proliferative diabetic retinopathy (PDR) subjects revealed that vitreous concentration of CA-I in PDR group was 15.3 and 8.2 times higher than that of non-diabetic and diabetic without retinopathy groups, respectively. In the rat, intravitreal injection of CA caused retinal vascular hyperpermeability through different mechanism form that of VEGF induced barrier breakdown. Authors postulated that in diabetic retinopathy, increased CA elevates intraocular pH which in turn activates kallikrein-kinin system and subsequent bradykinin receptor activation leads to BRB breakdown (Gao et al., 2007). Moreover, in streptozocin-induced diabetic rats, decreased kallikrein-binding protein level has been noted (Hatcher et al., 1997), which could increase the free kallikrein level. CA inhibitors are potential candidate of supplementary treatment option for diabetic macular edema. Actually in a pilot study with a few participants, acetazolamide, a CA inhibitor, showed partial effect in improving diabetic macular edema (Giusti et al., 2001).

3.6 Inflammation

It is now generally accepted that the pathogenesis of diabetic retinopathy involves low grade inflammation and vascular endothelial dysfunction (Gerhardinger et al., 2005; Joussen et al., 2004; van Hecke et al., 2005). Leukostasis of retinal microvasculature was consistently found from the early stage of diabetic retinopathy. Several experimental and clinical evidences indicated that leukostasis is one of the most important causative factors of typical diabetic microvascular pathologies such as microvascular acellularity, capillary drop-out and microaneurysm formation (Kim et al., 2005; Lutty et al., 1997; McLeod et al., 1995). Moreover, leukostasis in diabetic retinopathy is closely associated with BRB breakdown (Leal et al., 2007). In the diabetic retina, upregulation of VEGF and increased inducible NO synthase activity is involved in the expression of endothelial adhesion molecules like ICAM-1, VCAM-1 (Ishida et al., 2003; Leal et al., 2007; Nowak et al., 2008). Experimental study using ICAM knock-out mice revealed that adhesion molecule plays a key role in the endothelial dysfunction and barrier breakdown of diabetic retinopathy (Joussen et al., 2004).

Several inflammatory cytokines are participated in the breakdown of BRB in diabetes. Interleukin-1 (IL-1)β and tumor necrosis factor (TNF)-α are the representative inflammatory cytokines participate in the pathogenesis of diabetic retinopathy. Both in the vitreous humour and serum of patients with proliferative diabetic retinopathy, the level of IL-1β and TNF-α is increased (Demircan et al., 2006). The activity of caspase 1 which is a proteolytic enzyme involved in the production of IL-1β is also up-regulated in the retinas of diabetic patients (Mohr et al., 2002). IL-1β is a well known cytokine that induces barrier dysfunction through leukocyte recruitment in diverse pathologic condition. High concentration of glucose stimulates endothelial IL-1β over-expression and results in apoptosis of endothelial cell through the activation of NF-κB in vitro. Supplement of IL-1β caused retinal microvascular change resembling that of diabetic retinopathy (Kowluru & Odenbach, 2004) and inhibition of caspase-1/interleukin-1beta signaling with minocycline prevented vascular pathology of diabetic rat (Vincent & Mohr, 2007). TNF-α is also involved in the loss of retinal microvascular cells in diabetic retina (Behl et al., 2008). In bovine retinal endothelial cells, TNF-α disturbs the expression of tight junction proteins (claudin-5 and ZO-1) and subcellular localization of these proteins (Aveleira et al., 2010). In the TNF-α knock-out rat, diabetes associated retinal leukostasis, apoptosis of retinal microvascular cells and breakdown of BRB are significantly suppressed (Huang et al., 2011). Also in a diabetic rat, etanercept, a soluble tumor necrosis factor receptor (p75):Fc fusion protein (TNFR:Fc) effectively reduced leukostasis and breakdown of BRB (Joussen et al., 2002).

4. Clinical implication and current treatment modalities of diabetic inner BRB dysfunction: Diabetic macular edema

Macular edema which resulted from the dysfunctional BRB is the most common cause of visual disturbance in patients with nonproliferative diabetic retinopathy (NPDR). In addition to the disruption of inner BRB of the pre-existing retinal vasculature, the 'leaky' property of new vessels contributes to the macular edema in patients with proliferative diabetic retinopathy (PDR). Breakdown of BRB causes retention of fluid and plasma contents, such as lipoproteins within neural retina leading to retinal thickening. According to the data of Wisconsin epidemiologic study of diabetic retinopathy (WESDRP), the prevalence of diabetic macular edema ranges from 18 to 20% among the patients with diabetes (Klein et al., 1984a; Klein et al., 1984b).

After the reports of Early Treatment of Diabetic Retinopathy Study (ETDRS) focal/grid laser photocoagulation was the standard treatment method in diabetic macular edema. Stabilization or some improvement of vision was acquired in patients with macular edema who received laser photocoagulation. Although it is still the most cost-effective treatment modality in diabetic macular edema, some patients suffer from the post-treatment paracentral scotomas (Striph et al., 1988) and enlarging atrophic laser scars (Schatz et al., 1991). Although rare, vision threatening complications like choroidal neovascularization and subretinal fibrosis were also reported (Cunningham & Shons, 1979). Because of the refractory macular edema and complications of laser treatment, several pharmacological treatment modalities had been introduced. Further delineation on the exact mechanism of action is still needed, but intravitreal steroid injection is a powerful treatment option in diabetic macular edema. There are many in vitro and in vivo studies suggesting the mechanisms involved in the effect of corticosteroid treatment for diabetic macular edema. An in vitro study using bovine retinal endothelial cell monolayer showed that hydrocortisone treatment reduced monolayer permeability to water and solutes, increased tight junction proteins (ZO-1 and occludin) and reduced occludin phosphorylation (Antonetti et al., 2002). In experimental diabetic retina, corticosteroids demonstrated differential regulation of VEGF receptors (down-regulation of VEGFR-2 and up-regulation of VEGFR-1, a 'decoy' receptor) (Zhang et al., 2008), inhibitory effects on VEGF, ICAM-1 expression (Wang et al., 2008) and leukostasis (Tamura et al., 2005). Despite of the potential side effects like cataract and increased ocular pressure, intravitreal triamcinolone injection is one of the most commonly used treatment modality in diabetic retinopathy. More recently, several anti-VEGF agents are applicated in the treatment of diabetic macular edema. Several reports comparing the effectiveness of focal/grid laser photocoagulation, intravitreal triamcinolone injection and various anti-VEGF agents has been published (Diabetic Retinopathy Clinical Research Network, 2008; Soheilian et al., 2009), but more large scale studies with prolonged observation period are needed.

5. Possible therapeutic approach to diabetic retinopathy through BRB modulation

In addition to previously commented treatment modalities, diverse therapeutic agents had been suggested for the medical treatment of diabetic retinopathy through the modulation of inner BRB disruption. Clinical studies involving medical treatment of inner BRB dysfunction are summarized in table 1 and each therapeutic candidate is further delineated below.

Drug (Class)	Suggested mechanism	Clinical trials		
		Study	Population (N:enrolled/completed)	Result
Fenofibrate (Fibrate)	Inhibit VEGF production Reduce adhesion molecule level	FIELD study	Type 2 DM patients without requiring lipid modifying treatment (9795/9764)	Reduced the risk of ME which needs laser treatment
Lisinopril (ACE inhibitor)	Inhibit VEGF production	EUCLID	Non-hypertensive type 1 DM patients (530/354)	No significant effect on the retinopathy progression
Candesartan (AT1R blocker)	Inhibit VEGF production	DIRECT-prevent 1	Normoalbuminuric, normotensive type 1 DM patients (1421/1421)	Reduce the risk of retinopathy
		DIRECT-protect 1	Normoalbuminuric, normotensive type 1 DM patients (1905/1905)	No significant preventing effect on both retinopathy progression and ME development
		DIRECT-protect 2	Normoalbuminuric, type 2 DM (1905/1905)	
Telmisartan (AT1R blocker)	Reduce RAGE expression	Untitled (Nakamura et al., 2005)	Patients with essential hypertension (7/7)	Decrease serum levels of sRAGE
Ruboxistaurin (PKC inhibitor)	Blocking VEGF mediated tight junction dysregulation	PKC-DRS	Patients with moderate to severe NPDR (252/157)	No significant effect on both retinopathy progression and ME development Reduced the risk of MVL
		PKC-DRS2	Patients with moderate to severe NPDR (685/514)	Reduced the progression of ME into the center of macula and need for laser treatment for ME
		PKC-DMES	Patients with DME farther than 300 μm from central macula, an ETDRS retinopathy level from 20 to 47A (686/506)	Preventive effect on ME progression
Pimagedine (Aminoguanidine)	Lowering AGEs production	ACTION I trial	Patients with type 1 DM (690/472)	Significantly reduced the risk of three-step or greater progression of the retinopathy score

Abbreviations

ACTION I: A Clinical Trial In Overt Nephropathy of Type 1 Diabetics, AT1R: angiotensin II type 1 receptor, DIRECT: Diabetic Retinopathy Cardesartan Trials, ETDRS: Early Treatment of Diabetic Retinopathy Study, DM: diabetes mellitus, EUCLID: EURODIAB Controlled Trial of Lisinopril in Insulin-Dependent Diabetes Mellitus, FIELD: Fenofibrate Intervention and Event Lowering in Diabetes, FU: follow-up, ME: macular edema, MVL: moderate visual loss, PKC-DRS: PKC inhibitor diabetic retinopathy study, PKC-DMES: PKC inhibitor diabetic macular edema study, sRAGE: soluble form of RAGE.

Table 1. Possible medical therapeutic agent for the treatment of diabetic retinopathy through a modulation of inner BRB disruption

5.1 Fenofibrate

Because dyslipidemia is a well documented risk factor of diabetic macular edema and hard exudates deposition, lipid lowering treatment was expected to have benefit on these complications. The Fenofibrate Intervention and Event Lowering in Diabetes (FIELD) study group applicated fenofibrate, a peroxisome proliferator-activated receptor (PPAR)-α agonist which is widely used as lipid lowering agent in diabetic patients to reduce the risk of microvascular and macrovascular complications. PPAR-α agonist not only modulates lipid composition, but also inhibits the production of VEGF (Panigrahy et al., 2008) and reduces serum levels of adhesion molecule VCAM-1 and ICAM-1 (Rosenson et al., 2007) which are key components in the pathogenesis of BRB breakdown. Fenofibrate treatment demonstrated significant preventive effect on the hypoxia induced endothelial hyperpermeability of an in vitro BBB model (Mysiorek et al., 2009). In the type 2 diabetes patients without requiring lipid-modifying treatment, mean 5 years of fenofibrate (200 mg/day) treatment significantly reduced the risk of macular edema development which needs laser treatment (31% reduction) (Keech et al., 2007).

5.2 Blocking of the Retina-Angiotensin System (RAS)

In human eye, the local expression of RAS components: renin, angiotensin converting enzyme (ACE) and angiotensin has been reported (Wagner et al., 1996) and their activation in diabetic retinopathy (Danser et al., 1989) is well documented. Increasing evidences indicate that angiotensin II stimulates the expression of VEGF in vitro (Williams et al., 1995). In streptozotocin-induced diabetic animal, ACE inhibitor treatment inhibited retinal VEGF production and subsequent retinal vascular hyperpermeability associated with BRB breakdown (Kim et al., 2009). Moreover, among the patients with proliferative diabetic retinopathy, vitreous level of VEGF is significantly lower in patients receiving ACE-inhibition (Hogeboom van Buggenum et al., 2002). In diabetic hypertensive rat, treatment with candesartan, an angiotensin II receptor blocker effectively suppressed the vascular permeability across the BBB (Awad, 2006).

On these experimental bases, several RAS inhibiting agents had been applicated for the treatment of diabetic retinopathy. The EURODIAB Controlled Trial of Lisinopril in Insulin-Dependent Diabetes Mellitus (EUCLID) suggested that lisinopril, an ACE inhibitor could have benefit on the progression of diabetic retinopathy in patients with type 1 diabetes. However, the primary endpoint was the progression of diabetic retinopathy, and the protective effect does not showed statistical strength (Chaturvedi et al., 1998).

The Diabetic Retinopathy Cardesartan Trials (DIRECT) group has performed three separate randomized, double-blind, placebo-controlled clinical trials to evaluate the efficacy of candesartan on reducing the incidence (DIRECT-Prevent 1), progression of retinopathy in type 1 (DIRECT-Protect 1) (Chaturvedi et al., 2008) and the progression of retinopathy in type 2 diabetes patients (DIRECT-Protect 2) (Sjolie et al., 2008). In both DIRECT-Protect 1 and 2, the primary endpoint was progression of diabetic retinopathy, which was defined as three or more step deterioration of ETDRS level. Development of clinically significant macular edema (CSME), development of proliferative diabetic retinopathy or both were settled as secondary endpoint. Five years of candesartan treatment did showed significantly increased probability of diabetic retinopathy regression (34% increment) in type 2 diabetes patients, but there were no significant preventing effects on the progression of disease in both type 1 and 2 patients. Although it was not the primary endpoint, the incidence of CSME development was not affected by candesartan treatment.

5.3 Protein kinase C inhibitors

Since Ishii et al. (Ishii et al., 1996) demonstrated that LY333531, a selective inhibitor of PKC β-isoform could rescue diabetic animals from vascular dysfunction, several clinical studies on ruboxistaurin (orally active form of selective PKC β inhibitor: LY333531) use for diabetic retinopathy had been performed: the PKC inhibitor diabetic retinopathy study (PKC-DRS), the PKC inhibitor diabetic retinopathy study 2 (PKC-DRS2), the PKC inhibitor diabetic macular edema study (PKC-DMES). PKC-DRS is a phase 3, multicenter, double-masked, placebo controlled trial involving patients with moderate to severe NPDR, the endpoints of which are progression of diabetic retinopathy (equal to or greater than three-step worsening in the ETDRS scale), moderate vision loss (MVL: vision decrease of three or more lines on the ETDRS chart) and sustained MVL (SMVL: MVL in two consecutive visit 6 or more months apart). Oral administration of ruboxistaurin (32 mg/day) for more than 36 months showed no preventive effect on the diabetic retinopathy progression, but significantly delayed the occurrence of MVL and SMVL and reduced the risk of MVL to one-third of that in the placebo group (The Protein Kinase C beta Inhibitor Diabetic Retinopathy Study [PKC-DRS], 2005). According to PKC-DRS2, a following phase 3 clinical trial designed to evaluate visual outcome of ruboxistaurin treatment in patients with moderate to severe NPDR, administration of ruboxistaurin reduced a 3-year risk of SMVL from 9.1% to 5.5% (40% risk reduction). Moreover, ruboxistaurin reduced the progression of macular edema into the center of macula and need for laser treatment for macular edema (Aiello et al., 2006). PKC-DMES, an multicenter, double-masked, randomized placebo controlled trial the endpoint of which was progression to sight threatening macular edema or application of photocoagulation for diabetic macular edema, revealed partial effect of ruboxistaurin on the progression of diabetic macular edema to a more severe form in patients with diabetic macular edema (The Protein Kinase C beta inhibitor diabetic macular edema study [PKC-DMES], 2007).

5.4 Blockade of AGE-RAGE pathway

5.4.1 Lowering AGEs production

Aminoguanidine is a prototype drug for the prevention of diabetes-induced AGEs formation in vivo (Brownlee et al., 1986). The pharmacological mechanism of aminoguanidine involves inhibition of NO synthases and semicarbazide-sensitive amine oxidase. Hammes et al. insisted aminoguanidine treatment effectively inhibited the retinal arteriolar accumulation of AGEs, prevented abnormal endothelial proliferation and pericyte loss in diabetic rat. Acellular capillaries and microaneurysms, typical pathologic findings of diabetic retinopathy were also reduced significantly in the aminoguanidine treatment group (Hammes et al., 1991). Administration of aminoguanidine effectively attenuated cellular loss and microthrombus formation of retinal vessels also in diabetic spontaneous hypertensive rats (Hammes et al., 1994). In these reports, authors adapted in situ detection of advanced glycosylation-specific fluorescence for the quantification of AGEs, which might not be specific for AGEs, but also detect other oxidation products. Kern et al. found that aminoguanidine treatment effectively reduces pericyte loss, formation of microaneurysms and acellular capillaries, but inhibitory effect of retinal AGEs accumulation is not significant in diabetic dogs (Kern & Engerman, 2001). A randomized, placebo-controlled study in patients with type 1 diabetes mellitus showed that treatment with pimagedine, a kind of aminoguanidine significantly reduced the risk of three-step or greater progression of the retinopathy (ETDRS) score (Bolton et al., 2004). The exact pharmachologic mechanism of aminoguanidine in preventing diabetic retinopathy progression is still to be elucidated and more clinical trials are needed to clearly delineate the benefit of aminoguanidine treatment in diabetic retinopathy.

5.4.2 Lowering RAGE expression

Several commonly used therapeutic agents showed effects on the reduction of RAGE expression in vascular endothelial cell: thiazolidinediones (rosiglitazone and pioglitazone), calcium channel blocker (nifedipine), angiotensin II receptor blocker (telmisartan). Rosiglitazone and pioglitazone, kinds of thiazolidinediones, an anti-diabetic drug act by binding to peroxisome proliferator-activated receptors reduces basal and tumor necrosis factor-α stimulated expression of RAGE in cultured human umbilical vein endothelial cells. Decreased RAGE by thiazolidinediones results in subsequent inhibition of AGEs stimulated expression of pro-inflammatory protein (Marx et al., 2004). Nifedipine, a calcium channel blocker inhibits RAGE upregulation in AGEs treated human umbilical vein endothelial cells to reduce AGEs induced ROS production (Yamagishi & Takeuchi, 2004). Telmisartan, an angiotensin II receptor blocker inhibits RAGE expression in cultured human microvascular endothelial cells in vitro and decreases serum soluble form of RAGE level in patients with essential hypertension (Nakamura et al., 2005). In vivo studies evaluating the effect of those agents on the inner BRB breakdown in diabetic retinopathy are needed.

6. References

Abbott, N.J., Ronnback, L. & Hansson, E. (2006). Astrocyte-endothelial interactions at the blood-brain barrier. *Nat Rev Neurosci*, Vol.7, No.1, pp. 41-53, ISSN 1471-003X

Aiello, L.P., Avery, R.L., Arrigg, P.G., Keyt, B.A., Jampel, H.D., Shah, S.T., Pasquale, L.R., Thieme, H., Iwamoto, M.A. & Park, J.E., et al. (1994). Vascular endothelial growth factor in ocular fluid of patients with diabetic retinopathy and other retinal disorders. *N Engl J Med*, Vol.331, No.22, pp. 1480-1487, ISSN 0028-4793

Aiello, L.P., Bursell, S.E., Clermont, A., Duh, E., Ishii, H., Takagi, C., Mori, F., Ciulla, T.A., Ways, K., Jirousek, M., Smith, L.E. & King, G.L. (1997). Vascular endothelial growth factor-induced retinal permeability is mediated by protein kinase C in vivo and suppressed by an orally effective beta-isoform-selective inhibitor. *Diabetes*, Vol.46, No.9, pp. 1473-1480, ISSN 0012-1797

Aiello, L.P., Davis, M.D., Girach, A., Kles, K.A., Milton, R.C., Sheetz, M.J., Vignati, L. & Zhi, X.E. (2006). Effect of ruboxistaurin on visual loss in patients with diabetic retinopathy. *Ophthalmology*, Vol.113, No.12, pp. 2221-2230, ISSN 1549-4713

Akagi, Y., Kador, P.F., Kuwabara, T. & Kinoshita, J.H. (1983). Aldose reductase localization in human retinal mural cells. *Invest Ophthalmol Vis Sci*, Vol.24, No.11, pp. 1516-1519, ISSN 0146-0404

Antonetti, D.A., Barber, A.J., Hollinger, L.A., Wolpert, E.B. & Gardner, T.W. (1999). Vascular endothelial growth factor induces rapid phosphorylation of tight junction proteins occludin and zonula occluden 1. A potential mechanism for vascular permeability in diabetic retinopathy and tumors. *J Biol Chem,* Vol.274, No.33, pp. 23463-23467, ISSN 0021-9258

Antonetti, D.A., Barber, A.J., Khin, S., Lieth, E., Tarbell, J.M. & Gardner, T.W. (1998). Vascular permeability in experimental diabetes is associated with reduced endothelial occludin content: vascular endothelial growth factor decreases occludin in retinal endothelial cells. Penn State Retina Research Group. *Diabetes,* Vol.47, No.12, pp. 1953-1959, ISSN 0012-1797

Antonetti, D.A., Wolpert, E.B., DeMaio, L., Harhaj, N.S. & Scaduto R.C., Jr. (2002). Hydrocortisone decreases retinal endothelial cell water and solute flux coincident with increased content and decreased phosphorylation of occludin. *J Neurochem,* Vol.80, No.4, pp. 667-677, ISSN 0022-3042

Aveleira, C.A., Lin, C.M., Abcouwer, S.F., Ambrosio, A.F. & Antonetti, D.A. (2010). TNF-alpha signals through PKCzeta/NF-kappaB to alter the tight junction complex and increase retinal endothelial cell permeability. *Diabetes,* Vol.59, No.11, pp. 2872-2882, ISSN 1939-327X

Awad, A.S. (2006). Role of AT1 receptors in permeability of the blood-brain barrier in diabetic hypertensive rats. *Vascul Pharmacol,* Vol.45, No.3, pp. 141-147, ISSN 1537-1891

Barber, A.J. & Lieth, E. (1997). Agrin accumulates in the brain microvascular basal lamina during development of the blood-brain barrier. *Dev Dyn,* Vol.208, No.1, pp. 62-74, ISSN 1058-8388

Barber, A.J., Lieth, E., Khin, S.A., Antonetti, D.A., Buchanan, A.G. & Gardner, T.W. (1998). Neural apoptosis in the retina during experimental and human diabetes. Early onset and effect of insulin. *J Clin Invest,* Vol.102, No.4, pp. 783-791, ISSN 0021-9738

Behl, Y., Krothapalli, P., Desta, T., DiPiazza, A., Roy, S. & Graves, D.T. (2008). Diabetes-enhanced tumor necrosis factor-alpha production promotes apoptosis and the loss of retinal microvascular cells in type 1 and type 2 models of diabetic retinopathy. *Am J Pathol,* Vol.172, No.5, pp. 1411-1418, ISSN 1525-2191

Bergers, G. & Benjamin, L.E. (2003). Tumorigenesis and the angiogenic switch. *Nat Rev Cancer,* Vol.3, No.6, pp. 401-410, ISSN 1474-175X

Bolton, W.K., Cattran, D.C., Williams, M.E., Adler, S.G., Appel, G.B., Cartwright, K., Foiles, P.G., Freedman, B.I., Raskin, P., Ratner, R.E., Spinowitz, B.S., Whittier, F.C. & Wuerth, J.P. (2004). Randomized trial of an inhibitor of formation of advanced glycation end products in diabetic nephropathy. *Am J Nephrol,* Vol.24, No.1, pp. 32-40, ISSN 0250-8095

Brownlee, M., Vlassara, H., Kooney, A., Ulrich, P. & Cerami, A. (1986). Aminoguanidine prevents diabetes-induced arterial wall protein cross-linking. *Science,* Vol.232, No.4758, pp. 1629-1632, ISSN 0036-8075

Carmeliet, P., Dor, Y., Herbert, J.M., Fukumura, D., Brusselmans, K., Dewerchin, M., Neeman, M., Bono, F., Abramovitch, R., Maxwell, P., Koch, C.J., Ratcliffe, P., Moons, L., Jain, R.K., Collen, D. & Keshert, E. (1998). Role of HIF-1alpha in hypoxia-mediated apoptosis, cell proliferation and tumour angiogenesis. *Nature,* Vol.394, No.6692, pp. 485-490, ISSN 0028-0836

Chan-Ling, T. & Stone, J. (1992). Degeneration of astrocytes in feline retinopathy of prematurity causes failure of the blood-retinal barrier. *Invest Ophthalmol Vis Sci,* Vol.33, No.7, pp. 2148-2159, ISSN 0146-0404

Chaturvedi, N., Porta, M., Klein, R., Orchard, T., Fuller, J., Parving, H.H., Bilous, R. & Sjolie, A.K. (2008). Effect of candesartan on prevention (DIRECT-Prevent 1) and progression

(DIRECT-Protect 1) of retinopathy in type 1 diabetes: randomised, placebo-controlled trials. *Lancet*, Vol.372, No.9647, pp. 1394-1402, ISSN 1474-547X

Chaturvedi, N., Sjolie, A.K., Stephenson, J.M., Abrahamian, H., Keipes, M., Castellarin, A., Rogulja-Pepeonik, Z. & Fuller, J.H. (1998). Effect of lisinopril on progression of retinopathy in normotensive people with type 1 diabetes. The EUCLID Study Group. EURODIAB Controlled Trial of Lisinopril in Insulin-Dependent Diabetes Mellitus. *Lancet*, Vol.351, No.9095, pp. 28-31, ISSN 0140-6736

Chibber, R., Ben-Mahmud, B.M., Coppini, D., Christ, E. & Kohner, E.M. (2000). Activity of the glycosylating enzyme, core 2 GlcNAc (beta1,6) transferase, is higher in polymorphonuclear leukocytes from diabetic patients compared with age-matched control subjects: relevance to capillary occlusion in diabetic retinopathy. *Diabetes*, Vol.49, No.10, pp. 1724-1730, ISSN 0012-1797

Cunha-Vaz, J.G. (1978). Pathophysiology of diabetic retinopathy. *Br J Ophthalmol*, Vol.62, No.6, pp. 351-355, ISSN 0007-1161

Cunningham, B.L. & Shons, A.R. (1979). Free flap transfers in rats using an irradiated recipient site. *Br J Plast Surg*, Vol.32, No.2, pp. 137-140, ISSN 0007-1226

Danser, A.H., van den Dorpel, M.A., Deinum, J., Derkx, F.H., Franken, A.A., Peperkamp, E., de Jong P.T. & Schalekamp, M.A. (1989). Renin, prorenin, and immunoreactive renin in vitreous fluid from eyes with and without diabetic retinopathy. *J Clin Endocrinol Metab*, Vol.68, No.1, pp. 160-167, ISSN 0021-972X

Demircan, N., Safran, B.G., Soylu, M., Ozcan, A.A. & Sizmaz, S. (2006). Determination of vitreous interleukin-1 (IL-1) and tumour necrosis factor (TNF) levels in proliferative diabetic retinopathy. *Eye (Lond)*, Vol.20, No.12, pp. 1366-1369, ISSN 0950-222X

Dempsey, E.C., Newton, A.C., Mochly-Rosen, D., Fields, A.P., Reyland, M.E., Insel, P.A. & Messing, R.O. (2000). Protein kinase C isozymes and the regulation of diverse cell responses. *Am J Physiol Lung Cell Mol Physiol*, Vol.279, No.3, L429-438, ISSN 1040-0605

Diabetic Retinopathy Clinical Research Network. (2008). A randomized trial comparing intravitreal triamcinolone acetonide and focal/grid photocoagulation for diabetic macular edema. *Ophthalmology*, Vol.115, No.9, pp. 1447-1449, ISSN 1549-4713

Dohgu, S., Takata, F., Yamauchi, A., Nakagawa, S., Egawa, T., Naito, M., Tsuruo, T., Sawada, Y., Niwa, M. & Kataoka, Y. (2005). Brain pericytes contribute to the induction and up-regulation of blood-brain barrier functions through transforming growth factor-beta production. *Brain Res*, Vol.1038, No.2, pp. 208-215, ISSN 0006-8993

Enge, M., Bjarnegard, M., Gerhardt, H., Gustafsson, E., Kalen, M., Asker, N., Hammes, H.P., Shani, M., Fassler, R. & Betsholtz, C. (2002). Endothelium-specific platelet-derived growth factor-B ablation mimics diabetic retinopathy. *EMBO J*, Vol.21, No.16, pp. 4307-4316, ISSN 0261-4189

Esser, S., Lampugnani, M.G., Corada, M., Dejana, E. & Risau, W. (1998). Vascular endothelial growth factor induces VE-cadherin tyrosine phosphorylation in endothelial cells. *J Cell Sci*, Vol.111, No.Pt 13, pp. 1853-1865, ISSN 0021-9533

Fallier-Becker, P., Sperveslage, J., Wolburg, H. & Noell, S. (2011). The impact of agrin on the formation of orthogonal arrays of particles in cultured astrocytes from wild-type and agrin-null mice. *Brain Res*, Vol.1367, pp. 2-12, ISSN 1872-6240

Feng, Y., Venema, V.J., Venema, R.C., Tsai, N., Behzadian, M.A. & Caldwell, R.B. (1999). VEGF-induced permeability increase is mediated by caveolae. *Invest Ophthalmol Vis Sci*, Vol.40, No.1, pp. 157-167, ISSN 0146-0404

Ferrara, N., Gerber, H.P. & LeCouter, J. (2003). The biology of VEGF and its receptors. *Nat Med*, Vol.9, No.6, pp. 669-676, ISSN 1078-8956

Fosmark, D.S., Bragadottir, R., Stene-Johansen, I., Berg, J.P., Berg, T.J., Lund, T., Sandvik, L. & Hanssen, K.F. (2007). Increased vitreous levels of hydroimidazolone in type 2 diabetes patients are associated with retinopathy: a case-control study. *Acta Ophthalmol Scand,* Vol.85, No.6, pp. 618-622, ISSN 1395-3907

Frey, T. & Antonetti, D.A. (2011). Alterations to the Blood-Retinal Barrier in Diabetes: Cytokines and Reactive Oxygen Species. *Antioxid Redox Signal,* Vol.15, No.5, pp. 1271-1284, ISSN 1557-7716

Furuse, M., Fujita, K., Hiiragi, T., Fujimoto, K. & Tsukita, S. (1998). Claudin-1 and -2: novel integral membrane proteins localizing at tight junctions with no sequence similarity to occludin. *J Cell Biol,* Vol.141, No.7, pp. 1539-1550, ISSN 0021-9525

Gao, B.B., Clermont, A., Rook, S., Fonda, S.J., Srinivasan, V.J., Wojtkowski, M., Fujimoto, J.G., Avery, R.L., Arrigg, P.G., Bursell, S.E., Aiello, L.P. & Feener, E.P. (2007). Extracellular carbonic anhydrase mediates hemorrhagic retinal and cerebral vascular permeability through prekallikrein activation. *Nat Med,* Vol.13, No.2, pp. 181-188, ISSN 1078-8956

Gardner, T.W. (1995). Histamine, ZO-1 and increased blood-retinal barrier permeability in diabetic retinopathy. *Trans Am Ophthalmol Soc,* Vol.93, pp. 583-621, ISSN 0065-9533

Gardner, T.W., Lieth, E., Khin, S.A., Barber, A.J., Bonsall, D.J., Lesher, T., Rice, K. & Brennan, W.A., Jr. (1997). Astrocytes increase barrier properties and ZO-1 expression in retinal vascular endothelial cells. *Invest Ophthalmol Vis Sci,* Vol.38, No.11, pp. 2423-2427, ISSN 0146-0404

Garner, A. (1993). Histopathology of diabetic retinopathy in man. *Eye (Lond),* Vol.7, No.Pt 2, pp. 250-253, ISSN 0950-222X

Genuth, S., Sun, W., Cleary, P., Sell, D.R., Dahms, W., Malone, J., Sivitz, W. & Monnier, V.M. (2005). Glycation and carboxymethyllysine levels in skin collagen predict the risk of future 10-year progression of diabetic retinopathy and nephropathy in the diabetes control and complications trial and epidemiology of diabetes interventions and complications participants with type 1 diabetes. *Diabetes,* Vol.54, No.11, pp. 3103-3111, ISSN 0012-1797

Gerhardinger, C., Costa, M.B., Coulombe, M.C., Toth, I., Hoehn, T. & Grosu, P. (2005). Expression of acute-phase response proteins in retinal Muller cells in diabetes. *Invest Ophthalmol Vis Sci,* Vol.46, No.1, pp. 349-357, ISSN 0146-0404

Gerhardt, H. & Betsholtz, C. (2003). Endothelial-pericyte interactions in angiogenesis. *Cell Tissue Res,* Vol.314, No.1, pp. 15-23, ISSN 0302-766X

Giacco, F. & Brownlee, M. (2010). Oxidative stress and diabetic complications. *Circ Res,* Vol.107, No.9, pp. 1058-1070, ISSN 1524-4571

Giusti, C., Forte, R., Vingolo, E.M. & Gargiulo, P. (2001). Is acetazolamide effective in the treatment of diabetic macular edema? A pilot study. *Int Ophthalmol,* Vol.24, No.2, pp. 79-88, ISSN 0165-5701

Gonzalez-Mariscal, L., Tapia, R. & Chamorro, D. (2008). Crosstalk of tight junction components with signaling pathways. *Biochim Biophys Acta,* Vol.1778, No.3, pp. 729-756, ISSN 0006-3002

Greenberg, J.I., Shields, D.J., Barillas, S.G., Acevedo, L.M., Murphy, E., Huang, J., Scheppke, L., Stockmann, C., Johnson, R.S., Angle, N. & Cheresh, D.A. (2008). A role for VEGF as a negative regulator of pericyte function and vessel maturation. *Nature,* Vol.456, No.7223, pp. 809-813, ISSN 1476-4687

Gumbiner, B., Lowenkopf, T. & Apatira, D. (1991). Identification of a 160-kDa polypeptide that binds to the tight junction protein ZO-1. *Proc Natl Acad Sci U S A,* Vol.88, No.8, pp. 3460-3464, ISSN 0027-8424

Hammes, H.P., Brownlee, M., Edelstein, D., Saleck, M., Martin, S. & Federlin, K. (1994). Aminoguanidine inhibits the development of accelerated diabetic retinopathy in the spontaneous hypertensive rat. *Diabetologia*, Vol.37, No.1, pp. 32-35, ISSN 0012-186X

Hammes, H.P., Federoff, H.J. & Brownlee, M. (1995). Nerve growth factor prevents both neuroretinal programmed cell death and capillary pathology in experimental diabetes. *Mol Med*, Vol.1, No.5, pp. 527-534, ISSN 1076-1551

Hammes, H.P., Lin, J., Renner, O., Shani, M., Lundqvist, A., Betsholtz, C., Brownlee, M. & Deutsch, U. (2002). Pericytes and the pathogenesis of diabetic retinopathy. *Diabetes*, Vol.51, No.10, pp. 3107-3112, ISSN 0012-1797

Hammes, H.P., Martin, S., Federlin, K., Geisen, K. & Brownlee, M. (1991). Aminoguanidine treatment inhibits the development of experimental diabetic retinopathy. *Proc Natl Acad Sci U S A*, Vol.88, No.24, pp. 11555-11558, ISSN 0027-8424

Harhaj, N.S., Felinski, E.A., Wolpert, E.B., Sundstrom, J.M., Gardner, T.W. & Antonetti, D.A. (2006). VEGF activation of protein kinase C stimulates occludin phosphorylation and contributes to endothelial permeability. *Invest Ophthalmol Vis Sci*, Vol.47, No.11, pp. 5106-5115, ISSN 0146-0404

Hatcher, H.C., Ma, J.X., Chao, J., Chao, L. & Ottlecz, A. (1997). Kallikrein-binding protein levels are reduced in the retinas of streptozotocin-induced diabetic rats. *Invest Ophthalmol Vis Sci*, Vol.38, No.3, pp. 658-664, ISSN 0146-0404

Hogeboom van Buggenum, I.M., Polak, B.C., Reichert-Thoen, J.W., de Vries-Knoppert, W.A., van Hinsbergh, V.W. & Tangelder, G.J. (2002). Angiotensin converting enzyme inhibiting therapy is associated with lower vitreous vascular endothelial growth factor concentrations in patients with proliferative diabetic retinopathy. *Diabetologia*, Vol.45, No.2, pp. 203-209, ISSN 0012-186X

Hori, S., Ohtsuki, S., Hosoya, K., Nakashima, E. & Terasaki, T. (2004). A pericyte-derived angiopoietin-1 multimeric complex induces occludin gene expression in brain capillary endothelial cells through Tie-2 activation in vitro. *J Neurochem*, Vol.89, No.2, pp. 503-513, ISSN 0022-3042

Huang, H., Gandhi, J.K., Zhong, X., Wei, Y., Gong, J., Duh, E.J. & Vinores, S.A. (2011). TNFalpha is required for late BRB breakdown in diabetic retinopathy, and its inhibition prevents leukostasis and protects vessels and neurons from apoptosis. *Invest Ophthalmol Vis Sci*, Vol.52, No.3, pp. 1336-1344, ISSN 1552-5783

Huang, Q. & Yuan, Y. (1997). Interaction of PKC and NOS in signal transduction of microvascular hyperpermeability. *Am J Physiol*, Vol.273, No.5 Pt 2, pp. H2442-2451, ISSN 0002-9513

Iandiev, I., Pannicke, T., Reichenbach, A., Wiedemann, P. & Bringmann, A. (2007). Diabetes alters the localization of glial aquaporins in rat retina. *Neurosci Lett*, Vol.421, No.2, pp. 132-136, ISSN 0304-3940

Ishida, S., Usui, T., Yamashiro, K., Kaji, Y., Ahmed, E., Carrasquillo, K.G., Amano, S., Hida, T., Oguchi, Y. & Adamis, A.P. (2003). VEGF164 is proinflammatory in the diabetic retina. *Invest Ophthalmol Vis Sci*, Vol.44, No.5, pp. 2155-2162, ISSN 0146-0404

Ishii, H., Jirousek, M.R., Koya, D., Takagi, C., Xia, P., Clermont, A., Bursell, S.E., Kern, T.S., Ballas, L.M., Heath, W.F., Stramm, L.E., Feener, E.P. & King, G.L. (1996). Amelioration of vascular dysfunctions in diabetic rats by an oral PKC beta inhibitor. *Science*, Vol.272, No.5262, pp. 728-731, ISSN 0036-8075

Jiang, B.H., Rue, E., Wang, G.L., Roe, R. & Semenza, G.L. (1996). Dimerization, DNA binding, and transactivation properties of hypoxia-inducible factor 1. *J Biol Chem*, Vol.271, No.30, pp. 17771-17778, ISSN 0021-9258

Joussen, A.M., Poulaki, V., Le, M.L., Koizumi, K., Esser, C., Janicki, H., Schraermeyer, U., Kociok, N., Fauser, S., Kirchhof, B., Kern, T.S. & Adamis, A.P. (2004). A central role for inflammation in the pathogenesis of diabetic retinopathy. *FASEB J*, Vol.18, No.12, pp. 1450-1452, ISSN 1530-6860

Joussen, A.M, Poulaki, V., Mitsiades, N., Kirchhof, B., Koizumi, K., Dohmen, S. & Adamis, A.P. (2002). Nonsteroidal anti-inflammatory drugs prevent early diabetic retinopathy via TNF-alpha suppression. *FASEB J*, Vol.16, No.3, pp. 438-440, ISSN 1530-6860

Kaji, Y., Usui, T., Ishida, S., Yamashiro, K., Moore, T.C., Moore, J., Yamamoto, Y., Yamamoto, H. & Adamis, A.P. (2007). Inhibition of diabetic leukostasis and blood-retinal barrier breakdown with a soluble form of a receptor for advanced glycation end products. *Invest Ophthalmol Vis Sci*, Vol.48, No.2, pp. 858-865, ISSN 0146-0404

Keech, A.C., Mitchell, P., Summanen, P.A., O'Day, J., Davis, T.M., Moffitt, M.S., Taskinen, M.R., Simes, R.J., Tse, D., Williamson, E., Merrifield, A., Laatikainen, L.T., d'Emden, M.C., Crimet, D.C., O'Connell, R.L. & Colman, P.G. (2007). Effect of fenofibrate on the need for laser treatment for diabetic retinopathy (FIELD study): a randomised controlled trial. *Lancet*, Vol.370, No. 9600, pp. 1687-1697, ISSN 1474-547X

Kempen, J.H., O'Colmain, B.J., Leske, M.C., Haffner, S.M., Klein, R., Moss, S.E., Taylor, H.R. & Hamman, R.F. (2004). The prevalence of diabetic retinopathy among adults in the United States. *Arch Ophthalmol*, Vol.122, No.4, pp. 552-563, ISSN 0003-9950

Kern, T.S. & Engerman, R.L. (2001). Pharmacological inhibition of diabetic retinopathy: aminoguanidine and aspirin. *Diabetes*, Vol.50, No.7, pp. 1636-1642, ISSN 0012-1797

Kevil, C.G., Payne, D.K., Mire, E. & Alexander, J.S. (1998). Vascular permeability factor/vascular endothelial cell growth factor-mediated permeability occurs through disorganization of endothelial junctional proteins. *J Biol Chem*, Vol.273, No. 24, pp. 15099-15103, ISSN 0021-9258

Kim, I., Moon, S.O., Kim, S.H., Kim, H.J., Koh, Y.S. & Koh, G.Y. (2001). Vascular endothelial growth factor expression of intercellular adhesion molecule 1 (ICAM-1), vascular cell adhesion molecule 1 (VCAM-1), and E-selectin through nuclear factor-kappa B activation in endothelial cells. *J Biol Chem*, Vol.276, No.10, pp. 7614-7620, ISSN 0021-9258

Kim, J.H., Jun, H.O., Yu, Y.S. & Kim, K.W. (2010a). Inhibition of protein kinase C delta attenuates blood-retinal barrier breakdown in diabetic retinopathy. *Am J Pathol*, Vol.176, No.3, pp. 1517-1524, ISSN 1525-2191

Kim, J.H., Yu, Y.S., Cho, C.S. & Kim, K.W. (2009). Blockade of angiotensin II attenuates VEGF-mediated blood-retinal barrier breakdown in diabetic retinopathy. *J Cereb Blood Flow Metab*, Vol.29, No.3, pp. 621-628, ISSN 1559-7016

Kim, J.H., Yu, Y.S. & Kim, K.W. (2010b). Impaired retinal vascular development in anencephalic human fetus. *Histochem Cell Biol*, Vol.134, No.3, pp. 277-284, ISSN 1432-119X

Kim, S.Y., Johnson, M.A., McLeod, D.S., Alexander, T., Hansen, B.C. & Lutty, G.A. (2005). Neutrophils are associated with capillary closure in spontaneously diabetic monkey retinas. *Diabetes*, Vol.54, No.5, pp. 1534-1542, ISSN 0012-1797

Klein, R., Klein, B.E., Moss, S.E., Davis, M.D. & DeMets, D.L. (1984a). The Wisconsin epidemiologic study of diabetic retinopathy. II. Prevalence and risk of diabetic retinopathy when age at diagnosis is less than 30 years. *Arch Ophthalmol*, Vol.102, No.4, pp. 520-526, ISSN 0003-9950

Klein, R., Klein, B.E., Moss, S.E., Davis, M.D. & DeMets, D.L. (1984b). The Wisconsin epidemiologic study of diabetic retinopathy. III. Prevalence and risk of diabetic retinopathy when age at diagnosis is 30 or more years. *Arch Ophthalmol*, Vol.102, No.4, pp. 527-532, ISSN 0003-9950

Kowluru, R.A. & Odenbach, S. (2004). Role of interleukin-1beta in the development of retinopathy in rats: effect of antioxidants. *Invest Ophthalmol Vis Sci*, Vol.45, No.11, pp. 4161-4166, ISSN 0146-0404

Leal, E.C., Manivannan, A., Hosoya, K., Terasaki, T., Cunha-Vaz, J., Ambrosio, A.F. & Forrester, J.V. (2007). Inducible nitric oxide synthase isoform is a key mediator of leukostasis and blood-retinal barrier breakdown in diabetic retinopathy. *Invest Ophthalmol Vis Sci*, Vol.48, No.11, pp. 5257-5265, ISSN 0146-0404

Lee, S.W., Kim, W.J., Choi, Y.K., Song, H.S., Son, M.J., Gelman, I.H., Kim, Y.J. & Kim, K.W. (2003). SSeCKS regulates angiogenesis and tight junction formation in blood-brain barrier. *Nat Med*, Vol.9, No.7, pp. 900-906, ISSN 1078-8956

Leveen, P., Pekny, M., Gebre-Medhin, S., Swolin, B., Larsson, E. & Betsholtz, C. (1994). Mice deficient for PDGF B show renal, cardiovascular, and hematological abnormalities. *Genes Dev*, Vol.8, No.16, pp. 1875-1887, ISSN 0890-9369

Lin, W.L. (1988). Leakage of blood-retinal barrier due to damaging effect of protamine sulfate on the endothelium. *Acta Neuropathol*, Vol.76, No.4, pp. 427-431, ISSN 0001-6322

Lutty, G.A, Cao, J. & McLeod, D.S. (1997). Relationship of polymorphonuclear leukocytes to capillary dropout in the human diabetic choroid. *Am J Pathol*, Vol.151, No.3, pp. 707-714, ISSN 0002-9440

Marx, N., Walcher, D., Ivanova, N., Rautzenberg, K., Jung, A., Friedl, R., Hombach, V., de Caterina, R., Basta, G., Wautier, M.P. & Wautiers, J.L. (2004). Thiazolidinediones reduce endothelial expression of receptors for advanced glycation end products. *Diabetes*, Vol.53, No.10, pp. 2662-2668, ISSN 0012-1797

McLeod, D.S., Lefer, D.J., Merges, C. & Lutty, G.A. (1995). Enhanced expression of intracellular adhesion molecule-1 and P-selectin in the diabetic human retina and choroid. *Am J Pathol*, Vol.147, No.3, pp. 642-653, ISSN 0002-9440

Mizutani, M., Kern, T.S. & Lorenzi, M. (1996). Accelerated death of retinal microvascular cells in human and experimental diabetic retinopathy. *J Clin Invest*, Vol.97, No.12, pp. 2883-2890, ISSN 0021-9738

Mohr, S., Xi, X., Tang, J. & Kern, T.S. (2002). Caspase activation in retinas of diabetic and galactosemic mice and diabetic patients. *Diabetes*, Vol.51, No.4, pp. 1172-1179, ISSN 0012-1797

Murata, T., Ishibashi, T., Khalil, A., Hata, Y., Yoshikawa, H. & Inomata, H. (1995). Vascular endothelial growth factor plays a role in hyperpermeability of diabetic retinal vessels. *Ophthalmic Res*, Vol.27, No.1, pp. 48-52, ISSN 0030-3747

Mysiorek, C., Culot, M., Dehouck, L., Derudas, B., Staels, B., Bordet, R., Cecchelli, R., Fenart, L. & Berezowski, V. (2009). Peroxisome-proliferator-activated receptor-alpha activation protects brain capillary endothelial cells from oxygen-glucose deprivation-induced hyperpermeability in the blood-brain barrier. *Curr Neurovasc Res*, Vol.6, No.3, pp. 181-193, ISSN 1875-5739

Nagelhus, E.A., Veruki, M.L., Torp, R., Haug, F.M., Laake, J.H., Nielsen, S., Agre, P. & Ottersen, O.P. (1998). Aquaporin-4 water channel protein in the rat retina and optic nerve: polarized expression in Muller cells and fibrous astrocytes. *J Neurosci*, Vol.18, No.7, pp. 2506-2519, ISSN 0270-6474

Nakamura, K., Yamagishi, S., Nakamura, Y., Takenaka, K., Matsui, T., Jinnouchi, Y. & Imaizumi, T. (2005). Telmisartan inhibits expression of a receptor for advanced glycation end products (RAGE) in angiotensin-II-exposed endothelial cells and decreases serum levels of soluble RAGE in patients with essential hypertension. *Microvasc Res,* Vol.70, No.3, pp. 137-141, ISSN 0026-2862

Navarro, P., Ruco, L. & Dejana, E. (1998). Differential localization of VE- and N-cadherins in human endothelial cells: VE-cadherin competes with N-cadherin for junctional localization. *J Cell Biol,* Vol.140, No.6, pp. 1475-1484, ISSN 0021-9525

Newton, A.C. (1997). Regulation of protein kinase C. *Curr Opin Cell Biol,* Vol.9, No.2, pp. 161-167, ISSN 0955-0674

Nowak, M., Wielkoszynski, T., Marek, B., Kos-Kudla, B., Swietochowska, E., Sieminska, L., Kajdaniuk, D., Glogowska-Szelag, J. & Nowak, K. (2008). Blood serum levels of vascular cell adhesion molecule (sVCAM-1), intercellular adhesion molecule (sICAM-1) and endothelial leucocyte adhesion molecule-1 (ELAM-1) in diabetic retinopathy. *Clin Exp Med,* Vol.8, No.3, pp. 159-164, ISSN 1591-8890

Panigrahy, D., Kaipainen, A., Huang, S., Butterfield, C.E., Barnes, C.M., Fannon, M., Laforme, A.M., Chaponis, D.M., Folkman, J. & Kieran, M.W. (2008). PPARalpha agonist fenofibrate suppresses tumor growth through direct and indirect angiogenesis inhibition. *Proc Natl Acad Sci U S A,* Vol.105, No.3, pp. 985-990, ISSN 1091-6490

Pardridge, W.M. (1999). Blood-brain barrier biology and methodology. *J Neurovirol,* Vol.5, No.6, pp. 556-569, ISSN 1355-0284

Persidsky, Y., Ramirez, S.H., Haorah, J. & Kanmogne, G.D. (2006). Blood-brain barrier: structural components and function under physiologic and pathologic conditions. *J Neuroimmune Pharmacol,* Vol.1, No.3, pp. 223-236, ISSN 1557-1904

Qaum, T., Xu, Q., Joussen, A.M., Clemens, M.W., Qin, W., Miyamoto, K., Hassessian, H., Wiegand, S.J., Rudge, J., Yancopoulos, G.D. & Adamis, A.P. (2001). VEGF-initiated blood-retinal barrier breakdown in early diabetes. *Invest Ophthalmol Vis Sci,* Vol.42, No.10, pp. 2408-2413, ISSN 0146-0404

Rosenson, R.S., Wolff, D.A., Huskin, A.L., Helenowski, I.B. & Rademaker, A.W. (2007). Fenofibrate therapy ameliorates fasting and postprandial lipoproteinemia, oxidative stress, and the inflammatory response in subjects with hypertriglyceridemia and the metabolic syndrome. *Diabetes Care,* Vol.30, No.8, pp. 1945-1951, ISSN 1935-5548

Rungger-Brandle, E., Dosso, A.A. & Leuenberger, P.M. (2000). Glial reactivity, an early feature of diabetic retinopathy. *Invest Ophthalmol Vis Sci,* Vol.41, No.7, pp. 1971-1980, ISSN 0146-0404

Russ, P.K., Davidson, M.K., Hoffman, L.H., Haselton, F.R. (1998). Partial characterization of the human retinal endothelial cell tight and adherens junction complexes. *Invest Ophthalmol Vis Sci,* Vol.39, No.12, pp. 2479-2485, ISSN 0146-0404

Schatz, H., Madeira, D., McDonald, H.R. & Johnson, R.N. (1991). Progressive enlargement of laser scars following grid laser photocoagulation for diffuse diabetic macular edema. *Arch Ophthalmol,* Vol.109, No.11, pp. 1549-1551, ISSN 0003-9950

Shepro, D. & Morel, N.M. (1993). Pericyte physiology. *FASEB J,* Vol. 7, No.11, pp. 1031-1038, ISSN 0892-6638

Shimizu, F., Sano, Y., Haruki, H. & Kanda, T. (2011). Advanced glycation end-products induce basement membrane hypertrophy in endoneurial microvessels and disrupt the blood-nerve barrier by stimulating the release of TGF-beta and vascular endothelial growth factor (VEGF) by pericytes. *Diabetologia,* Vol.54, No.6, pp. 1517-1526, ISSN 1432-0428

Sjolie, A.K., Klein, R., Porta, M., Orchard, T., Fuller, J., Parving, H.H., Bilous, R. & Chaturvedi, N. (2008). Effect of candesartan on progression and regression of retinopathy in type

2 diabetes (DIRECT-Protect 2): a randomised placebo-controlled trial. *Lancet*, Vol.372, No.9647, pp. 1385-1393, ISSN 1474-547X

Soheilian, M., Ramezani, A., Obudi, A., Bijanzadeh, B., Salehipour, M., Yaseri, M., Ahmadieh, H., Dehghan, M.H., Azarmina, M., Moradian, S. & Peyman, G.A. (2009). Randomized trial of intravitreal bevacizumab alone or combined with triamcinolone versus macular photocoagulation in diabetic macular edema. *Ophthalmology*, Vol.116, No.6, pp. 1142-1150, ISSN 1549-4713

Sorbinil Retinopathy Trial Research Group. (1990). A randomized trial of sorbinil, an aldose reductase inhibitor, in diabetic retinopathy. *Arch Ophthalmol*, Vol.108, No.9, pp. 1234-1244, ISSN 0003-9950

Soriano, P. (1994). Abnormal kidney development and hematological disorders in PDGF beta-receptor mutant mice. *Genes Dev*, Vol.8, No.16, pp. 1888-1896, ISSN 0890-9369

Stitt, A.W., Bhaduri, T., McMullen, C.B., Gardiner, T.A. & Archer, D.B. (2000). Advanced glycation end products induce blood-retinal barrier dysfunction in normoglycemic rats. *Mol Cell Biol Res Commun*, Vol.3, No.6, pp. 380-388, ISSN 1522-4724

Stitt, A.W., Li, Y.M., Gardiner, T.A., Bucala, R., Archer, D.B. & Vlassara, H. (1997). Advanced glycation end products (AGEs) co-localize with AGE receptors in the retinal vasculature of diabetic and of AGE-infused rats. *Am J Pathol*, Vol.150, No.2, pp. 523-531, ISSN 0002-9440

Striph, G.G., Hart, W.M., Jr. & Olk, R.J. (1988). Modified grid laser photocoagulation for diabetic macular edema. The effect on the central visual field. *Ophthalmology*, Vol.95, No.12, pp. 1673-1679, ISSN 0161-6420

Tamura, H., Miyamoto, K., Kiryu, J., Miyahara, S., Katsuta, H., Hirose, F., Musashi, K. & Yoshimura, N. (2005). Intravitreal injection of corticosteroid attenuates leukostasis and vascular leakage in experimental diabetic retina. *Invest Ophthalmol Vis Sci*, Vol.46, No.4, pp. 1440-1444, ISSN 0146-0404

Thanabalasundaram, G., Pieper, C., Lischper, M. & Galla, H.J. (2010). Regulation of the blood-brain barrier integrity by pericytes via matrix metalloproteinases mediated activation of vascular endothelial growth factor in vitro. *Brain Res*, Vol.1347, pp. 1-10, ISSN 1872-6240

The Diabetic Retinopathy Study Research Group. (1987). Indications for photocoagulation treatment of diabetic retinopathy: Diabetic Retinopathy Study Report no. 14. *Int Ophthalmol Clin*, Vol.27, No.4, pp. 239-253, ISSN 0020-8167

The Protein Kinase C beta Inhibitor Diabetic Macular Edema Study Group. (2007). Effect of ruboxistaurin in patients with diabetic macular edema: thirty-month results of the randomized PKC-DMES clinical trial. *Arch Ophthalmol*, Vol.125, No.3, pp. 318-324, ISSN 0003-9950

The Protein Kinase C beta Inhibitor Diabetic Retinopathy Study Group. (2005). The effect of ruboxistaurin on visual loss in patients with moderately severe to very severe nonproliferative diabetic retinopathy: initial results of the Protein Kinase C beta Inhibitor Diabetic Retinopathy Study (PKC-DRS) multicenter randomized clinical trial. *Diabetes*, Vol.54, No.7, pp. 2188-2197, ISSN 0012-1797

van Hecke, M.V., Dekker, J.M., Nijpels, G., Moll, A.C., Heine, R.J., Bouter, L.M., Polak, B.C. & Stehouwer, C.D. (2005). Inflammation and endothelial dysfunction are associated with retinopathy: the Hoorn Study. *Diabetologia*, Vol.48, No.7, pp. 1300-1306, ISSN 0012-186X

Vincent, J.A. & Mohr, S. (2007). Inhibition of caspase-1/interleukin-1beta signaling prevents degeneration of retinal capillaries in diabetes and galactosemia. *Diabetes*, Vol.56, No.1, pp. 224-230, ISSN 0012-1797

Vinores, S.A., Van Niel, E., Swerdloff, J.L. & Campochiaro, P.A. (1993). Electron microscopic immunocytochemical demonstration of blood-retinal barrier breakdown in human diabetics and its association with aldose reductase in retinal vascular endothelium and retinal pigment epithelium. *Histochem J*, Vol.25, No.9, pp. 648-663, ISSN 0018-2214

Vlassara, H., Fuh, H., Makita, Z., Krungkrai, S., Cerami, A. & Bucala, R. (1992). Exogenous advanced glycosylation end products induce complex vascular dysfunction in normal animals: a model for diabetic and aging complications. *Proc Natl Acad Sci U S A*, Vol.89, No.24, pp. 12043-12047, ISSN 0027-8424

Wagner, J., Jan Danser, A.H., Derkx, F.H., de Jong, T.V., Paul, M., Mullins, J.J., Schalekamp, M.A. & Ganten, D. (1996). Demonstration of renin mRNA, angiotensinogen mRNA, and angiotensin converting enzyme mRNA expression in the human eye: evidence for an intraocular renin-angiotensin system. *Br J Ophthalmol*, Vol.80, No.2, pp. 159-163, ISSN 0007-1161

Wallow, I.H. & Geldner, P.S. (1980). Endothelial fenestrae in proliferative diabetic retinopathy. *Invest Ophthalmol Vis Sci*, Vol.19, No.10, pp. 1176-1183, ISSN 0146-0404

Wang, K., Wang, Y., Gao, L., Li, X., Li, M. & Guo, J. (2008). Dexamethasone inhibits leukocyte accumulation and vascular permeability in retina of streptozotocin-induced diabetic rats via reducing vascular endothelial growth factor and intercellular adhesion molecule-1 expression. *Biol Pharm Bull*, Vol.31, No.8, pp. 1541-1546, ISSN 0918-6158

Wang, W., Dentler, W.L. & Borchardt, R.T. (2001). VEGF increases BMEC monolayer permeability by affecting occludin expression and tight junction assembly. *Am J Physiol Heart Circ Physiol*, Vol.280, No.1, pp. H434-440, ISSN 0363-6135

Weidemann, A., Krohne, T.U., Aguilar, E., Kurihara, T., Takeda, N., Dorrell, M.I., Simon, M.C., Haase, V.H., Friedlander, M. & Johnson, R.S. (2010). Astrocyte hypoxic response is essential for pathological but not developmental angiogenesis of the retina. *Glia*, Vol.58, No.10, pp. 1177-1185, ISSN 1098-1136

Williams, B., Baker, A.Q., Gallacher, B. & Lodwick, D. (1995). Angiotensin II increases vascular permeability factor gene expression by human vascular smooth muscle cells. *Hypertension*, Vol.25, No.5, pp. 913-917, ISSN 0194-911X

Williams, J.M., Sr., de Juan, E., Jr. & Machemer, R. (1988). Ultrastructural characteristics of new vessels in proliferative diabetic retinopathy. *Am J Ophthalmol*, Vol.105, No.5, pp. 491-499, ISSN 0002-9394

Wistrand, P.J., Schenholm, M. & Lonnerholm, G. (1986). Carbonic anhydrase isoenzymes CA I and CA II in the human eye. *Invest Ophthalmol Vis Sci*, Vol.27, No.3, pp. 419-428, ISSN 0146-0404

Wolburg-Buchholz, K., Mack, A.F., Steiner, E., Pfeiffer, F., Engelhardt, B. & Wolburg, H. (2009). Loss of astrocyte polarity marks blood-brain barrier impairment during experimental autoimmune encephalomyelitis. *Acta Neuropathol*, Vol.118, No.2, pp. 219-233, ISSN 1432-0533

Wolburg, H., Noell, S., Wolburg-Buchholz, K., Mack, A. & Fallier-Becker, P. (2009). Agrin, aquaporin-4, and astrocyte polarity as an important feature of the blood-brain barrier. *Neuroscientist*, Vol.15, No.2, pp. 180-193, ISSN 1073-8584

Xia, P., Aiello, L.P., Ishii, H., Jiang, Z.Y., Park, D.J., Robinson, G.S., Takagi, H., Newsome, W.P., Jirousek, M.R. & King, G.L. (1996). Characterization of vascular endothelial growth factor's effect on the activation of protein kinase C, its isoforms, and endothelial cell growth. *J Clin Invest*, Vol.98, No.9, pp. 2018-2026, ISSN 0021-9738

Xia, P., Inoguchi, T., Kern, T.S., Engerman, R.L., Oates, P.J. & King, G.L. (1994). Characterization of the mechanism for the chronic activation of diacylglycerol-protein kinase C pathway in diabetes and hypergalactosemia. *Diabetes*, Vol.43, No.9, pp. 1122-1129, ISSN 0012-1797

Yamagishi, S., Amano, S., Inagaki, Y., Okamoto, T., Koga, K., Sasaki, N., Yamamoto, H., Takeuchi, M. & Makita, Z. (2002a). Advanced glycation end products-induced apoptosis and overexpression of vascular endothelial growth factor in bovine retinal pericytes. *Biochem Biophys Res Commun*, Vol.290, No.3, pp. 973-978, ISSN 0006-291X

Yamagishi, S., Amano, S., Inagaki, Y., Okamoto, T., Takeuchi, M. & Makita, Z. (2002b). Beraprost sodium, a prostaglandin I2 analogue, protects against advanced gycation end products-induced injury in cultured retinal pericytes. *Mol Med*, Vol.8, No.9, pp. 546-550, ISSN 1076-1551

Yamagishi, S., Hsu, C.C., Taniguchi, M., Harada, S., Yamamoto, Y., Ohsawa, K., Kobayashi, K. & Yamamoto, H. (1995). Receptor-mediated toxicity to pericytes of advanced glycosylation end products: a possible mechanism of pericyte loss in diabetic microangiopathy. *Biochem Biophys Res Commun*, Vol.213, No.2, pp. 681-687, ISSN 0006-291X

Yamagishi, S. & Takeuchi, M. (2004). Nifedipine inhibits gene expression of receptor for advanced glycation end products (RAGE) in endothelial cells by suppressing reactive oxygen species generation. *Drugs Exp Clin Res*, Vol.30, No.4, pp.169-175, ISSN 0378-6501

Yan, S.F., Ramasamy, R., Naka, Y. & Schmidt, A.M. (2003). Glycation, inflammation, and RAGE: a scaffold for the macrovascular complications of diabetes and beyond. *Circ Res*, Vol.93, No.12, pp. 1159-1169, ISSN 1524-4571

Yancopoulos, G.D., Davis, S., Gale, N.W., Rudge, J.S., Wiegand, S.J. & Holash, J. (2000). Vascular-specific growth factors and blood vessel formation. *Nature*, Vol.407, No.6801, pp. 242-248, ISSN 0028-0836

Zhang, X., Bao, S., Lai, D., Rapkins, R.W., Gillies, M.C. (2008). Intravitreal triamcinolone acetonide inhibits breakdown of the blood-retinal barrier through differential regulation of VEGF-A and its receptors in early diabetic rat retinas. *Diabetes*, Vol.57, No.4, pp. 1026-1033, ISSN 1939-327X

Zhang, Y. & Stone, J. (1997). Role of astrocytes in the control of developing retinal vessels. *Invest Ophthalmol Vis Sci*, Vol.38, No.9, pp. 1653-1666, ISSN 0146-0404

6

Fibrovascular Membranes Associated with PDR: Development of Molecular Targets by Global Gene Expression Profiling

Shigeo Yoshida, Keijiro Ishikawa, Mitsuru Arima,
Ryo Asato, Yukio Sassa and Tatsuro Ishibashi
Department of Ophthalmology, Kyushu University Graduate School of Medical Sciences, Fukuoka, Japan

1. Introduction

Diabetic retinopathy (DR) is one of the leading causes of decreased vision and blindness in industrialized countries (Bhavsar, 2002). Much of the retinal damage that characterizes advanced proliferative diabetic retinopathy (PDR) results from retinal neovascularization (Simo, et al., 2006). When the newly formed vessels are associated with fibrous proliferations that form fibrovascular membranes (FVMs) on the surface of the neuroretina, traction retinal detachments can develop, resulting in potentially severe loss of vision (Hiscott, et al., 2000).

FVMs are characterized by the migration and proliferation of various types of cells, e.g., retinal glial cells, fibroblasts, macrophages/monocytes, hyalocytes, laminocytes, and vascular endothelial cells. It has been postulated that the formation of FVMs represents a wound healing process (Hiscott, et al., 2000). To date, the factors regulating the development and progression of FVMs have not been fully determined. Moreover, despite improvements in vitreal surgical techniques, panretinal photocoagulavtion, and the use of intravitreal anti-VEGF drugs such as Ranibizumab, the prognosis for DR is still poor especially in advanced cases of PDR. It is therefore required to develop better treatments that are based on the pathogenesis of FVMs.

2. Conventional studies investigating the mechanisms of FVM formation

Earlier conventional studies investigating the molecular effects of FVM formation have focused mainly on one or a few molecules or pathways. Several molecules, e.g., vascular endothelial growth factor (VEGF), tumor necrosis factor-α (TNF- α), basic fibroblast growth factor (bFGF), intereleukin-8 (IL-8), apelin, tumor endothelial marker 7 (TEM7), monocyte chemoattractant protein-1 (MCP-1;CCL2), erythropoietin, angiopoietin-2, advanced glycation end product, nuclear factor kappa-B, and activator protein-1 have been detected in FVMs and/or vitreous fluid collected from patients with PDR (Simo, et al., 2006; Yoshida, et al., 1998; Yoshida, et al., 1999; Yoshida, et al., 2010; Watanabe, et al., 2005).

Retinal hypoxia is assumed to be the common mechanism which initiates a series of events leading to retinal neovascularization (Ishikawa, et al., 2010). Cellular inflammation is initiated at the blood-microvascular endothelial-cell interface, and leukocytic infiltration has been observed after retinal hypoxia. Several mediators of retinal neovascularization have been determined in well-established murine models of oxygen-induced retinopathy (OIR) (Smith, et al., 1994).

Chemokines, a family of structurally related cytokines involved in the activation and directed migration of leukocytes, may be pathophysiologically key mediators of inflammation (Singh, et al.). Two well-studied CC chemokines are MCP-1 and macrophage inflammatory protein-1α (MIP-1α;CCL3). Both MCP-1 and MIP-1α have been shown to mediate the recruitment of leukocytes and induction of neovascularization in several inflammatory diseases.

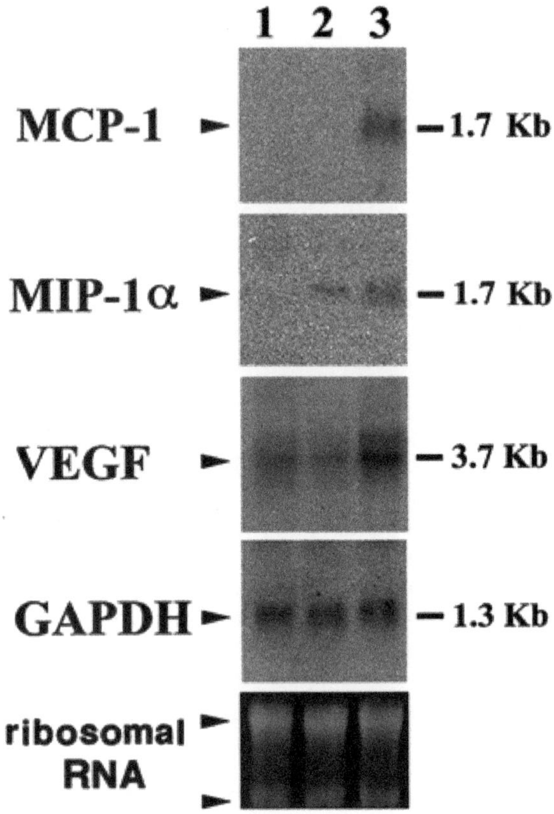

Fig. 1. Northern blot determination of mRNA expression of MCP-1, MIP-1α, and VEGF in murine OIR. Representative blots of three independent experiments are shown. Lane 1, Control retina (P12); lane 2, retina after 5 days exposure to hyperoxia (P12); lane 3, retina 12 h after hypoxia (P12.5). For control, the same blot was stripped and reprobed with GAPDH, and 18 S and 28 S ribosomal RNA were used for equal loading of RNA. Each lane contains 10 μg total RNA. Reproduced with permission from Yoshida et al. [17]

In order to determine the role played by MCP-1 and MIP-1α, we have investigated whether these chemokines can be induced in murine OIR (Singh, et al.). The expression of the mRNAs of MCP-1 and MIP-1α was very low or undetectable in the retinas of the normal controls and in P12 mice killed just 5 days after hyperoxia (Fig. 1). A dramatic increase in MCP-1 mRNA expression was observed 12 h after the onset of hypoxia. The profile of MIP-1α mRNA expression was similar to that of MCP-1 mRNA, except that a slight increase of MIP-1α mRNA was detected in the retinas of mice 5 days (P12) after hyperoxia.

In contrast to MCP-1 and MIP-1α, a steady level of VEGF mRNA expression was found in the retinas of control, normal mice (Fig. 1). Hyperoxia resulted in a significant down-regulation in the level of VEGF mRNA, and the subsequent hypoxia led to a significant up-regulation of VEGF expression compared with that in the control retinas.

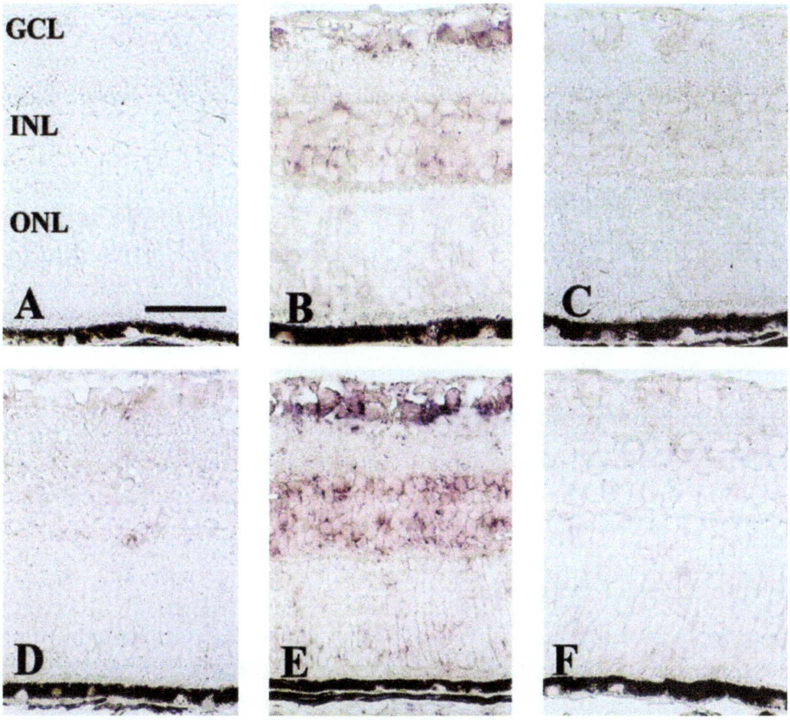

Fig. 2. In situ hybridization for MCP-1 and MIP-1α in the retinas of murine OIR. Hybridization was performed with antisense (A, B, D, E) or sense (C, F) probes specific for MCP-1 (A–C) and MIP-1α (D–F). A, D, Control normal retina (P12); B, C, E, and F, retina 12 h after hypoxia (P12.5). GCL, Ganglion cell layer; INL, inner-nuclear layer; ONL, outer-nuclear layer. Original bar = 50 μm. Reproduced with permission from Yoshida et al. [17]

In retinal hypoxia, the inner retina, which is supplied by retinal vessels, is hypoxic, whereas the outer retina, supplied by the choroidal vessels, is not. In situ hybridization for MCP-1 and MIP-1α showed a prominent increase of positive cells located in the inner retina 12 h after the hypxia (P12.5) in comparison to the lower level of staining in the nonhypoxic retinas of control mice (Fig. 2). The inner retinal layer where ganglion cells and astrocytes are located was the most prominent cellular site of MCP-1 and MIP-1α gene expression in the hypoxic inner retina. This suggests that MCP-1 and MIP-1α expressed in this region attract resident microglia, hyalocytes, and/or bone marrow-derived monocyte lineage cells (BM-MLCs) through the blood-retinal barrier toward the superficial layer of the retina where neovascularization occurs.

Among the environmental stimuli, gene expression by macrophages/BM-MLCs following hypoxia is becoming increasingly well-characterized to have angiogenic potential(Lewis, et al., 2007). In murine OIR, macrophages/BM-MLCs in the ischemic retina exhibited thicker and more distended processes compared with those in normal, control retinas (Ishikawa, et al., 2011). We assume that such "hypoxia-activated" BM-MLCs have the potential to produce an array of angiogenic cytokines and growth factors including TNF-α and VEGF, which can contribute to the progression of retinal neovascularization/revascularization. TNF-α is an angiogenic molecule produced by hypoxic monocytes/macrophages (Yun, et al., 1997) and is a likely mediator of retinal neovascularization/revascularization. It has been reported that TNF-α level is higher in patients with PDR(Limb, et al., 2001), and we have detected this molecule in the macrophages/BM-MLCs in murine OIR (Yoshida, et al., 2004). Moreover, we have demonstrated that TNF-α up-reguletes the production of IL-8, VEGF, bFGF, or MCP-1 in retinal vascular cells and/or glial cells adjacent to microvessels triggering neovascularization/revascularization in an autocrine or paracrine manner (Yoshida, et al., 2004; Yoshida, et al., 1997). These processes are likely to be important in promoting macrophages/ BM-MLCs-related retinal neovascularization/revascularization in hypoxic retinas.

3. Global gene expression profiling of FVMs

Despite earlier studies investigating the molecular effects of retinal hypoxia, the molecular events taking place in hypoxic retinas that may lead to retinal neovascularization remain undetermined. The recent technological advancements in genomics, such as advent of microarray technology, have opened up new avenues to identify all the genes and their products that are expressed in a particular tissue.

To determine the factors that are activated during retinal hypoxia, we performed a gene expression profiling of hypoxic retinas obtained from a murine OIR using gene microarray thechnology(Ishikawa, et al., 2010). Our analyses showed that retinal hypoxia were associated with specific changes in the patterns of gene expression. These alterations may reflect the postischemic inflammation, and subsequent neural and vascular remodeling, and pathologic neovascularization in retinas of murine OIR (Fig. 3).

Several genes reported to be involved in retinal hypoxia, such as *Vegfa*(Yoshida, et al., 2003), *Hif1a*(Ozaki, et al., 1999), and *Mip1a*(*Ccl3*)(Yoshida, et al., 2003), were also detected to be differentially expressed in the hypoxic retina in our study, confirming that our microarray analyses were trustworthy. Interestingly, the most up-regulated gene among the differentially-expressed genes in hypoxic retinas was the *Mip1β(Ccl4)* and not *Vegfa* and other chemokines.

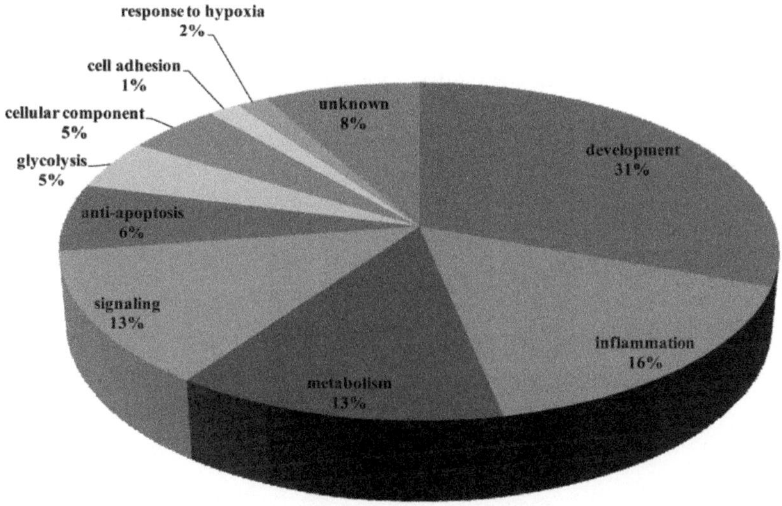

Fig. 3. Distribution of Gene Ontology terms in genes regulated by hypoxic retinas. Ontology of genes upregulated by hypoxia. Reproduced with permission from Ishikawa et al. [8]

MIP-1β (CCL4) is a member of the CC chemokine family that are characterized by their ability to direct migration of leukocytes into inflamed tissue. MIP-1β was first isolated from the culture medium of LPS-activated macrophages, and it recruited macrophages/microglia to sites of injury in patients with sepsis, arthritis, and systemic sclerosis. Because MIP-1β is not known to be a hypoxia-responsive gene in the retina, it may play more roles in hypoxic retinas than previously envisaged. Therefore, further studies are required to determine the role played by MIP-1β in hypoxia-induced retinal neovascularization/revascularization (Ishikawa, et al., 2011).

Expressed sequence tag (EST) analysis, another method of global gene expression profiling, permit the identification of genes expressed in particular tissues in a completely unambiguous manner (Wistow, 2006). ESTs may also reveal comprehensive data on transcript and gene variants. These represent important sources for the search for as yet incompletely characterised genes and pathways as exemplified by the NEIBank project in the eye research field (Wistow, 2006). We hypothesized that a comprehensive analysis of gene expression in FVMs may open up new avenues in enhancing our understanding of the formation of FVMs, and such an effort should lead to further advances in the surgical and medical treatment of FVMs (Yoshida, et al., 2010).

To overcome the limitation of the starting amount of RNA from the FVMs obtained from patients with PDR, We chose to employ Switching Mechanism at the 5′ end of RNA Transcript (SMART) technology, an exponential PCR-based technology. With this technology, we have successfully constructed a complementary DNA (cDNA) library from the FVMs and sequenced more than 2800 cDNAs (Yoshida, et al., 2010). We next performed sequence similarity searches to compare every EST to those in public databases. For ESTs with known gene matches in public databases, functional annotation was retrieved from the human cDNA database (Ensembl) and analysed by FatiGO.

Among the 625 non-redundant clusters, 515 (82%) matched Ensembl. The remaining 110 (17%) corresponded to potentially novel ESTs or untranslated sequences. Among those database-matched, 515 clusters were subdivided by functional subsets of genes related to ribosomal activity, oxidative phosphorylation, focal adhesion, cell adhesion, and other functions by FatiGO analysis (Fig. 4). This suggests that many subsets of functional genes are expressed in FVMs. Thus, there are many complex interactions among the molecules that are encoded by those genes. Among these, ferritin, light polypeptide (*FTL*) and metastasis associated lung adenocarcinoma transcript 1 (*MALAT1*) appeared to be the most abundant transcripts in the FVMs (Yoshida, et al., 2010).

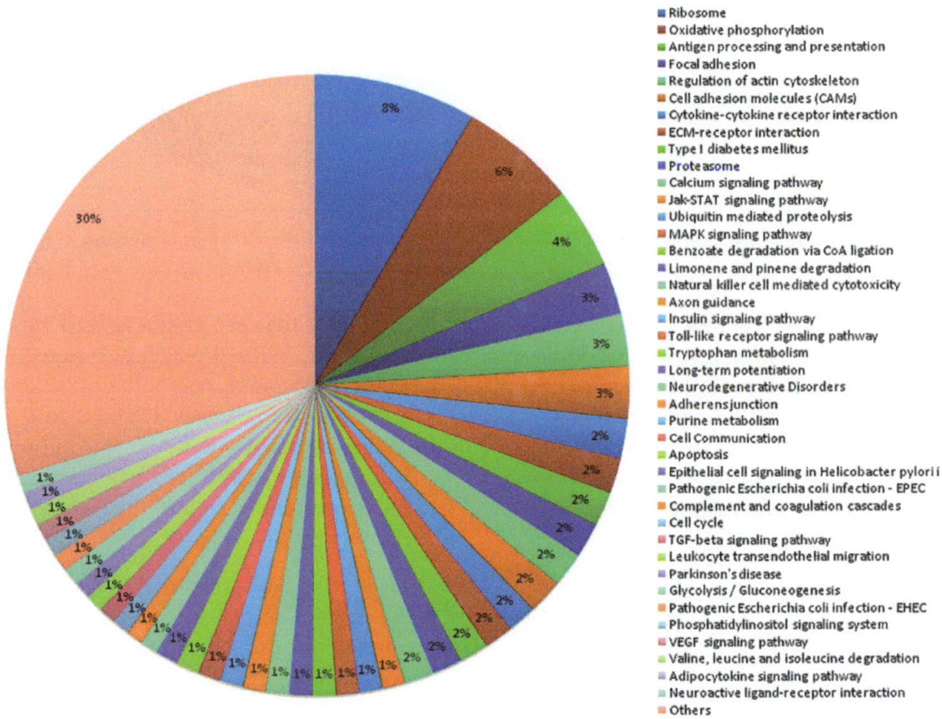

Fig. 4. The known human genes identified in the human fibrovascular membranes (FVMs) are grouped according to the Kyoto Encyclopedia of Genes and Genomes (KEGG) functional categories. Reproduced with permission from Yoshida et al. [20]

The importance of the production of extracellular matrix by FVMs is well recognized (Hiscott, et al., 1999). In agreement with this notion, functional annotation of ESTs determined that those genes related to cell adhesions and focal adhesions are highly expressed in FVMs. Until now, among the components in extracellular matrix, type II collagen, SPARC and FN, major components of the vitreous, are well-known molecules. However, our EST analysis demonstrated the expression of *COL1A2, COL3A1, MXRA8,* and others, in addition to *FN, SPARC* as cellular adhesion components. This indicates that cells that comprise the FVM actively produce a variety of adhesion molecules and are actively involved in cell migration and proliferation (Yoshida, et al., 2010).

4. Development of molecular targets by global gene expression profiling of FVMs

Recently, several trials of anti-VEGF therapy such as Ranibizmab have been applied on patients with intraocular neovascular diseases. However, undesirable side effects including brain and retinal vein occlusion have been reported (von Hanno, et al., 2010). Therefore, identifying the other molecular targets that can be treated less invasively is definitely still a goal. Because we were able to determine the existence of several potential factors other than VEGF by global gene expression profiling of FVMs (Yoshida, et al., 2010), we postulate that some of the extracted genes may be additional novel candidates for molecular targeting therapy. Among newly identified genes from FVMs, we found that tumor endothelial marker 7 (TEM7) and periostin were expressed more strongly in FVMs than in idiopatic epiretinal membranes (ERMs) (Yoshida, et al., 2011; Yamaji, et al., 2008). This led us to hypothesize that these two molecules play key roles in the maintenance and/or development of FVMs.

a. Tumor endothelial marker 7 (TEM7)

As described earlier, recent technological improvements in cellular fractionation and genomics have led to the identification of several markers preferentially expressed on vascular endothelial cells of human tumors (Nanda and St Croix, 2004). Among these markers, the tumor endothelial markers (TEMs) are a group of cell surface proteins preferentially expressed on the endothelial cells of various cancer cells.

Of these cell surface markers, TEM7, also known as plexin domain-containing 1 (PLXDC1), is especially attractive because it is the most abundant isoform among the TEMs. TEM7 protein is overexpressed in the neovascular vessels of human solid tumors such as lung, colon, and esophageal cancers (Nanda and St Croix, 2004). The full-length form of TEM7 has sequence characteristics of cell surface proteins, including signaling peptides, plexin-semaphorin-integrin (PSI) domain, and transmembrane domain(s). In addition, TEM7 is expressed as a complex pattern of transcripts derived by alternative splicing with potentially different activities and biological functions. These transcripts are predicted to be intracellular (TEM7-I), secreted (TEM7-S), or on the cell surface membrane (TEM7-M) of the endothelial cells of tumors.

We asked whether the mRNA of TEM7 is expressed in the neovascular endothelial cells of FVMs surgically removed from patients with PDR (Fig. 5) (Yamaji, et al., 2008). The mRNA of TEM7 was enhanced in 10 of 10 FVMs obtained from PDR patients but was barely detected in the five idiopathic ERMs (control). In addition, RT-PCR with specific primer pairs yielded multiple bands suggesting the presence of splice variants of TEM7 in the FVMs. The mRNAs of IL-8 were detected in 10 of 10 FVM specimens, VEGF in 8 of 10 FVM specimens, and VEGFR2 in 9 of 10 FVM specimens. In contrast to TEM7, these 3 angiogenic molecules were also upregulated in some of the control idiopathic ERMs (3 of 5, 3 of 5, and 2 of 5, respectively).

To determine the location of the protein of TEM7 in FVMs, we next double-stained the FVM sections with an anti-TEM7 monoclonal antibody (IM193), which specifically detects TEM7-M, and an antibody to CD34, an endothelial cell marker (Fig. 6). Consistent with previous results on the staining patterns of tumors with neovascularization (Nanda and St Croix, 2004), the antibody specifically labeled the neovascular endothelial cells in the FVMs (Fig. 6).

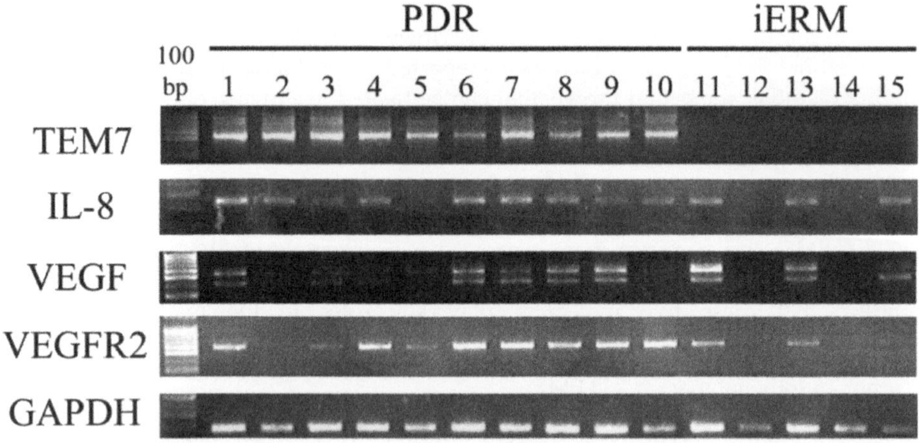

Fig. 5. RT-PCR analysis of TEM7, IL-8, VEGF, VEGFR2, and GAPDH in fibrovascular membranes derived from patients with proliferative diabetic retinopathy (PDR; patients 1–10) and in epiretinal membranes from eyes with idiopathic epiretinal membranes (iERMs; patients 11–15). After 35 cycles, 8 µL each sample was electrophoresed through a 2% Tris-acetate-EDTA agarose gel, and the fractionated products were stained with ethidium bromide. Note the distinct high expression of the mRNA of TEM7 in the fibrovascular membranes derived from patients with PDR compared with control iERMs. Reproduced with permission from Yamaji et al. [24]

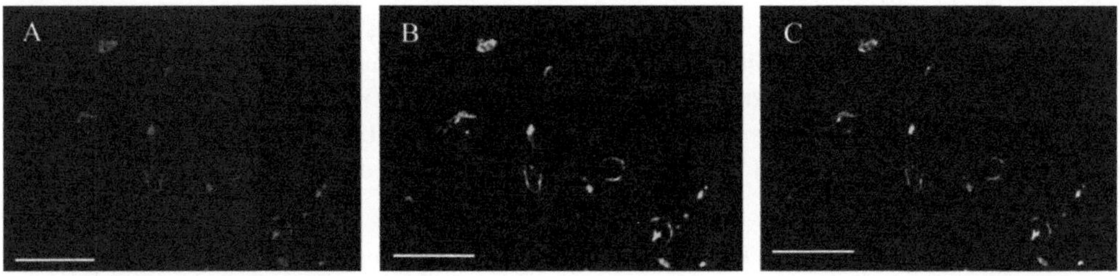

Fig. 6. Double staining for TEM7 and CD34 in the FVM. (A) Neovascular endothelial cells are visible after specific staining with CD34 in the FVM. (B) Specific staining for TEM7 in the same section shows an identical staining pattern. (C) Double staining for TEM7 and vascular endothelial cells in the same sample shows positive cells for both antibodies. The *yellow* staining is caused by the overlapping of the *red* and the *green* colors, showing colocalization of TEM7-M with the pan-endothelial marker CD34. Sale bars, 50 µm. Reproduced with permission from Yamaji et al. [24]

To determine a more exact location of the TEM7 protein within the neovascular endothelial cells, we performed immunoelectron microscopy using monoclonal anti-TEM7 antibody (IM193). Electron microscopy revealed that TEM7-M was expressed at the tight junctions and at the luminal surfaces of the vascular endothelial cells (Fig. 7)

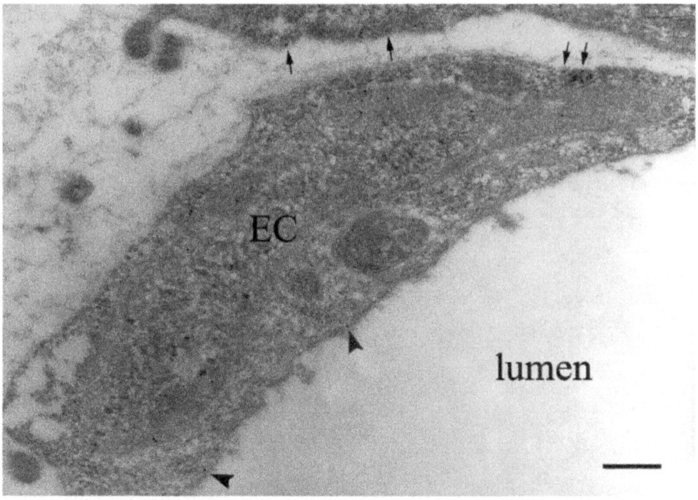

Fig. 7. TEM7 staining for transmission electron microscopy with IM193 antibody to detect TEM7-M. Staining is observed on the tight junctions (*arrows*) and on the luminal surfaces of endothelial cells (ECs; *arrowheads*). Scale bar, 200 nm. Reproduced with permission from Yamaji et al. [24]

Considerable effort has been invested recently to develop agents that block the formation of new blood vessels. For example, Bebacizumab, a selective VEGF inhibitor, was recently found to be effective in the regression of retinal and iris neovascularization secondary to PDR, but because of its cytostatic property, its effect may be limited to established vasculature. Therefore, it has become apparent that targeted destruction of the established vasculature is another option for therapeutic opportunities. In this regard, the presence of membrane-bound TEM7 on the luminal surfaces of neovascular endothelial cell is of interest (Fig. 7). Recently, cortactin, a monomeric protein that can be activated by external stimuli to promote polymerization and rearrangement of the actin cytoskeleton, and nidogen, a component of the basement membrane, were identified as proteins capable of binding to the extracellular region of TEM7 (Lee, et al., 2006; Nanda, et al., 2004). Because the retinal vessels are the only vessels that can be observed in situ, it may be possible to use a more selective ligand-based neovascular endothelial cell targeting strategy by delivering the bioactive molecules to the blood-retinal neovascular endothelial interface. For example, photodynamic therapy using such TEM7-binding partners labeled with photosensitive biomolecules may open new possibilities for a lower invasive therapy of retinal neovascularization.

b. Periostin

Periostin is a matricellular protein and is a member of the fasciclin family (Takeshita, et al., 1993). It contains an N-terminal secretory signal peptide, followed by a cysteine-rich domain, four internal homologous repeats, and a C-terminal hydrophilic domain (Horiuchi, et al., 1999). The high degree of structural and sequence homology of periostin with fasciclin 1 and transforming growth factor β–induced (TGFBI) suggests that periostin plays a role in cell adhesion and migration (Horiuchi, et al., 1999). In addition, periostin is expressed as a complex pattern of transcripts derived by alternative splicing with potentially different activities and biological functions (Yoshida, et al., 2011).

Periostin expression is altered in different diseases, including neoplasias, cardiovascular disease, and wound repair (Kanno, et al., 2008). Periostin is overexpressed in various human cancers such as pancreas, colon, ovary, oral squamous cell carcinoma, and lung, and its overexpression is correlated with the aggressiveness of the tumor and with poorer survival. Moreover, tumor cell lines engineered to overexpress periostin have accelerated the growth and higher angiogenic and metastatic potential in immunocompromised animals. In the heart, periostin plays a key role in the progression of cardiac valve complex degeneration by inducing angiogenesis and MMP production (Hakuno, et al., 2010). Periostin is also an element of bone marrow fibrosis and subepithelial fibrosis of bronchial asthma (Takayama, et al., 2006).

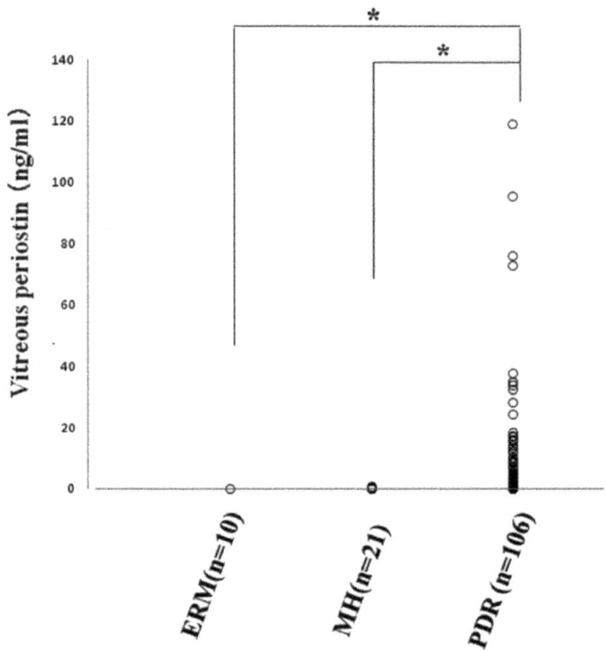

Fig. 8. Periostin levels in vitreous samples from eyes with nondiabetic (epiretinal membrane and macular hole) ocular diseases and eyes with proliferative diabetic retinopathy. ERM, epiretinal membrane. *$P < 0.001$. Reproduced with permission from Yoshida et al. [23]

We examined the amount of periostin in the 106 vitreous samples of patients with PDR collected during vitrectomy, and in the 31 vitreous samples obtained from patients during macular hole or ERM surgery (Yoshida, et al., 2011). We found that the concentration of periostin in the vitreous of patients with PDR was significantly higher than that in the vitreous of patients without PDR (Fig. 8). The concentration of periostin in the vitreous of patients with PDR was significantly correlated with the presence of FVMs but that of VEGF was not correlated (Yoshida, et al., 2011). The differences in the correlations between periostin and VEGF are probably because VEGF is upregulated in the retina at an earlier stage in response to hypoxia before the fromation of FVMs (Ishikawa, et al., 2010; Yoshida, et al., 2003).

Immunohistochemical analyses with the anti-periostin antibody revealed that periostin was expressed in the vascular pericytes that were α-SMA positive (Yoshida, et al., 2011). Periostin is reported to promote angiogenesis by an up-regulation of the VEGF receptor, Flk-1/KDR, by endothelial cells through an integrin αVβ3-focal adhesion kinase-mediated signaling pathway (Shao, et al., 2004). This suggests that periostin may play a role in promoting and/or maintaining vasculature in FVMs in a paracrine fashion. In addition, periostin was also expressed in myofibroblast-like cells in the stroma of FVMs (Yoshida, et al., 2011). It has been reported that a stable expression of a periostin in 293T cells causes the cells to undergo fibroblast-like transformation, and the cells expressing ectopic periostin increased cell migration, invasion, and adhesion (Yan and Shao, 2006). These findings suggest that periostin-expressing myofibroblast-like cells may play a role in the invasive properties of FVMs. Taken together, these results indicate that periostin may play specific roles in the formation and/or maintenance of FVMs.

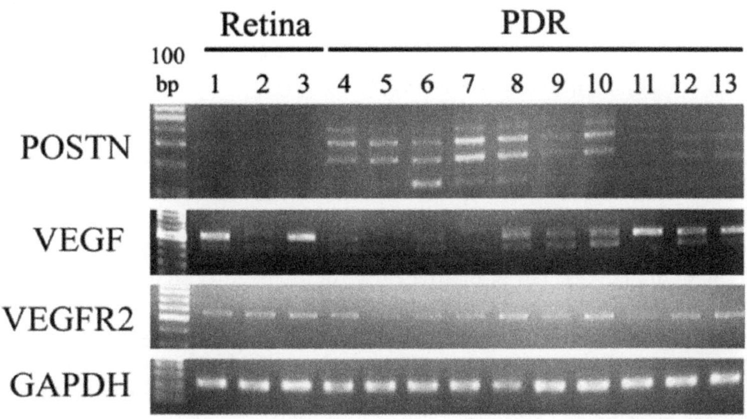

Fig. 9. RT-PCR analyses of periostin (POSTN), VEGF, VEGFR2, and GAPDH in FVMs derived from patients with proliferative diabetic retinopathy (PDR; *lanes 4–13*) and from control retinas (*lanes 1–3*). After 35 cycles, 8 μL each sample was electrophoresed through a 2% Tris-acetate-EDTA agarose gel, and the fractionated products were stained with ethidium bromide. Note the high expression of the mRNA of periostin with multiple bands in the FVMs derived from patients with PDR compared with control retinas. Reproduced with permission from Yoshida et al. [23]

Alternative splicing events occur within the C-terminal region of periostin, which is a key region that regulates cell invasiveness and metastasis (Shimazaki and Kudo, 2008). We confirmed that three spliced variants and the WT of human periostin were present in FVMs (Fig. 9) and that the periostin splice variant specifically regulated α-SMA gene expression (Yoshida, et al., 2011). It is suggested that the β strands within the C-terminal region may mediate binding interactions with other proteins such as FN or collagen. Because cell-specific isoform profiles and isoform-specific biological properties of periostin have been demonstrated (Shimazaki and Kudo, 2008), the existence of the different isoforms of periostin in FVMs may be used to vary the binding properties of periostin to other ECM proteins. This can then result in the deregulation of crucial cellular processes such as adhesion, proliferation, differentiation, and invasion. Unraveling the role of alternative splicing of periostin in the formation of FVMs may yield the basis for the development of isoform-specific molecular targeting therapeutic strategies.

5. Conclusion

By applying global gene expression technology to FVMs and hypoxic retinas, we have successfully identified novel genes that may play key roles in the formation and/or maintenance of FVMs. We believe that the transcriptome analyses performed in our studies may provide valuable information and thus should facilitate a wide range of future studies to establish tissue-specific molecular mechanisms associated with formation of FVMs.

As described earlier, recently-introduced anti-VEGF therapy on patients with intraocular neovascular diseases can reportedly accompany undesirable side effects such as brain and retinal vein occlusion. This was partly attributed to a steady level of VEGF expression in the normal retina, suggesting a role of VEGF in keeping normal homeostasis of the retina (Fig. 1) (Yoshida, et al., 2011). The manipulation of the VEGF pathway to inhibit pathologic neovascularization could result in unexpected disturbances of the normal homeostasis in the retina and thus should be approached carefully.

Because the vitreous concentrations of periostin were not significantly correlated with those of VEGF in the patients with PDR (Yoshida, et al., 2011), it may be inferred that periostin and VEGF do not act in a directly synchronized manner in the formation of FVMs. Moreover, in contrast to VEGF, periostin and TEM7 is assumed to be nonfunctional in normal retinas, in keeping with the very low levels of periostin in the normal control retinas (Fig. 9; (Yamaji, et al., 2008)). These results raise the possibility that the two molecules might be a potential therapeutic target to regulate "disease-specific" pathways in the formation of FVMs while minimizing the unfavorable side effects to the normal retina. Therefore, modulating the expression of periostin and/or TEM7 by antibodies or antisense oligonucleotides directed against the molecule could be a novel therapeutic strategy for inhibiting the progression of FVMs associated with PDR.

6. References

[1] Bhavsar, A.R. (2002) Diabetic retinopathy. The diabetes eye exam initiative. *Minn Med* 85, 46-7.

[2] Simo, R., Carrasco, E., Garcia-Ramirez, M., Hernandez, C. (2006) Angiogenic and antiangiogenic factors in proliferative diabetic retinopathy. *Curr Diabetes Rev* 2, 71-98.

[3] Hiscott, P., Wong, D., Grierson, I. (2000) Challenges in ophthalmic pathology: the vitreoretinal membrane biopsy. *Eye* 14 (Pt 4), 549-59.

[4] Yoshida, A., Yoshida, S., Khalil, A.K., Ishibashi, T., Inomata, H. (1998) Role of NF-kappaB-mediated interleukin-8 expression in intraocular neovascularization. *Invest Ophthalmol Vis Sci* 39, 1097-1106.

[5] Yoshida, A., Yoshida, S., Ishibashi, T., Kuwano, M., Inomata, H. (1999) Suppression of retinal neovascularization by the NF-kappaB inhibitor pyrrolidine dithiocarbamate in mice. *Invest Ophthalmol Vis Sci* 40, 1624-9.

[6] Yoshida, S., Ishikawa, K., Matsumoto, T., Yoshida, A., Ishibashi, T., Kono, T. (2010) Reduced concentrations of angiogenesis-related factors in vitreous after vitrectomy

in patients with proliferative diabetic retinopathy. *Graefes Arch Clin Exp Ophthalmol* 248, 799-804.

[7] Watanabe, D., Suzuma, K., Matsui, S., Kurimoto, M., Kiryu, J., Kita, M., Suzuma, I., Ohashi, H., Ojima, T., Murakami, T., Kobayashi, T., Masuda, S., Nagao, M., Yoshimura, N., Takagi, H. (2005) Erythropoietin as a retinal angiogenic factor in proliferative diabetic retinopathy. *N Engl J Med* 353, 782-92.

[8] Ishikawa, K., Yoshida, S., Kadota, K., Nakamura, T., Niiro, H., Arakawa, S., Yoshida, A., Akashi, K., Ishibashi, T. (2010) Gene expression profile of hyperoxic and hypoxic retinas in a mouse model of oxygen-induced retinopathy. *Invest Ophthalmol Vis Sci* 51, 4307-19.

[9] Smith, L.E., Wesolowski, E., McLellan, A., Kostyk, S.K., D'Amato, R., Sullivan, R., D'Amore, P.A. (1994) Oxygen-induced retinopathy in the mouse. *Invest Ophthalmol Vis Sci* 35, 101-111.

[10] Singh, R., Lillard, J.W., Jr., Singh, S. Chemokines: key players in cancer progression and metastasis. *Front Biosci (Schol Ed)* 3, 1569-82.

[11] Lewis, C.E., De Palma, M., Naldini, L. (2007) Tie2-expressing monocytes and tumor angiogenesis: regulation by hypoxia and angiopoietin-2. *Cancer Res* 67, 8429-32.

[12] Ishikawa, K., Yoshida, S., Nakao, S., Sassa, Y., Asato, R., Kohno, R., Arima, M., Kita, T., Yoshida, A., Ohichida, K., Ishibashi, T. (2011) Bone marrow-derived monocyte lineage cells recruited by MIP-1beta promote physiological revascularization in mouse model of oxygen-induced retinopathy *Lab Invest*, in press.

[13] Yun, J.K., McCormick, T.S., Villabona, C., Judware, R.R., Espinosa, M.B., Lapetina, E.G. (1997) Inflammatory mediators are perpetuated in macrophages resistant to apoptosis induced by hypoxia. *Proc Natl Acad Sci U S A* 94, 13903-8.

[14] Limb, G.A., Hollifield, R.D., Webster, L., Charteris, D.G., Chignell, A.H. (2001) Soluble TNF receptors in vitreoretinal proliferative disease. *Invest Ophthalmol Vis Sci* 42, 1586-91.

[15] Yoshida, S., Yoshida, A., Ishibashi, T. (2004) Induction of IL-8, MCP-1, and bFGF by TNF-alpha in retinal glial cells: implications for retinal neovascularization during post-ischemic inflammation. *Graefes Arch Clin Exp Ophthalmol* 242, 409-13.

[16] Yoshida, S., Ono, M., Shono, T., Izumi, H., Ishibashi, T., Suzuki, H., Kuwano, M. (1997) Involvement of interleukin-8, vascular endothelial growth factor, and basic fibroblast growth factor in tumor necrosis factor alpha-dependent angiogenesis. *Mol Cell Biol* 17, 4015-23.

[17] Yoshida, S., Yoshida, A., Ishibashi, T., Elner, S.G., Elner, V.M. (2003) Role of MCP-1 and MIP-1alpha in retinal neovascularization during postischemic inflammation in a mouse model of retinal neovascularization. *J Leukoc Biol* 73, 137-44.

[18] Ozaki, S., Johnson, L.V., Mullins, R.F., Hageman, G.S., Anderson, D.H. (1999) The human retina and retinal pigment epithelium are abundant sources of vitronectin mRNA. *Biochem Biophys Res Commun* 258, 524-9.

[19] Wistow, G. (2006) The NEIBank project for ocular genomics: data-mining gene expression in human and rodent eye tissues. *Prog Retin Eye Res* 25, 43-77.

[20] Yoshida, S., Ogura, A., Ishikawa, K., Yoshida, A., Kohno, R., Yamaji, Y., Ikeo, K., Gojobori, T., Kono, T., Ishibashi, T. (2010) Gene expression profile of fibrovascular membranes from patients with proliferative diabetic retinopathy. *Br J Ophthalmol* 94, 795-801.

[21] Hiscott, P., Sheridan, C., Magee, R.M., Grierson, I. (1999) Matrix and the retinal pigment epithelium in proliferative retinal disease. *Prog Retin Eye Res* 18, 167-90.

[22] von Hanno, T., Kinge, B., Fossen, K. (2010) Retinal artery occlusion following intravitreal anti-VEGF therapy. *Acta Ophthalmol* 88, 263-6.

[23] Yoshida, S., Ishikawa, K., Asato, R., Arima, M., Sassa, Y., Yoshida, A., Yoshikawa, H., Narukawa, K., Obika, S., Ono, J., Ohta, S., Izuhara, K., Kono, T., Ishibashi, T. (2011) Increased expression of periostin in vitreous and fibrovascular membranes obtained from patients with proliferative diabetic retinopathy. *Invest Ophthalmol Vis Sci* 52, 5670-8.

[24] Yamaji, Y., Yoshida, S., Ishikawa, K., Sengoku, A., Sato, K., Yoshida, A., Kuwahara, R., Ohuchida, K., Oki, E., Enaida, H., Fujisawa, K., Kono, T., Ishibashi, T. (2008) TEM7 (PLXDC1) in neovascular endothelial cells of fibrovascular membranes from patients with proliferative diabetic retinopathy. *Invest Ophthalmol Vis Sci* 49, 3151-7.

[25] Nanda, A., St Croix, B. (2004) Tumor endothelial markers: new targets for cancer therapy. *Curr Opin Oncol* 16, 44-9.

[26] Lee, H.K., Seo, I.A., Park, H.K., Park, H.T. (2006) Identification of the basement membrane protein nidogen as a candidate ligand for tumor endothelial marker 7 in vitro and in vivo. *FEBS Lett* 580, 2253-7.

[27] Nanda, A., Buckhaults, P., Seaman, S., Agrawal, N., Boutin, P., Shankara, S., Nacht, M., Teicher, B., Stampfl, J., Singh, S., Vogelstein, B., Kinzler, K.W., St Croix, B. (2004) Identification of a binding partner for the endothelial cell surface proteins TEM7 and TEM7R. *Cancer Res* 64, 8507-11.

[28] Takeshita, S., Kikuno, R., Tezuka, K., Amann, E. (1993) Osteoblast-specific factor 2: cloning of a putative bone adhesion protein with homology with the insect protein fasciclin I. *Biochem J* 294 (Pt 1), 271-8.

[29] Horiuchi, K., Amizuka, N., Takeshita, S., Takamatsu, H., Katsuura, M., Ozawa, H., Toyama, Y., Bonewald, L.F., Kudo, A. (1999) Identification and characterization of a novel protein, periostin, with restricted expression to periosteum and periodontal ligament and increased expression by transforming growth factor beta. *J Bone Miner Res* 14, 1239-49.

[30] Kanno, A., Satoh, K., Masamune, A., Hirota, M., Kimura, K., Umino, J., Hamada, S., Satoh, A., Egawa, S., Motoi, F., Unno, M., Shimosegawa, T. (2008) Periostin, secreted from stromal cells, has biphasic effect on cell migration and correlates with the epithelial to mesenchymal transition of human pancreatic cancer cells. *Int J Cancer* 122, 2707-18.

[31] Hakuno, D., Kimura, N., Yoshioka, M., Mukai, M., Kimura, T., Okada, Y., Yozu, R., Shukunami, C., Hiraki, Y., Kudo, A., Ogawa, S., Fukuda, K. (2010) Periostin advances atherosclerotic and rheumatic cardiac valve degeneration by inducing angiogenesis and MMP production in humans and rodents. *J Clin Invest* 120, 2292-306.

[32] Takayama, G., Arima, K., Kanaji, T., Toda, S., Tanaka, H., Shoji, S., McKenzie, A.N., Nagai, H., Hotokebuchi, T., Izuhara, K. (2006) Periostin: a novel component of subepithelial fibrosis of bronchial asthma downstream of IL-4 and IL-13 signals. *J Allergy Clin Immunol* 118, 98-104.

[33] Shao, R., Bao, S., Bai, X., Blanchette, C., Anderson, R.M., Dang, T., Gishizky, M.L., Marks, J.R., Wang, X.F. (2004) Acquired expression of periostin by human breast cancers promotes tumor angiogenesis through up-regulation of vascular endothelial growth factor receptor 2 expression. *Mol Cell Biol* 24, 3992-4003.

[34] Yan, W., Shao, R. (2006) Transduction of a mesenchyme-specific gene periostin into 293T cells induces cell invasive activity through epithelial-mesenchymal transformation. *J Biol Chem* 281, 19700-8.

[35] Shimazaki, M., Kudo, A. (2008) Impaired capsule formation of tumors in periostin-null mice. *Biochem Biophys Res Commun* 367, 736-42.

Part 2

Inflammation and Angiogenesis

7

Immunological Risk Factors for the Development and Progression of Diabetic Retinopathy

Katarzyna Zorena, Dorota Raczyńska, and Krystyna Raczyńska
Medical University of Gdańsk
Poland

1. Epidemiology

International epidemiological studies indicate that over the last 50 years there has been progressive raise in diabetes incidence. According to International Diabetes Federation (IDF) currently there are 284 millions of people affected by diabetes worldwide and IDF prognosis predicts that in 2030 this number for all countries and human races will reach 438 million which will account for 7.7% of global population (IDF Atlas, 2010). The highest prevalence of diabetes is in North America where it reached the level of 10.2% of adult population whereas in Europe the prevalence is 6.9% of population aged 20 to 79 years. Particularly worrying is constant increase in diabetes incidence of both type 1 (Patterson et al., 2009; Jarosz-Chobot et al., 2011) as well as type 2 (D'Adamo & Caprio, 2011) in developmental age population. As a consequence of increase in diabetes prevalence there is higher number of patients with microangiopathic complications including diabetic retinopathy (DR) in children and youth (Cho et al., 2011) and in adults (Rosenson et al., 2011). Chronic complications reduce the quality of life and are a main cause of disability. Diabetic retinopathy has become a leading reason for blindness and visual impairment in developed countries and is constantly increasing (Fong et al ., 2004). Nearly all patients with type 1 diabetes will develop some manifestation of DR, whereas in type 2 diabetic patients 80% of insulin- dependent patients and 50% of patients not requiring insulin therapy will have DR within 20 to 25 years following disease onset (Lamoureux & Wong, 2011). Among younger-onset patients with diabetes, the prevalence of any retinopathy was 8% at 3 years, 25% at 5 years, 60% at 10 years, and 80% at 15 years. The prevalence of proliferative diabetic retinopathy (PDR) was 0% at 3 years and increased to 25% at 15 years (National Health and Nutrition Examination Survey, 2006).

2. Pathomechanism of diabetic retinopathy

Although there is a high incidence of diabetic retinopathy, its pathogenesis still remains enigmatic. Before changes in the eye fundus become visible in ophtalmoscopic examination or fluorescein angiography, in immunohistopathological study there are already visible morphological changes in precapillary arterioles, capillaries and venules of diameter less than 100 μm. In initial stage of development of diabetic retinopathy there is thickening of basal membrane of small vessels, its narrowing and closure, disappearance of pericytes, weakening and distension of small vessel walls and, in consequence, formation of microaneurisms and endothelial cell proliferation. Additionally, the following take place: functional changes in capillaries, increase in their permeability and disruption of blood-retina barrier. As a result of enhanced vascular permeability, oedemas and haemorrhages appear in the retina. Moreover, the closure of retinal vessels leads to areas with loss of blood flow within retina, which causes its chronic ischaemia and hypoxia and subsequent increase in the production of growth factors that, in turn, induce angiogenesis, formation of arterio-venous anastomoses and proliferation of fibrous tissue within retina and optic nerve disc (Yoshida et al., 2004; Curtis et al., 2009; Roy et al., 2010; Lange et al. 2011). It is commonly accepted that hyperglycaemia plays crucial role in pathogenesis of diabetic angiopathy (Roy et al., 2010; Kowluru et al., 2010). Hyperglycaemia leads to the formation of advanced glycation end products (AGEs) which are durable, irreversible and their characteristic feature is to create cross-links between proteins which in turn affects flexibility of vessels (Wa et al., 2007; Roy et al., 2010; Yamagishi et al., 2011). It was proved that AGEs interaction with receptor for advanced glycation end products (RAGEs) plays a key role in development and progression of late diabetic complications (Thomas et al., 2011; Yamagishi et al., 2011; Zong et al., 2011). In multiple studies investigating diabetic retinopathy pathogenesis more and more attention is paid to inflammatory and angiogenic factors (Naldini et al., 2005; Maier et al., 2006; Campa et al, 2010; Praidou et al., 2010).

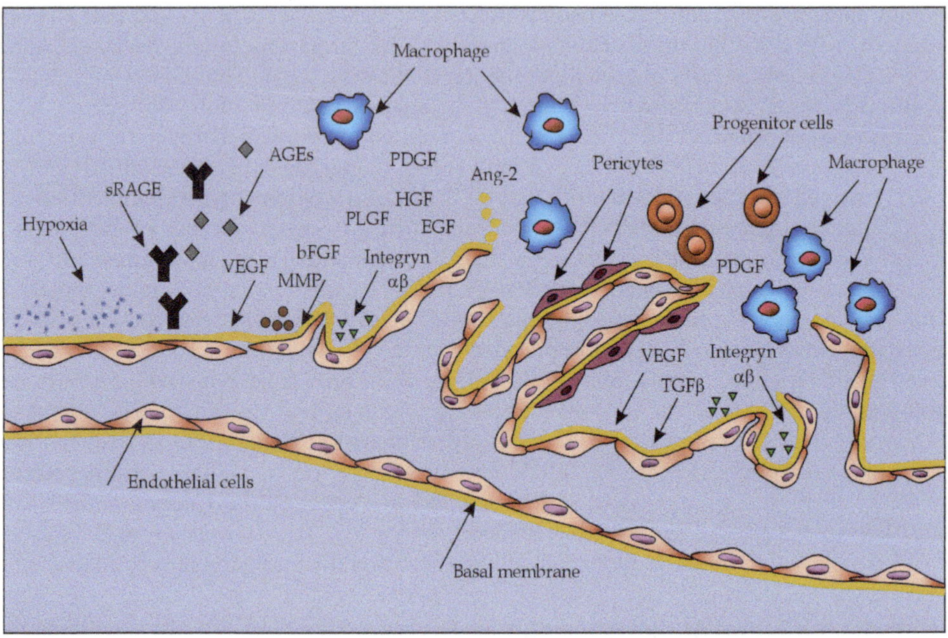

Fig. 1. The selected factors involved in the development and progression of diabetic retinopathy. AGEs - advanced glycation end products, RAGEs - receptor for advanced glycation end products, VEGF- vascular endothelial growth factor, IGF-I - insulin like growth factor, PLGF - placental growth factor, HGF – hepatocyte growth factor, PEDF - pigment epithelium derived factor, bFGF - basic fibroblast growth factor, TGF-β transforming growth factor beta, MMPs – metalloproteinases PDGF-platelet-derived growth factor , EGF-Epidermal growth factor, Ang-2 - Angiopoietin-2

In the eye of a healthy person endothelial cells are mitotically inactive thanks to pro-angiogenic and anti-angiogenic factors remaining in balance. Healthy organism maintains perfect equilibrium between angiogenesis modulators (Carmeliet, 2003; Kvanta, 2006). However in the case of hypoxia or inflammation this balance may be shifted towards neoangiogenesis (Kvanta, 2006; Campa et al., 2010). Eye angiogenesis is a complicated multi-stage process in which new vessels are created from existing ones (Kvanta, 2006; Curtis et al., 2009). This usually leads to significant loss of vision in patients with type 1 as well as type 2 diabetes (Rosenson et al., 2011; Durham & Herman, 2011). Results of studies conducted within last ten years proved that eye angiogenesis may involve choroid, cornea as well as retina (Kvanta, 2006; Caporali & Emanueli, 2011). During retinal angiogenesis newly formed vessels grow into vitreous where they may break and cause haemorrhage or retinal detachment. Fig. 1-3 shows three examples of a fundus of the eyes from normal and diabetic individuals.

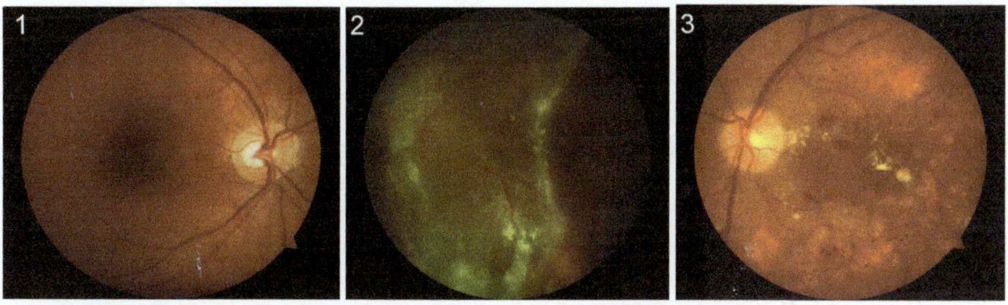

Fig. 2. Fundus photos of eyes from normal and diabetic individuals. 1. Normal fundus of the eye. 2. Proliferative diabetic retinopathy with tractional retinal detachment. 3. Diabetic retinopathy accompanied by macular oedema, status after argon laser therapy.

3. Inflammatory and angiogenic factors of diabetic retinopathy

3.1 Growth factors

3.1.1 Vascular Endothelial Growth Factor (VEGF)

VEGF is the most potent factor stimulating physiological and pathological angiogenesis. It is a 46-48 kD of molecular weight glycosylated homo-dimer produced by endothelial cells, macrophages, CD4 lymphocytes, plasmatic cells, myocytes, megakaryocytes as well as neoplasm cells (Ferrara et al., 2003, Ferrara, 2004). VEGF induces new blood vessel formation through binding to receptors. The VEGF family encompasses 6 proteins: VEGF-A,-B,-C,-D,-E and PLGF. Best known and most frequently used clinically is VEGF-A. There are also other VEGF isoforms known: VEGF121, VEGF145, VEGF148, VEGF162, VEGF165, VEGF183, VEGF189, VEGF206, with different amino acid chain length, ability to bind heparin, mitogenic activity and VEGF receptor affinity (Ferrara, 2004; Simó et al., 2006; Wirostko et al., 2008). VEGF stimulates proliferation and migration of endothelial cells and increases blood vessel permeability (Aiello et al, 1994; Wirostko et al., 2008). Furthermore it induces production of tissue collagenase and increases macrophage and monocytes chemotaxis. The authors (Matsumoto et al., 2002; Oh et al., 2010; Suzuki et al., 2011) demonstrated that VEGF increases monocyte chemoattractant protein-1 (MCP-1) mRNA expression. VEGF induces MCP-1 most likely through activation of transcription factors such as NFκB and AP-1 and signalling pathways dependent and independent from ERKs (Mohammad & Kowluru, 2010). It is known that pro-inflammatory protein MCP-1 is a potent attractant for monocytes and has been detected in the majority of patients with proliferative retinopathy. As it causes monocyte/ macrophage infiltration, it leads to vascular abnormalities (Czepluch et al., 2009; Zhang et al., 2009).The hypothesis that monocytes / macrophages participate in the pathogenesis of retinopathy is further supported by the results (Kataoka et al.,2011). The vitreous macrophages are attracted to the pathological vessels induced by retinal ischemia. In children and adolescents with T1DM there was a significant increase of VEGF levels in serum, not only in patients with type 1 diabetes and non-proliferative retinopathy, but also in patients in whom the ophthalmic examination showed no changes in the organ of sight (Chiarelli et al., 2000; Santilli et al., 2002; Zorena et al., 2007; Myśliwiec et al., 2008). Those findings suggest that VEGF may play a role in the development of vascular changes within the eye in children and adolescents already in first few years of disease when available diagnostic methods can't detect retinopathic changes. Furthermore, in other studies (Zorena et al., 2010) it has been noted that VEGF level has been higher in patients with hypertension, retinopathy and nephropathy compared to diabetic patients without hypertension although with retinopathy and nephropathy.In addition, there were no significant differences in VEGF levels between patients with T1DM group without hypertension, but with retinopathy and nephropathy compared to healthy controls group. Furthermore, how does hypertension lead to increased production of VEGF in children and adolescents with retinopathy is not fully known. It is believed that it is a multidirectional process. On one hand it is known that persistent hyperglycaemia leading to the elevation of HbA1c levels may lead to the production and accumulation of advanced glycation end products. Formation of AGEs promotes production of pro-inflammatory cytokines which may further initiate increase of VEGF levels and thus indirectly lead to the development of hypertension in T1DM (Gallego et al., 2008; Roy et al., 2010). It was shown that VEGF binds to VEGFR-2 receptor at the endothelial cell surface which leads to phosphorylation of transcription factors via MAPK (mitogen activated protein kinase) (Suzuma et al., 2001; Wirostko et al., 2008). As a consequence, there is increase in expression of adhesive molecules, cytokines, chemokines which in turn increase proliferation of endothelial cells and production of extracellular matrix with simultaneous impairment of its degradation. This leads to progressive fibrosis and closure of vessels' lumen and subsequently increases blood flow resistance. Higher resistance in vascular system results in further raise in VEGF production which in turn causes changes in structure and ratio of collagen to elastin which makes blood vessels stiffer and leads to increase in blood pressure (Iglesias-de la Cruz et al., 2002; Kvanta et al., 2006; Wirostko et al., 2008). Increased levels of VEGF has been detected in vitreous of adult patients with proliferative diabetic retinopathy (Maier et al., 2008; Marek et al., 2010; Lange et al., 2011). Moreover, it has been demonstrated that high level of VEGF in vitreous of patients with proliferative diabetic retinopathy has been associated with increased VEGF level in serum (Maier et al., 2008). The emerging new therapies based on application of anti VEGF gave promising results in treatment of proliferative diabetic retinopathy (Adamis et al,. 2006; Starita et al., 2007;. Hernández-DaMota et al., 2010; Engelbert et al., 2011). The first drug in this group was sodium pegaptanib (Macugen) with anti VEGF165 properties and has been administered intravitreally. Pegaptanib has been used as a treatment of both diabetic macular edema (DME) as well as PDR (Adamis et al., 2006; Querques et al., 2009; Hornan et al., 2010). After intravitreal injection of another VEGF-A inhibitor - ranibizumab (registered by FDA in June 2006 as a Lucentis) is good antiangiogenic with vision improvement in 95% of patients (Jorge et al., 2011; Rosenfeld et al., 2011).

3.1.2 Insulin like Growth Factor (IGF-I)

IGF-I is a polypeptide showing high similarity to insulin. Two different forms are distinguished: IGF-I and IGF-II. IGF-I circulates in blood in the form of IGF-binding protein (IGF-BP), probably inhibiting activity of free IGF. IGF-I is a pivotal growth factor secreted as a result of stimulation by human growth hormone. Both in vivo and in vitro studies indicate its anti-apoptotic and anti-inflammatory properties (Goes et al., 1996; Sukhanov et al., 2007; Sun et al., 2010). There are reports that IGF-I has protective actions in ischaemic rat kidney due to inhibition of inflammatory cytokine production (Goes et al., 1996) and anti-apoptotic in Parkinson disease via inhibition of GSK-3β signalling pathway (Sun et al., 2010). IGF-I exerts its protective actions also in central nervous system and cardiomyocytes (Sun et al., 2010). In premature babies a small concentration of IGF-I is a risk factor of retinopathy of prematurity (Pérez-Muñuzuri et al., 2010). IGF-I deficiency after birth may play a role in development and deterioration of neurological deficiencies in premature babies (Lofqvist et al., 2006). On the other hand in children and youth with T1DM and microangiopathy IGF-I levels have been found to be lower compared to group of patients without microangiopathy (Peczyńska et al., 2004). Furthermore, IGF-I levels were lowest in children with T1DM for over 10 years. Interestingly, the same group of children had raised VEGF levels in serum and the longer the duration of the disease, the higher were the levels (with maximum levels in patients with diabetes for over 10 years) (Chiarelli et al., 2000; Santilli et al., 2001; Peczyńska et al. 2004; Zorena et al., 2009). Also much lower IGF-I concentrations were found in adolescents with microangiopathy compared to diabetic patients without complications and healthy children (Wedrychowicz et al., 2005). However, IGFBP-1 levels in serum were much higher whereas IGFBP-3 were lower in patients with microangiopathy compared to those without complications. Thus circulating IGFBP-1 may play a role in development of diabetic complications while IGFBP-3 may be protective (Kielczewski et al., 2011). In adults with PDR, levels of IGF-I and VEGF in vitreous were significantly higher than in control group (Simo et al., 2002; Poulaki et al., 2004; Hartnett et al., 2009). Surprisingly there were no differences in levels of both factors in serum in each group. This effect could be explained by two mechanisms: higher concentration of IGF-I binding protein (IGFBP's) in vitreous may neutralize the increased IGF-I production or may lower the production of free IGF-I in tissues of diabetic patients (Simo et al., 2002). Additional evidence supporting IGF-I in PDR result from use of IGF-I inhibitors. Somatostatin and octreotide, a somatostatin analogue, inhibited IGF-I receptor (IGF-1R) phosphorylation and decreased VEGF production (Sall et al. 2004). Systemic inhibition of IGF-I signalling in a relevant animal model with a receptor-neutralizing antibody, or with inhibitors of PI-3 kinase (PI-3K), c-Jun kinase (JNK), or Akt, suppressed downstream signalling pathways, VEGF expression, ICAM-1 levels, leukostasis, and BRB breakdown. Intravitreal administration of IGF-I increased retinal factors AKT, JNK, HIF-1alpha, NF-κB, AP-1 activity, and VEGF levels. Haurigot et al., 2009 demonstrated that high intra-ocular concentration of IGF-I in retina is sufficient to activate processes leading to disruption of blood-retina barrier and increase in vascular permeability as a consequence of high expression of IGF-I in retina.

3.1.3 Placental Growth Factor (PLGF)

PLGF is a homodimer protein belonging to VEGF family, showing structural similarity to VEGF-A. Three PLGF isoforms have been described (PLGF-1,-2,-3). Those isoforms do not interact with VEGFR-2 but they bind to VEGFR-1 (Christinger et. al., 2004). PLGF has been recently isolated as a factor, stimulating neovascularization. Over the last decade, the direct or indirect pro angiogenic effect of PLGF was demonstrated during ischaemia, inflammation and wound healing. There are controversies regarding the pro-angiogenic activity of placental growth factor in diabetic retinopathy. In the eye, loss of PLGF does not hamper retinal development (Feeney et al., 2003) but impairs choroidal neovascularization (Rakic et al., 2003). Intravitreal injections of PLGF prevent oxygen-induced retinal ischaemia, without inducing neovascularization (Campochiaro et al., 2006). In animals' retinal cells only small amounts of PLGF have been detected. However, increased levels have been detected in eyes affected by advanced neovascularization in retina (Khaliq et al., 1998; Miyamoto et al., 2007).

3.1.4 Hepatocyte Growth Factor (HGF)

HGF is a pleiotropic factor derived from mesenchymal tissue regulating growth and migration of various cells. HGF is synthesized mainly in liver but also in lungs, kidney, smooth muscles and corneal endothelial cells (Stoker et al., 1987). It is secreted as a single chain precursor which is activated by proteolytic cleavage. Simó et al., 2006 have detected increased concentrations of both HGF as well as VEGF in vitreous of patients with PDR compared to patients with diabetes but without complications and healthy control group. However, they have not demonstrated relevant correlation between HGF and VEGF. Yoshida et al., 2010 investigating levels of angiopoietin-2 , HGF, bFGF, PDGF, TIMP-1 and TIMP-2 in the vitreous body of PDR patients before and after vitrectomy has shown a marked decrease of HGF as well as angiopoietin-2 levels in the vitreous body of PDR patients after vitrectomy.

3.1.5 Pigment Epithelium Derived Factor (PEDF)

PEDF also known as serpin F1 (SERPINF1), is a multifunctional secreted protein that has anti-angiogenic and neurotrophic functions. Found in vertebrates, this 50 kD protein holds promise in the treatment of such conditions as heart disease, cancer and choroidal neovascularization (Filleur et al., 2009). PEDF is secreted by many retinal cells including Müller cells, endothelial cells, pericytes, and pigment epithelium cells of retina (Doll et al., 2003; Barnstable et al., 2004; Tombran-Tink et al., 2010). Studies conducted on PEDF depleted mice, showed that lack of this gene results in serious abnormalities in both, cell differentiation as well as in retinal morphology (Doll et. al., 2003). In 2003 the first hypothesis emerged that PEDF may hamper angiogenesis by direct reduction of VEGF gene expression (Yamagishi et al., 2003). Most recent data confirm also that PEDF has direct effect on vascular endothelial growth factor receptor 1 (VEGFR-1) by increasing g-secretase complex activity (Cai et al., 2011). Activation of g-secretase leads directly to proteolytic cleavage within VEGFR-1 and C-end domain of receptor is removed which subsequently migrates from cell membrane into cytosol (Cai et al., 2006; Cai et al., 2011). Additionally, PEDF inhibits production of reactive oxygen species (ROS) and MCP-1 and furthermore, it neutralizes negative effects of AGE (Inagaki et al., 2003). Other studies suggest that transcription factor, NF-κB and Fas ligand and its receptor play a role in PEDF mechanism of action. Volpert et. al. 2002, proved that anti-FasL antibodies and application of inhibitors hampers PEDF action. PEDF may equally prevent cell apoptosis by activation of transcription factor NF-κB, as well as lead to programmed cell deaths via increasing Fas ligand expression (Volpert et al., 2002). Studies (Cai et al., 2006) have demonstrated that PEDF used in bovine retinal microvascular endothelial cells culture (BRMECs) did not affect their migration and formation of primary vessel canals. However, when an addition of PEDF had been preceded by application of VEGF then this factor reduced significantly proliferation and endothelial cells migration induced by VEGF. Studies evaluating the antiangiogenic properties of PEDF have also shown that exerts a modulating effect on the formation of new retinal blood vessels and promote angiogenesis in hypoxia (Barnstable et al., 2004; Elayappan et al., 2009; Subramanian et al., 2011).

3.1.6 Basic fibroblast Growth Factor (bFGF)

Fibroblast growth factors, or FGFs, are a family of growth factors involved in wound healing, embryonic development, and angiogenesis. There are two FGF distinguished: acidic (aFGF) and basic (bFGF), the latter being attributed to play the most significant role in angiogenesis. This factor has an ability to directly activate endothelial cells, it also affects proliferation, migration of endothelial cells and fibroblasts, induces proteolytic enzymes and synthesis of fibronectin, collagen, proteoglycans and hyaluronic acid (Shi et al., 2011). Synthesis of bFGF takes place in retina cells as well as in cornea and is activated by inflammation or a local injury (Polykandriotis et al., 2011). It has been suggested that bFGF exerts its paracrine effects on the eye by inhibition of apoptosis. Other studies have demonstrated that beta-FGF works via two pathways a calcium independent FGFR1 through PI 3-K, P70(S6K) and Akt to increased VEGF from the RPE and a calcium dependant FGFR2. The inhibition of those two pathways suppresses bFGF-induced choroidal endothelial cells proliferation (Rosenthal et al., 2005). Deissler et al., 2011, have discovered that VEGF165 but not bFGF is mainly responsible for changes in cell permeability observed in retinal endothelium.

3.1.7 Transforming Growth Factor beta (TGF-β)

TGF-β is a member of transforming growth factor family which has immunomodulatory function. It is secreted primarily by monocytes, macrophages, lymphocytes, and dendritic cells. This cytokine takes part in angiogenesis, stimulates synthesis and degeneration of extracellular matrix proteins, regulates induction of apoptosis and stimulates proliferation of mesenchymal cells.

TGF-β exists in three isoforms coded by different genes β1, β2, β3; best known is TGF- β1 (Bertolino et al., 2005; Orlova et al., 2011) . TGF-β is believed to be the most important ligand in the pathogenesis of fibrotic diseases in the eye. Such ocular fibrotic diseases include scarring in the cornea and conjunctiva, fibrosis in the corneal endothelium, post-cataract surgery fibrosis of the lens capsule, excess scarring of tissue around the extraocular muscles in the strabismus surgery and proliferative vitreoretinopathy (Saika et al., 2009; Sumioka et al., 2011; Hills et al., 2011). Those properties of TGF-β are confirmed in animal models (Yingchuan et al., 2010; Kowluru et al., 2010) as well as in patients with diabetic retinopathy (George et al., 2009; Abu El-Asrar et al., 2010). It is believed that TGF-β plays a role in pathogenesis of diabetic retinopathy via hyperglycaemia and inflammation. Kowluru et al., 2010 have reported that both the duration of the initial exposure to high glucose, and normal glucose that follows high glucose, are critical in determining the outcome of the alterations in the inflammatory mediators such as IL-1 beta, NF-kB, VEGF, TNF-α including with TGF-β in retinal.

3.1.8 Angiogenin

Angiogenin is a small protein that is implicated in angiogenesis. Angiogenin mRNA expression is detectable in epithelial cells, fibroblasts and blood cells (Tello-Montoliu et al., 2006). Higher level of angiogenin was observed in serum in children and adolescents with non-proliferative retinopathy as compared to the group of children and adolescents without DR (Chiarelli et al., 2002; Raczyńska K et al., 2008). Maier et al., 2006 have revealed that angiogenin level has been increasing in the vitreous in diabetic patients. Nevertheless it is suggested that the increased level was an effect of blood-retina barrier disruption and leakage of growth factors from blood vessels into eye (Maier et al., 2006). Lower levels of serum angiogenin was demostrated in patients with type 2 diabetes (Siebert et al., 2007; Siebert et al., 2010). Lower level of angiogenin but higher VEGF were found also in the vitreous of patients T1DM with PDR (Marek et al., 2011).

4. Cytokines

4.1 Interleukin 6 (IL-6)

Interleukin 6 has been well known as a pro-inflammatory cytokine. However, there is an increasing number of reports about its anti-inflammatory character (Sanchez et al., 2003; Sappington et al., 2006; Nandi et al., 2010). *In vitro* in presence of increased pressure and injury resulting from ischaemia, IL-6 inhibited apoptosis of retinal ganglion cells (Sanchez et al., 2003; Sappington et al.,2006). On the other hand (Dace et al., 2008) M1 macrophages prevented neovascularisation within retina due to high secretion of IL-6, IL-12 and IL-23. Although, majority of reports confirm its negative role in the onset and progression of diabetic retinopathy (Noma et al., 2009; Funk M et al., 2010; Koleva-Georgieva et al., 2011). IL-6 is produced mainly by macrophages, monocytes, lymphocytes T and B, while in the eye IL-6 is produced by keratocytes, Müller cells, pigmented epithelium, corneal epithelium, iris and ciliary body (Yoshida et al., 2001). IL-6 secretion is activated by hypoxia, AGEs, and PKC (protein kinase C) (Giacco & Brownlee, 2010; Adamiec-Mroczek et al., 2010; Lange et al., 20011). In children and adolescents with diabetic retinopathy, higher levels of IL-6 were demonstrated in serum (Lo Hui-Chen et al., 2004; Zorena et al., 2007; Myśliwiec et al., 2008 , Bradshaw et al., 2009). A significant increase in the level of IL-6 was found in PDR patients compared to NPDR and healthy children. Authors recorded significant gradation in the IL-6 increase when comparing healthy children, children with T1DM without abnormalities in the eyes, and diabetic children with non proliferative diabetic retinopathy. Higher IL-6 and TNF levels in diabetic children are attributed to worse metabolic balance and chronic inflammation (Zorena et al., 2007; Myśliwiec et al., 2008). Apart from IL-6 influence on the set and progression of diabetic retinopathy in young patients with diabetes, higher levels of VEGF and C-reactive protein were also found (Coulon at al., 2005; Zorena et al., 2007). Coulon et al., discovered in their studies that children with long standing diabetes and retinopathy as well as nephropathy had five times higher levels of CRP than patients with diabetes but without complications (Coulon et al., 2005). Authors concluded that high level of pro-inflammatory cytokines in long standing diabetes is a result of ongoing inflammatory process. In inflammatory conditions IL-6 levels in serum may increase even 100 times, therefore IL-6 is regarded as an early and sensitive but non-specific indicator of inflammatory process affecting the organism (Abrahamsson et al, 1997). High IL-6 levels have been observed also in patients with type 2 diabetes and retinopathy as compared to patients without retinopathy (JH Lee et al., 2008; Goldberg., 2009). Also in aqueous from eyes with diabetic macular edema (Funk et al. 2010) found to be significantly increased IL-6 and VEGF. When patients were given bevacizumab, it was noted that VEGF levels dropped below physiological levels. Oh et al., 2010, demonstrated positive correlation between the aqueous levels of IL-6 and macular thickness indicating that IL-6 may play a central role in the development of diabetic macular edema. Other studies concerned the increased levels of IL-6, TNF, ET-1 vWF, sE-selectin in vitreous detected in patients with type 2 diabetes and PDR (Adamiec-Mroczek et al., 2010). Furthermore, authors noted correlation between TNF-α, ET-1 and HbA1c suggesting that there is close relation between metabolic equilibrium and inflammatory factors in T2DM patients. Thus, those studies support pro-inflammatory and proangiogenic role of IL-6.

4.2 Interleukin 10 (IL- 10)

Several recent studies reported that local IL -10 production may lead to angiogenesis in retina. Studies demonstrated that IL-10 may polarize macrophages in proangiogenic direction (Apte RS., 2006, Kelly et al., 2007, Dance et al., 2008). In macrophages of C57BL/6 mice with induced retinopathy, there has been significantly higher proangiogenic cytokine gene expression. This hasn't been found in macrophages of mice with IL-10 -/- phenotype (Dace et al., 2008). In children and adolescents with long-standing type 1 diabetes more than 60% of patients with symptoms of diabetic retinopathy showed no activity of this cytokine in serum. IL-10 levels analysis in group of children with T1DM and various grades of diabetic complications in the eye suggests that higher secretion of IL-10 may protect from late complications (Myśliwiec et al., 2006). Also, there were no significant differences in the IL-10 levels in the vitreous of patients with proliferative retinopathy as compared to those without PDR (Hernandez et al., 2005). However in T2DM patients, IL-10 was progressively lower with more advanced retinopathy (JH Lee et al., 2008). Suzuki et al., 2011 demonstrated higher levels of IL-10 as well as positive correlation between IL-10 and VEGF in patients with PDR compared to those with central retinal vein occlusion (CRVO).

4.3 Interleukin 12

Interleukin 12 (IL 12) has been described initially as a factor stimulating natural cytotoxic cells and causing maturation of cytotoxic lymphocytes. Under physiological circumstances it is produced mainly by macrophage, dendritic cells, keratinocytes, granulocytes, and mast cells (Trinchieri, 1998). In vivo, it was demonstrated that IL-12 is a potent antiangiogenic cytokine and this effect is mediated through interferon-γ (Voest et al., 1995). Few studies conducted in recent years indicate that IL-12 does not affect *per se* endothelial cells, but just by IFN-γ (Voest et al., 1995). This in turn regulates production of second line chemokines via induction of protein (IP)-10 being recognized as the most important mediator for IL-12 in angiogenesis activation (Sgadari et al., 1996). Furthermore, another report suggests that inhibition of IL-12 production may be mediated by natural killer cells (NK) (Ghiringhelli et al., 2006). A significantly lower IL-12 level but higher TNF and VEGF levels were found in a group of children and adolescents with diabetes and NPDR as compared to a group of patients without DR (Zorena et al., 2007). Another study (Zorena et al., 2008) reported imbalance between pro and antiangiogenic factors in serum of children and adolescents with long term T1DM. This imbalance was demonstrated between TNF-α and IL-12. It has been observed that patients who had both low TNF-α and IL-12 levels did not develop diabetic complications like retinopathy or nephropathy. However, when patients had high level of TNF-α and absent IL-12 they developed microangiopathic complications. Shift in balance towards TNF-α promotes late diabetic complications. Loss of equilibrium between pro and antiangiogenic actions of TNF-α and IL-12 underpins late diabetic complications. Applied monoclonal antibody against p40 subunit of IL-12 - Uteskinumab gave positive results in a patient with Crohn's disease (Sansó Sureda et al., 2011).

4.4 Tumor Necrosis Factor alpha (TNF-α)

TNF-α is one of most important inflammatory cytokines. It is produced primarily by monocytes and macrophages on which it exerts its endo-, para- and autocrine actions. It stimulates cytotoxic properties of monocytes and macrophages and simultaneously is a mediator of cytotoxicity. Its biological effects depends strongly on quantity and intensity of TNF-α secretion. Apart from taking part in inflammatory processes it also plays important role in neovascularisation (Wilson &Balkwill, 2002). TNF-α exerts versatile effects due to its ability to induce synthesis of other cytokines functionally related to TNF-α, extracellular matrix proteins, monocyte and fibroblast chemotaxis modulation and also influences the expression of adhesive molecules in retinal vessels (Doganay et al.,2002; Naldini & Carraro, 2005). Teflon implants soaked in 3.5 ng TNF-α and implanted into rat cornea caused a visible growth of new blood vessels after 7 days (Fajardo et al., 1992). A similar effect was achieved on chicken embryo membranes (Hooper et al., 2005). However, (Patterson et al., 1996) showed an antiangiogenic action of TNF-α using human endothelial cells. The authors showed that incubation of those cells with known proangiogenic factor VEGF for 24h augmented their proliferative activity more than two fold, whereas 12h pre-incubation abolished this effect. However, TNF-α alone revealed a weak cytotoxic effect towards endothelial cells. Inhibition of endothelial cell proliferation by TNF-α was associated with reduction in VEGFR-2 (KDR/Flt-1) receptor mRNA transcription level which depends on dose and the duration of cytokines. Low concentrations of TNF-α can trigger signalling pathways through p55 and p75 receptor, but in high concentrations only through p55 (Bigda et al., 1994). In young patients with newly diagnosed diabetes increased activity of TNF-α has been demonstrated (Myśliwiec et al, 2006). High levels of TNF-α have been detected also in type 1 diabetic children and adolescents with non-proliferative retinopathy (Myśliwiec et al, 2006, Zorena et al. 2007). TNF-α may become a relevant indicator of development and risk of diabetic retinopathy. Similar observations were made in adult patients with PDR (Gustavsson et al., 2008; Koleva-Georgieva et al., 2011). Levels of TNF-α in vitreous of Type 2 diabetic patients with PDR were higher than those found in control group. Furthermore a correlation between TNF-α and HbA1c is observed, suggesting that there is a close relation between glycaemic control and inflammatory factors in T2DM patients (Adamiec-Mroczek et al., 2008; Lee JH, 2008). TNFRI and TNFRII receptors' levels in vitreous of patients with PDR and proliferative vitreoretinopathy were much higher than in patients with perforation in macula (Limb et al., 2001). Attempts are being made to block TNF-α actions with monoclonal antibodies (Sfikkakis et al., 2010; Giganti et al., 2010; Biswas et al., 2010). In randomized studies, the intravenous use of infliximab has improved visual acuity in patients with diabetic macular edema (DME) (Sfikakis et al., 2010).

Etanercept is a soluble TNF-α receptor that acts as competitive inhibitor blocking effects of TNF-α binding to cells. Etanercept reduced leukocyte adherence in retinal blood vessels of diabetic rats for 1 week as compared to control. Etanercept did not reduce retinal VEGF levels, but it inhibited blood-retinal barrier breakdown and NF-κB activation in the diabetic retina (Joussen et al., 2002; Zheng et al., 2004).

5. Adipocytokines

5.1 Leptin

Leptin was discovered as a first adipocytokine in 1994 (Zhang Y et al., 1994). Team of researchers (Ates et al., 2008) have found relationship between leptin and retinal vein occlusion. The authors suggest that leptin may play a role in pathogenesis of retinal vein occlusion probably by influencing vessel wall homeostasis. In diabetes, leptin may affect angiogenesis process by induction of vascular endothelial growth factor (VEGF) and suppression of pigment epithelium derived factor (PEDF) and also production of intracellular reactive oxygen species (ROS) in retinal vascular endothelial cells. (Gariano et al. 2000, Yamagishi et al., 2003). However, in other studies the authors reported no association between leptin and the development and progression of retinopathy (Sari et al., 2010).

5.2 Adiponectin

Adiponectin is a 28 kD protein and its structure is similar to TNF-α, collagen VIII and IX and C1q molecule of complement. As demonstrated in vitro adiponectin exerts antyaterogenne, by inhibiting the adhesion of monocytes to endothelial cells and the transformation of macrophages into foam cells (Diez & Iglesias, 2003; Tan et al., 2004; Abi Khalil et al., 2011). Zhou et al., 2011 demonstrated that adiponectin hampers monocytes adhesion to endothelial cells in blood vessel walls by reduction in adhesive protein expression. The study also reported that adiponectin inhibits macrophages transformation into foam cells, reduces smooth muscle proliferation, increases NO synthesis and stimulates angiogenesis. Several studies present adiponectin as an anti-inflammatory cytokine (Matzuzawa et al., 2005; Goldberg et al., 2009; Zhou et al., 2011). In vitro studies revealed that TNF-α inhibits adiponectin gene expression through inhibition of nuclear factor NFκB, which is activated by adiponectin. Increasing insulin resistance and growth of adipose tissue increases TNF-alpha expression leading to a decrease of adiponectin concentration (Savino et al., 2008). Additional studies have shown that adiponectin directly stimulates the production of IL10 by macrophages and decreases the production of proinflammatory cytokines TNF-α and IL6 (Wulster-Radcliffe et al., 2004, Kumada et al., 2004, Kollias et al., 2011, Zhou et al., 2011). Adiponectin inhibits adhesive molecules expression in endothelial cells and also production of cytokines in macrophages thus reduces the inflammatory process which is present in early stages of atherosclerosis and microangiopathy (Diez & Iglesias, 2003; Goldberg et al., 2009). Increase in adiponectin level in serum is thought to be a response to endothelium damage (Schalwijk et al., 2006; Goldberg et al, 2009).Correlation was found between severity of diabetic retinopathy and adiponectin in patients with T1DM and T2DM (Frystyk et al., 2005; Zietz et al., 2008; Kato et al., 2008).

6. Chemokines

6.1 Stromal Cell-Derived Factor (SDF-1)

SDF-1 is a small cytokine of the chemokines family (C-X-C motif) or a ligand 12 (CXCL12). SDF-1 plays an important role in the angiogenesis by recruiting endothelial progenitor cells from bone marrow (Unoki et al, 2010). In the animal model it has been shown that VEGF, SDF-1 alpha and CXCR-4 all play part in the development of diabetic retinopathy. An increase in SDF-1 alpha expression has been observed, and it correlated with the duration of the disease(Lin et al., 2009) as well as with the level of pro-inflammatory cytokines IL-6 and IL-8 (Otsuka et al, 2010). An increase in SDF-1 concentration in the vitreous has been observed also in patients with proliferative retinopathy, the more pronounced, the more acute had been the disease course (Meleth et al., 2005; Chen et al., 2008).

6.2 Monocyte Chemotactic Protein-1 (CCL2/MCP-1)

Chemokine (C-C motif) ligand 2 (CCL2) is a small cytokine belonging to the CC chemokine family that is also known as monocyte chemotactic protein-1 (MCP-1) and small inducible cytokine A2. CCL2 is a monomeric polypeptide, with a molecular weight of approximately 13kD (Yoshimura & Leonard., 1992). The cell surface receptors that bind CCL2 are CCR2 and CCR4 (Xia & Sui.,2009). MCP-1, as well as its interaction with CCR2, plays a pivotal role in mediating persistent mononuclear phagocyte infiltration that leads to chronic inflammatory (Romagnani et al., 2004). Inhibition of CCL2-CCR2 signalling blocks the recruitment of inflammatory monocytes, inhibits metastasis in vivo and prolongs the survival of tumour-bearing mice (Qian et al., 2011). Also, MCP-1 has been recognized as an angiogenic chemokine (Strieter et al.,2005). In vivo angiogenesis assays showed that MCP-1-induced angiogenesis was as potent as that induced by vascular endothelial growth factor (VEGF). The angiogenic effect of MCP-1 was completely inhibited by a VEGF inhibitor, suggesting that MCP-1-induced angiogenesis is mediated through pathways involving VEGF (Kim et al., 2005). In young patients with long term diabetes and microangiopathy levels of CCL2/MCP-1 were higher than in those without microangiopathy (Zorena et al., 2010). The authors suggest active role of this chemokine in onset and development of diabetic retinopathy. Increased level of CCL2/MCP-1 was higher also in the vitreous of adult patients in PDR. (Hernandez et al., 2005; Abu El-Asrar et al., 2006). The aqueous levels of MCP-1, IP-10, IL-8, and VEGF were higher in the eyes of diabetic patients than in the eyes of non-diabetic subjects. The aqueous levels of MCP-1 and IP-10 were elevated in the eyes with severe NPDR and PDR compared to eyes with less severe DR and eyes of non-diabetic subjects (Oh et al., 2010).

7. Matrix metalloproteinases (MMPs) and metalloproteinase inhibitors (TIMP)

7.1 Metalloproteinases (MMPs)

Increased levels of metalloproteinases such as MMP-2, MMP-9 and MMP-14 have been demonstrated in early stages of retinopathy (Giebel et al., 2005). It has been demonstrated that high glucose increases the production of MMP-9 in retina cells (Kovluru et al., 2010; Mohammad & Kowluru, 2011). Increased level of MMPs leads to faster degradation of basement membrane proteins thereby increasing permeability. Pericyte apoptosis and basement membrane changes result in dilatation of capillaries and formation of microaneurisms. These conditions impair blood flow and in consequence lead to ischaemia in the retina. Disruption of physiological blood-retina barrier leads to formation of hard exudates. Retinal hypoxia worsens abnormalities in MMP/TIMP system caused by hyperglycaemia leading to excessive production of basement membrane material and proliferation of pathological capillaries. During retinal hypoxia the production of growth factors including VEGF increases, which stimulates metalloproteinases expression in extracellular matrix. It has been noted that in proliferative retinopathy the MMP-2 and MMP-9 activity increases (Jacqueminet et al., 2006, Kowluru et al., 2010).

7.2 Tissue inhibitor of matrix metalloproteinase 3 (TIMP-3)

Tissue inhibitor of matrix metalloproteinase 3 (TIMP-3) belongs to zinc (Zn) binding endopeptidases group which takes part in remodelling and degradation of extracellular matrix. In the eye TIMP-3 is closely related to Bruch's membrane and regulates angiogenesis (Janssen et al., 2008). Analysis of micromatrix demonstrated that out of investigated metalloproteinases and its inhibitors: MMP1, MMP2, MMP11, MMP14, MMP25, TIMP1, TIMP2, TIMP3 and TIMP4 which were present in pericytes, only TIMIP3 mRNA may play role in impairment of microcirculation in diabetic retinopathy (Barth et al., 2007).

8. Conclusion

In developed countries diabetic retinopathy has become the most prevalent cause of blindness and loss of visual acuity, and its incidence is on the rise. Occurrence and progression of diabetic retinopathy may be a result of activation of immunological cells in the metabolic imbalance of the disease. Late diabetic complications may also reflect the ongoing autoimmunological process that started already in the *prediabetic* period. It has been proved that plasma levels of pro-inflammatory/pro-angiogenic factors was higher in patients with proliferative retinopathy than in those with diabetes but without morphological changes in the eye fundus. Moreover, high concentrations of VEGF, TNF-α, IL-6 has been found not only in plasma but also in the vitreous of PDR patients. High hopes have been placed on the use of monoclonal antibodies anti-VEGF and anti-TNF. Particularly etanercept, bevacizumab and ranibizumab have been used to prevent ocular neovascularisation. However only concomitant use of several therapeutic methods is regarded as effective in achieving plausible results in treatment of proliferative retinopathy.

9. References

Abrahamsson J, Påhlman M, Mellander L. (1997). Interleukin 6, but not tumour necrosis factor-alpha, is a good predictor of severe infection in febrile neutropenic and non-neutropenic children with malignancy. *Acta Paediatr.*, 86(10):1059-64.

Abi Khalil C, Mohammedi K, Aubert R, Abou Jaoude E, Travert F, Hadjadj S, Fumeron F, Roussel R, Marre M.(2011). Hyperadiponectinemia is independent of kidney function, diabetes duration, and control in type 1 diabetic patients without microangiopathy. *J Clin Endocrinol Metab.*,96(3):E485-7

Abu El-Asrar A.M., Struyf S., Kangave D. (2006). Chemokines in proliferative diabetic retinopathy and proliferative vitreoretinopathy. *Eur Cytokine Netw*, 17, 155-65.

Abu El-Asrar AM, Missotten L, Geboes K. (2010). Expression of advanced glycation end products and related molecules in diabetic fibrovascular epiretinal membranes. *Clin Experiment Ophthalmol.*, 38(1):57-64; .

Adamiec-Mroczek J, Oficjalska-Młyńczak J. (2008). Assessment of selected adhesion molecule and proinflammatory cytokine levels in the vitreous body of patients with type 2 diabetes--role of the inflammatory-immune process in the pathogenesis of proliferative diabetic retinopathy. *Graefes Arch Clin Exp Ophthalmol*, 246(12):1665-70

Adamiec-Mroczek J, Oficjalska-Młyńczak J, Misiuk-Hojło M. (2010). Roles of endothelin-1 and selected proinflammatory cytokines in the pathogenesis of proliferative diabetic retinopathy: Analysis of vitreous samples. *Cytokine*, (49) 3: 269-74

Adamis AP, Altaweel M, Bressler NM, Cunningham Jr ET, Davis MD, Goldbaum M (2006). Changes in retinal neovascularization after pegaptanib (Macugen) therapy in diabetic individuals. *Ophthalmology.*;113:23–8.

Aiello LP, Avery RL, Arrigg PG, Keyt BA, Jampel HD, Shah ST, Pasquale LR, Thieme H, Iwamoto MA, Park JE, et al. (1994). Vascular endothelial growth factor in ocular fluid of patients with diabetic retinopathy and other retinal disorders. *N Engl J Med* 331: 1480–1487.

Apte RS, Richter J, Herndon J, Ferguson TA. (2006). Macrophages inhibit neovascularization in a murine model of age-related macular degeneration. *PLoS Med.* 3:e310.

Ates O, Keles M, Bilen H, Kiziltunc A, Kocer I, Kulacoglu DN, Türkeli M, Baykal O. (2008). Increased serum levels of leptin in retinal vein occlusion. *Tohoku J Exp Med.*, 215(4):373-6.

Barnstable C, Tombran-Tink J. (2004). Neuroprotective and antiangiogenic actions of PEDF in the eye: molecular targets and therapeutic potential. *Prog. Retin Eye Res.*, 23: 561–577

Barth JL, Yu Y, Song W, Lu K, Dashti A, Huang Y, Argraves WS, Lyons TJ. (2007). Oxidised, glycated LDL selectively influences tissue inhibitor of metalloproteinase-3 gene expression and protein production in human retinal capillary pericytes. *Diabetologia*, 10: 2200-8.

Bertolino P, Deckers M, Lebrin F, Ten Dijke P. (2005). Transforming growth factor-β signal transduction in angiogenesis and vascular disorders. *Chest*, 128(6 Suppl):585S-590S.

Bigda J, Beletsky C, Brakebusch Y. (1994). Dual role of the p75 tumor necrosis factor (TNF) receptor in TNF cytotoxicity. *J Exp Med,* 180, 2, 445-460

Biswas NR, Das GK, Dubey AK. (2010). Monoclonal antibodies in ophthalmology. *Nepal Med Coll J.,*12(4):264-71.

Bradshaw EM, Raddassi K, Elyaman W, Orban T, Gottlieb PA, Kent SC, Hafler DA. (2009). Monocytes from patients with type 1 diabetes spontaneously secrete proinflammatory cytokines inducing Th17 cells. *J Immunol,* 183(7):4432-9

Campa C, Costagliola C, Incorvaia C, Sheridan C, Semeraro F, De Nadai K, Sebastiani A, Parmeggiani F. (2010). Inflammatory mediators and angiogenic factors in choroidal neovascularization: pathogenetic interactions and therapeutic implications. *Mediators Inflamm.* pii: 546826

Campochiaro PA. (2006). Potential applications for RNAi to probe pathogenesis and develop new treatments for ocular disorders. *Gene Ther.,*13(6):559–562

Caporali A, Emanueli C. (2011). MicroRNA regulation in angiogenesis. *Vascul Pharmacol,* Jul 14. [Epub ahead of print]

Cai J, Jiang WG, Grant MB, Boulton M. (2006). Pigment epithelium-derived factor inhibits angiogenesis via regulated intracellular proteolysis of vascular endothelial growth factor receptor 1. *J. Biol. Chem,* 281: 3604–3613

Cai J, Wu L, Qi X, Li Calzi S, Caballero S, Shaw L, Ruan Q, Grant MB, Boulton ME. (2011). PEDF Regulates Vascular Permeability by a γ-Secretase-Mediated Pathway. *PLoS One.* 6(6):e21164

Carmeliet P. (2003). Angiogenesis in health and disease. *Nat Med,* 9: 653–660.

Chen L, Lü L, Li Y, Huang X, Zhang J, Li S. (2008). Vitreous levels of stromal cell-derived factor-1 and vascular endothelial growth factor in diabetic retinopathy. *Yan Ke Xue Bao,* 24(1):6-8

Chiarelli F, Spagnoli A, Basciani F, Tumini S, Mezzetti A, Cipollone F, Cuccurullo F, Morgese G, Verrotti A. (2000). Vascular endothelial growth factor (VEGF) in children, adolescents and young adults with type 1 diabetes mellitus: relation to glycaemic control and microvascular complications. *Diabet Med,* 17(9):650-6.

Chiarelli F, Pomilo M, Mohn A, Tumini S, Verrotti A, Mezzetti A, Cipollone F, Wasniewska M, Morgese G, Spagnoli A. (2002). Serum angiogenin concentrations in young patients with diabetes mellitus. *Eur J Clin Invest,* 32(2):110-4.

Cho YH, Craig ME, Hing S, Gallego PH, Poon M, Chan A, Donaghue KC (2011). Microvascular complications assessment in adolescents with 2- to 5-yr duration of type 1 diabetes from 1990 to 2006. *Pediatr Diabetes* [Epub ahead of print] Article by DOI 10.1111/j.1399-5448.2011.00762

Christinger HW, Fuh G, de Vos AM, Wiesmann C. (2004). The crystal structure of placental growth factor in complex with domain 2 of vascular endothelial growth factor receptor-1. *J Biol Chem,* 279:10382–10388

Coulon J, Willems D, Dorchy H. (2005). Increase in C-reactive protein plasma levels during diabetes in infants and young adults. *Presse Med.,*34(2 Pt 1):89-93.

Curtis TM, Gardiner TA, Stitt AW. (2009). Microvascular lesions of diabetic retinopathy: clues towards understanding pathogenesis? *Eye (Lond),* 23(7):1496-508

Czepluch FS, Zweigle B, Waltenberger J. (2009). Chemotaxis analysis of circulating monocytes in patients with a recent acute coronary syndrome. *Atherosclerosis.* 204(1):304-8

D'Adamo E, Caprio S. (2011). Type 2 diabetes in youth: epidemiology and pathophysiology. *Diabetes Care*. 34 Suppl 2:S161-5.

Dace DS, Apte RS. (2008). Effect of senescence on macrophage polarization and angiogenesis. *Rejuvenation Res*.11(1):177-85

Dace DS, Khan AA, Kelly J, Apte RS. (2008). Interleukin-10 promotes pathological angiogenesis by regulating macrophage response to hypoxia during development. *pLoS ONE*; 3(10):e3381.

Deissler HL, Deissler H, Lang GE. (2011). Inhibition of vascular endothelial growth factor (VEGF) is sufficient to completely restore barrier malfunction induced by growth factors in microvascular retinal endothelial cells. *Br J Ophthalmol*, 95(8):1151-6

Diez J, Iglesias P. (2003). The role of novel adipocyte -derived hormone adiponectin in human disease. *Eur J Endocrinol*, 148,288-293

Doganay S, Evereklioglu C, Turkoz ERH, Sevinc A, Mehmet N, Savli H. (2002). Comparision of serum NO, TNFα, IL-1β, sIL-2R, IL-6 and IL-8 levels with grades of retinopathy in patients with diabetes mellitus. *Eye*,16:163-70.

Doll J.A., Stellmach V.M., Bouck N.P., Bergh A.R., Lee C., Abramson L.P., Cornwell M.L., Pins M.R., Borensztajn J., Crawford S.E. (2003). Pigment epithelium-derived factor regulates the vasculature and mass of the prostate and pancreas. *Nat. Med.*, 9: 774-780

Durham JT, Herman IM. (2011). Microvascular modifications in diabetic retinopathy. *Curr Diab Rep*.;11(4):253-64.

Elayappan B, Ravinarayannan H, Pasha SP, Lee KJ, Gurunathan S (2009). PEDF inhibits VEGF- and EPO- induced angiogenesis in retinal endothelial cells through interruption of PI3K/Akt phosphorylation. *Angiogenesis*,12(4):313-24.

Engelbert M, Zweifel SA. and Freund KB. (2010;2011). Long-term follow-up for type 1 (subretinal pigment epithelium) neovascularisation using a modified "treat and extend" dosing regimen of intravitreal antivascular endothelial growth factor therapy, *Retina*, 30(9):1368-75. Erratum in: *Retina*. 2011 Jan;31(1):208.

Fajardo LF Kwan HH, Kowalski J, Prionas SD, Allison AC. (1992). Dual role of tumor necrosis factor-alpha in angiogenesis. *Am J Pathol*,140(3):539.

Feeney SA, Simpson DA, Gardiner TA, Boyle C, Jamison P, et al. (2003). Role of vascular endothelial growth factor and placental growth factors during retinal vascular development and hyaloid regression. *Invest Ophthalmol Vis Sci*.;44(2):839–847

Ferrara N, Gerber HP, LeCouter J. (2003). The biology of VEGF and its receptors. *Nat Med*. 2003;9:669–676

Ferrara N. (2004). Vascular endothelial growth factor: basic science and clinical progress. *Endocr Rev*, 25: 581-611.

Filleur S, Nelius T, de Riese W, Kennedy RC (2009). Characterization of PEDF: a multi-functional serpin family protein. *J. Cell. Biochem*, 106: 769–75

Folkman J (1971): Tumour angiogenesis: therapeutic implications. *N Engl J Med*, 285: 1182–1185.

Fong, D.S. Aiello, L.P. Ferris F.L. III and Klein R. (2004). Diabetic retinopathy, *Diabetes Care* 27, pp. 2540–2553

Frystyk J, Tarnow L, Hansen TK, Parving HH, Flyvbjerg A. (2005). Increased serum adiponectin levels in type 1 diabetic patients with microvascular complications. *Diabetologia*. 48(9):1911-8

Funk M, Schmidinger G, Maar N, Bolz M, Benesch T, Zlabinger GJ, Schmidt-Erfurth UM. (2010). Angiogenic and inflammatory markers in the intraocular fluid of eyes with diabetic macular edema and influence of therapy with bevacizumab. *Retina.* 30(9):1412-9.

Gallego PH, Craig ME, Hing S, Donaghue KC (2008).. Role of blood pressure in development of early retinopathy in adolescents with type 1 diabetes: prospective cohort study. *BMJ,* 337: a918.

Gariano R, Nath A, D'Amico D. (2000). Elevation of vitreous leptin in diabetic retinopathy and retinal detachment. *Invest Ophthalmol Vis Sci,* 41: 3576-81.

George B, Chen S, Chaudhary V, Gonder J, Chakrabarti S. (2009). Extracellular matrix proteins in epiretinal membranes and in diabetic retinopathy. *Curr Eye Res.* Feb;34(2):134-44.

Gerhardinger C, McClure KD, Romeo G, Podesta F, Lorenzi M. (2001). IGF-I mRNA and signaling in the diabetic retina. *Diabetes.* 50: 175–183.

Ghiringhelli F, Menard C, Martin F, Zitvogel L (2006). The role of regulatory T cells in the control of natural killer cells: relevance during tumor progression. *Immunol Rev,* 214: 229-238.

Giacco F, Brownlee M. (2010). Oxidative stress and diabetic complications. *Circ Res.,*107(9):1058-70

Giebel SJ, Menicucci G, McGuire PG, Das A.(2005). Matrix metalloproteinases in early diabetic retinopathy and their role in alteration of the blood-retinal barrier. *Lab Invest,* 85(5):597-607.

Giganti M, Beer PM, Lemanski N, Hartman C, Schartman J, Falk N. (2010). Adverse events after intravitreal infliximab (Remicade). *Retina.* 30(1):71-80.

Goes N, Urmson J, Vincent D, Ramassar V, Halloran PF. (1996). Effect of recombinant human insulin- like growth factor-1 on the inflammatory response to acute renal injury. *J. Am. Soc. Nephrol.,* 7, 710-720.

Goldberg RB. (2009). Cytokine and cytokine-like inflammation markers, endothelial dysfunction, and imbalanced coagulation in development of diabetes and its complications. *J Clin Endocrinol Metab.*94(9):3171-82.

Gustavsson C, Agardh E, Bengtsson B, Agardh CD. (2008). TNF-alpha is an independent serum marker for proliferative retinopathy in type 1 diabetic patients. *J Diabetes Complications,* 22(5):309-16.

Hartnett ME, Tinkham N, Paynter L, Geisen P, Rosenberg P, Koch G, Cohen KL. (2009). Aqueous vascular endothelial growth factor as a predictor of macular thickening following cataract surgery in patients with diabetes mellitus. *Am J Ophthalmol.*148(6):895-901.e

Haurigot V, Villacampa P, Ribera A, Llombart C, Bosch A, Nacher V, Ramos D, Ayuso E, Segovia JC, Bueren JA, Ruberte J, Bosch F.(2009). Increased intraocular insulin-like growth factor-I triggers blood-retinal barrier breakdown. *J Biol Chem.* 284(34):22961-9

Hernández-Da Mota and Nuñez-Solorio S.M. (2010). Experience with intravitreal bevacizumab as a preoperative adjunct in 23-G vitrectomy for advanced proliferative diabetic retinopathy, *Eur. J. Ophthalmol.* 20, pp. 1047–1052

Hernández C, Segura RM, Fonollosa A, Carrasco E, Francisco G, Simó R. (2005). Interleukin-8, monocyte chemoattractant protein-1 and IL-10 in the vitreous fluid of patients with proliferative diabetic retinopathy. *Diabet Med.* 22, 719-22.

Hills CE, Squires PE. (2011). The role of TGF-β and epithelial-to mesenchymal transition in diabetic nephropathy. *Cytokine Growth Factor Rev*, 2011 Jul 12. [Epub ahead of print]

Hooper LC, Chin MS, Detrick B, Hooks JJ. (2005). Retinal degeneration in experimental coronavirus retinopathy (ECOR) is associated with increased TNF-alpha, soluble TNFR2 and altered TNF-alpha signaling. *J Neuroimmunol.* 166(1-2):65-74.

Hornan D, Edmeades N, Krishnan R, Khan J, Lochhead J. (2010). Use of pegaptanib for recurrent and non-clearing vitreous haemorrhage in proliferative diabetic retinopathy. *Eye (Lond).* 24:1315–9.

Iglesias-de la Cruz MC, Ziyadeh FN, Isono M, Kouahou M, Han DC, Kalluri R (2002). Effects of high glucose and TGF-beta1 on the expression of collagen IV and vascular endothelial growth factor in mouse podocytes. *Kidney Int.,* 62: 901–913.

Imai D, Yoneya S, Gehlbach PL, Wei LL, Mori K. (2005). Intraocular gene transfer of pigment epithelium-derived factor rescues photoreceptors from light-induced cell death. *J Cell Physiol.* 202(2):570-8.

Inagaki Y, Yamagishi S, Okamoto T, Takeuchi M, Amano S. (2003). Pigment epitheliumderived factor prevents advanced glycation end products-induced monocyte chemoattractant protein-1 production in microvascular endothelial cells by suppressing intracellular reactive oxygen species generation. *Diabetologia;* 46: 284-7.

IDF Atlas . http://www.diabetesatlas.org/

Jacqueminet S, Ben Abdesselam O, Chapman MJ, Nicolay N, Foglietti MJ, Grimaldi A, Beaudeux JL. (2006). Elevated circulating levels of matrix metalloproteinase-9 in type 1 diabetic patients with and without retinopathy. *Clin Chim Acta.* 367(1-2):103-7

Janssen A, Hoellenriegel J, Fogarasi M, Schrewe H, Seeliger M, Tamm E, Ohlmann A, May CA, Weber BH, Stöhr H. (2008). Abnormal vessel formation in the choroid of mice lacking tissue inhibitor of metalloprotease-3. *Invest Ophthalmol Vis Sci.* 7: 2812-2

Jarosz-Chobot P, Polanska J, Szadkowska A, Kretowski A, Bandurska-Stankiewicz E, Ciechanowska M, Deja G, Mysliwiec M, Peczynska J, Rutkowska J, Sobel-Maruniak A, Fichna P, Chobot A, Rewers M.(2011). Rapid increase in the incidence of type 1 diabetes in Polish children from 1989 to 2004, and predictions for 2010 to 2025. *Diabetologia,* 54(3):508-15.

Jorge R, Oliveira RS, Messias A, Almeida FP, Strambe ML, Costa RA, Scott IU. (2011). Ranibizumab for retinal neovascularization. *Ophthalmology,* 118(5):1004-1004.e1.

Joussen AM, Poulaki V, Mitsiades N, Kirchhof B, Koizumi K, Döhmen S, Adamis AP. (2002),. Nonsteroidal anti-inflammatory drugs prevent early diabetic retinopathy via TNF-alpha suppression. *FASEB J.*16(3):438-40

Kataoka K, Nishiguchi KM, Kaneko H, van Rooijen N, Kachi S, Terasaki H. (2011). The roles of vitreal macrophages and circulating leukocytes in retinal neovascularization. *Invest Ophthalmol Vis Sci.* 52(3):1431-8.

Kato K, Osawa H, Ochi M, Kusunoki Y, Ebisui O, Ohno K, Ohashi J, Shimizu I, Fujii Y, Tanimoto M, Makino H. (2008). Serum total and high molecular weight adiponectin levels are correlated with the severity of diabetic retinopathy and nephropathy. *Clin Endocrinol (Oxf).* 68(3):442-9.

Kelly J, Ali Khan A, Yin J, Ferguson TA, Apte RS. (2007). Senescence regulates macrophage activation and angiogenic fate at sites of tissue injury in mice. *J Clin Invest.* 117: 3421-3426.

Khaliq A, Foreman D, Ahmed A, Weich H, Gregor Z, McLeod D Boulton M. (1998). Increased expression of placenta growth factor in proliferative diabetic retinopathy. *Lab Invest.* 78, 109-16.

Kielczewski JL, Hu P, Shaw LC, Li Calzi S, Mames RN, Gardiner TA, McFarland E, Chan-Ling T, Grant MB. (2011) Novel protective properties of IGFBP-3 result in enhanced pericyte ensheathment, reduced microglial activation, increased microglial apoptosis, and neuronal protection after ischemic retinal injury. *Am J Pathol.* 178:1517-28.

Kim MY, Byeon CW, Hong KH, Han KH, Jeong S. (2005). Inhibition of angiogenesis by the MCP-1 (monocyte chemoattractant protein-1) binding peptide. *FEBS Lett.* 579: 1597-601.

Koleva-Georgieva DN, Sivkova NP, Terzieva D. (2011). Serum inflammatory cytokines IL-1beta, IL-6, TNF-alpha and VEGF have influence on the development of diabetic retinopathy. *Folia Med (Plovdiv).* 53(2):44-50.

Kollias A, Tsiotra PC, Ikonomidis I, Maratou E, Mitrou P, Kyriazi E, Boutati E, Lekakis J, Economopoulos T, Kremastinos DT, Dimitriadis G, Raptis SA. (2011). Adiponectin levels and expression of adiponectin receptors in isolated monocytes from overweight patients with coronary artery disease. *Cardiovasc Diabetol,* 1;10:14.

Kowluru RA, Zhong Q, Kanwar M. (2010). Metabolic memory and diabetic retinopathy: role of inflammatory mediators in retinal pericytes. *Exp Eye Res.*90(5):617-23

Kumada M, S. Kihara, O. Noriyuki, H. Kobayashi, Y. Okamoto, K. Ohashi, K. Maeda, H. Nagarentani, K. Kishida, N. Maeda, A. Nagasawa, T. Funahashi, Matsuzawa Y. (2004). Adiponectin specifically increased tissue inhibitor of metalloproteinase-1 through interleukin-10 expression in human macrophages, *Circles 109,* 2046– 2049.

Kvanta A. (2006). Ocular angiogenesis: The role of growth factors. *Acta phthalmol Scand;* 84: 282-288.

Lamoureux EL, Wong TY. (2011). Diabetic retinopathy in 2011: further insights from new epidemiological studies and clinical trials. *Diabetes Care,* 34(4):1066-7.

Lange CA, Stavrakas P, Luhmann UF, de Silva DJ, Ali RR, Gregor ZJ, Bainbridge JW. (2011). Intraocular Oxygen Distribution in Advanced Proliferative Diabetic Retinopathy. Am J Ophthalmol. [Epub ahead of print]

Lee JH, Lee W, Kwon OH, Kim JH, Kwon OW, Kim KH, Lim JB. (2008). Cytokine profile of peripheral blood in type 2 diabetes mellitus patients with diabetic retinopathy. *Ann Clin Lab Sci.*38(4):361-7.

Limb G, Hollifield R, Webster L, Charteris D, Chignell A. (2001). Soluble TNF receptors in vitreoretinal proliferati−ve disease. *Invest Ophthalmol Vis Sci,* 142, 1586–1591.

Lin A, Lei M, Xie X, Xu H. (2009). Expression and meaning of pro-angiogenic factors in retinopathy of diabetic rats. *Zhong Nan Da Xue Xue Bao Yi Xue Ban.* 34(12):1243-50

Lo Hui-Chen, Lin Su-Chen, Wang Yu-Mei. (2004). The relationship among serum cytokines, chemokine, nitric oxide, and leptin in children with type 1 diabetes mellitus. *Clin Bioch,* 37: 666-72

Löfqvist C, Engström E, Sigurdsson J, Hård AL, Niklasson A, Ewald U, Holmström G, Smith LE, Hellström A. (2006). Postnatal head growth deficit among premature infants parallels retinopathy of prematurity and insulin-like growth factor-1 deficit. *Pediatrics,* 117, 1930-1938.

Losso JN, Truax RE, Richard G. (2010). Trans-resveratrol inhibits hyperglycemia-induced inflammation and connexin downregulation in retinal pigment epithelial cells. *J Agric Food Chem.* 58(14):8246-52.

Maier R., Weger M., Haller-Schober E.M., El-Shabrawi Y., Theisl A., Barth A., Aigner R. (2006). Haas A Application of multiplex cytometric bead array technology for the measurement of angiogenic factors in the vitreous. *Mol Vis.*12:1143-7.

Maier R, Weger M, Haller-Schober EM, El-Shabrawi Y, Wedrich A, Theisl A, Aigner R, Barth A, Haas A. (2008). Multiplex bead analysis of vitreous and serum concentrations of inflammatory and proangiogenic factors in diabetic patients. *Mol Vis.*14:637-43.

Marek N, Myśliwiec M, Raczyńska K, Zorena K, Myśliwska J, Trzonkowski P. (2010) Increased spontaneous production of VEGF by CD4+ T cells in type 1 diabetes. *Clin Immunol.*137:261-70.

Marek N, Raczyńska K, Siebert J, Myśliwiec M, Zorena K, Myśliwska J, Reiwer-Gostomska M, Trzonkowski P. (2011). Decreased angiogenin concentration in vitreous and serum in proliferative diabetic retinopathy. *Microvasc Res*, 82(1):1-5.

Matsumoto Y, Takahashi M, Ogata M. Relationship between glycoxidation and cytokines in the vitreous of eyes with diabetic retinopathy. Jpn J Ophthalmol. 2002 Jul-Aug;46(4):406-12.

Matzuzawa Y. (2005). Adiponectin: identification, physiology and clinical relevance in metabolic and vascular disease. *Atheroscler Suppl* ; 6:7-14.

Meleth AD, Agrón E, Chan CC, Reed GF, Arora K, Byrnes G, Csaky KG, Ferris FL 3rd, Chew EY. (2005). Serum inflammatory markers in diabetic retinopathy. *Invest Ophthalmol Vis Sci.* 46(11):4295-301.

Miyamoto N, de Kozak Y, Jeanny JC, Glotin A, Mascarelli F, Massin P, BenEzra D, Behar-Cohen F. (2007). Placental growth factor-1 and epithelial haemato-retinal barrier breakdown: potential implication in the pathogenesis of diabetic retinopathy. *Diabetologia.* 50(2):461-70

Mohammad G, Kowluru RA. (2010). Matrix metalloproteinase-2 in the development of diabetic retinopathy and mitochondrial dysfunction. *Lab Invest.* 90(9):1365-72.

Mohammad G, Kowluru RA. (2011). Diabetic retinopathy and signaling mechanism for activation of matrix metalloproteinase-9. *J Cell Physiol.* doi: 10.1002/jcp.22822.

Myśliwiec M, Balcerska A, Zorena K, Myśliwska J, Nowacka M, Lipowski P, Raczyńska K. (2006). Selected immunologic and biochemical risk factors of the retinopathy and nephropathy development in children with diabetes mellitus type 1. *Endokrynologia, Diabetologia i Choroby Przemiany Materii Wieku Rozwojowego.* 4: 269-273.

Myśliwiec M, Zorena K, Balcerska A, Myśliwska J, Lipowski P, Raczyński K. (2006). The activity of N-acetyl-beta-D-glucosaminidase and tumor necrosis factor-alpha at early stage of diabetic retinopathy development in type 1 diabetes mellitus children. *Clinical Biochemistry* 39: 851-856.

Myśliwiec M, Balcerska A, Zorena K, Myśliwska J, Lipowski P, Raczyńska K. (2008). The role of vascular endothelial growth factor, tumor necrosis factor alpha and interleukin-6 in pathogenesis of diabetic retinopathy. Diabetes Research and Clinical Practice; 79:141-146.

Naldini A, Carraro F. (2005). Role of inflammatory mediators in angiogenesis. Curr Drug Targets Inflamm Allergy.

Nandi D, Mishra MK, Basu A, Bishayi B. (2010). Protevtive effects of interleukin-6 in lipopolisacharide (LPS)-induced experimental endotoxemia are linked to alteration in hepatic anti-oxidant enzymes and endogenous cytokines. *Immunobiology*, 215:443-451.

National Health and Nutrition Examination Survey 1999–2002. (2006). Prevalence of diabetes and impaired fasting glucose in adults in the U.S. population. *Diabetes Care*, 29:1263–1268.

Noma H, Funatsu H, Mimura T, Harino S, Hori S. (2009). Vitreous levels of interleukin-6 and vascular endothelial growth factor in macular edema with central retinal vein occlusion. *Ophthalmology*, 116(1):87-93.

Oh IK, Kim SW, Oh J, Lee TS, Huh K. (2010). Inflammatory and angiogenic factors in the aqueous humor and the relationship to diabetic retinopathy. *Curr Eye Res*.35(12):1116-27.

Orlova VV, Liu Z, Goumans MJ, Ten Dijke P. (2011). Controlling angiogenesis by two unique TGF-β type I receptor signaling pathways. *Histol Histopathol*. 26(9):1219-30.

Otsuka H, Arimura N, Sonoda S, Nakamura M, Hashiguchi T, Maruyama I, Nakao S, Hafezi-Moghadam A, Sakamoto T. (2010). Stromal cell-derived factor-1 is essential for photoreceptor cell protection in retinal detachment. *Am J Pathol*.177(5):2268-77

Patterson C, Parrella MA, Endege WO, Yoshizumi M, Lee Mu-En, Haber E. *(1996)*, Dowregulation of Vascular Endothelial Growth Factor Receptors by Tumor Necrosis Factor-alpha in Cultured Human Vascular Endothelial Cells. *J Clin Invest. 98,2, 490-96.*

Patterson CC, Dahlquist GG, Gyürüs E, Green A, Soltész G (2009) EURODIAB Study Group. Incidence trends for childhood type 1 diabetes in Europe during 1989-2003 and predicted new cases 2005-20: a multicentre prospective registration study. *Lancet* 373:2027-3

Peczyńska J, Urban M, Urban B, Głowińska B, Florys B. (2004). Assessment of growth factor levels in adolescents with type 1 diabetes mellitus and the beginning of diabetic microangiopathy. *Pediatr Endocrinol Diabetes Metab*, 10(1):41-8.

Pérez-Muñuzuri A, Fernández-Lorenzo JR, Couce-Pico ML, Blanco-Teijeiro MJ, Fraga-Bermúdez JM. (2010). Serum levels of IGF1 are a useful predictor of retinopathy of prematurity. *Acta Paediatr*, 99(4):519-25

Polykandriotis E, Arkudas A, Beier JP, Dragu A, Rath S, Pryymachuk G, Schmidt VJ, Lametschwandtner A, Horch RE, Kneser U. (2011). The impact of VEGF and bFGF on vascular stereomorphology in the context of angiogenic neo-arborisation after vascular induction. *J Electron Microsc* (Tokyo).

Poulaki V, Joussen AM, Mitsiades N, Mitsiades CS, Iliaki EF, Adamis AP. (2004). Insulin-like growth factor-I plays a pathogenetic role in diabetic retinopathy. *Am J Pathol.* 165(2):457-69.

Praidou A, Androudi S, Brazitikos P, Karakiulakis G, Papakonstantinou E, Dimitrakos S. (2010). Angiogenic growth factors and their inhibitors in diabetic retinopathy. *Curr Diabetes Rev*, 6(5):304-12

Querques G, Bux AV, Martinelli D, Iaculli C, Noci ND. (2009). Intravitreal pegaptanib sodium (Macugen) for diabetic macular oedema. *Acta Ophthalmol*.;87:623–30

Raczyńska K, Zorena K, Myśliwska J, Myśliwiec M, Raczyńska-Woźniak D, Balcerska A. (2008). Analysis of the Pro-Angiogenic Factor Influencing the Development of

Retinopathy in Children with Diabetes Mellitus Type 1. *Polish Journal of Environmental Studies,* Vol.17, 1A: 132-136.

Rakic JM, Lambert V, Devy L, Luttun A, Carmeliet P, et al. (2003). Placenta growth factor, a member of the VEGF Family, contribute to the development of choroidal neovascularization. *Invest Ophthalmol Vis Sci.* 44(7):3186–3193.

Romagnani P, Lasagni L, Annunziato F, Serio M, Romagnani S, (2004) CXC chemokines: the regulatory link between inflammation and angiogenesis. *Trends Immunol,* 25, 201-9

Rosenfeld PJ. (2011). Bevacizumab versus ranibizumab for AMD. N Engl J Med. 2011 May 19;364(20):1966-7. Epub

Rosenthal R, Malek G, Salomon N, Peill-Meininghaus M, Coeppicus L, Wohlleben H, Wimmers S, Bowes Rickman C, Strauss O. (2005). The fibroblast growth factor receptors, FGFR1 and FGFR2, mediate two independent signalling pathways in human retinal pigment epithelial cells. *Biochem. Biophys. Res. Commun.* 337, 241–247.

Rosenson RS, Fioretto P, Dodson PM. (2011). Does microvascular disease predict macrovascular events in type 2 diabetes? Atherosclerosis. [Epub ahead of print]

Roy S, Trudeau K, Roy S, Behl Y, Dhar S, Chronopoulos A. (2010). New insights into hyperglycemia-induced molecular changes in microvascular cells. *J Dent Res* 89:116-27

Saika S, Yamanaka O, Okada Y, Tanaka S, Miyamoto T, Sumioka T, Kitano A, Shirai K, Ikeda K. (2009). TGF beta in fibroproliferative diseases in the eye. Front Biosci (Schol Ed). 1:376-90.

Sall JW, Klisovic DD, O'Dorisio MS, Katz SE. (2004). Somatostatin inhibits IGF-1 mediated induction of VEGF in human retinal pigment epithelial cells. *Exp Eye Res.* 79(4):465-76.

Sanchez RN, Chan CK, Garg S, Kwong JM, Wong MJ, Sadun AA, Lam TT. (2003). Interleukin-6 in retinal ischemia reperfusion injury in rats. *Invest Ophtalmol Vis Sci.* 44:4006-4011.

Sansó Sureda A Rocamora Durán V Sapiña Camaró A Royo Escosa V Bosque López MJ. (2011). Ustekinumab in a patient with Crohn's disease and anti-TNF-α-induced psoriasis. *Gastroenterol Hepatol.* [Epub ahead of print]

Santilli F, Spagnoli A, Mohn A, Tumini S, Verrotti A, Cipollone F, Mezzetti A, Chiarelli F. (2001). Increased vascular endothelial growth factor serum concentrations may help to identify patients with onset of type 1 diabetes during childhood at risk for developing persistent microalbuminuria. *J Clin Endocrinol Metab.* 86(8):3871-6.

Sappington RM, Calkins DJ. (2006). Pressure-induced regulation of IL-6 in retinal glial cells: involvement of the ubiquitin/proteasome pathway and NFkappaB. *Invest Ophthalmol Vis Sci.* 47(9):3860-9.

Sari R, Balci MK, Apaydin C. (2010). The relationship between plasma leptin levels and chronic complication in patients with type 2 diabetes mellitus. *Metab Syndr Relat Disord.* 8(6):499-503.

Savino F. (2008). Adiponectin: an intriguing hormone for paediatricians. *Acta Pediatr,* 97:701-705.

Schalwijk CG, Chaturvedi N, Schram M. (2006). Adiponectin is inversely associated with renal function in type 1 diabetic patients. *J Endocrinol Metab* 91: 129-135

Sfikakis PP, Grigoropoulos V, Emfietzoglou I, Theodossiadis G, Tentolouris N, Delicha E, Katsiari C, Alexiadou K, Hatziagelaki E, Theodossiadis PG. (2010). Infliximab for diabetic macular edema refractory to laser photocoagulation: a randomized, double-blind, placebo-controlled, crossover, 32-week study. *Diabetes Care.* 33(7):1523-8

Sgadari C, Angiolillo AL, Tosato G. (1996). Inhibition of angiogenesis by interleukin-12 is mediated by the interferon-inducible protein 10. *Blood* ,87:3877–82.

Shi C, Lu J, Wu W, Ma F, Georges J, Huang H, Balducci J, Chang Y, Huang Y. (2011). Endothelial Cell-Specific Molecule 2 (ECSM2) Localizes to Cell-Cell Junctions and Modulates bFGF-Directed Cell Migration via the ERK-FAK Pathway. *PLoS One,* 6(6):e21482

Siebert J, Reiwer-Gostomska M, Myśliwska J, Marek N, Raczyńska K, Glasner L.(2010). Glycemic control influences serum angiogenin concentrations in patients with type 2 diabetes.*Diabetes Care.* 33:1829-30

Siebert J, Reiwer-Gostomska M, Babinska Z, Myśliwska J, Myśliwski A, Skopińska - Różewska E, Sommer E, Skopiński P. (2007). Low serum angiogenin level concentrations in patients with type 2 diabetes. *Diabetes Care,* 30 :3086–3087

Simó R, Carrasco E, García-Ramírez M, Hernández C. (2006). Angiogenic and antiangiogenic factors in proliferative diabetic retinopathy. *Curr Diabetes Rev;* 2: 71-98.

Simo R, Lecube A, Segura RM, Garcia Arumi J, Hernandez C. (2002). Free insulin growth factor-I and vascular endothelial growth factor in the vitreous fluid of patients with proliferative diabetic retinopathy. *Am J Ophthalmol,* 134: 376–382.

Starita M. Patel, Katz B. and Adamis A.P. (2007). Vascular endothelial growth factor and the potential therapeutic use of pegaptanib (macugen) in diabetic retinopathy, *Dev. Ophthalmol.* 39 pp. 122–148

Stoker M, Gherardi E, Perryman M, Gray J. (1987). Scatter factor is a fibroblast-derived modulator of epithelial cell mobility. *Nature,* 327:239–242.

Strieter RM, Burdick MD, Gomperts BN, Belperio JA, Keane MP (2005). CXC chemokines in angiogenesis. *Cytokine Growth Factor Rev.*16: 593-609.

Subramanian P, Crawford SE, Becerra SP. (2011). Assays for the antiangiogenic and neurotrophic serpin pigment epithelium-derived factor. *Methods Enzymol.* 499:183-204.

Sukhanov S, Higashi Y, Shai SY, Vaughn C, Mohler J, Li Y, Song YH, Titterington J, Delafontaine P. (2007). IGF-1 reduces inflammatory responses, suppresses oxidative stress, and decreases atherosclerosis progression in ApoE-deficient mice. *Arterioscler Thromb Vasc Biol.* 27(12):2684-90.

Sumioka T, Fujita N, Kitano A, Okada Y, Saika S. (2011). Impaired angiogenic response in the cornea of mice lacking tenascin C. *Invest Ophthalmol Vis Sci.* 52(5):2462-7.

Sun X, Huang L, Zhang M, Sun S, Wu Y. (2010). Insulin like growth factor-1 prevents 1-mentyl-4-phenylphyridinium-induced apoptosis in PC12 cells through activation of glycogen synthase kinase-3beta. *Toxicology.* 271(1-2):5-12

Suzuma I, Hata Y, Clermont A, Pokras F, Rook SL, Suzuma K. (2001) Cyclic stretch and hypertension induce retinal expression of vascular endothelial growth factor and vascular endothelial growth factor receptor-2: potential mechanisms for exacerbation of diabetic retinopathy by hypertension. *Diabetes,* 50: 444–454.

Suzuki Y, Nakazawa M, Suzuki K, Yamazaki H, Miyagawa Y. (2011). Expression profiles of cytokines and chemokines in vitreous fluid in diabetic retinopathy and central retinal vein occlusion. *Jpn J Ophthalmol.* 55(3):256-63.

Tan KC, Xu A, Chow WS, Lam MC, Ai VH, Tam SC, Lam KS. (2004). Hypoadiponectinemia is associated with impaired endothelium-depentend vasodilation. *Journal of Clin Endocrinol and Metabolism.* 100: 2473- 2476.

Tello-Montoliu A, Patel JV, Lip GY. (2006). Angiogenin: a review of the pathophysiology and potential clinical applications. *J Thromb Haemost,* 4(9):1864-74.

Thomas MC, Söderlund J, Lehto M, Mäkinen VP, Moran JL, Cooper ME, Forsblom C, Groop PH. (2011). ; on behalf of the FinnDiane Study Group. Soluble receptor for AGE (RAGE) is a novel independent predictor of all-cause and cardiovascular mortality in type 1 diabetes. *Diabetologia.* [Epub ahead of print]

Tombran-Tink J. (2010). PEDF in angiogenic eye diseases. *Curr Mol Med.* 10(3):267-78.

Trinchieri, G. (1998). *Int. Rev. Immunol,* 16(3-4), 365-396.

Unoki N, Murakami T, Nishijima K, Ogino K, van Rooijen N, Yoshimura N (2010). SDF-1/CXCR4 contributes to the activation of tip cells and microglia in retinal angiogenesis.. Invest Ophthalmol Vis Sci..,51: 3362-7

Voest EE, Kenyon BM, O'Reilly MS, Truitt G, D'Amato RJ, Folkman J. (1995). Inhibition of angiogenesis in vivo by interleukin 12. *J Natl Cancer Inst.* 87:581–6.

Volpert O.V., Zaichuk T., Zhou W., Reiher F., Ferguson T.A., Stuart P.M., Amin M., Bouck N.P. (2002). Inducer-stimulated Fas targets activated endothelium for destrustion by anti-angiogenic thrombospndin-1 and pigment epithelium-derived factor. *Nat. Med.,* 8: 349-357

Wa C, Cerny RL, Clarke WA, Hage DS. (2007). Characterization of glycation adducts on human serum albumin by matrix-assisted laser desorption/ionization time-of-flight mass spectrometry. *Clin Chim Acta* 385: 48-60

Wedrychowicz A, Dziatkowiak H, Nazim J, Sztefko K. (2005). Insulin-like growth factor-1 and its binding proteins, IGFBP-1 and IGFBP-3, in adolescents with type-1 diabetes mellitus and microalbuminuria. *Horm Res.* 63(5):245-5

Wilson, J.; Balkwill, F (2002). *Semin. Cancer Biol,* 12(2), 113-120.

Wirostko B, Wong TY, Simo´ R. (2008). Vascular endothelial growth factor and diabetic complications. *Prog Retin Eye Res,* 27: 608–621.

Wulster-Radcliffe MC, K.M. Ajuwon, J. Wang, J.A. Christian, M.E. Spurlock, (2004). Adiponectin differentially regulates cytokines in procine macrophages. *Biochem. Biophys. Res. Commun,* 316. 924– 929.

Xia M, Sui Z. (2009). Recent developments in CCR2 antagonists. *Expert Opin Ther Pat* 19: 295–303

Yamagishi S, Amano S., Inagaki Y., Okamoto T., Takeuchi M., Inoue H. (2003). Pigment epithelium-derived factor inhibits leptin-induced angiogenesis by suppressing vascular endothelial growth factor gene expression through anti-oxidative properties. Microvasc. Res, 65: 186-190.

Yamagishi SI, Maeda S, Matsui T, Ueda S, Fukami K, Okuda S. (2011). Role of advanced glycation end products (AGEs) and oxidative stress in vascular complications in diabetes. *Biochim Biophys Acta.* Apr 1. [Epub ahead of print]

Yingchuan F, Chuntao L, Hui C, Jianbin H. (2010). Increased Expression of TGF-beta1 and Smad 4 on Oxygen-Induced Retinopathy in Neonatal Mice. *Adv Exp Med Biol.* 664:71-7.

Yoshida S, Yoshida A, Ishibashi T. (2004). Induction of IL-8, MCP-1, and bFGF by TNF-alpha in retinal glial cells: implications for retinal neovascularization during post-ischemic inflammation. *Graefes Arch Clin Exp Ophthalmol.* 242(5):409-13.

Yoshida S, Ishikawa K, Matsumoto T, Yoshida A, Ishibashi T, Kono T. (2010). Reduced concentrations of angiogenesis-related factors in vitreous after vitrectomy in patients with proliferative diabetic retinopathy. *Graefes Arch Clin Exp Ophthalmol.* 248(6):799-804

Yoshida S, Sotozono C, Ikeda T, Kinoshita S. (2001). Interleukin−6 [IL−6] production by cytokine−stimulated human Müller cells. *Curr Eye Res.*, 22, 341–347.

Yoshimura T, Leonard EJ. (1992). Human monocyte chemoattractant protein-1: structure and function. *Cytokines.* 4:131-52.

Zhang Y, Proenca R, Maffei M, Barone M, Leopold L, Friedman JM , 1994. Positional cloning of the mouse obese gene and its human homologue. *Nature,* 372: 425–432.

Zhang W, Rojas M, Lilly B, Tsai NT, Lemtalsi T, Liou GI, Caldwell RW, Caldwell RB. (2009). NAD(P)H oxidase-dependent regulation of CCL2 production during retinal inflammation. *Invest Ophthalmol Vis Sci.*50: 3033-40

Zheng L, Szab C and Kern TS. (2004) "Poly(ADP-ribose) polymerase is involved in the development of diabetic retinopathy via regulation of nuclear factor-κB," *Diabetes,* 53: 2960–2967.

Zietz B, Buechler C, Kobuch K, Neumeier M, Schölmerich J, Schäffler A. (2008). Serum levels of adiponectin are associated with diabetic retinopathy and with adiponectin gene mutations in Caucasian patients with diabetes mellitus type 2. *Exp Clin Endocrinol Diabetes.* 116(9):532-6

Zhou Y, Wei Y, Wang L, Wang X, Du X, Sun Z, Dong N, Chen X. (2011). Decreased adiponectin and increased inflammation expression in epicardial adipose tissue in coronary artery disease. *Cardiovasc Diabetol.* 12;10(1):2.

Zong H, Ward M, Stitt AW.(2011). AGEs, RAGE, and Diabetic Retinopathy. *Curr Diab Rep.*;11(4):244-52.

Zorena K, Myśliwska J, Myśliwiec M, Balcerska A, Hak Ł, Lipowski P, Raczyńska K. (2007). Serum TNF-Alpha Level Predicts Nonproliferative Diabetic Retinopathy in Children. *Mediators Inflamatation.* 1, 92196.

Zorena K, Myśliwska J, Myśliwiec M, Balcerska A, Lipowski P, Raczyńska K (2007). Interleukin-12, vascular endothelial growth factor and tumor necrosis factor-alpha in the process of neoangiogenesis of diabetic retinopathy in children. *Klin Oczna,* 109(4-6):155-9.

Zorena K, Myśliwska J, Myśliwiec M, Balcerska A, Raczyńska-Woźniak D, Raczyńska K. (2007). Inflammatory and angiogenic factors in children with diabetic retinopathy. *Family Med. Prim. Care Rev.* 4: 1007-1010.

Zorena K, Myśliwska J, Myśliwiec M, Balcerska A, Lipowski P, Raczyńska K. (2008). Interleukin 12 and Tumor Necrosis Factor-α equilibrium is prerequisite for clinical course free from late complications in type 1 diabetes mellitus children. *Scandinavian Journal Immunology,* 67, 2, 204-8.

Zorena K, Myśliwska J, Myśliwiec M, Balcerska A, Lipowski P, Raczyńska-Woźniak D, Raczyńska K. (2009). Modulatory factors responsible for neoangiogenesis in young patients with long-standing diabetes mellitus type 1. *Recent Patents Endocr. Metabol. Immun. Drug Disc.*vol. 3, nr 2, 144-149.

Zorena K, Myśliwiec M, Myśliwska J, Balcerska A, Wiśniewski P, Kula M, Raczyńska D. (2010). The status of the CCL2/MCP-1 and CXCL10/IP-10 chemokines in children and youths with type 1 diabetes mellitus. *Pediatric Endocrinology*, 4: 9-18.

Zorena K, Myśliwska J, Myśliwiec M, Rybarczyk-Kapturska K, Malinowska E, Wiśniewski P, Raczyńska K. (2010). Association between vascular endothelial growth factor and hypertension in children and adolescents type I diabetes mellitus. *J Hum Hypertens*, 24(11):755-62

8

Inflammation and Diabetic Retinopathy

Hongbin Lü
*Department of Ophthalmology,
Affiliated Hospital of Luzhou Medical College, Sichuan Province,
China*

1. Introduction

Diabetic retinopathy (DR) is the leading cause of blindness in working-age individuals. There is increasing evidence that established risk factors for DR, including duration of diabetes, hyperglycemia, and hypertension, only explain a limited amount of the variance in the risk of DR. Furthermore, the underlying pathogenesis of DR remains inadequately understood. Diabetes causes metabolic and physiologic abnormalities in the retina, and these changes suggest a role for inflammation in the development of DR. These changes include up regulation of isoforms of nitric oxide synthase (iNOS), cyclooxygenases (COX)-2, intercellular adhesion molecule 1 (ICAM-1), vascular endothelial growth factor (VEGF), nuclear factor kappa B (NF-κB), increased production of nitric oxide, prostaglandin E2, interleukin (IL)- 1β, and cytokines, as well as increased permeability and leukostasis.

Using selective pharmacologic inhibitors or genetically modified animals, an increasing number of therapeutic approaches have been identified that significantly inhibit development of at least the early stages of diabetic retinopathy, especially occlusion and degeneration of retinal capillaries. A common feature of a number of these therapies is that they inhibit production of inflammatory mediators. The concept that localized inflammatory processes play a role in the development of diabetic retinopathy is relatively new, but evidence that supports the hypothesis is accumulating rapidly. The focus of this chapter is on the inflammatory nature of many of the molecular and cellular processes leading to this vascular damage, as well as on the pathologic neovascularization that often accompanies it. Finally, clinical findings validating the role of inflammation in DR are described.

2. An inflammation in the early performance of diabetic retinopathy

Diabetic retinopathy classically has been regarded as a disease of the retinal microvasculature, and the natural history of the disease has been divided into an early, nonproliferative (or background) stage, and a later, proliferative stage. It is becoming appreciated also that cells of the neuroretina also are affected in diabetes. A number of metabolic or molecular abnormalities that are characteristic of inflammation have been detected in retinas of diabetic animals or patients, or in retinal cells exposed to elevated concentrations of glucose. Histologically, vascular lesions in the early stages of diabetic retinopathy in man and animals are characterized by the presence of saccular capillary microaneurysms, pericyte deficient capillaries, and obliterated and degenerate capillaries. These degenerate capillaries are not perfused, and so increases in their frequency represent reductions in retinal perfusion.

Capillary occlusion and degeneration initially occurs in single, isolated capillaries, and has no clinical importance when only few capillaries have become nonperfused. As more and more capillaries become occluded, however, retinal perfusion likely decreases, at least locally. Mechanisms believed to contribute to the degeneration of retinal capillaries in diabetes include occlusion of the vascular lumen by white blood cells or platelets, death of capillary cells secondary to biochemical abnormalities within the vascular cells themselves, or capillary cell death secondary to products generated by other nearby cells (such as neurons or glia). All species studied today have been found to show degeneration of retinal capillaries as well as death of pericytes and endothelial cells, but microaneurysms are not commonly found in rodent models of diabetic retinopathy. Inflammation is a nonspecific response to injury that includes a variety of functional and molecular mediators, including recruitment and activation of leukocytes. Inflammation typically has beneficial effects on an acute basis, but can have undesirable effects if persisting chronically. The increased expression of many inflammatory proteins is regulated at the level of gene transcription through the activation of proinflammatory transcription factors, including NF-κB. These proinflammatory transcription factors are activated and play a critical role in amplifying and perpetuating the inflammatory process. Transcription factors associated with production of proinflammatory mediators include NF-κB, activator protein 1 (AP-1), specificity protein 1 (Sp1), peroxisome proliferator-activated receptors (PPARs) and other members of the nuclear receptor superfamily. Proinflammatory proteins (including COX-2, interleukin-1, tumor necrosis factor alpha) can contribute to cell damage and death in tissues including brain and retina, at least in part via activation of NF-κB (Fig.1.).

2.1 NF-κB

NF-κB is a widely expressed inducible transcription factor that is an important regulator of many genes involved in mammalian inflammatory and immune responses, proliferation and apoptosis. Evidence in support of an important role of NF-κB in the pathogenesis of early stages of diabetic retinopathy is twofold. First, inhibition of proteins whose expression is regulated by NF-κB (such as iNOS and ICAM) inhibit diabetes-induced degeneration of retinal capillaries. Second, compounds known to inhibit NF-κB likewise inhibit the development of the retinopathy. For example, several different antioxidants which inhibit the development of capillary degeneration and pericyte loss in retinas of diabetic rats also inhibit the diabetes-induced activation of retinal NF-κB. Likewise, low-intermediate doses of salicylates (aspirin, sodium salicylate, and sulfasalazine) which inhibited NF-κB activation in retinas of diabetic rats, also inhibited expression of inflammatory mediators like iNOS and ICAM-1, and capillary degeneration and pericyte loss in those animals. Aspirin is known to inhibit also production of prostaglandins, but salicylate and sulfasalazine have much less of this activity, suggesting that the common action of these 3 salicylates to inhibit retinopathy in diabetes was not primarily mediated by inhibition of prostaglandins.

Our experiments showed that Ubiqutin-proteasome system can influence the occurrence and development of DR by regulating NF-κB and IκB expression. Application of MG 132, ubiqutin-proteasome inhibitor, can inhibit the ubiquitination of IκB degradation, and block the activation of NF-κB, which may play an early intervention role in DR.

2.2 iNOS

iNOS expression is regulated at least in part by NF-κB. Interestingly, experimental sympathectomy itself increases gene and protein expression of iNOS in retinas of nondiabetic rats, suggesting that loss of sympathetic activity, such as which occurs in diabetes, might contribute to the upregulation of this inflammatory protein in the retina. In retinas of diabetic animals, increased levels of nitric oxide products (nitrotyrosine, nitrite, nitrate) have been reported. Upregulation of iNOS has been found in retinas of experimental diabetic rodents and patients in most studies. Diabetes-induced alterations inexpression of other isoforms of nitric oxide synthase also have been reported. A possible role of iNOS in the pathogenesis of diabetic retinopathy is suggested by the studies of aminoguanidine. Aminoguanidine is a relatively selective inhibitor of iNOS, and has been found to inhibit the diabetes-induced increase nitric oxide production and iNOS expression in retina. Aminoguanidine also has been found to inhibit the development of the microvascular lesions of diabetic retinopathy in diabetic dogs, rats, and mice. Nevertheless, aminoguanidine also has other effects, so this therapy does not absolutely prove a role of iNOS in the pathogenesis of the retinopathy. The role of iNOS in the development of the early stages of diabetic retinopathy recently has been investigated directly using mice genetically deficient in iNOS. In that study, wildtype diabetic mice developed the expected degeneration of retinal capillaries, as well as increase in leukostasis and superoxide generation. In contrast, diabetic mice deficient in iNOS did not develop these structural or functional abnormalities. eNOS expression also has been reported to be elevated in the retinas in the diabetic rats, and it has been suggested that eNOS might play a role in the development of diabetes-induced leukostasis and/or retinopathy. This posibility has not been experimentally addressed due, in part, to the hypertension that results in the absence of eNOS, as well as a lack of specific inhibitors of the enzyme.

2.3 Cyclooxygenases

COX-2 expression is regulated at least in part by NF-κB. In retinas of diabetic animals, induction of COX-2 as well as increased production of prostaglandins has been reported. Researchers have shown that PGE_2 production by retinas from diabetic rats was significantly inhibited by celecoxib (a selective COX-2 inhibitor), but not by a COX-1 inhibitor, suggesting that COX-2 is primarily responsible for the diabetes-induced increase in retinal production of PGE_2 in diabetic rats. Inhibition of COX-2 has been reported to inhibit the diabetes-induced upregulation of retinal prostaglandins and VEGF, the increase in retinal vessel permeability and leukostasis, and the death of retinal endothelial cells cultured in diabetic-like concentrations of glucose. The COX-2 inhibitor, Meloxicam, also reduced eNOS levels, inhibited NF-κB activation in the diabetic retina, and modestly, but significantly, reduced TNFα levels in the retina. Its effect on histologic lesions of diabetic retinopathy was not studied. Less selective COX inhibitors have inhibited the development of the retinopathy in diabetic dogs and rodents, as well as the increase in vascular permeability in diabetic rodents. Nepafenac is an inhibitor of cyclooxygenases that can be applied in eye drops. It was found to inhibit diabetes-induced prostaglandin production and leukocyte adhesion in retinal vessels of diabetic rats, and the diabetes-induced increase in the number of TUNEL-positive capillary cells, acellular capillaries, and pericyte ghosts in the retina.

Micro RNAs (miRNAs) are a class of highly conserved, small non-coding RNAs that powerfully regulate gene expression at the posttranscriptional level. A growing number of reports have established a link between miRNAs and DR in recent years. Kovacs B et al. proposed upregulation of NF-κB-, VEFG-, and p53- responsive miRNAs constituted key miRNA signatures, reflecting ongoing pathologic changes of early DR. But the exact roles of miRNAs in DR are still unknown. Our teams are still devoting the study of differentially expressed miRNA of human retinal capillary endothelial cells in high glucose environment by miRNA gene chip.(Table 1,2)

miRNAs	倍数	miRNAs	倍数
hsa-miR-886-5p	4.73	hsa-miR-93	2.18
hsa-miR-147b	4.52	hsa-miR-148b	2.17
hsa-miR-886-3p	3.62	hsa-miR-455-3p	2.17
hsa-miR-18a	2.92	hsa-miR-130b	2.16
hsa-miRPlus-F1147	2.74	hsa-miR-1265	2.14
hsa-miR-200a	2.69	hsa-let-7f	2.14
hsa-miR-185	2.63	hsa-miR-195	2.11
hsa-miR-155	2.58	hsa-miR-19b	2.09
hsa-miR-106b	2.42	hsa-miR-320b	2.09
hsa-miR-320c	2.28	hsa-miR-505*	2.05
hsa-miR-320d	2.28	hsa-miR-151-3p	2.05
hsa-miR-10a	2.28	hsa-miR-20a	2.04
hsa-miR-1913	2.25	hsa-miR-98	2.03
hsa-miR-374b	2.24	hsa-miR-500	2.02
hsa-miR-29a*	2.23	hsa-let-7d	2.02
		hsa-miR-101	2.02

Table 1. The up-regulated miRNA（Fold change>2) A: Normal control group B: High glucose group

miRNAs	倍数
hsa-miR-483-3p	0.16
hsa-miRPlus-E1238	0.23
hsa-miR-365*	0.23
hsa-miR-943	0.26
hsa-miR-1908	0.29
hsa-miR-3202	0.33
hsa-miR-1246	0.36
hsa-miRPlus-E1077	0.36
hsa-miRPlus-E1285	0.38
hsa-miRPlus-F1099	0.44
hsa-miR-491-3p	0.44
hsa-miR-765	0.45
hsa-miRPlus-F1155	0.46
hsa-miRPlus-E1153	0.48
hsa-miRPlus-F1026	0.48
hsa-miR-513a-5p	0.49
hsa-miR-1264	0.49
hsa-miRPlus-E1133	0.49

Table 2. The down-regulated miRNAs(Fold change<0.5) A: Normal control group B: High glucose group

3. Leukocyte activation and endothelial cell injury

Attraction and adhesion of leukocytes to the vascular wall are important components of inflammatory processes. This leukostasis has been found to be significantly increased in retinas of diabetic animals, and might contribute to the capillary nonperfusion in diabetic retinopathy. Leukocyte stiffness has been reported to be increased in diabetes (decreased filterability) and to contribute to the development of capillary nonperfusion in retinal vessels. A second line of evidence shows that abnormal leukocyte adherence to retinal vessels in diabetes occurs via adhesion molecules.

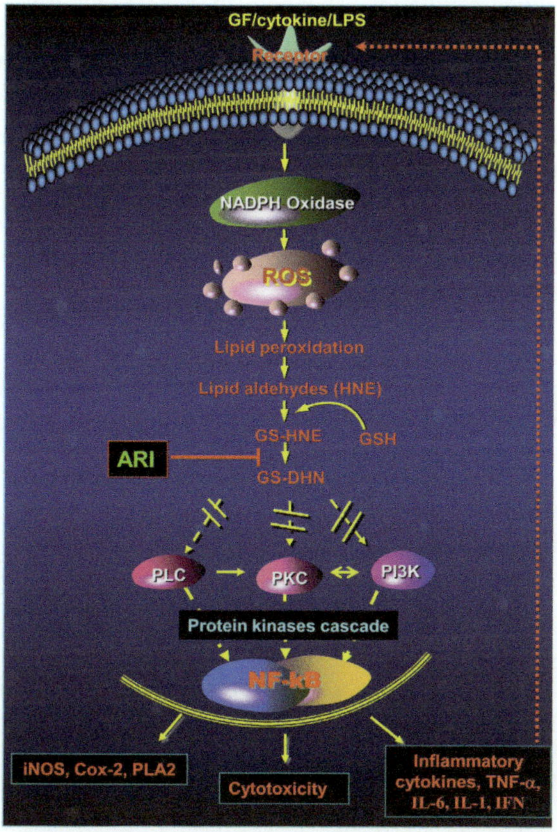

Fig. 1.Role of aldose reductase in mediation of inflammatory signals. Cytokines, growth factors (GF), and lipopolysaccharide (LPS) cause oxidative stress via generation of ROS which forms toxic lipid aldehydes such as HNE by lipid peroxidation. HNE being highly electrophilic conjugates with cellular glutathione (GSH) spontaneously or catalyzed by GST to form GS-HNE. The reduced products of GS-aldehydes, GS-DHN, transduce inflammatory signaling via cascade of protein kinases leading to activation of NF- κ B. Activation of NF- κ B transcribes genes responsible for various inflammatory pathologies. (Reproduced from Int J Biochem Cell Biol. 2010 January ; 42(1): 17–20. doi:10.1016/j.biocel.2009.09.009.)

Diabetes increases expression of ICAM-1 in retinas of animals and humans and interaction of this adhesion molecule on retinal endothelia with the CD18 adhesion molecule on monocytes and neutrophils contributes to the diabetes-induced increase in leukostasis within retinal vessels. Leukostasis has been postulated to be a factor in death of retinal endothelial cells in diabetes. Using in situ perfusion methods, evidence consistent with capillary occlusion secondary to leukostasis has been observed in occasional retinal vessels, but it is unclear whether this occurred in vivo or was an artifact caused by the perfusion in vitro. Retinas from diabetic mice lacking ICAM-1 and CD18 are protected from the development of diabetes-induced increase in leukostasis, vascular permeability, and degeneration of retinal capillaries, showing these proteins to be important in the development of early stages of diabetic retinopathy. Whether their role in the development of the retinal disease results from capillary occlusion or some other mechanism, however, has not been explored.

In experimental studies employing rodent models of diabetes, diabetic retinal vascular leakage, capillary nonperfusion, and endothelial cell damage are temporally and spatially correlated with a low-level leukocyte influx and persistent retinal leukostasis. This leukostasis is mediated by retinal upregulation of ICAM-1, together with an increased expression of its cognate integrin ligands on neutrophils. Subsequently, endothelial cell injury and death result from Fas/FasL-mediated apoptosis.

In response to this injury, the endothelium maintains a sustained high rate of cell division, which is believed to result in exhaustion of its regenerative capacity. This stress is further exacerbated by a diabetes-induced defect in the ability of endothelial precursor cells to repair the damaged vasculature. While the vascular damage is primarily a function of infiltrating leukocytes, DR is also associated with ischemic neovascularization, a process that is amplified by the influx of macrophages.

4. Causes of inflammation

4.1 Vascular Endothelial Growth Factor (VEGF)

VEGF is a proinflammatory molecule that plays a well-recognized role in neovascularization and in increased permeability. VEGF expression is regulated largely by hypoxia, but it also accumulates in the retina early in diabetes, before any retinal hypoxia is yet apparent. It is produced by multiple cell types in the retina in diabetes, including ganglion cells, Müller cells, and pericytes. Repeated injections of high concentrations of VEGF in the eyes of non-diabetic monkeys result in retinal changes which in some ways resemble those in the early stages of diabetic retinopathy, including vascular tortuosity and microaneurysms.

4.2 Tumor Necrosis Factor-α (TNF-α)

The levels of several proinflammatory cytokines including IL-1β, TNF-α, IL-6, and IL-8 are increased in the vitreous of patients with proliferative diabetic retinopathy and in retinas from diabetic rodents. Inflammation is one of the processes implicated in the apoptosis of retinal cells , and TNF-α is considered as an important mediator of apoptosis of retinal endothelial cells in diabetes.

Evidence supporting a role for TNF-α in DR comes from studies demonstrating elevations of TNF-α in ocular fibrovascular membranes, platelets, and plasma or serum of patients with DR. Vitreous elevations in TNF-α in patients with proliferative DR were reported in one study, although another study found no difference in the vitreous levels of TNF-α between those with proliferative DR and those with noninflammatory retinopathies. The susceptibility to diabetic retinopathy has been associated with TNF-α gene polymorphism and expression of HLA-DR3 and HLA-DR4 phenotypes. In addition, TNF-α is found in the extracellular matrix, endothelium, and vessel walls of fibrovascular tissue of eyes with proliferative diabetic retinopathy.

Eternacept is a soluble TNF-α receptor that acts as competitive inhibitor to block effects of TNF-α binding to cells. Eternacept reduced leukocyte adherence in retinal blood vessels of diabetic rats for 1 week compared to control. Eternacept did not reduce retinal VEGF levels, but it inhibited blood-retinal barrier breakdown and NF-κB activation in the diabetic retina.

4.3 Inter-cellular Adhesion Molecule 1 (ICAM-1)

White blood cells bind to ICAM-1 on the surface of endothelial cells as a component of a multistep process leading to adherence of the white blood cell to the endothelial wall. ICAM-1 is a peptide known to mediate leukocyte adhesion and transmigration. ICAM-1 may be operative in the stasis observed in diabetic retinopathy, because ICAM-1 immunoreactivity is increased in the diabetic retinal vasculature of humans.

ICAM-1 is upregulated by several stimuli, including VEGF, PARP activation, oxidative stress, and dylipidemia, at least in part by NF-κB.

4.4 Endothelin-1(ET-1)

ET-1 is one of the strongest vasoconstrictive factors. The DAG/PKC pathway determines blood flow dysregulation by decreasing endothelial NOS activity and/or increasing the synthesis of ET-1. Observations indicate that the participation of endothelin in coagulation disorders is also essential for the development of proliferative diabetic retinopathy (PDR). Some studies point out the fact that thrombosis in the rat microcirculation and a DIC-like process in the rabbit circulation develop under the influence of ET-1. An important element in the development of this disturbance is the documented mitogen-activated protein (MAPK kinase)-dependent ET-1 production. Another study has found that the molecular function of ET-1 and PKC is predicted. According to this study, different pathways can be derived from ET-1 and PKC; however, ET-1–PKC produces the same pathway as PKC. This could mean that the interaction between ET-1 and PKC results in increased activity of the PKC pathway but does not generate any new pathway.

4.5 IL-6

Clinical reports show that IL-6 in the vitreous fluid increases not only in uveitis but also in diabetic retinopathy, retinal vein occlusion, and retinal detachment. Research with experimental animals has shown that diffusible factors, IL-6 and other proteins in the IL-6 family, such as leukemia inhibitory factor (LIF) and ciliary neurotrophic factor (CNTF), are expressed in the retina. Both IL-6 and LIF are found in Müller glial cells, and CNTF is found in the retinal ganglion cells and astrocytes around the vessels. These endogenous IL-6 family proteins are upregulated during inflammation and function to promote pathogenesis of the vascular system.

IL-6 family proteins use cytokine-specific receptors to activate a transmembrane receptor, gp130, which then recruits Janus kinase (JAK) to activate transcription factor signal transducer and activator of transcription 3 (STAT3). STAT3 then regulates various molecules at the transcriptional level, including suppressor of cytokine signaling 3 (SOCS3). SOCS3 acts as a negative feedback modulator of STAT3 by inhibiting JAK and subsequent STAT3 activation. In the retina, SOCS3 is expressed in the photoreceptor cells, Müller glial cells, and retinal ganglion cells, and it inhibits STAT3 activation in these cells. Since STAT3 activation induces further STAT3-activating factors, such as the IL-6 family ligands, the balance between STAT3 activation and SOCS3 level is one of the key determinants of an inflammatory reaction.

5. Anti-inflammatory and effects of anti-inflammatory drug treatment

5.1 Glucocorticoid

Glucocorticoids are well-established anti-inflammatory compounds that may be effective in reversing or preventing the progression of macular edema, and are currently under investigation as a therapy for diabetic retinopathy. Glucocorticoids are effective at reversing VEGF-induced permeability in animal models. In addition to the anti-inflammatory effect of glucocorticoids, our laboratory has demonstrated that these steroids also induce the synthesis and assembly of tight junctions and the dephosphorylation of occluding commensurate with a reduction in endothelial permeability. Recent work revealed the presence of a novel enhancer element unlike the canonical glucocorticoid response element, in the occludin promoter that controls glucocorticoid responsiveness of this gene (manuscript submitted). Future studies may reveal more specific means to control expression of the tight junction proteins and barrier properties.

5.2 Nonsteroidal anti-inflammatory drugs

Nonsteroidal anti-inflammatory drugs (NSAIDs) are one of the most commonly prescribed classes of medications worldwide. Aspirin and other chemically related compounds, used systemically for many decades for their analgesic, antipyretic, and anti-inflammatory properties, have more recently been prepared in topical ophthalmic formulations. As such, they have proven useful to enhance mydriasis, reduce postoperative inflammation, and prevent and treat cystoid macular edema (CME) associated with cataract surgery. In addition, they can be used to decrease pain and photophobia after refractive surgery and to alleviate itching associated with allergic conjunctivitis.The development of NSAIDs that preferentially inhibit COX-2 provides the potential for relieving pain and inflammation without the adverse effects of COX-1 blockade, but the advantages of this approach have been questioned. Although COX-2 inhibitors may reduce gastro-intestinal toxicity, they appear to have equivalent nephrotoxicity to conventional NSAIDs.

5.3 VEGF drugs for VEGF in the PDR

Both clinical and preclinical findings have implicated VEGF in the pathophysiology of diabetic retinopathy. The VEGF family, which includes VEGF-A, VEGF-B, VEGF-C, VEGF-D, VEGF-E and placental growth factor, plays an important role in angiogenesis and vascular permeability.

Three anti-VEGF pharmacologic agents are currently available commercially. Pegaptanib is a paginated aptamer that targets the VEGF165 isoform. It has been shown to inhibit VEGF's endothelial mitogen activity and its vascular permeability effects. The US Food and Drug Administration (FDA) has approved Macugen for the treatment of neovascular AMD. The VEGF Inhibition Study in Ocular Neovascularization (VISION) trial established its safety and efficacy in neovascular AMD. Ranibizumab is a recombinant, humanized antibody fragment that binds all isoforms of VEGF, whereas bevacizumab (Avastin, Genentech, Inc.) is a recombinant, full-length, humanized antibody that also binds all VEGF isoforms. Lucentis is currently FDA-approved for neovascular AMD, while Avastin is used on an off-label basis for a variety of ophthalmic conditions. Large clinical trials of Avastin are currently underway for AMD, DME, and vein occlusions, but the safety and efficacy of Avastin for intraocular use remains to be demonstrated.

6. Conclusions

Acquired visual impairment of DR is the consequence of diabetic blood-retinal barrier breakdown. Peroxisome proliferator-activated receptor-gamma excitomotor (PPAR-γ), rosiglitazone, lessened much more of the pericytes, and decreased the number of proliferative endothelial cells with the lower permeability value of the blood-retinal barrier in our DM model rats research, induced by streptozotocin (STZ).

Diabetic retinopathy is a common microvascular complication in the eyes of diabetic individuals. Besides its serious threat to vision, the presence of retinopathy also signifies an excess risk of morbidity and mortality attributable to systemic micro and macrovascular disease. Numerous defects that develop in retinas as a result of diabetes are consistent with diabetes-induced inflammatory response in that tissue. These inflammatory changes apparently are important in the pathogenesis of diabetic retinopathy, since inhibition of this inflammatory cascade at any of multiple steps can inhibit the early stages of diabetic retinopathy in animals. Findings of diabetes induced inflammatory changes, generally, in the human eye also, are consistent with the postulate that inflammatory processes contribute to the development of diabetic retinopathy. The evidence in diabetic animals is sufficient to warrant further investigations of the role of inflammation in the development of diabetic retinopathy in patients.

7. References

[1] T. S. Kern. Contributions of Inflammatory Processes to the Development of the Early Stages of Diabetic Retinopathy. Experimental Diabetes Research . 2007; 2007: 95103

[2] A. Sima, W. X. Zhang, P. V. Cherian, et al., Impaired visual evoked potential and primary axonopathy of the optic nerve in the diabetic BB/W-rat, Diabetologia, vol. 35, no. 7, pp. 602–607, 1992.

[3] M. Kamijo, P. V. Cherian, and A. A. F. Sima, The preventive effect of aldose reductase inhibition on diabetic optic neuropathy in the BB/W-rat, Diabetologia, vol. 36, no. 10, pp.893–898, 1993.

[4] H. P. Hammes, H. J. Federoff, and M. Brownlee, Nerve growth factor prevents both neuroretinal programmed cell death and capillary pathology in experimental diabetes,Molecular Medicine, vol. 1, no. 5, pp. 527–534, 1995.

[5] L. E. Swenarchuk, L. E. Whetter, and A. P. Adamis, The Role of Inflammation in the pathophysiology of diabetic retinopathy, Contemporary Diabetes, 2008, 2, Part 2, 303-331
[6] R. Ehrlich, A. Harris, T. A. Ciulla, et al., 2010.Diabetic macular oedema: physical, physiological and molecular factors contribute to this pathological process. Acta Ophthalmol. 88, 279e291.
[7] A. J. Barber, E. Lieth, S. A. Khin, et al., 1998.Neural apoptosis in the retina during experimental and human diabetes. Early onset and effect of insulin. J. Clin. Invest. 102, 783e791.
[8] Kern, T.S., Barber, A.J., 2008. Retinal ganglion cells in diabetes. J. Physiol. 15,4401e4408.
[9] A. Scott, M. B. Powner, P. Gandhi, Astrocyte-Derived Vascular Endothelial Growth Factor Stabilizes Vessels in the Developing Retinal Vasculature, PLoS ONE, July 2010, Vol.5,Issue 7, e11863
[10] H. Sone, Y. Kawakami, Y. Okuda, et al., Ocular vascular endothelial growth factor levels in diabetic rats are elevated before observable retinal proliferative changes, Diabetologia,vol. 40, no. 6, pp. 726–730, 1997.
[11] B. Gerhardinger, L. F. Brown, S. Roy, et al., Expression of vascular endothelial growth factor in the human retina and in nonproliferative diabetic retinopathy, American Journal of Pathology, vol. 152, no. 6, pp. 1453–1462, 1998.
[12] Y. Segawa, Y. Shirao, S.-I. Yamagishi, et al., Upregulation of retinal vascular endothelial growth factor mRNAs in spontaneously diabetic rats without ophthalmoscopic retinopathy.A possible participation of advanced glycation end products in the development of the early phase of diabetic retinopathy, Ophthalmic Research, vol. 30, no. 6, pp. 333–339, 1998.
[13] M. J. Tolentino, J. W. Miller, E. S. Gragoudas, et al., Intravitreous injections of vascular endothelial growth factor produce retinal ischemia and microangiopathy in an adult primate,Ophthalmology, vol. 103, no. 11, pp. 1820–1828, 1996.
[14] M. J. Tolentino, D. S. McLeod, M. Taomoto, et al., Pathologic features of vascular endothelial growth factor-induced retinopathy in the nonhuman primate, American Journal of Ophthalmology, vol. 133,no. 3, pp. 373–385, 2002.
[15] G. A. Limb, A. H. Chignell, W. Green, et al. (1996) Distribution of TNF alpha and its reactive vascular adhesion molecules in fibrovascular membranes of proliferative diabetic retinopathy. Br. J. Ophthalmol. 80, 168.173
[16] K. Hawrami, G. A. Hitman, M. Rema, et al., Ramachandran, A.,and Mohan, V. (1996) An association in non-insulin-dependent diabetes mellitus subjects between susceptibility to retinopathy and tumor necrosis factor polymorphism. Hum. Immunol.46, 49.54
[17] A. M. Joussen, V. Poulaki, N. Mitsiades, et al., Nonsteroidal anti-inflammatory drugs prevent early diabetic retinopathy via TNF-α suppression, The FASEB Journal, vol. 16, no. 3,pp. 438–440, 2002.
[18] C. Harada, A. Okumura, K. Namekata, et al., Role of monocyte chemotactic protein-1 and nuclear factor κB in the pathogenesis of proliferative diabetic retinopathy, Diabetes Research and Clinical Practice, vol. 74, no. 3, pp. 249–256,2006.
[19] T. A. Springer, Adhesion receptors of the immune system. Nature, (London) 346, 425–434,1990.
[20] F. W. Luscinskas, M. I. Cybulsky, J. M.Kiely, et al., (1991) J. Immunol. 146, 1617–1625.
[21] K. Miyamoto, S. Khosrof, S.-E. Bursell, et al., Prevention of leukostasis and vascular leakage in streptozotocin-induced diabetic retinopathy via intercellular adhesion

molecule-1 inhibition, Proceedings of the National Academy of Sciences of the United States of America, vol. 96, no. 19, pp. 10836–10841,1999.

[22] S. Chen, M. D. Apostolova, M. G. Cherian, et al., Interaction of endothelin-1 with vasoactive factors in mediating glucose-induced increased permeability in endothelial cells. Lab Invest 2000; 80:1311–21.

[23] D. Bednarska-Chabowska, R. Adamiec, W. Rychlik-Golema, et al., Selected problems of endothelial functions. I. The role of endothelium in maintaining the hematological and circulatory balance. Pol Merkur Lek 2002; 12(70):322–7.

[24] E. C. Eringa, C. D. Stehouwer, G. P. Nieuw Amerongen, et al., Vasoconstrictor effects of insulin in skeletal muscle arterioles are mediated by ERK1/2 activation in endothelium. Am J Physiol Heart Circ Physiol 2004; 287:H2043–8.

[25] V. Wiwanitki, Endothelin-1 and protein kinase C co-expression in the pathogenesis of diabetic retinopathy. Journal of Diabetes and Its Complications November 2007,Volume 21, Issue 6 , pp 359-362,

[26] B. D. Kuppermann, M. S. Blumenkranz, J. A. Haller, et al. Randomized controlled study of an intravitreous dexamethasone drug delivery system in patients with persistent macular edema. Arch Ophthalmol 2007; 125(3):309–17.

[27] J. L. Edelman, D. Lutz, M. R. Castro. Corticosteroids inhibit VEGF-induced vascular leakage in a rabbit model of blood-retinal and blood-aqueous barrier breakdown. Exp Eye Res 2005; 80(2):249–58.

[28] D. A. Antonetti, E. B. Wolpert, L. DeMaio, et al. Hydrocortisone decreases retinal endothelial cell water and solute flux coincident with increased content and decreased phosphorylation of occludin. J Neurochem 2002; 80:667–77.

[29] M. A. El Asrar, D. Maimone, P. H. Morse, et al., Cytokines in the vitreous of patients with proliferative diabetic retinopathy, American Journal of Ophthalmology, vol. 114, no. 6, pp. 731–736, 1992.

[30] H. Funatsu, H. Yamashita, T. Ikeda, et al., Vitreous levels of interleukin-6 and vascular endothelial growth factor are related to diabetic macular edema, Ophthalmology, vol. 110, no. 9, pp. 1690–1696, 2003.

[31] H. Noma, H. Funatsu, M. Yamasaki et al., Pathogenesis of macular edema with branch retinal vein occlusion and intraocular levels of vascular endothelial growth factor and interleukin-6, American Journal of Ophthalmology, vol. 140,no. 2, pp. 256–261, 2005.

[32] B. Kenarova, L. Voinov, C. Apostolov, et al., Levels of some cytokines in subretinal fluid in proliferative vitreoretinopathy and rhegmatogenous retinal detachment, European Journal of Ophthalmology, vol. 7, no. 1,pp. 64–67, 1997.

[33] M. Nakatani, T. Seki, Y. Shinohara et al., Pituitary adenylate cyclase-activating peptide (PACAP) stimulates production of interleukin-6 in rat Muller cells, Peptides, vol. 27, no. 7, pp.1871–1876, 2006.

[34] C. Neophytou, A. B. Vernallis, A. Smith, et al.,Muller-cell-derived leukaemia inhibitory factor arrests rod photoreceptor differentiation at a postmitotic pre-rod stage of development, Development, vol. 124, no. 12, pp. 2345–2354,1997.

[35] A. Müller, T. G. Hauk, M. Leibinger, et al., Exogenous CNTF stimulates axon regeneration of retinal ganglion cells partially via endogenous CNTF,Molecular and Cellular Neuroscience, vol. 41, no. 2, pp. 233–246, 2009.

[36] N. Nagai, Y. Oike, K. Noda et al., Suppression of ocular inflammation in endotoxin-induced uveitis by blocking the angiotensin II type 1 receptor, Investigative Ophthalmology and Visual Science, vol. 46, no. 8, pp. 2925–2931, 2005.

[37] X. Wang, P. Lupardus, S. L. LaPorte, et al.,Structural biology of shared cytokine receptors, Annual Review of Immunology, vol. 27, pp. 29–60, 2009.
[38] A. Yoshimura, Regulation of cytokine signaling by the SOCS and Spred family proteins, Keio Journal of Medicine, vol. 58, no. 2, pp. 73–83, 2009.
[39] Y. Ozawa, K. Nakao, T. Kurihara et al., Roles of STAT3/SOCS3 pathway in regulating the visual function and ubiquitinproteasome-dependent degradation of rhodopsin during retinal inflammation, Journal of Biological Chemistry, vol. 283,no. 36, pp. 24561–24570, 2008.
[40] Y. Ozawa, K. Nakao, T. Shimazaki et al., SOCS3 is required to temporally fine-tune photoreceptor cell differentiation, Developmental Biology, vol. 303, no. 2, pp. 591–600, 2007.
[41] H. Ogura, M. Murakami, Y. Okuyama et al., Interleukin-17 promotes autoimmunity by triggering a positive-feedback loop via interleukin-6 induction, Immunity, vol. 29, no. 4, pp.628–636, 2008.
[42] B. J. Baker, L. N. Akhtar, and E. N. Benveniste, SOCS1 and SOCS3 in the control of CNS immunity, Trends in Immunology, vol. 30, no. 8, pp. 392–400, 2009.
[43] Y. Ozawa, K. Nakao, T. Shimazaki et al., Downregulation of STAT3 activation is required for presumptive rod photoreceptor cells to differentiate in the postnatal retina, Molecular and Cellular Neuroscience, vol. 26, no. 2, pp. 258–270, 2004.
[44] T. Kurihara, Y. Ozawa, K. Shinoda et al., Neuroprotective effects of angiotensin II type 1 receptor (AT1R) blocker,telmisartan, via modulating AT1R and AT2R signaling in retinal inflammation, Investigative Ophthalmology and Visual Science, vol. 47, no. 12, pp. 5545–5552, 2006.
[45] M. Sasaki, Y. Ozawa, T. Kurihara et al., Neuroprotective effect of an antioxidant, lutein, during retinal inflammation, Investigative Ophthalmology&Visual Science, vol. 50, no. 3, pp.1433–1439, 2009.
[46] S. J. Kim, A. J. Flach, and L. M. Jampol., Nonsteroidal Anti-inflammatory Drugs in Ophthalmology, SURVEY OF OPHTHALMOLOGY VOLUME 55 _ NUMBER 2 _ MARCH–APRIL 2010
[47] D. S. cLeod, D. J. Lefer, C. Merges, et al. (1995) Enhanced expression of intracellular adhesion molecule-1 and P-selectin in the diabetic human retina and choroid. Am J Pathol 147:642–653
[48] C. Bell, E. Lynam, D. J. Landfair, et al. (1999) Oligonucleotide NX1838 inhibits VEGF165-mediated cellular responses in vitro. In Vitro Cell Dev Biol Anim 35:533–54
[49] E. S. Gragoudas, A. P. Adamis, E. T. Jr. Cunningham, et al., VEGF Inhibition Study in Ocular Neovascularization Clinical Trial Group (2004) Pegaptanib for neovascular agerelated macular degeneration. N Engl J Med 351:2805–2816
[50] WU Yan, Lü Hong-Bin, et al.(2010), Effect of MG 132 on expression of NF-κB and IκB in early period diabetic retinopathy in rats, Recent Advances in Ophthalmology. vol30,no.5,pp.441-444
[51] JIANG Ling, LIAO Hong-xia, WU Yan, Lü Hong-Bin, et al. (2010), Effects of peroxisome proliferator-activated receptor-gamma excitomotor on blood-retinal barrier in rat with diabetic retinopathy, Chinese Ophthalmic Research, vol28, no11, pp.1054-1058
[52] Beatrix Kovacs, Stephen Lumayag, Colleen Cowan, Shunbin Xu. MicroRNAs in Early Diabetic Retinopathy in Streptozotocin-induced Diabetic Rats. Invest Ophthalmol Vis Sci, Apr 2011; 10.1167/iovs.10-6879

9

Inflammation and Angiogenesis in Diabetic Retinopathy

Ying Yang, Ying Zhang and Yiping Li
Department of Endocrinology and Metabolism,
Yunnan Province 2nd Hospital,
Kunming,
PR China

1. Introduction

Diabetic retinopathy (DR) is a significant cause of global blindness; a major cause of blindness in the world.There is emerging evidence that retinopathy is initiated and propagated by inflammation and angiogenesis. Increased cytokines and growth factors, in conjunction with redox stress, contribute to the development and progression of DR of abnormalities of endothelial cells and pericytes in DR.

The four traditional metabolic pathways involved in the development of DR include: increased polyol pathway flux, advanced glycation end-product formation, activation of protein kinase Cisoforms and hexosamine pathway flux. These pathways individually and synergistically contribute to angiogenic growth factors, anti-angiogenic factors resulting in significant microvascular blood retinal barrier remodeling. The pathways are associated with inflammation and angiogenesis,either. Preventing or delaying the blindness associated with these intersecting abnormal metabolic pathways may be approached through strategies targeted to reduction of tissue inflammation. Understanding these abnormal metabolic pathways and the accompanying inflammation and angiogenesis mayprovide both the clinician and researcher a new concept of approaching this complicated disease process.

2. Diabetic Retinopathy (DR)

DR is associated with the following structural features: basement membrane (BM) thickening, pericyte loss,microaneurysms, intraretinal microvascular abnormalities(IRMA), diabetic macular edema (DME) and pre-retinal neovascularization,processes which can lead to blindness through hemorrhage and tractional retinal detachment[1]. Retinal endothelial cells (EC) are supported and sealed by a nearly equal number of pericytes in the retinal optic nerve fiber, inner and outer plexiform and choroidal layers creating a blood retinal barrier (BRB) of closed capillaries[1, 2].

The vascular disruptions of DR/DME are characterized by abnormal vascular flow, disruptions in permeability,and/or closure or nonperfusion of capillaries.

A hallmark of early DR is the change in the structure and cellular composition of the microvasculature[3].

In early stages of DME, breakdown of the inner blood-retinal barrier may occur, resulting in accumulation of extracellular fluid in the macula[4,5].Pericytes are essential cellular components in the regulation of retinal capillary perfusion, and damage to these cells in diabetes leads to altered retinal hemodynamics, including abnormal autoregulation of retinal blood flow[6]. Loss of retinal pericytes represents another early microaneurysm formation[7-9].

There is evidence that retinal leukostasis may also play an important role in the pathogenesis of DR. Leukocytes possess large cell volume, high cytoplasmic rigidity, a natural tendency to adhere to the vascular endothelium, and a capacity to generate toxic superoxide radicals and proteolytic enzymes[10]. In diabetes,there is increased retinal leukostasis, which affects retinal endothelial function, retinal perfusion, angiogenesis, and vascular permeability. And, leukocytes in diabetes are less deformable, a higher proportion are activated, and they may be involved in capillary nonperfusion, endothelial cell damage, and vascular leakage in the retinal microcirculation[10]. A study showed that diabetic vascular leakage and nonperfusion are temporally and spatially associated with retinal leukostasis in streptozotocin induced diabetic rats[11]. There are many capillary occlusions by leukocytes and capillary dropout or degeneration associated with leukocytes in the diabetic retina[10]. Serial acridine orange leukocyte fluorography and fluorescein angiography(FA) show trapped leukocytes directly associated with areas of downstream nonperfusion in the diabetic retinal microcirculation[10].

A number of proangiogenic, angiogenic and antiangiogenic factors are involved in the pathogenesis and progression of diabetic retinal disease, Vascular Endothelial Growth Factor (VEGF) being one of the most important. Other growth factors, which are known to participate in the pathogenesis of the disease, are: Platelet Derived Growth Factor (PDGF), Fibroblast Growth Factor (FGF), Hepatocyte Growth Factor (HGF), Transforming Growth Factor (TGF), Placental Endothelial Cell Growth Factor (PlGF), Connective Tissue Growth Factor (CTGF). Other molecules that are involved in the disease mechanisms are: intergrins, angiopoietins, protein kinase C (PKC), ephrins, interleukins, leptin, angiotensin, monocyte chemotactic protein (MCP), vascular cell adhesion molecule (VCAM), tissue plasminogen activator (TPA), and extracellular matrix metalloproteinases (ECM-MMPs).

3. Vascular Endothelial Growth Factor (VEGF)

The VEGFs are a family of proteins that are mitogenic for vascular endothelial cells and increase vascular permeability. VEGF is important in fetal vascular development,with VEGF levels diminishing after birth. VEGF is expressed by retinal glial cells[12] and vascular endothelial cells[13]. VEGF is secreted by numerous ocular cell types[14], and increased levels of VEGF have been detected in ocular fluids of patients with proliferative diabetic retinopathy[15]. In vivo, administration of neutralizing VEGF antibodies to experimental animals reverses high-glucose–induced vascular hyperpermeability[16], which is an early manifestation of endothelial dysfunction in diabetic patients[17].

VEGF expression is regulated largely by hypoxia, but it also accumulates in the retina early in diabetes, before any retinal hypoxia is yet apparent [18-20]. It is produced by multiple cell types in the retina in diabetes, including ganglion cells, Mueller cells, and pericytes. Repeated injections of high concentrations of VEGF in the eyes of nondiabetic monkeys result in retinal changes which in some ways resemble those in the early stages of diabetic retinopathy, including vascular tortuosity and microaneurysm[21, 22]. Genetic factors are important in the pathogenesis of DR; there is a clear association of increased expression of VEGF with DR as well as numerous VEGF polymorphisms that are linked to increased VEGF levels and DR.[23] Their result has demonstrated that the development of different stages of diabetic retinopathy is closely correlated with an increased VEGF level in the retina[24].Clinical trials using anti-VEGF therapies are showing promising results against stages of diabetic retinopathy[25].

VEGF is a potent vascular permeability factor, and VEGF upregulation has been linked to neovascular eye diseases including diabetic retinopathy[23]. VEGF-induced neovascular changes have previously been demonstrated on animal models based on increasing VEGF levels through implants[26], recombinant adenovirus-mediated VEGF expression[27, 28], or transgenic technologies[29, 30].

In the eye, one of the earliest signs of diabetic retinopathy is retinal capillary occlusion, blocking blood flow and generating capillary-free areas[31]. Hypoxic conditions could develop in these capillary-free areas, and this in turn could induce the upregulation of angiogenic factor production, such as VEGF and intercellular adhesion molecules[32, 33]. The increased concentration of angiogenic factors would then cause vascular changes including vascular dilatations, tortuous blood vessels, microaneurysms, and endothelial cell proliferation. Subsequently,over an extended period of time, these changes could result in the development of poorly matured leaky vessels[34, 35].Previous histological studies have demonstrated a strong correlation between endothelial cell proliferation, pericyte loss, and the development of microaneurysm[36]. Incidentally, VEGF, which is a known factor of endothelial cell proliferation, has also been shown to promote pericyte detachment and loss[37].

Troglitazone and rosiglitazone, another thiazolidinediones (TZD), increase VEGF mRNA levels in 3T3-L1 adipocytes.Although increased VEGF may be beneficial for subjects with macroangiopathy and troglitazone is currently not available for clinical use, vascular complications, especially diabetic retinopathy, must be followed with great caution in subjects treated with TZD [38].

Federico et al[39] tested selective PPARα and PPARγ synthetic agonists potential ability to stimulate neoangiogenesis in well-established in vitro and in vivo assays. They found that specific and selective activation of PPARα and PPARγ leads to increased production of VEGF, a prototypical angiogenic agent, and formation of endothelial tubules when endothelial cells are co-cultured with interstitial cells. In vivo, PPARα and PPARγ synthetic agonists stimulate angiogenesis in the mouse corneal neovascularization assay, whereas fibrates and TZDs are unable to induce angiogenesis in the same experimental setting. PPARα- and PPARγ-angiogenic process is associated with increased expression of VEGF and increased phosphorylation of endothelial nitric oxide (NO) synthase(eNOS) and Akt. Finally, it may be inhibited by blocking VEGF activity. The ability of PPARa and PPARγ agonists to induce neoangiogenesis might have important implications for the clinical and therapeutic management of type 2 diabetes[39].

4. Pigmented Epithelial Derived Factor (PEDF)

PEDF is a member of the serine protease inhibitor (serpin) superfamily with neurotrophic and antiangiogenic properties, and a decreased level of PEDF in the eye is important in the pathogenesis of proliferative DR[40]. In the retina, angiogenesis is regulated by two counterbalancing systems: angiogenic stimulators, such as VEGF, and angiogenic inhibitors, such as angiostatin and pigment epithelium–derived factor (PEDF)[40].

PEDF is a natural extracellular component of the retina and has been found in the vitreous and aqueous humors. Decreased levels of PEDF were reported in the ocular fluids of patients with angiogenic eye diseases[41]. PEDF has potent antiangiogenic activity in retinal EC growth and migration and suppressed ischemia-induced retinal neovascularization[42].

Pericyte loss is one of the earliest hallmarks of DR and an important reason for pericyte loss is reactive oxygen species (ROS)[43]. In DR, PEDF has a novel benefit since PEDF protects retinal pericytes against oxidative stress-induced injury through its anti-oxidative properties, which might slow the development of diabetic retinopathy[43].PEDF protects against high glucose or ROS induced pericyte apoptosis and dysfunction through its anti-oxidative properties via induction of glutathione[44].

Guoquan et al[45] compared susceptibilities of Sprague Dawley(SD) and Brown Norway(BN) rats with ischemia-induced retinal neovascularization. They found that the hyperoxia-treated BN rats showed a significant reduction in retinal PEDF and a substantial increase of VEGF at both the protein and RNA levels, resulting in an increased VEGF-to-PEDF ratio. The results suggested that BN rats developed more severe retinal neovascularization, which correlated with a greater increase of the VEGF-to-PEDF ratio in BN than in SD rats[45].

PEDF, a potent inhibitor of angiogenesis, has been found to be involved in the pathogenesis of PDR[46, 47]. It is well known that there are quite a few stimulators and inhibitors of angiogenesis in the eye; among them, VEGF has been identified as a primary angiogenic stimulator[48] and PEDF as a major angiogenic inhibitor[47]. The time course of the VEGF-to-PEDF ratio change correlated with the development and progression of retinal neovascularization. The VEGF-to-PEDF ratio represented a dynamic balance between angiogenic stimulators and inhibitors; and disturbance of the balance played a key role in the pathogenesis of DR[45, 49, 50]. In vitro study revealed that lowering of the VEGF-to-PEDF mRNA ratio could inhibit the migration of uveal melanoma cells[51].

Additionally, PEDF induces the ERK signal cascade which contributes to retinal pigment epithelial cell cytoprotection against oxidative stress[52]. Thus, retinal cells including the BRB capillaries and their supportive and protective pericytes may possess a system capable of efficiently responding to PEDF[43, 44].

Retinal ischemia induces intraocular neovascularization,presumably by stimulating the expression of angiogenic growth factors and by inhibiting the release of antiangiogenic cytokines[53, 54]. Vitreal levels of angiogenic growth factors have been shown to be directly associated with the degree of retinal angiogenesis[15, 55]. PEDF protects cerebellar granule cells against neurotoxic agents[56] and is also called early population doubling level cDNA-1 (EPC-

1), reflecting its upregulation during cell cycle arrest (G0) in young but not in senescent cultured fibroblasts[57].

PEDF has been shown to be a highly effective inhibitor of angiogenesis in animal and cell culture models. The production of PEDF was decreased by hypoxia[47], which is also a central pathogenic stimulus in PDR. Immunoneutralization of PEDF diminished the ability of cadaveric human vitreous to inhibit migration of endothelial cells, thereby demonstrating that a loss of PEDF is functionally important in mediating angiogenic properties of human vitreous ex vivo. Most importantly, systemically administered PEDF prevented aberrant blood vessel growth in a murine model of ischemia-induced retinopathy[58].

PEDF has been shown to be a major antiangiogenic growth factor in the mammalian eye. Joachim[41] et al analyzed the in vivo regulation of PEDF in patients with and without hypoxic eye disease. Their data strongly support the concept that retinal angiogenesis is induced by loss of the major angiogenesis inhibitor in the eye, PEDF, in combination with an increased expression of angiogenic growth factors such as VEGF. These findings suggest that substitution of angiogenesis inhibitors may be an effective approach in the treatment of PDR[41].

In the study of Zhi[59] et al ,diabetic rats and control animals were randomly assigned to receive perindopril or vehicle for 24 weeks, and bovine retinal capillary endothelial cells (BRECs) were incubated with normal or high glucose with or without perindopril. The results showed the VEGF-to-PEDF ratio was increased in the retina of diabetic rats; perindopril lowered the increased VEGF-to-PEDF ratio in diabetic rats and ameliorated the retinal damage. In BRECs, perindopril lowered the hyperglycemia-induced elevation of VEGF-to-PEDF ratio by reducing mitochondrial ROS and the decreased ROS production was a result of perindopril induced upregulation of PPARY and UCP-2 expression[59].

Although VEGF is the major factor in the initiation of advanced stages of diabetic retinopathy, it is increasingly recognized that PlGF is a significant factor in promoting the aberrant angiogenesis characteristic of a variety of pathological states.

5. Adiponectin (ADPN)

The adipocyte derived factor ADPN is an insulin sensitivity activator, and is correlated to retinal redox stress and remodeling in metabolic syndrome and T2DM. Low levels of serum ADPN levels were found to be correlated with the severity of retinopathy[60]. Insulin-sensitizing agents reduce pathological retinal microvessel formation through ADPN mediated modulation of tumor necrosis factor alpha (TNF α) production[61]. ADPN' s effect on diabetic retinopathy is not clear. However, ADPN induces eNO production by stimulating phosphorylation and activation of eNOS. ADPN inhibits specific binding of oxidized LDL and its uptake by macrophages. ADPN possesses anti-inflammatory properties and thus may negatively modulate the process of atherogenesis[62, 63].

In the early phase of diabetic retinopathy, hyperglycemia initiates endothelial cell injury, retinal vessel loss, and ischemia,as well as changes in leukocyte adhesion to the vascular endothelium[64, 65]. These conditions subsequently lead to the overproduction of various proangiogenic factors and proinflammatory cytokines, which, in turn, promotes abnormal neovascular changes[66].The primary goal for treatment of ischemic retinopathy is to preserve vision through the inhibition of abnormal neovascularization and vascular damage.

Adiponectin is a circulating adipose-derived cytokine with antiinflammatory properties[67, 68].In animal models,adiponectin deficiency is associated with the increased inflammatory responses under conditions of stresses including overnutrition and ischemic insult[69, 70]. In addition, adiponectin has been shown to protect against the development of various diseases including detrimental cardiac and vascular remodeling,ischemic stroke and increased albuminuria[69, 71-74]. In human populations, circulating adiponectin levels inversely correlate with the inflammatory marker C-reactive protein levels in blood stream[67, 75, 76]. Low plasma adiponectin levels are associated with the increased prevalence of type 2 diabetes and its macrovascular complications including ischemic heart disease[63, 67, 77].

Clinical studies regarding the relationship between plasma adiponectin level and retinopathy in diabetes have been inconclusive[78, 79]. Higuchi et al investigated whether adiponectin affects the retinal vascularization and inflammation in a mouse model of ischemia-induced retinopathy.When neonatal mice were subjected to ischemia-induced retinopathy, pathological retinal neovascularization during ischemia was exacerbated in adiponectin-knockout (APN-KO) mice compared with wild-type mice. APN-KO mice also exhibited increased leukocyte adhesion and tumor necrosis factor (TNF)-a expression in hypoxic retina. Adenovirus-mediated overexpression of adiponectin attenuated hypoxia-induced pathological retinal neovascularization by 35% in wild-type mice and by 40% in APN-KO mice and leukostasis by 64% in wild-type mice and by 75% in APN-KO mice, which were associated with reduced TNF-a production. TNF-a blockade diminished the enhanced pathological neovascularization in APN-KO mice, and the inhibitory effects of adiponectin overexpression on retinal neovascularization and leukocyte adhesion were abolished in mice lacking TNF-a. These data provide evidence that adiponectin protects against retinal vessel injury following pathological stimuli through modulation of TNF-a inflammatory responses[80].

ADPN suppresses adverse effects of inflammatory cytokines and reduces oxidative stress induced by oxidized LDL or high glucose in EC[62, 63]. ADPN inhibits VEGF-stimulated human coronary artery EC migration via cAMP/PKA dependent signaling including VEGF-induced generation of ROS, which implicates it as an important role in vascular processes associated with diabetes. Because ADPN is known to act as an antioxidant, anti-inflammatory, antiapoptotic and antifibrotic protein then its low levels may predispose it to a loss of any or all of the above known protective features of ADPN and directly or indirectly affect the capillary BRB including the pericyte. Importantly, ADPN may be used in the future as an early candidate biomarker of DR in CMS and T2DM.

6. Leptin

Not all patients with poor control of diabetes over long periods of time, develop retinopathy, suggesting the involvement of other mechanisms. The adipose tissue is an important endocrine organ that secretes many biologically active substances such as free fatty acids, adiponectin, and interleukin (IL)-6. They are collectively termed adipocytokines[81]. Leptin is one of adipocytokines, acting directly on the hypothalamus, thereby regulating food intake and energy expenditure[82]. The leptin receptor (Ob-R) is a single transmembrane protein that belongs to the gp130 family of cytokine receptor superfamily. The leptin receptor has several alternatively spliced isoforms, one of which, a biologically active Ob-Rb isoform, is expressed not only in the hypothalamus but also in a variety of peripheral tissues, suggesting the direct action of leptin in the periphery. The peripheral actions of leptin include the activation of platelet aggregation , the modulation of immune function[83], and the stimulation of vascular endothelial cell proliferation and angiogenesis[84, 85]. Upon binding to Ob-Rb, leptin has been shown to activate signal transducers and activators of transcription (STAT).

A study has revealed that plasma leptin concentrations are elevated significantly in patients with proliferative diabetic retinopathy relative to those with nonproliferative retinopathy[86]. Furthermore, vitreous leptin concentrations are higher in patients with proliferative diabetic retinopathy or retinal detachment[87].

Using the retinopathy of prematurity model, a mouse model of ischemia-induced retinal neovascularization, Eri Suganami [88]et al have demonstrated more pronounced retinal neovascularization in 17-day-old transgenic mice overexpressing leptin than in age-matched wild-type littermates. Leptin receptor expression was also detected in primary cultures of porcine retinal endothelial cells, where it upregulated VEGF mRNA expression. This effect was thought to be mediated at least partly through the activation of signal transducers and activators of transcription(STAT)3, because adenoviral transfection of the dominant negative form of STAT3 abolished the leptin-induced upregulation of VEGF mRNA expression in retinal endothelial cells. This study provides evidence that leptin stimulates the ischemia-induced retinal neovasucularization possibly through the upregulation of endothelial VEGF[88].

7. Insulin-like Growth Factor-1 (IGF-1)

Similar to VEGF, the activation of IGF-1 also increases PKC activation, so IGF-1 may be regulated by oxidative stress via the PKC pathway[89]. Retinal IGF-1 mRNA levels are lower in the human and diabetic rat when compared to age matched non-diabetic controls[90] and IGF-1 can have direct mitogenic effects on retinal EC[60].IGF-1 can stimulate glucose transport into retinal microvascular EC via activation of PKC and can modulate the expression and activity of VEGF[91].

Growth hormone and IGF-I have been suspected of playing a role in the progression of diabetic retinopathy. In a previous era, hypophysectomy was shown to lead to regression of proliferative retinopathy in a study of 100 patients[92]. Similarly, diabetic dwarfs with low systemic IGF-I levels due to growth hormone deficiency have a reduced incidence of proliferative DR compared with age- and sex matched diabetic patients. Such observations have raised interest in the use of growth hormone–inhibitory and antiproliferative somatostatin analogs to treat severe proliferative DR, however, a growth hormone receptor antagonist, pegvisomant, failed to induce regression of neovascularization [93]. This negative result may have occurred because the treatment was initiated too late; treatment may need to have started prior to the development of proliferative DR. In another small-scale trial (23 patients), octreotide (a somatostatin analog) treatment reduced the requirement for laser photocoagulation compared with conventional treatment in patients with either severe NPDR or early proliferative DR [94]. Over the 15-month study, only1 of 22 octreotide-treated patients required photocoagulation compared with 9 of 24 conventionally treated patients.

8. Interleukin-1 Beta (IL-1β)

Levels of the proinflammatory cytokine, IL-1β , are known to be increased in retinas from diabetic rats[95-97]. Intravitreal injection of IL-1β or exposure of retinal endothelial cells to the cytokine in vitro was shown to be capable of causing degeneration of retinal capillary endothelial cells[98], but the relevance of these findings to capillary degeneration in vivo is not clear because the levels of IL-1β likely were pharmacologically high. The role of IL-1β in the pathogenesis of diabetic retinopathy recently has been more directly studied using diabetic mice in whom the enzyme responsible for IL-1β production was inhibited or in whom the IL-1β receptor was deleted. IL-1β is the predominant product of caspase-1, and the biological activity of IL-1β is mediated by binding to the cell surface receptor, IL-1R1. Activity of caspase-1 is increased in retinas of diabetic mice, galactosefed mice, and diabetic humans, and in retinal Müller cells incubated in elevated glucose concentration[99]. Inhibition of caspase-1 using minocycline inhibited the diabetes induced increase in IL-1β and decreased degeneration of retinal capillaries in those animals[95]. Likewise, inhibition of IL-1β signaling using IL-1β receptor knock-out mice protected the animals from diabetes-induced retinal pathology at 7 months duration of diabetes[95]. The results indicate that activation of caspase-1 and subsequent production of IL-1β play an important role in the development of diabetes induced retinal pathology. One known action of IL-1β is to activate NF-κ B.

IL-1β gene expression is known to reside in EC and glial cells and its expression is significantly upregulated in high glucose conditions allowing for BRB allowing inflammatory cells to increase their migration across the BRB[98].

IL-1β is known to increase the expression of VEGF in retinal EC, and induces the expression of various genes whose promoters are regulated through complex interactions with NFκB[100]. IL-1β has been found to be increased in streptozotocin diabetic rat models[98] and IL-1β accelerates apoptosis in retinal capillary cells, specifically pericytes,through activation of NFκB, which is exacerbated by high glucose conditions[101]. NFκβ is a key regulator of antioxidant enzymes and can initiate transcription of genes involved in apoptosis and additionally increases downstream inflammatory cytokines[101]. Importantly, IL-1β activation—stimulation results in the translocation of NFκB from its cytosolic compartment to the nucleus where it initiates apoptotic genes and downstream inflammatory cytokines[101].

Additionally, IL-1β is considered as one of the most potent stimuli for inducible NOS (iNOS), contributing to ongoing inflammation via induction of iNOS protein and augmentation of its activity[98]. IL-1β receptor antagonism (IL-1 βra) in the retina and IL-1βhave been shown to interfere with the development of not only diabetic retinopathy but also pancreatic islet inflammation and beta cell apoptosis in humans with T2DM[102].

9. Interleukin-6 (IL-6)

The IL-6 cytokine shares common characteristics with VEGF, in that both are induced by hypoxia and hyperglycemia, and both play a role in vascular inflammation, permeability and angiogenesis[103]. Human studies have demonstrated that both VEGF and IL-6 were elevated in aqueous humor of patients with DR and even higher in those with proliferative DR indicating that VEGF and IL-6 play important roles in the development of DR[104]. Even peripheral blood levels of IL-6 and TNF α were elevated in humans with DR with the highest elevations found in those with proliferative DR[105]. It has been shown that the AngII-induced vascular alterations involved activation of NAD(P)H oxidase, IL-6, and increases in VEGF expression and further,that deletion of IL-6 prevented these effects of vascular inflammation in DR[106].

10. Monocyte Chemoattractant Protein (MCP-1)

MCP-1 contributes to the recruitment of inflammatory cells (monocytes/monocyte derived macrophage/microglia) in injured tissue and ROS injury may play a role in DR and retinal detachment[107]. MCP-1 is a potential angiogenic factor in the proliferative phase of DR and is associated with proliferation DR[107].Hyperglycemia increases the expression of MCP-1 in vascular EC[63] and AGE-induced ROS generation induced the MCP-1 gene and mRNA expression[63]. Recently, aqueous samples in humans with DR have revealed higher levels of MCP-1 and VEGF when compared to nondiabetic subjects and authors further state that inflammatory changes may precede the development of neovascularization in proliferative DR[108].

11. Vascular Cell Adhesion Molecule (VCAM)

Many specific growth factors mediate angiogenic process of diabetic retinopathy. VCAM-1, a member of the immunoglobulin supergene family of cellular adhesion molecules, is involved in the recruitment of leukocytes, their adhesion to vascular endothelium, and their subsequent migration into surrounding tissue. Interestingly, the expression of VCAM-1 has been found in epiretinal membranes from diabetic patients with PDR[109, 110]. In addition, it has been demonstrated that VCAM-1 promotes angiogenesis both in vitro and in vivo[111, 112].Olson et al. detected increased serum levels of VCAM-1 in diabetic patients with PDR[113]. Moreover, circulating levels of various adhesion molecules increase in patients with progressively worsening retinopathy, presumably as a result of shedding from both activated leukocytes and injured epithelium. However, systemic levels of VCAM-1 do not reflect the local production of VCAM-1 by the retina. Vitrectomy fluid samples obtained from diabetic patients with PDR are currently being used to explore indirectly

the retinal synthesis of several proteins, including growth factors, cytokines, and adhesion molecules. Two previous studies demonstrated that soluble VCAM-1 is increased in the vitreous cavity of diabetic patients with PDR compared with the vitreous of patients undergoing macular hole repair[114]or from cadaveric eyes[15].

12. Connective Tissue Growth Factor (CTGF)

The tissue repair process is regulated by a number of polypeptides including cytokines and growth factors. CTGF is a 38-kDa cysteinerich polypeptide that was originally identified from conditioned medium of human umbilical vein endothelial cells (HUVECs)[115]. CTGF, considered to be a downstream mediator of transforming growth factor-ß(TGF- ß)[116, 117], is indicated to induce the production of extracellular matrix,such as collagen and fibronectin, and to cause fibrosis[118]. One study have shown that CTGF is overexpressed in the membranes of eyes with PDR[119], suggesting that CTGF might be involved in the pathogenesis of PVR and PDR. In addition, A study revealed that CTGF is overexpressed also in the vitreous with PVR and PDR and additionally demonstrated that various types of vitreoretinal cells could be the sources of CTGF[120].

Furthermore, CTGF has been recently indicated to be one of the regulators of angiogenesis. In vitro, CTGF has been demonstrated to have proangiogenic effects on Human umbilical vein endothelial cell[121] and bovine aortic endothelial cells (BAECs)[122], and in vivo, CTGF has been indicated to induce angiogenesis in rat corneal pocket implants[123] and to be involved in tumor angiogenesis[124] and choroidal neovascularization[125, 126]

In the study of Takeshi et al, they demonstrated CTGF also stimulated the synthesis of fibronectin by hyalocytes and BRPEs without significant effect on collagen gel contraction by these cells. And CTGF promoted VEGF gene expression by hyalocytes and BRPEs. There was no significant correlation between the concentrations of CTGF and VEGF. These findings indicate that CTGF appears to be involved in the formation of proliferative membranes without direct regulation of their cicatricial contraction in the pathogenesis of proliferative vitreoretinal diseases. It is possible that CTGF has indirect effects by modulating the expression of VEGF[127].

13. Retinal Intercellular Adhesion Molecule-1 (ICAM-1) and CD18

The retinal vasculature of diabetic humans contains increased numbers of leukocytes, a finding that coincides with the increased expression of ICAM-1 in retinal vasculature[128]. The phenomenon is also present in diabetic animal models and occurs whether the diabetes is spontaneous in nature or is induced[11, 129, 130]. The increased density of leukocytes in the retinal vasculature begins as early as 1 week following the onset of experimental diabetes and results in injury to the endothelium via a FasL-mediated mechanism; a process that leads to breakdown of the BRB [131, 132]. Retinal ischemia is a second sight-threatening diabetic complication. Histolopathological analyses have shown that areas of angiographic non-perfusion in vivo frequently co-localize to regions full of acellular capillaries, that is, basement membrane tubes devoid any viable endothelial cells or pericytes[133].

The leukocytes that adhere to the diabetic retinal vasculature use specific adhesion molecules such as the integrin ligand CD18, which forms the invariable portion of the heterodimers Mac-1(CD11a/CD18) and LFA-1 (CD11b/CD18)[134]. Leukocytes use CD18 to tether themselves to intercellular adhesion molecule-1 (ICAM-1) on the surface of diabetic retinal vasculature.

A work has established the role of CD18/ICAM-1 leukocyte adhesion in the pathogenesis of early diabetes-induced leukostasis and blood-retinal barrier breakdown[131]. The study of Antonia et al also showed that retinal leukostasis increased within days of developing diabetes and correlated with the increased expression of retinal intercellular adhesion molecule-1 (ICAM-1) and CD18[135]. Mice deficient in the genes encoding for the leukocyte adhesion molecules CD18 and ICAM-1 were studied in two models of diabetic retinopathy with respect to the long-term development of retinal vascular lesions. CD18−/− and ICAM-1−/− mice demonstrated significantly fewer adherent leukocytes in the

retinal vasculature at 11 and 15 months after induction of diabetes with STZ. And this condition is associated with fewer damaged endothelial cells and lesser vascular leakage.

Galactosemia of up to 24 months causes pericyte and endothelial cell loss and formation of acellular capillaries. However, these changes are significantly reduced in CD18- and ICAM-1-deficient mice. Basement membrane thickening of the retinal vessels is increased in long-term galactosemic animals independent of the genetic strain. Thus,the chronic, low-grade subclinical inflammation is responsible for many of the signature vascular lesions of diabetic retinopathy.These data highlight the central and causal role of adherent leukocytes in the pathogenesis of diabetic retinopathy[135].

Attraction and adhesion of leukocytes to the vascular wall are important components of inflammatory processes. This leukostasis has been found to be significantly increased in retinas of diabetic animals, and might contribute to the capillary nonperfusion in diabetic retinopathy. Leukocyte stiffness has been reported to be increased in diabetes (decreased filterability) and to contribute to the development of capillary nonperfusion in retinal vessels [136, 137]. Diabetes increases expression of ICAM-1 in retinas of animals [11]and interaction of this adhesion molecule on retinal endothelia with the CD18 adhesion molecule on monocytes and neutrophils contributes to the diabetes-induced increase in leukostasis within retinal vessels[11]. Leukostasis has been postulated to be a factor in death of retinal endothelial cells in diabetes[131].

White blood cells bind to ICAM-1 on the surface of endothelial cells as a component of a multistep process leading to adherence of the white blood cell to the endothelial wall[11].This leukostasis is known to be increased in retinal blood vessels in diabetes, and this process is mediated via ICAM-1[11]. ICAM-1 is upregulated by several stimuli, including VEGF, PARP activation, oxidative stress, and dylipidemia[138-141], at least in part by NF-κ B.Genetically modified C57B1/6J mice have been used to explore the roles of ICAM-1 and its ligand on white blood cells (CD18) in the pathogenesis of diabetes-induced retinal vascular disease[135].

14. NF-κB

NF-κ B is a widely expressed inducible transcription factor that is an important regulator of many genes involved in mammalian inflammatory and immune responses, proliferation and apoptosis. NF-κ B is composed of homodimers and heterodimers, the most abundant and best-studied form in mammalian cells consisting of the p65 and p50 subunits. Diabetes has been found to cause migration of the p65 subunit into the nucleus of retinal pericytes[101], and of the p50 subunit into nuclei of retinal endothelial cells, pericytes, ganglion cells, and cells of the inner nuclear layer[142].

Evidence in support of an important role of NF-κ B in the pathogenesis of early stages of diabetic retinopathy is twofold. First, inhibition of proteins whose expression is regulated by NF-κ B (such as iNOS and ICAM) inhibit diabetes induced degeneration of retinal capillaries (described below).Second, compounds known to inhibit NF-κ B likewise inhibit the development of the retinopathy. For example, several different antioxidants which inhibit the development of capillary degeneration and pericyte loss in retinas of diabetic rats[143] also inhibit the diabetes-induced activation of retinal NF-κ B[138].Likewise, low-intermediate doses of salicylates (aspirin, sodium salicylate, and sulfasalazine) which inhibited NF-κ B activation in retinas of diabetic rats, also inhibited expression of inflammatory mediators like iNOS and ICAM-1, and capillary degeneration and pericyte loss in those animals[143, 144]. Aspirin is known to inhibit also production of prostaglandins, but salicylate and sulfasalazine have much less of this activity, suggesting that the common action of these salicylates to inhibit retinopathy in diabetes was not primarily mediated by inhibition of prostaglandins.

15. *iNOS*

Inducible isoform of nitric oxide synthase(iNOS) expression is regulated at least in part by NF-κ B. Interestingly, experimental sympathectomy itself increases gene and protein expression of iNOS in retinas of nondiabetic rats[145], suggesting that loss of sympathetic activity, such as which occurs in diabetes, might contribute to the upregulation of this inflammatory protein in the retina.

In retinas of diabetic animals, increased levels of nitric oxide products (nitrotyrosine, nitrite, nitrate) have been reported[144-146]. Upregulation of iNOS has been found in retinas of experimental diabetic rodents and patients in most studies[145-152]. Diabetes-induced alterations in expression of other isoforms of nitric oxide synthase also have been reported[153, 154]. A possible role of iNOS in the pathogenesis of diabetic retinopathy is suggested by the studies of aminoguanidine. Aminoguanidine is a relatively selective inhibitor of iNOS[155-158], and has been found to inhibit the diabetes-induced increase nitric oxide production and iNOS expression in retina[145].

Aminoguanidine also has been found to inhibit the development of the microvascular lesions of diabetic retinopathy in diabetic dogs[159]and rats[160].The role of iNOS in the development of the early stages of diabetic retinopathy recently has been investigated directly using mice genetically deficient in iNOS[161]. In that study, wildtype diabetic mice developed the expected degeneration of retinal capillaries, as well as increase in leukostasis and superoxide generation. In contrast, diabetic mice deficient in iNOS did not develop these structural or functional abnormalities.

16. Fas

Fas levels are increased in retinas of diabetic rats[132, 162]. Blocking FasL in vivo has been shown to prevent endothelial cell damage, vascular leakage, and platelet accumulation in diabetes, suggesting that the Fas/FasL system might contribute to the diabetes-induced damage that contributes to the development of the retinopathy[132], but its role in the development of retinal histopathology has not been assessed.

17. Angiopoietin-1

Angiopoietin-1 has been found to have anti-inflammatory actions, including inhibition of vascular permeability and adhesion protein expression[163]. When administered intravitreally to diabetic rats, angiopoietin-1 normalized blood-retinal barrier function, leukostasis and endothelial injury, and inhibited upregulation of retinal VEGF and ICAM-1mRNA and protein[164].

18. Hepatocyte Growth Factor (HGF)

HGF in the etiopathogenesis of PDR remains to be elucidated. A lot of studies[165-169] have found high intravitreous concentrations of HGF in patients with PDR. In the present study, we consider all these confounding factors in order to evaluate the vitreous levels of HGF in patients with PDR and to investigate its relationship with VEGF and retinopathy activity. A total of 28 diabetic patients with PDR, in whom a vitrectomy was performed, were included in the study. Thirty nondiabetic patients with other conditions requiring vitrectomy but in whom the retina was not directly affected by neovascularization served as a control group. Patients in whom intravitreous hemoglobin was detectable by spectophotometry were excluded. HGF and VEGF were determined by enzyme-linked immunosorbent assay. Vitreal levels of both VEGF and HGF were higher in diabetic patients with PDR than in the control group. These differences remained highly significant after adjusting for serum levels. To explore the influence of the breakdown of the blood-retinal barrier and, in consequence, the increased serum diffusion that occurs in PDR patients, the levels of both HGF and VEGF were normalized for total vitreal protein concentration. After correcting for total vitreous protein concentration, the ratio of VEGF to vitreal proteins remained significantly higher in diabetic patients with PDR than in the control group, respectively. However, the ratio of HGF to vitreal proteins was lower in diabetic patients than in nondiabetic control subjects. The lower intravitreous levels of HGF obtained after correcting for intravitreal proteins in patients with PDR in comparison with nondiabetic control subjects suggest that serum diffusion largely explains the differences detected in the intravitreous HGF levels between these groups. The vitreous concentrations of VEGF were higher in patients with active PDR than in patients with quiescent PDR. By contrast, vitreous HGF was not related to PDR activity[170].

19. Angiotensin II

Angiogenesis, the growth of new vessels, is a physiologic process that occurs under normal conditions. During these processes, angiogenesis is well regulated by a balance of positive and negative factors. However, in various disease states, such as tumor progression, inflammation, and diabetic retinopathy, deregulated overactive angiogenesis contributes to disease progression[171].Recent reports suggest that receptor tyrosine kinases (RTKs) of endothelial cells play a major role in both physiological and pathological angiogenesis[171, 172]. Two distinct RTK subfamilies are characterized by their abundant expression of endothelium. One subfamily consists of VEGF receptors Flt-1/VEGF-R1, Flk-1/VEGF-R2, and Flt-4/VEGF-R3[173-175]. VEGF, also known as vascular permeability factor, is an endothelial cell-specific mitogen that induces angiogenesis and increases vasopermeability[171].

The other endothelium-specific RTK subfamily is the Tie receptor family, consisting of Tie1 and Tie2[176]. Tie1-null mice die in utero with defects that may implicate the hemodynamics of transcapillary fluid exchange[177, 178]. Similarly, Tie2-knockout mice die from day 9.5 to 10.5, because of immature vessels and lack of microvessel formation[178, 179]. Unlike the VEGF receptor–knockout mouse[180], the number of endothelial cells was normal, and tubular formation was detected in Tie2-knockout mice. A mutation in Tie2 in humans was reported to cause venous malformations, which are typically an imbalance of endothelial cells and smooth muscle cells[181]. These findings suggest that the Tie2 system has a role in endothelialstromal cell communication and in maturation and stabilization of vascular structures.

Ligands for the Tie2 receptor have been identified as angiopoietin (Ang)-1 and Ang2 [182, 183] and, more recently,Ang3 and Ang4[184]. Ang1 phosphorylates Tie2 in cultured endothelial cells[182], whereas Ang2 does not induce phosphorylation of Tie2, but rather inhibits the Ang1-induced phosphorylation of Tie2 in vascular endothelial cells[183].Ang2-overexpressing transgenic mice die with vascular defects similar to Tie2- or Ang1-knockout mice[178, 185]. These observations suggest that Ang2 acts as a natural antagonist of Tie2 by blocking receptor activation by Ang1[183]. Recently, wide expression of Tie2 in the quiescent vasculature of adult tissues was reported[186]. A study using a corneal angiogenesis model revealed that Ang1 and Ang2 facilitates VEGF-induced neovascularization; Ang1 promotes vascular network maturation, whereas Ang2 initiates neovascularization[187].These data support the idea that angiopoietins/Tie2 may have a role not only in embryonic angiogenesis, but also in postnatal angiogenesis.

The renin-angiotensin system (RAS) is known to be a key factor in the cardiovascular homeostasis that regulates blood pressure and fluid electrolyte balance[188]. RAS abnormalities have also been reported to play a role in the progression of diabetic retinopathy[189]. Angiotensin II has been reported to regulate cell growth by inducing several growth factors[190-192]. In 1998 and 2000, Atsushi Otani et al reported that Angitensin II potentiates VEGF-mediated angiogenic activities through upregulation of VEGF-R2 expression in bovine retinal endothelial cells (BRECs) and upregulation of VEGF in bovine retinal pericytes (BRPs) [193, 194]. As RAS played a major role in the retinal angiogenic abnormalities associated with diabetes, Atsushi Otani et al investigated the effect of angiotensin II (AII) on Ang1 and Ang2 expression in cultured bovine retinal endothelial cells(BRECs). Their results showed that AII stimulated Ang2 but not Ang1 mRNA expression in a dose- and time-dependent manner. This response was inhibited completely by angiotensin type 1 receptor (AT1) antagonist. AII increased the transcription of Ang2 mRNA, but did not change the half-life. Protein kinase C (PKC) inhibitor completely inhibited AIIinduced Ang2 expression, and the mitogen-activated protein kinase (MAPK) inhibitor also inhibited it. In addition, the upregulation of Ang2 in an AII-induced in vivo rat corneal neovascularization model was also confirmed. These data suggest that AII stimulates Ang2 expression through AT1 receptor-mediated PKC and MAPK pathways in BREC, and AII may play a novel role in retinal neovascularization[195].

20. Glial cell-derived cytokines

BRB is a biological unit of retinal vessels with a well-differentiated network, including glial cells such as astrocytes and Müller cells, maintaining the retinal microenvironment and low permeability. The substantial apparatus of the BRB is a barrier comprised of tight junctions between the capillary endothelial cells that strictly regulate the paracellular pathways between the cells[196]. BRB breakdown is closely associated with a number of retinal diseases such as diabetic retinopathy, which is characterized by vascular leakage due to increased vascular permeability in its early pathogenesis[197].

Hich is believed to be a critical factor in the development of diabetic retinopathy[12, 15, 48]. However, the molecular pharmacology that directly inhibits activated VEGF has not been proven to satisfactorily block microangiopathy in diabetic retinopathy[198, 199]. Glial cell line–derived neurotrophic factor (GDNF) was originally identified as a neurotrophic differentiation factor for dopaminergic neurons in the central nervous system and retina.The certain advanced glycation end products could increase the vascular permeability of the BRB in vitro by the induction of VEGF and reduction of GDNF expression from glial cells have been demonstrated, suggesting that phenotypic alteration of glial cells in diabetes is responsible for the BRB breakdown[200-202].

The vitamin A metabolite all-*trans* retinoic acid (ATRA) is a potent regulator of cell differentiation and an essential signaling molecule in embryonic development and throughout life. A study has shown that ATRA can differentiate pluripotent embryonal carcinoma cells into neuronal and glial tissues and that it plays an important role in the induction of GDNF responsiveness in these cells[203]. Nami Nishikiori et al demonstrated that retinoic acid receptor (RAR)a stimulants preferentially act on glial cells, resulting in the enhanced expression of glial cell line-derived neurotrophic factor (GDNF) through recruitment of the RARa-driven trans-acting coactivator to the 5′-flanking region of the gene promoter. Conversely, RARa decreases expression of VEGF/vascular permeability factor. These gene expression alterations causally limit vascular permeability by modulating the tight junction function of capillary endothelium in a paracrine manner in vitro. The phenotypic transformation of glial cells mediated by RARa is sufficient for significant reductions of vascular leakage in the diabetic retina, suggesting that RARa antagonizes the loss of tight junction integrity induced by diabetes. These findings reveal that glial cell-derived cytokines such as GDNF and VEGF regulate BRB function, implying that the glial cell can be a possible therapeutic target in diabetic retinopathy[204].

21. References

[1] Miwa K, Nakamura J, Hamada Y, Naruse K, Nakashima E, Kato K, et al. The role of polyol pathway in glucose-induced apoptosis of cultured retinal pericytes. Diabetes Res Clin Pract. 2003; 60(1): 1-9.

[2] Yang Y, Hayden MR, Sowers S, Bagree SV, Sowers JR. Retinal redox stress and remodeling in cardiometabolic syndrome and diabetes. Oxid Med Cell Longev. 2010; 3(6): 392-403.

[3] Sims DE. The pericyte--a review. Tissue Cell. 1986; 18(2): 153-74.

[4] Ferris FL, 3rd, Patz A. Macular edema. A complication of diabetic retinopathy. Surv Ophthalmol. 1984; 28 Suppl: 452-61.

[5] Antcliff RJ, Marshall J. The pathogenesis of edema in diabetic maculopathy. Semin Ophthalmol. 1999; 14(4): 223-32.

[6] Ciulla TA, Harris A, Latkany P, Piper HC, Arend O, Garzozi H, et al. Ocular perfusion abnormalities in diabetes. Acta Ophthalmol Scand. 2002; 80(5): 468-77.

[7] Cogan DG, Toussaint D, Kuwabara T. Retinal vascular patterns. IV. Diabetic retinopathy. Arch Ophthalmol. 1961; 66: 366-78.

[8] Kuwabara T, Cogan DG. Retinal vascular patterns. VI. Mural cells of the retinal capillaries. Arch Ophthalmol. 1963; 69: 492-502.

[9] Speiser P, Gittelsohn AM, Patz A. Studies on diabetic retinopathy. 3. Influence of diabetes on intramural pericytes. Arch Ophthalmol. 1968; 80(3): 332-7.

[10] Miyamoto K, Ogura Y. Pathogenetic potential of leukocytes in diabetic retinopathy. Semin Ophthalmol. 1999; 14(4): 233-9.

[11] Miyamoto K, Khosrof S, Bursell SE, Rohan R, Murata T, Clermont AC, et al. Prevention of leukostasis and vascular leakage in streptozotocin-induced diabetic retinopathy via intercellular adhesion molecule-1 inhibition. Proc Natl Acad Sci U S A. 1999; 96(19): 10836-41.

[12] Murata T, Nakagawa K, Khalil A, Ishibashi T, Inomata H, Sueishi K. The relation between expression of vascular endothelial growth factor and breakdown of the blood-retinal barrier in diabetic rat retinas. Lab Invest. 1996; 74(4): 819-25.
[13] Levy AP, Levy NS, Wegner S, Goldberg MA. Transcriptional regulation of the rat vascular endothelial growth factor gene by hypoxia. J Biol Chem. 1995; 270(22): 13333-40.
[14] Miller JW, Adamis AP, Aiello LP. Vascular endothelial growth factor in ocular neovascularization and proliferative diabetic retinopathy. Diabetes Metab Rev. 1997; 13(1): 37-50.
[15] Aiello LP, Avery RL, Arrigg PG, Keyt BA, Jampel HD, Shah ST, et al. Vascular endothelial growth factor in ocular fluid of patients with diabetic retinopathy and other retinal disorders. N Engl J Med. 1994; 331(22): 1480-7.
[16] Tilton RG, Kawamura T, Chang KC, Ido Y, Bjercke RJ, Stephan CC, et al. Vascular dysfunction induced by elevated glucose levels in rats is mediated by vascular endothelial growth factor. J Clin Invest. 1997; 99(9): 2192-202.
[17] Leinonen H, Matikainen E, Juntunen J. Permeability and morphology of skeletal muscle capillaries in type 1 (insulin-dependent) diabetes mellitus. Diabetologia. 1982; 22(3): 158-62.
[18] Sone H, Kawakami Y, Okuda Y, Sekine Y, Honmura S, Matsuo K, et al. Ocular vascular endothelial growth factor levels in diabetic rats are elevated before observable retinal proliferative changes. Diabetologia. 1997; 40(6): 726-30.
[19] Gerhardinger C, Brown LF, Roy S, Mizutani M, Zucker CL, Lorenzi M. Expression of vascular endothelial growth factor in the human retina and in nonproliferative diabetic retinopathy. Am J Pathol. 1998; 152(6): 1453-62.
[20] Segawa Y, Shirao Y, Yamagishi S, Higashide T, Kobayashi M, Katsuno K, et al. Upregulation of retinal vascular endothelial growth factor mRNAs in spontaneously diabetic rats without ophthalmoscopic retinopathy. A possible participation of advanced glycation end products in the development of the early phase of diabetic retinopathy. Ophthalmic Res. 1998; 30(6): 333-9.
[21] Tolentino MJ, Miller JW, Gragoudas ES, Jakobiec FA, Flynn E, Chatzistefanou K, et al. Intravitreous injections of vascular endothelial growth factor produce retinal ischemia and microangiopathy in an adult primate. Ophthalmology. 1996; 103(11): 1820-8.
[22] Tolentino MJ, McLeod DS, Taomoto M, Otsuji T, Adamis AP, Lutty GA. Pathologic features of vascular endothelial growth factor-induced retinopathy in the nonhuman primate. Am J Ophthalmol. 2002; 133(3): 373-85.
[23] Yang Y, Andresen BT, Yang K, Zhang Y, Li X, Wang H. Association of vascular endothelial growth factor -634C/G polymorphism and diabetic retinopathy in type 2 diabetic Han Chinese. Exp Biol Med (Maywood). 2010; 235(10): 1204-11.
[24] Rakoczy PE, Brankov M, Fonceca A, Zaknich T, Rae BC, Lai CM. Enhanced recombinant adeno-associated virus-mediated vascular endothelial growth factor expression in the adult mouse retina: a potential model for diabetic retinopathy. Diabetes. 2003; 52(3): 857-63.
[25] Montero JA, Ruiz-Moreno JM, Correa ME. Intravitreal anti-VEGF drugs as adjuvant therapy in diabetic retinopathy surgery. Curr Diabetes Rev. 2011; 7(3): 176-84.

[26] Kenyon BM, Voest EE, Chen CC, Flynn E, Folkman J, D'Amato RJ. A model of angiogenesis in the mouse cornea. Invest Ophthalmol Vis Sci. 1996; 37(8): 1625-32.
[27] Anglade E, Csaky KG. Recombinant adenovirus-mediated gene transfer into the adult rat retina. Curr Eye Res. 1998; 17(3): 316-21.
[28] Spilsbury K, Garrett KL, Shen WY, Constable IJ, Rakoczy PE. Overexpression of vascular endothelial growth factor (VEGF) in the retinal pigment epithelium leads to the development of choroidal neovascularization. Am J Pathol. 2000; 157(1): 135-44.
[29] Okamoto N, Tobe T, Hackett SF, Ozaki H, Vinores MA, LaRochelle W, et al. Transgenic mice with increased expression of vascular endothelial growth factor in the retina: a new model of intraretinal and subretinal neovascularization. Am J Pathol. 1997; 151(1): 281-91.
[30] Ohno-Matsui K, Hirose A, Yamamoto S, Saikia J, Okamoto N, Gehlbach P, et al. Inducible expression of vascular endothelial growth factor in adult mice causes severe proliferative retinopathy and retinal detachment. Am J Pathol. 2002; 160(2): 711-9.
[31] Hata Y, Nakagawa K, Ishibashi T, Inomata H, Ueno H, Sueishi K. Hypoxia-induced expression of vascular endothelial growth factor by retinal glial cells promotes in vitro angiogenesis. Virchows Arch. 1995; 426(5): 479-86.
[32] Aiello LP, Northrup JM, Keyt BA, Takagi H, Iwamoto MA. Hypoxic regulation of vascular endothelial growth factor in retinal cells. Arch Ophthalmol. 1995; 113(12): 1538-44.
[33] Yan Q, Li Y, Hendrickson A, Sage EH. Regulation of retinal capillary cells by basic fibroblast growth factor, vascular endothelial growth factor, and hypoxia. In Vitro Cell Dev Biol Anim. 2001; 37(1): 45-9.
[34] Connolly DT. Vascular permeability factor: a unique regulator of blood vessel function. J Cell Biochem. 1991; 47(3): 219-23.
[35] Esser S, Wolburg K, Wolburg H, Breier G, Kurzchalia T, Risau W. Vascular endothelial growth factor induces endothelial fenestrations in vitro. J Cell Biol. 1998; 140(4): 947-59.
[36] Lu M, Amano S, Miyamoto K, Garland R, Keough K, Qin W, et al. Insulin-induced vascular endothelial growth factor expression in retina. Invest Ophthalmol Vis Sci. 1999; 40(13): 3281-6.
[37] Pettersson A, Nagy JA, Brown LF, Sundberg C, Morgan E, Jungles S, et al. Heterogeneity of the angiogenic response induced in different normal adult tissues by vascular permeability factor/vascular endothelial growth factor. Lab Invest. 2000; 80(1): 99-115.
[38] Emoto M, Anno T, Sato Y, Tanabe K, Okuya S, Tanizawa Y, et al. Troglitazone treatment increases plasma vascular endothelial growth factor in diabetic patients and its mRNA in 3T3-L1 adipocytes. Diabetes. 2001; 50(5): 1166-70.
[39] Biscetti F, Gaetani E, Flex A, Aprahamian T, Hopkins T, Straface G, et al. Selective activation of peroxisome proliferator-activated receptor (PPAR)alpha and PPAR gamma induces neoangiogenesis through a vascular endothelial growth factor-dependent mechanism. Diabetes. 2008; 57(5): 1394-404.
[40] Becerra SP. Structure-function studies on PEDF. A noninhibitory serpin with neurotrophic activity. Adv Exp Med Biol. 1997; 425: 223-37.

[41] Spranger J, Osterhoff M, Reimann M, Mohlig M, Ristow M, Francis MK, et al. Loss of the antiangiogenic pigment epithelium-derived factor in patients with angiogenic eye disease. Diabetes. 2001; 50(12): 2641-5.

[42] Duh EJ, Yang HS, Suzuma I, Miyagi M, Youngman E, Mori K, et al. Pigment epithelium-derived factor suppresses ischemia-induced retinal neovascularization and VEGF-induced migration and growth. Invest Ophthalmol Vis Sci. 2002; 43(3): 821-9.

[43] Amano S, Yamagishi S, Inagaki Y, Nakamura K, Takeuchi M, Inoue H, et al. Pigment epithelium-derived factor inhibits oxidative stress-induced apoptosis and dysfunction of cultured retinal pericytes. Microvasc Res. 2005; 69(1-2): 45-55.

[44] Yamagishi S, Inagaki Y, Amano S, Okamoto T, Takeuchi M, Makita Z. Pigment epithelium-derived factor protects cultured retinal pericytes from advanced glycation end product-induced injury through its antioxidative properties. Biochem Biophys Res Commun. 2002; 296(4): 877-82.

[45] Gao G, Li Y, Fant J, Crosson CE, Becerra SP, Ma JX. Difference in ischemic regulation of vascular endothelial growth factor and pigment epithelium--derived factor in brown norway and sprague dawley rats contributing to different susceptibilities to retinal neovascularization. Diabetes. 2002; 51(4): 1218-25.

[46] Patel JI, Tombran-Tink J, Hykin PG, Gregor ZJ, Cree IA. Vitreous and aqueous concentrations of proangiogenic, antiangiogenic factors and other cytokines in diabetic retinopathy patients with macular edema: Implications for structural differences in macular profiles. Exp Eye Res. 2006; 82(5): 798-806.

[47] Dawson DW, Volpert OV, Gillis P, Crawford SE, Xu H, Benedict W, et al. Pigment epithelium-derived factor: a potent inhibitor of angiogenesis. Science. 1999; 285(5425): 245-8.

[48] Pierce EA, Avery RL, Foley ED, Aiello LP, Smith LE. Vascular endothelial growth factor/vascular permeability factor expression in a mouse model of retinal neovascularization. Proc Natl Acad Sci U S A. 1995; 92(3): 905-9.

[49] Gao G, Li Y, Zhang D, Gee S, Crosson C, Ma J. Unbalanced expression of VEGF and PEDF in ischemia-induced retinal neovascularization. FEBS Lett. 2001; 489(2-3): 270-6.

[50] Chen H, Jia W, Xu X, Fan Y, Zhu D, Wu H, et al. Upregulation of PEDF expression by PARP inhibition contributes to the decrease in hyperglycemia-induced apoptosis in HUVECs. Biochem Biophys Res Commun. 2008; 369(2): 718-24.

[51] Yang H, Xu Z, Iuvone PM, Grossniklaus HE. Angiostatin decreases cell migration and vascular endothelium growth factor (VEGF) to pigment epithelium derived factor (PEDF) RNA ratio in vitro and in a murine ocular melanoma model. Mol Vis. 2006; 12: 511-7.

[52] Tsao YP, Ho TC, Chen SL, Cheng HC. Pigment epithelium-derived factor inhibits oxidative stress-induced cell death by activation of extracellular signal-regulated kinases in cultured retinal pigment epithelial cells. Life Sci. 2006; 79(6): 545-50.

[53] King GL, Suzuma K. Pigment-epithelium-derived factor--a key coordinator of retinal neuronal and vascular functions. N Engl J Med. 2000; 342(5): 349-51.

[54] Spranger J, Hammes HP, Preissner KT, Schatz H, Pfeiffer AF. Release of the angiogenesis inhibitor angiostatin in patients with proliferative diabetic

retinopathy: association with retinal photocoagulation. Diabetologia. 2000; 43(11): 1404-7.
[55] Meyer-Schwickerath R, Pfeiffer A, Blum WF, Freyberger H, Klein M, Losche C, et al. Vitreous levels of the insulin-like growth factors I and II, and the insulin-like growth factor binding proteins 2 and 3, increase in neovascular eye disease. Studies in nondiabetic and diabetic subjects. J Clin Invest. 1993; 92(6): 2620-5.
[56] Taniwaki T, Hirashima N, Becerra SP, Chader GJ, Etcheberrigaray R, Schwartz JP. Pigment epithelium-derived factor protects cultured cerebellar granule cells against glutamate-induced neurotoxicity. J Neurochem. 1997; 68(1): 26-32.
[57] Pignolo RJ, Cristofalo VJ, Rotenberg MO. Senescent WI-38 cells fail to express EPC-1, a gene induced in young cells upon entry into the G0 state. J Biol Chem. 1993; 268(12): 8949-57.
[58] Stellmach V, Crawford SE, Zhou W, Bouck N. Prevention of ischemia-induced retinopathy by the natural ocular antiangiogenic agent pigment epithelium-derived factor. Proc Natl Acad Sci U S A. 2001; 98(5): 2593-7.
[59] Zheng Z, Chen H, Ke G, Fan Y, Zou H, Sun X, et al. Protective effect of perindopril on diabetic retinopathy is associated with decreased vascular endothelial growth factor-to-pigment epithelium-derived factor ratio: involvement of a mitochondria-reactive oxygen species pathway. Diabetes. 2009; 58(4): 954-64.
[60] Kato K, Osawa H, Ochi M, Kusunoki Y, Ebisui O, Ohno K, et al. Serum total and high molecular weight adiponectin levels are correlated with the severity of diabetic retinopathy and nephropathy. Clin Endocrinol (Oxf). 2008; 68(3): 442-9.
[61] Higuchi A, Ohashi K, Shibata R, Sono-Romanelli S, Walsh K, Ouchi N. Thiazolidinediones reduce pathological neovascularization in ischemic retina via an adiponectin-dependent mechanism. Arterioscler Thromb Vasc Biol. 2010; 30(1): 46-53.
[62] Ouchi N, Kihara S, Arita Y, Nishida M, Matsuyama A, Okamoto Y, et al. Adipocyte-derived plasma protein, adiponectin, suppresses lipid accumulation and class A scavenger receptor expression in human monocyte-derived macrophages. Circulation. 2001; 103(8): 1057-63.
[63] Ouchi N, Kihara S, Arita Y, Maeda K, Kuriyama H, Okamoto Y, et al. Novel modulator for endothelial adhesion molecules: adipocyte-derived plasma protein adiponectin. Circulation. 1999; 100(25): 2473-6.
[64] Sheetz MJ, King GL. Molecular understanding of hyperglycemia's adverse effects for diabetic complications. JAMA. 2002; 288(20): 2579-88.
[65] Spranger J, Pfeiffer AF. New concepts in pathogenesis and treatment of diabetic retinopathy. Exp Clin Endocrinol Diabetes. 2001; 109 Suppl 2: S438-50.
[66] Gariano RF, Gardner TW. Retinal angiogenesis in development and disease. Nature. 2005; 438(7070): 960-6.
[67] Ouchi N, Kihara S, Funahashi T, Matsuzawa Y, Walsh K. Obesity, adiponectin and vascular inflammatory disease. Curr Opin Lipidol. 2003; 14(6): 561-6.
[68] Scherer PE, Williams S, Fogliano M, Baldini G, Lodish HF. A novel serum protein similar to C1q, produced exclusively in adipocytes. J Biol Chem. 1995; 270(45): 26746-9.

[69] Shibata R, Sato K, Pimentel DR, Takemura Y, Kihara S, Ohashi K, et al. Adiponectin protects against myocardial ischemia-reperfusion injury through AMPK- and COX-2-dependent mechanisms. Nat Med. 2005; 11(10): 1096-103.
[70] Maeda N, Shimomura I, Kishida K, Nishizawa H, Matsuda M, Nagaretani H, et al. Diet-induced insulin resistance in mice lacking adiponectin/ACRP30. Nat Med. 2002; 8(7): 731-7.
[71] Kubota N, Terauchi Y, Yamauchi T, Kubota T, Moroi M, Matsui J, et al. Disruption of adiponectin causes insulin resistance and neointimal formation. J Biol Chem. 2002; 277(29): 25863-6.
[72] Sharma K, Ramachandrarao S, Qiu G, Usui HK, Zhu Y, Dunn SR, et al. Adiponectin regulates albuminuria and podocyte function in mice. J Clin Invest. 2008; 118(5): 1645-56.
[73] Shibata R, Ouchi N, Kihara S, Sato K, Funahashi T, Walsh K. Adiponectin stimulates angiogenesis in response to tissue ischemia through stimulation of amp-activated protein kinase signaling. J Biol Chem. 2004; 279(27): 28670-4.
[74] Nishimura M, Izumiya Y, Higuchi A, Shibata R, Qiu J, Kudo C, et al. Adiponectin prevents cerebral ischemic injury through endothelial nitric oxide synthase dependent mechanisms. Circulation. 2008; 117(2): 216-23.
[75] Matsushita K, Yatsuya H, Tamakoshi K, Wada K, Otsuka R, Zhang H, et al. Inverse association between adiponectin and C-reactive protein in substantially healthy Japanese men. Atherosclerosis. 2006; 188(1): 184-9.
[76] Engeli S, Feldpausch M, Gorzelniak K, Hartwig F, Heintze U, Janke J, et al. Association between adiponectin and mediators of inflammation in obese women. Diabetes. 2003; 52(4): 942-7.
[77] Kumada M, Kihara S, Sumitsuji S, Kawamoto T, Matsumoto S, Ouchi N, et al. Association of hypoadiponectinemia with coronary artery disease in men. Arterioscler Thromb Vasc Biol. 2003; 23(1): 85-9.
[78] Matsuda M, Kawasaki F, Yamada K, Kanda Y, Saito M, Eto M, et al. Impact of adiposity and plasma adipocytokines on diabetic angiopathies in Japanese Type 2 diabetic subjects. Diabet Med. 2004; 21(8): 881-8.
[79] Yilmaz MI, Sonmez A, Acikel C, Celik T, Bingol N, Pinar M, et al. Adiponectin may play a part in the pathogenesis of diabetic retinopathy. Eur J Endocrinol. 2004; 151(1): 135-40.
[80] Higuchi A, Ohashi K, Kihara S, Walsh K, Ouchi N. Adiponectin suppresses pathological microvessel formation in retina through modulation of tumor necrosis factor-alpha expression. Circ Res. 2009; 104(9): 1058-65.
[81] Matsuzawa Y, Funahashi T, Nakamura T. Molecular mechanism of metabolic syndrome X: contribution of adipocytokines adipocyte-derived bioactive substances. Ann N Y Acad Sci. 1999; 892: 146-54.
[82] Friedman JM, Halaas JL. Leptin and the regulation of body weight in mammals. Nature. 1998; 395(6704): 763-70.
[83] Mantzoros CS. The role of leptin in human obesity and disease: a review of current evidence. Ann Intern Med. 1999; 130(8): 671-80.
[84] Sierra-Honigmann MR, Nath AK, Murakami C, Garcia-Cardena G, Papapetropoulos A, Sessa WC, et al. Biological action of leptin as an angiogenic factor. Science. 1998; 281(5383): 1683-6.

[85] Bouloumie A, Drexler HC, Lafontan M, Busse R. Leptin, the product of Ob gene, promotes angiogenesis. Circ Res. 1998; 83(10): 1059-66.
[86] Uckaya G, Ozata M, Bayraktar Z, Erten V, Bingol N, Ozdemir IC. Is leptin associated with diabetic retinopathy? Diabetes Care. 2000; 23(3): 371-6.
[87] Gariano RF, Nath AK, D'Amico DJ, Lee T, Sierra-Honigmann MR. Elevation of vitreous leptin in diabetic retinopathy and retinal detachment. Invest Ophthalmol Vis Sci. 2000; 41(11): 3576-81.
[88] Suganami E, Takagi H, Ohashi H, Suzuma K, Suzuma I, Oh H, et al. Leptin stimulates ischemia-induced retinal neovascularization: possible role of vascular endothelial growth factor expressed in retinal endothelial cells. Diabetes. 2004; 53(9): 2443-8.
[89] Yano K, Bauchat JR, Liimatta MB, Clemmons DR, Duan C. Down-regulation of protein kinase C inhibits insulin-like growth factor I-induced vascular smooth muscle cell proliferation, migration, and gene expression. Endocrinology. 1999; 140(10): 4622-32.
[90] Matsuzawa Y. Therapy Insight: adipocytokines in metabolic syndrome and related cardiovascular disease. Nat Clin Pract Cardiovasc Med. 2006; 3(1): 35-42.
[91] DeBosch BJ, Baur E, Deo BK, Hiraoka M, Kumagai AK. Effects of insulin-like growth factor-1 on retinal endothelial cell glucose transport and proliferation. J Neurochem. 2001; 77(4): 1157-67.
[92] Sharp PS, Fallon TJ, Brazier OJ, Sandler L, Joplin GF, Kohner EM. Long-term follow-up of patients who underwent yttrium-90 pituitary implantation for treatment of proliferative diabetic retinopathy. Diabetologia. 1987; 30(4): 199-207.
[93] Growth Hormone Antagonist for Proliferative Diabetic Retinopathy Study Group.The effect of a growth hormone receptor antagonist drug on proliferative diabetic retinopathy. Ophthalmology. 2001; **108**(12): 2266-72.
[94] The effect of a growth hormone receptor antagonist drug on proliferative diabetic retinopathy. Ophthalmology. 2001; 108(12): 2266-72.
[95] Grant MB, Mames RN, Fitzgerald C, Hazariwala KM, Cooper-DeHoff R, Caballero S, et al. The efficacy of octreotide in the therapy of severe nonproliferative and early proliferative diabetic retinopathy: a randomized controlled study. Diabetes Care. 2000; 23(4): 504-9.
[96] Vincent JA, Mohr S. Inhibition of caspase-1/interleukin-1beta signaling prevents degeneration of retinal capillaries in diabetes and galactosemia. Diabetes. 2007; 56(1): 224-30.
[97] Krady JK, Basu A, Allen CM, Xu Y, LaNoue KF, Gardner TW, et al. Minocycline reduces proinflammatory cytokine expression, microglial activation, and caspase-3 activation in a rodent model of diabetic retinopathy. Diabetes. 2005; 54(5): 1559-65.
[98] Kowluru RA, Odenbach S. Role of interleukin-1beta in the development of retinopathy in rats: effect of antioxidants. Invest Ophthalmol Vis Sci. 2004; 45(11): 4161-6.
[99] Kowluru RA, Odenbach S. Role of interleukin-1beta in the pathogenesis of diabetic retinopathy. Br J Ophthalmol. 2004; 88(10): 1343-7.
[100] Mohr S, Xi X, Tang J, Kern TS. Caspase activation in retinas of diabetic and galactosemic mice and diabetic patients. Diabetes. 2002; 51(4): 1172-9.
[101] Fan F, Stoeltzing O, Liu W, McCarty MF, Jung YD, Reinmuth N, et al. Interleukin-1beta regulates angiopoietin-1 expression in human endothelial cells. Cancer Res. 2004; 64(9): 3186-90.

[102] Romeo G, Liu WH, Asnaghi V, Kern TS, Lorenzi M. Activation of nuclear factor-kappaB induced by diabetes and high glucose regulates a proapoptotic program in retinal pericytes. Diabetes. 2002; 51(7): 2241-8.

[103] Dinarello CA, Donath MY, Mandrup-Poulsen T. Role of IL-1beta in type 2 diabetes. Curr Opin Endocrinol Diabetes Obes. 2010; 17(4): 314-21.

[104] Yu JG, Javorschi S, Hevener AL, Kruszynska YT, Norman RA, Sinha M, et al. The effect of thiazolidinediones on plasma adiponectin levels in normal, obese, and type 2 diabetic subjects. Diabetes. 2002; 51(10): 2968-74.

[105] Zhou L, Sun H, Xu J, Kang J. [Level of vascular endothelial growth factor and interleukin-6 in aqueous humor in diabetic retinopathy patients.]. Yan Ke Xue Bao. 2010; 25(1): 26-30.

[106] Lee JH, Lee W, Kwon OH, Kim JH, Kwon OW, Kim KH, et al. Cytokine profile of peripheral blood in type 2 diabetes mellitus patients with diabetic retinopathy. Ann Clin Lab Sci. 2008; 38(4): 361-7.

[107] Rojas M, Zhang W, Lee DL, Romero MJ, Nguyen DT, Al-Shabrawey M, et al. Role of IL-6 in angiotensin II-induced retinal vascular inflammation. Invest Ophthalmol Vis Sci. 2010; 51(3): 1709-18.

[108] Nakazawa T, Hisatomi T, Nakazawa C, Noda K, Maruyama K, She H, et al. Monocyte chemoattractant protein 1 mediates retinal detachment-induced photoreceptor apoptosis. Proc Natl Acad Sci U S A. 2007; 104(7): 2425-30.

[109] Oh IK, Kim SW, Oh J, Lee TS, Huh K. Inflammatory and angiogenic factors in the aqueous humor and the relationship to diabetic retinopathy. Curr Eye Res. 2010; 35(12): 1116-27.

[110] Tang S, Le-Ruppert KC, Gabel VP. Expression of intercellular adhesion molecule-1 (ICAM-1) and vascular cell adhesion molecule-1 (VCAM-1) on proliferating vascular endothelial cells in diabetic epiretinal membranes. Br J Ophthalmol. 1994; 78(5): 370-6.

[111] Limb GA, Chignell AH, Green W, LeRoy F, Dumonde DC. Distribution of TNF alpha and its reactive vascular adhesion molecules in fibrovascular membranes of proliferative diabetic retinopathy. Br J Ophthalmol. 1996; 80(2): 168-73.

[112] Ferrara N. Leukocyte adhesion. Missing link in angiogenesis. Nature. 1995; 376(6540): 467.

[113] Koch AE, Halloran MM, Haskell CJ, Shah MR, Polverini PJ. Angiogenesis mediated by soluble forms of E-selectin and vascular cell adhesion molecule-1. Nature. 1995; 376(6540): 517-9.

[114] Olson JA, Whitelaw CM, McHardy KC, Pearson DW, Forrester JV. Soluble leucocyte adhesion molecules in diabetic retinopathy stimulate retinal capillary endothelial cell migration. Diabetologia. 1997; 40(10): 1166-71.

[115] Barile GR, Chang SS, Park LS, Reppucci VS, Schiff WM, Schmidt AM. Soluble cellular adhesion molecules in proliferative vitreoretinopathy and proliferative diabetic retinopathy. Curr Eye Res. 1999; 19(3): 219-27.

[116] Bradham DM, Igarashi A, Potter RL, Grotendorst GR. Connective tissue growth factor: a cysteine-rich mitogen secreted by human vascular endothelial cells is related to the SRC-induced immediate early gene product CEF-10. J Cell Biol. 1991; 114(6): 1285-94.

[117] Grotendorst GR. Connective tissue growth factor: a mediator of TGF-beta action on fibroblasts. Cytokine Growth Factor Rev. 1997; 8(3): 171-9.
[118] Blom IE, Goldschmeding R, Leask A. Gene regulation of connective tissue growth factor: new targets for antifibrotic therapy? Matrix Biol. 2002; 21(6): 473-82.
[119] Leask A, Holmes A, Abraham DJ. Connective tissue growth factor: a new and important player in the pathogenesis of fibrosis. Curr Rheumatol Rep. 2002; 4(2): 136-42.
[120] Hinton DR, Spee C, He S, Weitz S, Usinger W, LaBree L, et al. Accumulation of NH2-terminal fragment of connective tissue growth factor in the vitreous of patients with proliferative diabetic retinopathy. Diabetes Care. 2004; 27(3): 758-64.
[121] Kita T, Hata Y, Kano K, Miura M, Nakao S, Noda Y, et al. Transforming growth factor-beta2 and connective tissue growth factor in proliferative vitreoretinal diseases: possible involvement of hyalocytes and therapeutic potential of Rho kinase inhibitor. Diabetes. 2007; 56(1): 231-8.
[122] Kireeva ML, Latinkic BV, Kolesnikova TV, Chen CC, Yang GP, Abler AS, et al. Cyr61 and Fisp12 are both ECM-associated signaling molecules: activities, metabolism, and localization during development. Exp Cell Res. 1997; 233(1): 63-77.
[123] Shimo T, Nakanishi T, Kimura Y, Nishida T, Ishizeki K, Matsumura T, et al. Inhibition of endogenous expression of connective tissue growth factor by its antisense oligonucleotide and antisense RNA suppresses proliferation and migration of vascular endothelial cells. J Biochem. 1998; 124(1): 130-40.
[124] Babic AM, Chen CC, Lau LF. Fisp12/mouse connective tissue growth factor mediates endothelial cell adhesion and migration through integrin alphavbeta3, promotes endothelial cell survival, and induces angiogenesis in vivo. Mol Cell Biol. 1999; 19(4): 2958-66.
[125] Shimo T, Nakanishi T, Nishida T, Asano M, Sasaki A, Kanyama M, et al. Involvement of CTGF, a hypertrophic chondrocyte-specific gene product, in tumor angiogenesis. Oncology. 2001; 61(4): 315-22.
[126] He S, Jin ML, Worpel V, Hinton DR. A role for connective tissue growth factor in the pathogenesis of choroidal neovascularization. Arch Ophthalmol. 2003; 121(9): 1283-8.
[127] Watanabe D, Takagi H, Suzuma K, Oh H, Ohashi H, Honda Y. Expression of connective tissue growth factor and its potential role in choroidal neovascularization. Retina. 2005; 25(7): 911-8.
[128] Kita T, Hata Y, Miura M, Kawahara S, Nakao S, Ishibashi T. Functional characteristics of connective tissue growth factor on vitreoretinal cells. Diabetes. 2007; 56(5): 1421-8.
[129] McLeod DS, Lefer DJ, Merges C, Lutty GA. Enhanced expression of intracellular adhesion molecule-1 and P-selectin in the diabetic human retina and choroid. Am J Pathol. 1995; 147(3): 642-53.
[130] Schroder S, Palinski W, Schmid-Schonbein GW. Activated monocytes and granulocytes, capillary nonperfusion, and neovascularization in diabetic retinopathy. Am J Pathol. 1991; 139(1): 81-100.
[131] Miyamoto K, Hiroshiba N, Tsujikawa A, Ogura Y. In vivo demonstration of increased leukocyte entrapment in retinal microcirculation of diabetic rats. Invest Ophthalmol Vis Sci. 1998; 39(11): 2190-4.

[132] Joussen AM, Murata T, Tsujikawa A, Kirchhof B, Bursell SE, Adamis AP. Leukocyte-mediated endothelial cell injury and death in the diabetic retina. Am J Pathol. 2001; 158(1): 147-52.

[133] Joussen AM, Poulaki V, Mitsiades N, Cai WY, Suzuma I, Pak J, et al. Suppression of Fas-FasL-induced endothelial cell apoptosis prevents diabetic blood-retinal barrier breakdown in a model of streptozotocin-induced diabetes. FASEB J. 2003; 17(1): 76-8.

[134] Kohner EM, Henkind P. Correlation of fluorescein angiogram and retinal digest in diabetic retinopathy. Am J Ophthalmol. 1970; 69(3): 403-14.

[135] Barouch FC, Miyamoto K, Allport JR, Fujita K, Bursell SE, Aiello LP, et al. Integrin-mediated neutrophil adhesion and retinal leukostasis in diabetes. Invest Ophthalmol Vis Sci. 2000; 41(5): 1153-8.

[136] Joussen AM, Poulaki V, Le ML, Koizumi K, Esser C, Janicki H, et al. A central role for inflammation in the pathogenesis of diabetic retinopathy. FASEB J. 2004; 18(12): 1450-2.

[137] Harris AG, Skalak TC, Hatchell DL. Leukocyte-capillary plugging and network resistance are increased in skeletal muscle of rats with streptozotocin-induced hyperglycemia. Int J Microcirc Clin Exp. 1994; 14(3): 159-66.

[138] Kelly LW, Barden CA, Tiedeman JS, Hatchell DL. Alterations in viscosity and filterability of whole blood and blood cell subpopulations in diabetic cats. Exp Eye Res. 1993; 56(3): 341-7.

[139] Zheng L, Szabo C, Kern TS. Poly(ADP-ribose) polymerase is involved in the development of diabetic retinopathy via regulation of nuclear factor-kappaB. Diabetes. 2004; 53(11): 2960-7.

[140] Lu M, Perez VL, Ma N, Miyamoto K, Peng HB, Liao JK, et al. VEGF increases retinal vascular ICAM-1 expression in vivo. Invest Ophthalmol Vis Sci. 1999; 40(8): 1808-12.

[141] Hubbard AK, Rothlein R. Intercellular adhesion molecule-1 (ICAM-1) expression and cell signaling cascades. Free Radic Biol Med. 2000; 28(9): 1379-86.

[142] Chen W, Jump DB, Grant MB, Esselman WJ, Busik JV. Dyslipidemia, but not hyperglycemia, induces inflammatory adhesion molecules in human retinal vascular endothelial cells. Invest Ophthalmol Vis Sci. 2003; 44(11): 5016-22.

[143] Zheng L, Howell SJ, Hatala DA, Huang K, Kern TS. Salicylate-based anti-inflammatory drugs inhibit the early lesion of diabetic retinopathy. Diabetes. 2007; 56(2): 337-45.

[144] Kowluru RA, Tang J, Kern TS. Abnormalities of retinal metabolism in diabetes and experimental galactosemia. VII. Effect of long-term administration of antioxidants on the development of retinopathy. Diabetes. 2001; 50(8): 1938-42.

[145] Kowluru RA, Engerman RL, Case GL, Kern TS. Retinal glutamate in diabetes and effect of antioxidants. Neurochem Int. 2001; 38(5): 385-90.

[146] Du Y, Smith MA, Miller CM, Kern TS. Diabetes-induced nitrative stress in the retina, and correction by aminoguanidine. J Neurochem. 2002; 80(5): 771-9.

[147] Abu El-Asrar AM, Desmet S, Meersschaert A, Dralands L, Missotten L, Geboes K. Expression of the inducible isoform of nitric oxide synthase in the retinas of human subjects with diabetes mellitus. Am J Ophthalmol. 2001; 132(4): 551-6.

[148] Du Y, Sarthy VP, Kern TS. Interaction between NO and COX pathways in retinal cells exposed to elevated glucose and retina of diabetic rats. Am J Physiol Regul Integr Comp Physiol. 2004; 287(4): R735-41.

[149] Carmo A, Cunha-Vaz JG, Carvalho AP, Lopes MC. Nitric oxide synthase activity in retinas from non-insulin-dependent diabetic Goto-Kakizaki rats: correlation with blood-retinal barrier permeability. Nitric Oxide. 2000; 4(6): 590-6.
[150] do Carmo A, Lopes C, Santos M, Proenca R, Cunha-Vaz J, Carvalho AP. Nitric oxide synthase activity and L-arginine metabolism in the retinas from streptozotocin-induced diabetic rats. Gen Pharmacol. 1998; 30(3): 319-24.
[151] Kowluru RA. Retinal metabolic abnormalities in diabetic mouse: comparison with diabetic rat. Curr Eye Res. 2002; 24(2): 123-8.
[152] Kowluru RA, Engerman RL, Kern TS. Abnormalities of retinal metabolism in diabetes or experimental galactosemia VIII. Prevention by aminoguanidine. Curr Eye Res. 2000; 21(4): 814-9.
[153] Kowluru RA. Effect of reinstitution of good glycemic control on retinal oxidative stress and nitrative stress in diabetic rats. Diabetes. 2003; 52(3): 818-23.
[154] Joussen AM, Poulaki V, Qin W, Kirchhof B, Mitsiades N, Wiegand SJ, et al. Retinal vascular endothelial growth factor induces intercellular adhesion molecule-1 and endothelial nitric oxide synthase expression and initiates early diabetic retinal leukocyte adhesion in vivo. Am J Pathol. 2002; 160(2): 501-9.
[155] Park JW, Park SJ, Park SH, Kim KY, Chung JW, Chun MH, et al. Up-regulated expression of neuronal nitric oxide synthase in experimental diabetic retina. Neurobiol Dis. 2006; 21(1): 43-9.
[156] Tilton RG, Pugliese G, LaRose LS, Faller AM, Chang K, Province MA, et al. Discordant effects of the aldose reductase inhibitor, sorbinil, on vascular structure and function in chronically diabetic and galactosemic rats. J Diabet Complications. 1991; 5(4): 230-7.
[157] Corbett JA, Tilton RG, Chang K, Hasan KS, Ido Y, Wang JL, et al. Aminoguanidine, a novel inhibitor of nitric oxide formation, prevents diabetic vascular dysfunction. Diabetes. 1992; 41(4): 552-6.
[158] Hasan K, Heesen BJ, Corbett JA, McDaniel ML, Chang K, Allison W, et al. Inhibition of nitric oxide formation by guanidines. Eur J Pharmacol. 1993; 249(1): 101-6.
[159] Misko TP, Moore WM, Kasten TP, Nickols GA, Corbett JA, Tilton RG, et al. Selective inhibition of the inducible nitric oxide synthase by aminoguanidine. Eur J Pharmacol. 1993; 233(1): 119-25.
[160] Kern TS, Engerman RL. Pharmacological inhibition of diabetic retinopathy: aminoguanidine and aspirin. Diabetes. 2001; 50(7): 1636-42.
[161] Kern TS, Tang J, Mizutani M, Kowluru RA, Nagaraj RH, Romeo G, et al. Response of capillary cell death to aminoguanidine predicts the development of retinopathy: comparison of diabetes and galactosemia. Invest Ophthalmol Vis Sci. 2000; 41(12): 3972-8.
[162] Zheng L, Du Y, Miller C, Gubitosi-Klug RA, Ball S, Berkowitz BA, et al. Critical role of inducible nitric oxide synthase in degeneration of retinal capillaries in mice with streptozotocin-induced diabetes. Diabetologia. 2007; 50(9): 1987-96.
[163] Joussen AM, Poulaki V, Mitsiades N, Kirchhof B, Koizumi K, Dohmen S, et al. Nonsteroidal anti-inflammatory drugs prevent early diabetic retinopathy via TNF-alpha suppression. FASEB J. 2002; 16(3): 438-40.

[164] Gamble JR, Drew J, Trezise L, Underwood A, Parsons M, Kasminkas L, et al. Angiopoietin-1 is an antipermeability and anti-inflammatory agent in vitro and targets cell junctions. Circ Res. 2000; 87(7): 603-7.

[165] Joussen AM, Poulaki V, Tsujikawa A, Qin W, Qaum T, Xu Q, et al. Suppression of diabetic retinopathy with angiopoietin-1. Am J Pathol. 2002; 160(5): 1683-93.

[166] Nishimura M, Ikeda T, Ushiyama M, Nanbu A, Kinoshita S, Yoshimura M. Increased vitreous concentrations of human hepatocyte growth factor in proliferative diabetic retinopathy. J Clin Endocrinol Metab. 1999; 84(2): 659-62.

[167] Katsura Y, Okano T, Noritake M, Kosano H, Nishigori H, Kado S, et al. Hepatocyte growth factor in vitreous fluid of patients with proliferative diabetic retinopathy and other retinal disorders. Diabetes Care. 1998; 21(10): 1759-63.

[168] Canton A, Burgos R, Hernandez C, Mateo C, Segura RM, Mesa J, et al. Hepatocyte growth factor in vitreous and serum from patients with proliferative diabetic retinopathy. Br J Ophthalmol. 2000; 84(7): 732-5.

[169] Umeda N, Ozaki H, Hayashi H, Kondo H, Uchida H, Oshima K. Non-paralleled increase of hepatocyte growth factor and vascular endothelial growth factor in the eyes with angiogenic and nonangiogenic fibroproliferation. Ophthalmic Res. 2002; 34(1): 43-7.

[170] Mitamura Y, Takeuchi S, Matsuda A, Tagawa Y, Mizue Y, Nishihira J. Hepatocyte growth factor levels in the vitreous of patients with proliferative vitreoretinopathy. Am J Ophthalmol. 2000; 129(5): 678-80.

[171] Simo R, Lecube A, Garcia-Arumi J, Carrasco E, Hernandez C. Hepatocyte growth factor in the vitreous fluid of patients with proliferative diabetic retinopathy: its relationship with vascular endothelial growth factor and retinopathy activity. Diabetes Care. 2004; 27(1): 287-8.

[172] Risau W. Mechanisms of angiogenesis. Nature. 1997; 386(6626): 671-4.

[173] Hanahan D. Signaling vascular morphogenesis and maintenance. Science. 1997; 277(5322): 48-50.

[174] Millauer B, Wizigmann-Voos S, Schnurch H, Martinez R, Moller NP, Risau W, et al. High affinity VEGF binding and developmental expression suggest Flk-1 as a major regulator of vasculogenesis and angiogenesis. Cell. 1993; 72(6): 835-46.

[175] Joukov V, Pajusola K, Kaipainen A, Chilov D, Lahtinen I, Kukk E, et al. A novel vascular endothelial growth factor, VEGF-C, is a ligand for the Flt4 (VEGFR-3) and KDR (VEGFR-2) receptor tyrosine kinases. EMBO J. 1996; 15(7): 1751.

[176] de Vries C, Escobedo JA, Ueno H, Houck K, Ferrara N, Williams LT. The fms-like tyrosine kinase, a receptor for vascular endothelial growth factor. Science. 1992; 255(5047): 989-91.

[177] Sato TN, Qin Y, Kozak CA, Audus KL. Tie-1 and tie-2 define another class of putative receptor tyrosine kinase genes expressed in early embryonic vascular system. Proc Natl Acad Sci U S A. 1993; 90(20): 9355-8.

[178] Puri MC, Rossant J, Alitalo K, Bernstein A, Partanen J. The receptor tyrosine kinase TIE is required for integrity and survival of vascular endothelial cells. EMBO J. 1995; 14(23): 5884-91.

[179] Sato TN, Tozawa Y, Deutsch U, Wolburg-Buchholz K, Fujiwara Y, Gendron-Maguire M, et al. Distinct roles of the receptor tyrosine kinases Tie-1 and Tie-2 in blood vessel formation. Nature. 1995; 376(6535): 70-4.

[180] Dumont DJ, Gradwohl G, Fong GH, Puri MC, Gertsenstein M, Auerbach A, et al. Dominant-negative and targeted null mutations in the endothelial receptor tyrosine kinase, tek, reveal a critical role in vasculogenesis of the embryo. Genes Dev. 1994; 8(16): 1897-909.

[181] Shalaby F, Rossant J, Yamaguchi TP, Gertsenstein M, Wu XF, Breitman ML, et al. Failure of blood-island formation and vasculogenesis in Flk-1-deficient mice. Nature. 1995; 376(6535): 62-6.

[182] Vikkula M, Boon LM, Carraway KL, 3rd, Calvert JT, Diamonti AJ, Goumnerov B, et al. Vascular dysmorphogenesis caused by an activating mutation in the receptor tyrosine kinase TIE2. Cell. 1996; 87(7): 1181-90.

[183] Davis S, Aldrich TH, Jones PF, Acheson A, Compton DL, Jain V, et al. Isolation of angiopoietin-1, a ligand for the TIE2 receptor, by secretion-trap expression cloning. Cell. 1996; 87(7): 1161-9.

[184] Maisonpierre PC, Suri C, Jones PF, Bartunkova S, Wiegand SJ, Radziejewski C, et al. Angiopoietin-2, a natural antagonist for Tie2 that disrupts in vivo angiogenesis. Science. 1997; 277(5322): 55-60.

[185] Oh SJ, Jeltsch MM, Birkenhager R, McCarthy JE, Weich HA, Christ B, et al. VEGF and VEGF-C: specific induction of angiogenesis and lymphangiogenesis in the differentiated avian chorioallantoic membrane. Dev Biol. 1997; 188(1): 96-109.

[186] Suri C, Jones PF, Patan S, Bartunkova S, Maisonpierre PC, Davis S, et al. Requisite role of angiopoietin-1, a ligand for the TIE2 receptor, during embryonic angiogenesis. Cell. 1996; 87(7): 1171-80.

[187] Wong AL, Haroon ZA, Werner S, Dewhirst MW, Greenberg CS, Peters KG. Tie2 expression and phosphorylation in angiogenic and quiescent adult tissues. Circ Res. 1997; 81(4): 567-74.

[188] Asahara T, Chen D, Takahashi T, Fujikawa K, Kearney M, Magner M, et al. Tie2 receptor ligands, angiopoietin-1 and angiopoietin-2, modulate VEGF-induced postnatal neovascularization. Circ Res. 1998; 83(3): 233-40.

[189] Dzau VJ. Molecular biology of angiotensin II biosynthesis and receptors. Can J Cardiol. 1995; 11 Suppl F: 21F-6F.

[190] Chaturvedi N, Sjolie AK, Stephenson JM, Abrahamian H, Keipes M, Castellarin A, et al. Effect of lisinopril on progression of retinopathy in normotensive people with type 1 diabetes. The EUCLID Study Group. EURODIAB Controlled Trial of Lisinopril in Insulin-Dependent Diabetes Mellitus. Lancet. 1998; 351(9095): 28-31.

[191] Naftilan AJ, Pratt RE, Dzau VJ. Induction of platelet-derived growth factor A-chain and c-myc gene expressions by angiotensin II in cultured rat vascular smooth muscle cells. J Clin Invest. 1989; 83(4): 1419-24.

[192] Delafontaine P, Lou H. Angiotensin II regulates insulin-like growth factor I gene expression in vascular smooth muscle cells. J Biol Chem. 1993; 268(22): 16866-70.

[193] Tomita H, Egashira K, Ohara Y, Takemoto M, Koyanagi M, Katoh M, et al. Early induction of transforming growth factor-beta via angiotensin II type 1 receptors contributes to cardiac fibrosis induced by long-term blockade of nitric oxide synthesis in rats. Hypertension. 1998; 32(2): 273-9.

[194] Otani A, Takagi H, Suzuma K, Honda Y. Angiotensin II potentiates vascular endothelial growth factor-induced angiogenic activity in retinal microcapillary endothelial cells. Circ Res. 1998; 82(5): 619-28.

[195] Otani A, Takagi H, Oh H, Suzuma K, Matsumura M, Ikeda E, et al. Angiotensin II-stimulated vascular endothelial growth factor expression in bovine retinal pericytes. Invest Ophthalmol Vis Sci. 2000; 41(5): 1192-9.

[196] Otani A, Takagi H, Oh H, Koyama S, Honda Y. Angiotensin II induces expression of the Tie2 receptor ligand, angiopoietin-2, in bovine retinal endothelial cells. Diabetes. 2001; 50(4): 867-75.

[197] Sawada N, Murata M, Kikuchi K, Osanai M, Tobioka H, Kojima T, et al. Tight junctions and human diseases. Med Electron Microsc. 2003; 36(3): 147-56.

[198] Frank RN. Diabetic retinopathy. N Engl J Med. 2004; 350(1): 48-58.

[199] Ng EW, Shima DT, Calias P, Cunningham ET, Jr., Guyer DR, Adamis AP. Pegaptanib, a targeted anti-VEGF aptamer for ocular vascular disease. Nat Rev Drug Discov. 2006; 5(2): 123-32.

[200] Comer GM, Ciulla TA. Pharmacotherapy for diabetic retinopathy. Curr Opin Ophthalmol. 2004; 15(6): 508-18.

[201] Miyajima H, Osanai M, Chiba H, Nishikiori N, Kojima T, Ohtsuka K, et al. Glyceraldehyde-derived advanced glycation end-products preferentially induce VEGF expression and reduce GDNF expression in human astrocytes. Biochem Biophys Res Commun. 2005; 330(2): 361-6.

[202] Igarashi Y, Chiba H, Utsumi H, Miyajima H, Ishizaki T, Gotoh T, et al. Expression of receptors for glial cell line-derived neurotrophic factor (GDNF) and neurturin in the inner blood-retinal barrier of rats. Cell Struct Funct. 2000; 25(4): 237-41.

[203] Igarashi Y, Utsumi H, Chiba H, Yamada-Sasamori Y, Tobioka H, Kamimura Y, et al. Glial cell line-derived neurotrophic factor induces barrier function of endothelial cells forming the blood-brain barrier. Biochem Biophys Res Commun. 1999; 261(1): 108-12.

[204] Thang SH, Kobayashi M, Matsuoka I. Regulation of glial cell line-derived neurotrophic factor responsiveness in developing rat sympathetic neurons by retinoic acid and bone morphogenetic protein-2. J Neurosci. 2000; 20(8): 2917-25.

[205] Nishikiori N, Osanai M, Chiba H, Kojima T, Mitamura Y, Ohguro H, et al. Glial cell-derived cytokines attenuate the breakdown of vascular integrity in diabetic retinopathy. Diabetes. 2007; 56(5): 1333-40.

Part 3

Clinical Aspects of Diabetic Retinopathy and Retinal Functions

10

Diabetic Macular Edema

Christina Antonopoulos and Manju Subramanian
Boston University School of Medicine
USA

1. Introduction

Diabetic macular edema represents one of the most important causes of visual morbidity in diabetes mellitus. The National Diabetes Information Clearinghouse estimates the prevalence of diabetes mellitus types 1 and 2 at 11.3% of the population above the age of 20, with an annual incidence of 1.9 million cases in the United States alone. In this population, the prevalence of diabetic macular edema is estimated at 30% of patients inflicted by the disease for 20 years or more. Diabetes mellitus is the leading cause of preventable blindness owing to both diabetic macular edema and complications of proliferative diabetic retinopathy (NDIC 2011). Thus once can expect that diabetic macular edema is a common entity in any Retina specialty practice with serious implications for vision loss if not treated in a timely and appropriate manner. Based on the critical findings of the Early Treatment in Diabetic Retinopathy Study, the standard of care has been focal laser photocoagulation therapy along with strong recommendations for strict blood glucose and blood pressure control. However since then, the spectrum of therapies for diabetic macular edema has expanded and continues to evolve. The use of steroid therapy and anti-vascular endothelial growth factor biologics have been compared to focal laser photocoagulation in order to establish more treatment options with equivalent efficacy and safety.

The following chapter is a comprehensive review of the basic pathophysiology, symptomatology, clinical findings, diagnostic methods, indications for intervention, and treatment modalities of diabetic macular edema. Careful attention is given to the review of treatment modalities, including steroid therapy, Anti-VEGF pharmacotherapy (sister drugs Lucentis (ranibizumab) and Avastin (bevacizumab)) and surgical techniques. A literature review is also summarized comparing these methods to focal laser photocoagulation therapy. Thus this chapter is designed to give the reader a fuller understanding of the diabetic macular edema as a clinical entity and how it can be addressed so as to preserve vision.

2. Pathophysiology

Diabetic macular edema is a microvascular complication of diabetes mellitus with serious implications for vision loss. The central pathophysiologic event is retinal capillary incompetence and leakage. Several biochemical hypotheses exist to explain the damage to retinal capillary constituents in diabetes mellitus. Prolonged hyperglycemia has been implicated in direct injury to retinal capillary endothelial cell and pericytes and to a decline in cell division (Engerman 1987). Cells in the body produce energy from the metabolism of glucose. The sorbitol (or polyol) pathway concurrently employs aldose reductase to reduce unused glucose to sorbitol (Brownlee 2001). Under normal circumstances cells metabolize glucose primarily via glycolysis, particularly because at a physiologic serum concentration, aldose reductase has a low affinity for glucose. However, high serum glucose concentrations can saturate the glycolysis pathway, making excess glucose molecules available for reduction to sorbitol by the avidly-binding aldose reductase. Excessive activation of the sorbitol pathway in hyperglycemia results in an accumulation of sorbitol in the intracellular space which has been considered toxic to cells, in particular to retinal capillary endothelial cells and pericytes (Brownlee 2001).

Retinal capillary walls normally consist of a succinct network of endothelial cells and mural pericytes, which exist in a deliberate one-to-one ratio. In the 1950s, Kuwabara and Cogan developed Trypsin digest studies in retinal tissue of diabetic human subjects, which made possible the close examination of the retinal vasculature by light microscopy (Kuwabara 1960). These retinal digest studies were the first of their kind to demonstrate the key pathologic events of diabetic retinopathy. The biochemical derangements of diabetes mellitus cause a preferential loss of pericytes, identified histologically as empty "balloon-like spaces" or "ghost cells" along retinal capillary walls (Kuwabara 1960). Immunologic studies have demonstrated that mural pericytes contain properties that make them structurally analogous to the smooth muscle layer of larger scale blood vessels. The contractile nature and tonus of pericytes contribute to the structural integrity of the retinal capillary wall (Herman 1985). Therefore, a loss of mural pericytes may cause focal weakening and saccular dilatation of retinal capillaries, identified biomicroscopically as microaneurysms. Microaneurysms are readily detected on close fundoscopic examination and by fluorescein angiography and are one of the earliest signs of nonproliferative diabetic retinopathy (Freidenwald 1950). They are visually indistinguishable from dot intraretinal hemorrhages and thus represent areas of focal retinal vasculature incompetence.

The breakdown of the inner blood retinal barrier at the level of the retinal capillary endothelial cells likewise contributes to capillary incompetence. This breakdown largely occurs with an opening of tight junctions, or *zonulae occludentes,* between adjacent endothelial cells (Green 1985). The pathophysiologic outcome of inner blood retinal barrier compromise and abnormally permeable microaneurysms is an unchecked leakage of erythrocytes, plasma, and lipoproteins into the retinal interstitium. Retinal edema results once this fluid leakage overwhelms the capacity of the retinal pigment epithelial pump to remove it. The sequelae of vascular incompetence and retinal edema include (1) precipitation of serum lipoproteins in the retinal interstitium, causing a disruption of the delicate retinal architecture and (2) retinal arteriolar closure, resulting in focal retinal ischemia (Ryan 1989).

Retinal arteriolar closure characterizes a more advanced stage of nonproliferative retinopathy and carries more serious implications for widespread retinal ischemia and progression to proliferative disease (Ryan 1989). Several mechanisms of arteriolar occlusion have been hypothesized, implicating both intraluminal and extraluminal forces. Firstly, erythrocyte and platelet agglutination and defective fibrinolysis may cause intraluminal occlusion of arterioles (Little 1981) Endothelial cell basement membrane thickening, a general histologic characteristic of diabetes mellitus, potentially causes luminal narrowing and occlusion. The accumulation of interstitial fluid and protein leads to increased tissue oncotic pressure and tissue turgor which may cause vascular closure by means of direct compression (Ryan 1989). Macular ischemia resulting from closure of retinal capillaries and arterioles may exacerbate concurrent macular edema.

Deformational macular edema caused by tractional membranes on the retinal surface is often observed in diabetic retinopathy either alone or in the presence of underlying diabetic macular edema (Clarkson 1977). Epiretinal membranes and a taut posterior hyaloid are the most common examples of tractional membranes. Epiretinal membranes are fibrocellular membranes caused by the migration and proliferation of retinal glial cells along the retinal surface. Their origin can be idiopathic or as a consequence of diabetic retinopathy or retinal vascular disorders. Depending on their severity, epiretinal membranes can cause retinal distortion and tractional retinal edema that is evident on both fundoscopy and fluorescein angiography (as cystoid macular edema). Epiretinal membranes can thus exacerbate underlying DME. The posterior hyaloid face of the vitreous can likewise cause deformational macular edema by exerting antero-posterior forces on the macula, as observed in the vitreomacular traction (VMT) syndrome. This is an idiopathic condition characterized by abnormal adhesion of the posterior hyaloid to the macula. As seen with epiretinal membranes, there may be tractional edema causing leakage in the macula and from the optic nerve head on fluorescein angiography (Hikichi 1995). Several hypotheses have attempted to explain the VMT syndrome: (1) Glycation of the vitreous: abnormal crosslinking of cortical vitreous in systemic hyperglycemic with tractional adherence to the macula causing a secondary deformation of retinal architecture (Dillinger 2004); (2) sequestration of pro-inflammatory factors or compounds in the pre-macular area by the posterior hyaloid that increase vascular permeability (Dillinger 2004); (3) frank, idiopathic contraction of the posterior hyaloid face with resultant deformational edema (Figueroa 2008).

The metabolic derangements of diabetes mellitus take a serious toll on the smallest constituents of the retinal vasculature. These early changes eventually manifest themselves on a macroscopic level, causing a generalized dysfunction of the blood retinal barrier, pathologic retinal edema, retinal vascular compromise and closure, tissue ischemia, and the potential for serious loss of visual acuity.

3. Clinical considerations

Macular edema is the terminology applied when careful fundoscopic examination reveals retinal thickening (with or without retinal exudates) within two disc diameters of the central macula. It may be observed at any stage of diabetic retinopathy, from minimal background diabetic retinopathy to active proliferative disease. The classic signs of background (nonproliferative) diabetic retinopathy are dot-blot hemorrhages, microaneurysms, hard exudates, and cotton wool spots. Dot-blot hemorrhages are intraretinal hemorrhages located in the outer retinal layers that directly result from incompetent retinal capillaries. Small, dot hemorrhages may be clinically indistinguishable from microaneurysms; whereas "blot" hemorrhages tend to be larger with indistinct borders located in the outer plexiform layer. Hard exudates are discrete, often confluent, yellow-white intraretinal accumulations of precipitated serum lipid. Their presence is likewise strong evidence of retinal capillary leakage. Cotton wool spots are thusly named due to their fluffy, white appearance in the retina. They represent foci of ischemic retinal whitening in areas of retinal capillary closure. Cotton wool spots may resolve over time without necessarily promoting retinal neovascularization. However, a high density of cotton wool spots in any single area may suggest more severe underlying ischemia and a greater risk of progression to proliferative disease.

Macular edema may exist in several forms, each of which require specific treatment strategies and may vary greatly in terms of visual prognosis. Macular edema is primarily characterized as focal or diffuse. Focal macular edema represents retinal thickening involving localized areas of the macula, usually from a single microaneurysm or of clusters of them. Focal edema is often in the form of a microaneurysm with a surrounding circinate ring of precipitated hard exudates (or plasma lipoproteins), which delineates edematous from non-edematous retina (Gass 1987). Plasma lipoproteins most commonly accumulate in the outer plexiform layer but may be deposited in the subretinal space causing an independent decline in vision if the fovea is involved. Diffuse macular edema corresponds to a more generalized retinal capillary incompetence with extensive fluid leakage in the macula. Additionally, although not generally considered an element of diabetic macular edema (DME), incompetence in the outer blood-retinal barrier has been implicated in diffuse edema (Bresnick 1986). Experimental animal models have suggested that loss of retinal pigment epithelial cell tight junctions and RPE necrosis in diabetes mellitus possibly lead to abnormal permeability from the choroid (Kirber 1980). This often leads to cystoid macular edema and is not necessarily associated with exudates. Both eyes are usually symmetrically affected, demonstrating the same severity of edema and visual acuity. Systemic factors such as glycemic control, blood pressure, and fluid retention status may alter the clinical appearance of diffuse macular edema, with periodic resolution and exacerbation even without therapeutic intervention (Ryan 1989).

Recently, the use of the terminology "focal" versus "diffuse" diabetic macular edema has come under scrutiny. Some critics of this terminology have argued that it is not precise as there may be great overlap between these two entities in terms of visual morbidity, management options, and prognosis. More accurate descriptors should ideally include information regarding the following characteristics: location and extent of edema, central foveal involvement or sparing, and the extent and location of associated exudation (Browning 2008).

Macular edema is a common cause of visual acuity loss, particularly in the context of poorly controlled blood glucose levels. However, vision can be preserved for months to years even with clinically significant diabetic macular edema. Thus the presence of excellent visual acuity does not contraindicate treatment of diabetic macular edema. In the majority of cases, macular edema does eventually lead to a decline in visual acuity, which is potentially reversible if the edema is successfully treated once the diagnosis is made. Chronic DME can cause a profound disruption of the retinal architecture. Cystoid maculopathy, characterized by retinal degeneration and atrophy in the macula, is typically resistant to even aggressive therapy and holds a poor visual prognosis.

A consequence of retinal capillary and arteriolar closure in diabetic retinopathy is the disruption of the fine capillary network surrounding the fovea (Hayreh 2008). The end stage of retinal vascular incompetence, capillary and arteriolar closure is macular ischemia, which results from compromised oxygen delivery in the macula (Hayreh 2008). Retinal edema and exudation in DME will increase the length of the pathway for diffusion of oxygen in to the vessel-devoid foveal avascular zone (Hayreh 2008). The inability to sustain the oxygen demands of this tissue will invariably have visual consequences, particularly once breakdown of the perifoveal capillary network is documented angiographically. Visual acuity is generally not affected until the diameter of the foveal avascular zone (usually 500 microns) exceeds 1000 microns (Ryan 1989). However, once this occurs, irreversible loss of visual acuity can be expected. Macular ischemia will compound diabetic macular edema; thus, when coexistent, it is often difficult to determine which has a greater effect on visual acuity. Such eyes tend to have poorer general prognosis, with a blunted response to focal laser therapy.

4. Clinical assessment

The characteristics of diabetic macular edema are best assessed by a combination of slit lamp biomicroscopy, fundus photography, fluorescein angiography, and more recently optical coherence tomography (OCT). The basic pathophysiologic lesions discussed above may be readily apparent in the posterior pole on fundoscopic examination with contact or noncontact lenses. Macular edema is detected as a thickening in the retinal layers with stereoscopic, binocular viewing. Mild retinal edema may escape detection whereas frank macular edema is typically quite apparent, particularly with coexisting intraretinal hemorrhage and hard exudate. Stereoscopic fundus photographs have been the standard method of quantifying diabetic macular edema in clinical trials (Davis 2008).

In ophthalmoscopically normal eyes, early changes in diabetic retinopathy may be detected by fluorescein angiography. A fluorescein angiogram is obtained when information about the structure and integrity of the retinal circulation is needed. However, it should not be used specifically to evaluate for the presence of DME. Fluorescein dye (a green vegetable-based dye) is injected into a vein in the antecubital fossa and a series of timed photographs are taken of the fundi. As previously stated, diabetic macular edema is a disease of retinal capillary incompetence with leakage of serum and blood products into the retinal interstitium. While fluorescein is largely bound to protein and the surface of erythrocytes in the blood column, approximately 20% of molecules are unbound (Richard 2008). Therefore, in the setting of inner blood retinal barrier compromise, there will be an egress of fluorescein into the retinal interstitium. The earliest evidence of this in background diabetic retinopathy is leakage from retinal microaneurysms, detectable as early punctate hyperfluorescence in the posterior pole. Macular edema is demonstrated as expanding hyperfluorescence from punctate foci in mid and late phases of the study. When cystoid macular edema is present, the leakage may be in a petaloid pattern.

Time domain and spectral domain optical coherence tomography (OCT) are newer imaging modalities commonly employed in the evaluation of diabetic macular edema. OCT provides qualitative cross-sectional images and retinal thickness maps as well as quantitative thickness estimates of the central macular subfield. The use of OCT as a diagnostic tool in diabetic macular edema has been investigated. Officially, the diagnosis of diabetic macular edema is made by specific fundoscopic criteria established by the ETDRS. Recent studies have compared OCT to fundus photography in order to validate the role of the former in diagnosing DME. For example, a 2008 study by the Diabetic Retinopathy Clinical Research Network demonstrated a moderate correlation between retinal thickness measurements rendered by time domain OCT (Zeiss Stratus OCT3) and area of retinal thickening determined by stereoscopic fundus photographs (Davis 2008). Furthermore, the authors report that OCT may be more sensitive than fundus photographs in measuring the change in retinal thickness over time and, in particular, after treatment of DME. While visual acuity itself remains the most important correlate of the severity of diabetic macular edema, this study demonstrated only a weak correlation between OCT retinal thickness estimates and visual acuity. Nevertheless, the group concluded that OCT is an acceptable method of quantifying diabetic macular edema and suggested the possibility of its use in future clinical trials evaluating the efficacy of treatment modalities. Furthermore, the use of OCT to guide focal laser photocoagulation therapy was suggested in a prospective interventional comparative study comparing it with fluorescein angiogram-guided treatment (Gallego-Pinazo 2011).

OCT has become an indispensible imaging study in the early detection of diabetic macular edema and in the assessment of treatment response. OCT is likewise helpful in the diagnosis of tractional forces impacting macula edema such as epiretinal membranes and vitreomacular abnormalities, which are not as easily assessed by fundoscopy. Prior to such imaging techniques assessment of vitreomacular traction was certainly less accurate.

5. Management

The Early Treatment in Diabetic Retinopathy Study (ETDRS), sponsored by the National Eye Institute in 1979, was a benchmark in the management of diabetic macular edema (ETDRS 1985). The ETDRS was a large-scale, multicenter, randomized clinical trial designed to investigate whether early treatment of macular edema by focal argon laser photocoagulation could prevent moderate visual loss, defined as a loss of three lines of vision or a doubling of the visual angle. Eyes with macular edema in the setting of mild to moderate nonproliferative diabetic retinopathy with a visual acuity of 20/40 or worse were recruited and divided into two treatment groups: immediate versus delayed focal laser photocoagulation. The standard technique and parameters of focal laser therapy were detailed by the ETDRS as follows: a laser spot size of 50-100 microns and duration of 0.10 seconds to focal microaneurysms observed with contact lens fundoscopy. When the macular edema is more diffuse, a grid pattern of similar parameters may be applied. Laser burns are titrated to a slight graying of the treated retina (ETDRS 1985; ETDRS 1987). Based on three years of follow-up data, the ETDRS concluded that immediate focal photocoagulation halved the rate of moderate visual loss. When patients were stratified in terms of severity of initial macular edema, the benefit of immediate focal laser therapy was maximized in patients with "clinically significant macular edema" (CSME). As such, the ETDRS defined CSME, which is characterized as follows:

- retinal edema located at or within 500 microns of the foveal center
- hard exudates at or within 500 microns of the foveal center if associated with thickening of adjacent retina
- a zone of retinal thickening larger than 1 disc area within 1 disc diameter of the foveal center (ETDRS 1985)

This treatment strategy implies that is that macular edema which does not satisfy the above characteristics may be closely observed clinically until the criteria are satisfied (ETDRS 1987).

Subclinical macular edema (SCME) is a term used to describe macular edema in which fluid or leakage is detected on optical coherence tomography or fluorescein angiography, but not detected clinically on examination, or if detected on examination, did not meet the definition of CSME as defined by the ETDRS. This has been quantified as a central retinal subfield thickness ranging from 200 to 300 microns (by third generation Zeiss Stratus OCT). A recent retrospective case-controlled study compared type II diabetics with SCME to age, sex, and disease duration-matched controls without macular edema (defined as central subfield thickness <200 microns). This study aimed to identify the risk factors and relative risk for progression to CSME from SCME. It found that a prior history of CSME, advancing age and graded increases in central retinal thickness over time increased the likelihood of progression to CSME in patients with sublinical edema (Bhavsar 2011).

Further analysis of ETDRS data revealed that eyes with center-involving CSME (i.e. intraretinal fluid involving the fovea) versus eyes with CSME without central involvement (i.e. encroaching upon but sparing fixation) demonstrated a differential response to focal laser therapy (ETDRS 1985). The ETDRS presented data indicating that treatment of center-involving CSME resulted in a 67% decrease in the rate of visual loss (defined as 15 or more letter at three years). However, the treatment of center-sparing CSME resulted in only an approximate 45% decrease in the rate of visual loss. The ETDRS was not designed to determine the most appropriate timing for focal laser therapy. However, based on its conclusions, immediate focal laser photocoagulation is recommended in both morphologies of CSME.

The management of diabetic macular edema has expanded since publication of the ETDRS findings. At present, treatment options are quite broad, incorporating proven and new therapies (or combinations of them), each designed to target a central pathophysiologic mechanism of the disease. Three proven methods exist to decrease the long-term risk of vision loss from DME, namely (1) tight blood sugar control (proven in Diabetes Control and Complications Trial (DCCT) and United Kingdom Prospective Diabetes Study (UKPDS)); (2) blood pressure control (UKPDS); and (3) focal laser photocoagulation therapy (ETDRS) (ETDRS 1985; DCCT 1983; UKPDS 1998).

Observation with encouragement of tight glycemic and blood pressure control is an option, particularly in subclinical macular edema (SCME). While spontaneous resolution of macular edema with excellent control of systemic risk factors is entirely possible, observation of patients deemed at high risk for clinical worsening is not advisable. In fact, the ETDRS did recommend focal laser therapy for macular edema outside 500 microns of fixation in the context of poor glycemic control (ETDRS 1985).

5.1 Focal laser photocoagulation therapy

Since the findings of ETDRS, focal laser photocoagulation remains the standard of care for the treatment of diabetic macular edema. The effects of focal laser in controlling macular edema are relatively long-lasting, demonstrated at up to three years. However, as was reported by the ETDRS, only 17% of eyes with baseline vision of worse than 20/40 experienced modest visual improvement, and a certain proportion of patients did not respond to focal laser therapy at all (ETDRS 1985). It is generally accepted that diffuse DME or cystoid macular edema in fixation precludes treatment by focal laser by virtue of its location. The more severe entities of DME have served as an impetus in the search for adjunctive or stand-alone pharmacotherapy in the treatment of diabetic macular edema.

5.2 Steroid agents

Steroid agents were an earlier first-line pharmacotherapy for diabetic macular edema. Triamcinolone acetonide and its newer, unpreserved formulation (for intravitreal injection) have been used as adjuncts of focal laser or stand-alone alternatives. The utility of peribulbar and intravitreal steroid injections has been established in the management of intraocular inflammation and cystoid macular edema secondary to non-infectious uveitis. (Kok, 2005); (Tanner, 1995). As such, attention was turned to employ this method as a possible treatment for DME. Initial efficacy studies conducted between 2001 and 2002 demonstrated a short-term therapeutic effect of a randomly selected 4 mg dose of intravitreal triamcinolone injection in DME, and its use became widespread despite a lack of data from randomized, prospective clinical trials assessing efficacy or possible adverse effects (Jonas 2001; Martidis 2002).

Peribulbar triamcinolone has likewise been employed as a treatment modality for diabetic macular edema. Peribulbar injection is commonly delivered at a dosage of 20 – 40 mg of triamcinolone acetonide (40mg/1ml) solution to one of three potential peribulbar locations: (1) anterior subconjunctival or subtenons; (2) posterior subtenons; (3) retrobulbar. Its hypothesized mechanism of action in treating diabetic macular edema involves a combination of decreasing retinal vascular permeability by downregulation of VEGF expression and decreasing leukostasis in retinal capillaries (Kern 2007).

A review of the literature reveals inconsistent reports of the efficacy of peribulbar steroid injection in treating DME. One retrospective study reported the efficacy of 40mg/1 ml posterior subtenons triamcinolone injection in eyes with DME and moderate vision loss (defined as a mean visual acuity of 20/80). Twenty-two percent of enrolled patients maintained a three or more line improvement in vision at 12 months (Bakri 2005). One study that compared posterior subtenons triamcinolone to placebo/sham injection in eyes with a mean visual acuity of 20/160 and fairly recalcitrant macular edema found no statistically significant improvement in visual acuity or decline in central retinal thickness (Entezari 2005). Another study enrolled patients with only mild diabetic macular edema and a mean visual acuity of 20/25. This study employed three arms to compare stand-alone peribulbar (anterior and posterior subtenons) therapy with focal laser photocoagulation therapy and a combination injection-laser therapy. After 34 weeks of follow-up, there was no conclusive improvement in visual acuity or decrement in central macular thickness in any of the treatment arms. However, a statistical trend indicated a decrease in the likelihood of re-injection if the injection was followed in the short term by focal laser (Chew 2007). A retrospective uncontrolled study reported that intravitreal triamcinolone was superior to a posterior subtenons delivery of the drug (Ozdek 2006).

In September 2008, the Diabetic Retinopathy Clinical Research Network published the two-year results of a multi-center, large scale, randomized clinical trial directly comparing the efficacy of focal laser therapy and intravitreal triamcinolone injections (1mg and 4 mg dosages) with visual acuity and central retinal thickness as primary outcome variables (Figueroa 2008). The original study population met strict inclusion and exclusion criteria and had a wide range of visual acuity and DME severity. The findings of this study declared a short-term benefit of 4 mg triamcinolone over the other groups at four months, no clear benefit of any modality at 12 months, and a clear benefit of focal laser over either steroid dosage at two years in terms of improvement in mean visual acuity. Retinal thickness parameters generally paralleled the trends in visual acuity in this study. Adverse effects, including cataract formation and intraocular pressure increase, were monitored during this study. Intravitreal steroids demonstrated higher rates of cataract formation. Importantly, the reversal of efficacy of focal laser over intravitreal steroid over two years was not confounded by cataract formation (Figueroa 2008). The identical three-year follow-up data were reported by this group in 2009 (Beck RW 2009). Thus focal laser therapy was proven to have a lasting effect on vision with a much safer side effect profile when compared to varying dosages of intravitreal triamcinolone acetonide.

5.3 Anti-Vascular Endothelial Growth Factor (VEGF) agents

The newest therapy in diabetic macular edema comprises biologic agents engineered to target the root cause of retinal vascular permeability, namely VEGF expression. VEGF-A is a known regulator protein of angiogenesis, vascular permeability, and pro-inflammatory activity (Murugeswari 2008; Roberts 1995). It binds VEGFR1 and VEGFR2 receptors and is upregulated primarily in response to tissue ischemia, inflammation, pH changes, and hormone growth factors (Penn 2008). Ranibizumab and bevacizumab are sister molecules of humanized murine monoclonal antibodies with affinity for binding VEGF isoforms. Ranibizumab (or Lucentis) is a humanized anti-VEGF-A recombinant Fab fragment (molecular weight 48 kDa), which binds all isoforms of VEGF A. Bevacizumab (or Avastin) is a full-length humanized antibody to VEGF-A (molecular weight 149 kDa) that binds all VEGF isoforms. Similar to triamcinolone acetonide, the delivery of both drugs is by intravitreal injection. Ranibizumab (or Lucentis) gained attention after approval by the United States Food and Drug administration in the management of exudative age-related macular edema (ARMD) in 2006. Bevacizumab (or Avastin) was initially approved as adjunctive chemotherapy of metastatic colon cancer and has been widely used in an off-label fashion in the treatment of exudative ARMD. These drugs have likewise been applied to treat macular edema secondary to diabetic retinopathy and retinal vein occlusions.

The efficacy of the anti-VEGF agents in diabetic macular edema has been the subject of several recent investigations. Arevalo and colleagues report efficacy data from the Pan-

American Collaborative Retina study group (Arevalo 2007). This retrospective interventional multicenter study evaluated the retinal thickness and ETDRS acuity data of 80 consecutive patients receiving intravitreal Avastin injections for center-involving diabetic macular edema in eyes not previously treated with focal laser. Eyes received at least one Avastin injection (either 1.25mg or 2.50mg) with smaller percentages of patients requiring a second or third injection over a six-month period (on average every 11 to 13 weeks). The group reported a favorable decline in OCT retinal thickness and visual acuities that were stable if not improved from baseline (Arevalo 2007). The 24-month extension of this study supported the six-month findings. Patients who received on average 5.8 injections of single or double dose Avastin demonstrated a partial resolution of macular edema and maintained, if not improved, upon baseline visual acuity (Arevalo 2009). To date, there has been no formal large-scale phase III randomized control trial for the efficacy of anti-VEGF agents in diabetic macular edema.

Additional studies have emerged to compare the efficacy of anti-VEGF therapy to focal laser photocoagulation in DME. The Bevacizumab or Laser Therapy (or BOLT) study was a prospective, randomized phase II clinical trial and a first of its kind to compare anti-VEGF therapy to focal laser therapy (Michaelidis 2010). The study randomized 80 eyes to receive either intravitreal bevacizumab injections (1.25mg/0.50ml) or macula laser therapy (MLT) group. Bevacizumab injections were given every six weeks for the first three months followed by as needed thereafter. Focal laser was offered initially and every four months as needed. Injected eyes received a minimum of three and maximum of nine injections, whereas the focal laser eyes received a minimum of one and maximum of four treatments in the 12-month study period. The primary outcome measure was ETDRS visual acuity. The study reported a statistically significant difference in mean ETDRS visual acuity in the bevacizumab group (61.3±10.4) as compared to the MLT group (50.0±16.6, $P = 0.0006$). Patients in the bevacizumab group were 5.1 times as likely to gain at least 10 ETDRS letters. Analogously, data on central retinal thickness showed a larger decrease from baseline in the bevacizumab group than the focal laser group. The BOLT study suggested that intravitreal bevacizumab therapy should be considered as a first choice in the management of center-involving DME. However, its use must be undertaken prudently in the setting of excellent visual acuity, as intravitreal injection is not without risk of complications.

5.4 Surgical management

Identification of vitreomacular traction (as in VMT syndrome) highlights the possible utility of pars plana vitrectomy in eliminating at least one factor that exacerbates diabetic macular edema. This was formally evaluated by the Diabetic Retinopathy Clinical Research network in a prospective cohort study (Haller 2010). This study was the first of its kind to systematically evaluate the effect of pars plana vitrectomy on visual acuity and retinal thickness outcomes in patients with diabetic macular edema who demonstrated vitreomacular traction on time-domain (Stratus) OCT. The study evaluated one eye from 87 diabetic patients with moderate visual loss (defined in the study as VA ranging from 20/63 - 20/400), a central retinal subfield thickness of >300 microns (by Stratus OCT), and evidence by OCT of vitreomacular traction (as assessed by the clinician). These eyes underwent standard pars plana vitrectomy and were followed at 3, 6, and 12 months. Six-month data from the study has been published. Care was taken to eliminate confounding factors with strict exclusion criteria. This study revealed that pars plana vitrectomy for eyes with DME and VMT quantitatively decreased the degree of macular edema. However, the visual acuity outcomes were less predictable in that study patients exhibited both an improvement (38%, 10 letters or more) or a decrement (22%, 10 letters or more). A major weakness of this study was the lack of a control group to demonstrate the natural course of eyes with vitreomacular traction (which the authors deemed unethical). Given the variability in operative outcomes of vitrectomy for vitreomacular traction in diabetic macular edema, this treatment modality requires further investigation.

6. Conclusion

With the increasing incidence of all types of diabetes mellitus in the United States and worldwide, diabetic macular edema will continue to represent a widespread cause of visual morbidity. A solid understanding of the basic pathophysiologic mechanisms of this disease is critical in the clinical evaluation, severity assessment, appropriate treatment selection, and effective patient counseling. Strict glycemic and blood pressure control are the most effective methods of treating DME, as they directly target the root cause of the problem: hyperglycemia, hypertension, microvascular damage and retinal vessel incompetence. Focal laser photocoagulation therapy is an advantageous, though time-limited, treatment that remains the standard of care for DME. More recent therapies have targeted the inflammatory pathways of this disease on a molecular level and have shown promising results. There is a role of surgical intervention when tractional membranes are believed to exacerbate macular edema. Further study is required to establish which of the available treatment modalities are superior. At present, successful treatment of diabetic macular edema requires thorough patient education, counseling, and compliance such that a mutually acceptable treatment protocol can be established and pursued.

7. References

Arevalo JF, *et al.* Primary intravitreal bevacizumab (Avastin) for diabetic macular edema: results from the Pan-American Collaborative Retina Study Group at 6-month follow-up. Ophthalmology 2007;114(4):743-750.

Arevalo JF, *et al.* Primary intravitreal bevacizumab (Avastin) for diabetic macular edema: results from the Pan-American Collaborative Retina Study Group at 24 months. Ophthalmology 2009; 116(8):1488-1497.

Bakri SJ, Kaiser P. Posterior subtenon triamcinolone acetonide for refractory diabetic macular edema: a randomized clinical trial. Eur J Ophthalmol 2005;139:290-4.

Beck RW, Edwards AR, Aiello LP, et al. Three-year follow up of a randomized trial comparing focal/grid photocoagulation and intravitreal triamcinolone of diabetic macular edema. Ophthalmol 2009; 127(3):245-251.

Bhavsar KV, Subramanian ML. Risk factors for progression of subclinical diabetic macular edema. Br J Ophthalmol . 2011;95(5):671-4.

Bresnick GH. Diabetic macular edema: a review. Ophthalmology 1986;93:989-997.

Browning J, *et al.* Diabetic Macular Edema: What is Focal and What is Diffuse?. Am J Ophthalmol 2008: 146(5): 649 – 655.

Brownlee M. Biochemistry and molecular cell biology of diabetic complications. Nature 414 (6865): 813–820.

Chew E, Strauber S, Beck R, et al. A randomized trial of peribulbar triamcinolone acetonide with and without focal photocoagulation for mild diabetic macular edema: a pilot study. Ophthalmol 2007;114(6):1190-1196.

Clarkson JG, Green WR, Massof D. A histologic review of 168 cases of preretinal membrane. Am J Ophthalmol.84:1,1977.

Davis M, Bressler S, Aiello L, et al. Comparison of time-domain OCT and fundus photographic assessments of retinal thickening in eyes with diabetic macular edema. Invest Ophthalmol Vis Sci. 2008;49(5):1745-1752.

Diabetes Control and Complications Trial Research Group. The effect of intensive treatment of diabetes on the development and progression of long-term complications in insulin-dependent diabetes mellitus. N Engl J Med 1993;329:977-86.

Dillinger P, Mester U. Vitrectomy with removal of the internal limiting membrane in chronic diabetic macular oedema. Graefes Arch Clin Exp Ophthalmol 2004;242:630-7.

Engerman RL, Pfaffenbach D, Davis MD. Cell turnover of capillaries. Lab Invest 1967 17:738-743.

Entezari M, Ahmadieh H, Dehghan MH, et al. Posterior sub-tenon triamcinolone for refractory diabetic macular edema: a randomized clinical trial. Am J Ophhtalmol 2005;139:240-9.

Early treatment Diabetic Retinopathy Study research group. Photocoagulation for diabetic macular edema. Early Treatment Diabetic retinopathy Study Report Number 1. Arch Ophthalmol 1985;103:1796-1806.

Early Treatment Diabetic Retinopathy Study Research Group: Treatment techniques and clinical guidelines for photocoagulation of diabetic macular edema. Early Treatment Diabetic Retinopathy study report number 2. Ophthalmology 1987;103:1796-806.

Figueroa MS, Contreras I, Noval S. Surgical and anatomical outcomes of pars plana vitrectomy of diffuse nontractional diabetic macular edema. Retina 2008;242:630-7.

Figueroa MS, Regueras A, Bertrand J, et al. A randomized trial comparing intravitreal triamcinolone acetonide and focal/grid photocoagulation for diabetic macular edema. Ophthalmol 2008;115(9):1447-1450.

Friedenwald JS. Diabetic retinopathy. Am J Ophthalmol 1950; 3:1187-1199.

Gallego-Pinazo R, *et al.* Macular laser photocoagulation guided by spectral-domain optical coherence tomography versus fluorescein angiography for diabetic macular edema. Clin Ophthalmol 2011:5 613-617.

Gass DM. Stereoscopic atlas of macular diseases diagnosis and treatment, Vol 2. C.V. Mosby Copmany, Washington, DC. 1987.

Green, WR. Retina. In Spencer, WH, ed: Ophthalmic pathology: an atlas and textbook, vol 2. WB Saunders Co, Philadelphia. 1985.

Haller JA, Qin H, Ante RS, et al. Vitrectomy outcomes in eyes with diabetic macular edema and vitreomacular traction. Ophthalmology 2010;117(6)1087-1093.

Hayreh SS. Role of retinal hypoxia in diabetic macular edema: a new concept. Graefes Arch Clin Exp Ophthalmol 2008: 246: 353-361.

Hikichi T, Yohida A, Trempe CL. Course of vitreomacular traction syndrome. Am J Ophthalmol. 1995;119:55-61.

Herman IM, D'Amore PA. Microvascular pericytes contain muscle and nonmuscle actins. J Cell Biol 1985;101:43-52.

Jonas JB, Sofker A. Intraocular injection of crystalline cortisone as adjunctive treatment of diabetic macular edema. Am J Ophthalmol 2001;132:425-7.

Kern TS. Contributions of inflammatory processes to the development of the early stages of diabetic retinopathy. Exp Diabetes Res 2007;2007:95-103.

Kirber WM, Nchols CW, Grimes PA, *et al.* A permeability defect of the retinal pigment epithelium occurrence in early streozocin diabetes. Arch Ophthalmol 1980;98:725-728.

Kok H, Lau C, Maycock N, et al. Outcome of intravitreal triamcinolone in uveitis. Ophthalmology 2005; 112(11):1916.e1-7.

Kuwabara T, Cogan DG. Studies of retinal vascular patterns. Part I. Normal architecture, Arch Ophthalmol 1960;64:904-911.

Little HL. Alterations in blood elements in the pathogenesis of diabetic retinopathy. Ophthalmology 1981; 88:647-654.

Martidis A, Duker JS, Greenberg PA, et al. Intravitreal triamcinolone for refractory diabetic macular edema. Ophthalmology 2002;109:920-7.

Michaelidis K, Kaines A, Hamilton RD, *et al.* A prospective randomized trial of intravitreal bevacizumab or laser therapy in the management of diabetic macular edema (BOLT) study) 12-month data: report 2. Ophthalmology 2010;117:1078-1086.

Murugeswari P, Shukla D, Rajendran A, *et al.* Proinflammatory cytokines and angiogenic and antiangiogenic factors in vitreous ofpatients with proliferative diabetic retinopathy and Eales' disease. Retina 2008; 28:8170824.

National Diabetes Information Clearinghouse 2011 (available at http://diabetes.niddk.nih.gov/dm/pubs/statistics/#fast)

Ozdek S, Bahceci UA, Gurelik G, Hasanreisoglu B. Posterior subtenon and intravitreal triamcinolone acetonide for diabetic macular edema. J Diabetes Complications 2006;20:246-51.

Penn JS, Madan A, Caldwell RB *et al.* Vascular endothelial growth factor in eye disease. Prog Retin Eye Res 2008; 27:331-371.

Richard, G. Fluorescein and ICG Angiography Textbook and Atlas. George Thieme Verlag: Stuttgart. 1998. 102-108.

Roberts WG, Palade GE. Increased microvascular permeability and endothelial fenestration induced by vascular endothelial growth factor. J Cell Sci 1995;108:2369-2379.

Ryan SJ. The Retina, Vol 2. C.V. Mosby Company, Baltimore. 1989.

Tanner V, Kanski JJ, Frith PA. Posterior Sub-Tenon's triamcinolone injections in the treatment of uveitis. Eye. 1998; 12 (Pt 4): 679-85.

UK Prospective Diabetes Study (UKPDS) Group. Intensive blood-glucose control with suphonylureas or insulin compared with conventional treatment and risk of complications in patients with type 2 diabetes (UKPDS 33). Lancet 1998;352:837-53.

11

Optical Coherence Tomography Findings in Diabetic Macular Edema

Desislava Koleva-Georgieva
University Eye Clinic, University Hospital"St. George", Plovdiv
Bulgaria

1. Introduction

Diabetic macular edema (DME) is one of the main causes of visual impairment in patients with diabetic retinopathy (Williams et al., 2004). The common diagnostic tools for assessing macular edema are stereo-ophthalmoscopy and fluorescein angiography. Stereoscopic examination of the fundus at the slit-lamp or on stereoscopic color fundus photographs is the standard method, as defined by the Early Treatment Diabetic Retinopathy Study (ETDRS), for evaluating macular thickening and for starting treatment when the clinical significant macular edema level has been reached (ETDRS Report Number 10, 1991). Fluorescein angiography is a complementary method for further detecting vascular leakage. However, these methods are subjective and seem to be insensitive for small changes in retinal thickness (Hee et al., 1995; Shahidi et al., 1991). In 1991 a revolutionary device was introduced in ophthalmology - optical coherence tomography (OCT) - and it dramatically improved the diagnosis of macular pathology (Huang et al., 1991). OCT provides detailed information about retinal microstructure and measures retinal thickness with high precision and reproducibility (Diabetic Retinopathy Clinical Research Network [DRCRN], 2007; Paunescu et al., 2004; Polito et al., 2005; Puliafito et al., 1995). The recently introduced spectral-domain OCT (SD OCT) machines have numerous improvements that enhance our ability to examine retinal microstructure and obtain more reliable measurements.

2. OCT principles and interpretation

2.1 OCT principles

OCT is a modern imaging technique for non-invasive and non-contact "in vivo" examination of the retina and the vitreoretinal interface on cross-section images or on a 3D image reconstruction, and for objective measurement of retinal thickness (Hee et al., 1995; Huang et al., 1991; Schuman et al., 2004). Its high resolution (5-10μm) is unobtainable for any other device. The operating principle resembles echography, but instead of ultrasound a low-coherent light signal is used. The first OCT devices are referred to as time-domain OCT (TD OCT). TD OCT technology relies on an optical technique known as Michelson low coherence interferometry (Shuman et al., 2004). The image acquisition and thickness measurements are achieved by detecting the echo time delay of the backreflected or backscattred light from internal retinal structures while it interferes with the light that has traveled a known path length. This is obtained by moving a reference mirror and the signal collection is a function of time (Brancato & Lumbroso, 2004; Schumann et al., 2004).

In the past few years SD OCT technology was introduced. At present there are two techniques for SD OCT. The first uses a spectrometer for detecting and measuring the light spectrum returning from tissue and a stationary reference mirror. Here mathematical operations, called Fourier transforms, are used. Thus SD OCT is also referred to as Fourier-domain OCT. As this technology allows detecting all echoes of backreflected light simultaneously and there are no moving parts, the imaging speed and resolution of SD OCT are higher than those of TD OCT (Podoleanu, 2005; van Velthoven et al., 2007). The second SD OCT technique is called "swept source-OCT". It uses a light source in which the emission wavelength is tuned rapidly over a broad wavelength range (Choma et al., 2003; Podoleanu, 2005). The main advantages of SD OCT over TD OCT are the increased imaging speed, the higher resolution and sensitivity, the possibility of obtaining a 3D retinal image reconstruction, more reliable thickness measurements and topographic retinal analyses.

2.2 OCT interpretation

The interpretation of OCT is based on analysis of various qualitative and quantitative data (Brancato & Lumbroso, 2004; Schuman et al., 2004). Before performing these analyses, an assessment of the OCT scan quality has to be made and the presence of scan artifacts has to be detected, since they can lead to retinal thickness measurement errors and false conclusions. The artifacts may be operator-induced (defocusing, depolarization and out of range image), patient-induced (off-center fixation resulting in incorrectly centered retinal thickness maps, blink and motion artifacts) or may be due to the limitations of the imaging technique (TD OCT has lower imaging speed and frequent blink and motion artifacts). All these artifacts have been recognized to cause breakdown in the performance of the segmentation software and thus leading to incorrect automated retinal thickness measurements (Ho et al., 2009; Ray et al., 2005; Sadda et al., 2006). Several studies have pointed out that segmentation breakdown may also be possible in high quality scans if there are pathological features such as full-thickness macular hole, pigment epithelial detachment, subretinal fluid, retinal fibrosis and hard exudates (Domalpally et al., 2009; Ho et al., 2009; Krebs et al., 2009; Sadda et al., 2006). The presence of media opacities (cataract, vitreous hemorrhage, ect.) and low signal intensity (low signal-to-noise ratio) may also induce segmentation breakdown. Although much progress has been made in improving the accuracy of the segmentation software, and the SD OCT devices perform better than the TD OCT, segmentation breakdown still occurs with the current SD OCT software. There is possibility of manual correction, but still it is time consuming and not always feasible in clinical settings. At this point it seems prudent to note this limitation of the current OCT software. Thus, until improvement in the segmentation algorithm is available, the clinician may minimize possible diagnostic and therapeutic errors when working with the current OCT devices by anticipating and recognizing automated retinal thickness measurement errors.

2.2.1 OCT characteristics of normal macular morphology

The interpretation of qualitative data is based on analyzing tissue reflectivity. As OCT has histological correspondence (Toth et al., 1997), the interpretation of the OCT image seems to be quite intuitive. However, it should be always remembered that OCT technology depicts tissue reflectivity. It is dependent on tissue optical properties, i.e. microscopic variations in the refractive index of subcellular structures, and on the amount of light signal absorbed by the overlying tissues (Brancato & Lumbroso, 2004; Schumann et al., 2004). Normal macular histology is divided into 10 distinct layers: inner limiting membrane (ILM), nerve fiber layer (NFL), ganglion cell layer (GCL), inner plexiform layer (IPL), inner nuclear layer (INL), outer plexiform layer (OPL), outer nuclear layer (ONL), external limiting membrane (ELM), rod and cone layer, and retinal pigment epithelium layer (RPE), (fig.1). They are formed by 4 cell types: RPE, photoreceptors, bipolar and ganglion cells. The reflectivity of the various layers is represented in the OCT scans by the so called false colors (a color coded way - white and red for high reflectivity, and blue and black for low reflectivity). The ILM is the first detected layer on the OCT scan, due to the contrast between the non-reflective vitreous and the reflective retina. Immediately behind it lies the NFL. It consists of horizontal axonal structures of high optical reflectivity and is depicted on OCT scans by red color. The NFL is thicker on the nasal side, because of the density of the papillomacular bundle. The plexiform layers are of medium reflectivity and appear yellow on the scans. The nuclear layers (GCL, INL and ONL) are of low optical reflectivity and appear as blue-black. The GCL is thickest in the parafoveal area. In the fovea there is thinning of the retina with absence of the inner layers and an increase in thickness of the ONL. It is easily recognized on the scans by its characteristic depression. The RPE, which contains melanin, is highly reflective and is the outermost red layer on the OCT scan. Behind it is the medium reflective choriocapillaris.

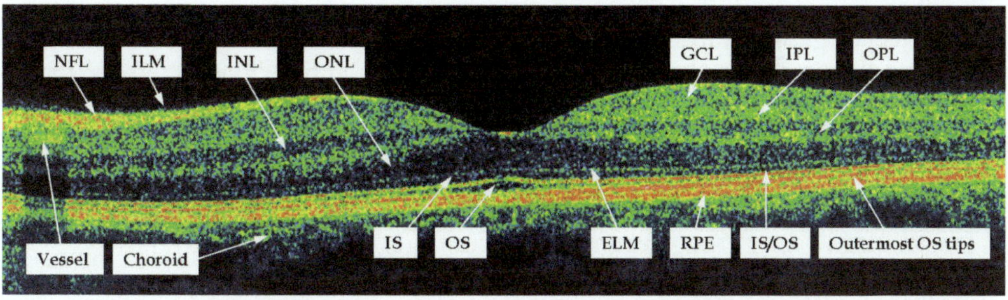

Fig. 1. Normal macular structure - SD OCT representation of retinal layers: inner limiting membrane (ILM), nerve fiber layer (NFL), ganglion cell layer (GCL), inner plexiform layer (IPL), inner nuclear layer (INL), outer plexiform layer (OPL), outer nuclear layer (ONL), external limiting membrane (ELM), inner segments (IS) and outer segments (OS) of the photoreceptors, IS/OS junction (IS/OS), and the retinal pigment epithelium layer (RPE).

In front of the RPE on Stratus TD OCT scans and on SD OCT scans there is another highly reflective (red) layer - it is the boundary between the inner segments (IS) and the outer segments (OS) of the photoreceptors. On TD OCT two highly reflective lines in the outer retina are visualized (as described above). On SD OCT there are three highly reflective lines in the outer retina - the innermost being the IS/OS junction, the outermost being the RPE, and the middle one is described to be the outermost tips of the OS, containing discs, rich in rhodopsin (Ooto et al., 2010; Srinivasan et al., 2006). On SD OCT despite these three highly reflective layers, a forth thinner high-to-medium reflective line is also visible in front of the

IS/OS layer and it represents the ELM. If an OCT scan intersects a retinal blood vessel it can be identified by the increased reflectivity and shadowing of the deeper structures.

2.2.2 OCT interpretation – qualitative analysis (morphology and reflectivity)

While performing qualitative analysis one should simultaneously perform morphological examination (changes in retinal profile - surface and posterior layers, and presence of abnormal structures) and reflectivity examination (hyper-reflectivity, hypo-reflectivity, and shadowing effects) (Brancato & Lumbroso, 2004). Pathological changes in retinal surface contour may represent disappearance of the normal foveal depression (in macular edema). Steepening of the foveal contour may be associated with epiretinal membranes, macular pseudoholes or lamellar holes. OCT can distinguish between lamellar holes, pseudoholes or various stages of full thickness macular holes. Pathological changes in posterior layers may be RPE detachments (form steep angles with the choriocapillaris) and neurosensory retinal detachments (form shallow angles with the RPE and protrude less). Retinal drusen produce wavy undulations of the pigment epithelium line. Abnormal intraretinal structures may be cotton wool spots (superficial hyper-reflective nodules with indistinct margins in the NFL), hard exudates (round numerous or plaque-like hyper-reflective spots usually in the inner layers, shadowing the deeper structures), choroidal neovascular membranes (nodular or rounded fusiform hyper-reflective structures in front of the RPE, or sometimes visualized as localized thickening of the RPE, choriocapillaris and OS, usually associated with edema or serous retinal detachment), fibrous scars (hyper-reflective structures in the outer retina that deform reduced in thickness retinal layers).

Retinal pathological features can be associated with changes in optical properties of the tissue and thus be detected on the OCT scan as changes in reflectivity. While performing this reflectivity analysis one should always remember that the reflectivity displayed on the scan is a result from the tissue reflectivity, the amount of light absorbed by overlying structures, and the amount of light that reaches the sensor after it has been further attenuated by interposing tissues. Thus care is required in interpreting OCT images when media opacities, poor alignment of the OCT instrument while imaging, high astigmatism or poorly centered intraocular implants are present, as these may reduce signal intensity.

Pathological features that can be hyper-reflective are: epiretinal and thick vitreal membranes, cotton wool spots, hard exudates, thick hemorrhages, retinal fibrosis, RPE hyperplasia or pigmented choroidal nevi, neovascular membranes, atrophy of the retina and RPE (the later cause increased reflectivity of the underlying choroid). Reduced reflectivity (hypo-reflectivity) is most often caused by fluid accumulation: intraretinal edema (it may be associated with formation of optically non-reflective cystoid spaces), or subretinal edema (serous neuroepithelial retinal detachment, serous pigment epithelial detachment). Hypo-reflectivity may also be present in retinal and RPE atrophy or RPE hypopigmentation, where along with tissue hypo-reflectivity there is increase of the reflectivity of the underlying choroid.

2.2.3 OCT interpretation – quantitative analysis

The quantitative analysis is a very important part of OCT interpretation. Quantitative measurements of retinal thickness, volume, and a variety of structures (i.e. retinal morphometry) provide objective information for diagnosing disease, tracking disease progress, and evaluating response to therapy. The availability of highly reproducible and repeatable retinal thickness measurements (DRCRN, 2007; Paunescu et al., 2004; Puliafito et al., 1995) is prerequisite for early diagnosis of macular edema.

Retinal thickness and volume are automatically calculated by the computer software and are displayed in numerical values (table format) or in color coded topographic retinal thickness maps. Retinal thickness is calculated for central fixation point, 9 ETDRS-like macular regions and total macular thickness. Retinal volume is displayed for 9 ETDRS-like macular regions and total macular volume (not all OCT devices display volume). The 9 ETDRS-like macular regions consist of one central circle of 500 µm radius (the foveal region), an inner and outer ring, each divided into four quadrants. The topographic color coded retinal thickness map (white and red for high thickness values, and blue for low thickness values) provides more graphic information that can be compared directly to the fundus image.

The automatic calculation of retinal thickness is dependent on a computer image-processing algorithm called segmentation. It allows automatic detection of the inner and outer retinal boundaries. After that automatic calculation of the measurements between these boundaries is performed (Schuman et al., 2004). At this point several important notes have to be made. First, in TD OCT the retinal thickness topographic map is displayed after interpolation of the measured retinal thickness form 6 radial cross-section scans (overall 6x512=3072 A-scans, or 6x128=768 A-scans for the entire macular area). The interpolation may miss pathologic areas with increased/decreased thickness between the 6 radial lines. In SD OCT retinal thickness topographic map is displayed after performing measurements from a great number of A-scans (27 000 A-scans for Cirrus HD-OCT (Carl Zeiss Meditec) and Spectral OCT/SLO (OPKO/OTI), 40 000 A-scans for Spectralis (Heidelberg Engineering), and over 50 000 A-scans for high resolution OCT devices). Thus retinal thickness measurement with SD OCT provides more precise and reliable data. Second, the different OCT devices have different segmentation algorithms, and there is published evidence of significant differences between TD OCT and SD OCT, as well as between different SD OCT machines (Han et al., 2009; Leung et al., 2008; Wolf-Schnurrbusch et al., 2009). The difference is mainly caused by the way of delineating the outer retinal boundary (at the level of the first, second or third hyper-reflective line in the outer retina). Thus measurements from different OCT devices cannot be compared in studies, as well as in the follow-up of patients in clinical settings. Third, the segmentation algorithm may not perform correctly in the presence of scan artifacts or particular pathological features and lead to thickness measurement errors (as described in 2.2.OCT interpretation).

The data base for normal retinal thickness should be different for the different OCT devices. There are a lot of studies on retinal thickness measurements in healthy eyes, and their number is even increasing with the introduction of new OCT machines. Normal values for the central point and foveal thickness according to several studies, using TD OCT and SD OCT are presented on table 1. The diversity of data for normal eyes seems to be much more confusing, than helpful. There is a general trend of measuring higher values of retinal thickness with more refined OCT technology. All measurements with SD OCT have higher values than measurements with TD OCT. The greater axial resolution of SD OCT (5-6 µm) compared to TD OCT (10 µm) and the higher precision of the software may explain the difference between TD OCT and SD OCT. The differences among the several types of SD OCT devices may also be significant and are due to the segmentation of the outer retinal boundary. The presented data on table 1 also suggest differences even in measurements with identical OCT devices. This may be due to the specific characteristics and composition of the examined populations - age, gender, race, refraction, ect.

Study	Number of examined eyes	OCT device	CFP	Fovea
Hee et al., 1995	20	Time-domain OCT prototype	147 ± 17	-
Hee et al., 1998	73	Time-domain OCT prototype	152 ± 21	174 ± 18
Otani et al., 1999	10	Time-domain OCT 1	133 ± 9	-
Schaudig et al., 2000	25	Time-domain OCT 1	152 ± 17	-
Massin et al., 2002	60	Time-domain OCT 1	146 ± 20	170 ± 18
Paunescu et al., 2004	10	Time-domain OCT 3 (Stratus)	164 ± 21	204 ± 20
Chan A et al., 2006	37	Taim-domain OCT 3 (Stratus)	182 ± 23	212 ± 20
Bressler et al., 2008	97	Time-domain OCT 3 (Stratus)	166 ± 23	201 ± 22
Kelty PJ et al., 2008	83	Time-domain OCT 3 (Stratus)	-	205 ± 27
El-Ashry et al., 2008	200	Time-domain OCT 3 (Stratus)	173 ± 23	203 ± 24
Leung CK et al., 2008	35	Time-domain OCT 3 (Stratus) Spectral OCT - Topcon 3D OCT	155 ± 16 -	196 ± 17 216 ± 12
Huang et al., 2009	32	Time-domain OCT 3 (Stratus) Spectral OCT - RTVue-100	164 ± 26 175 ± 17	193 ± 22 208 ± 21
Wolf-Schnurrbusch UEK et al., 2009	20	Time-domain OCT 3 (Stratus) Spectral OCT: Spectralis OCT Spectral OCT/SLO Cirrus HD OCT SOCT Copernicus RTVue-100	- - - - - -	213 ± 19 288 ± 16 243 ± 25 276 ± 17 246 ±23 245 ± 28
Koleva-Georgieva et al, 2010	39	Spectral OCT/SLO	176 ± 17	198 ± 21
Grover S et al., 2010	36	Time-domain OCT 3 (Stratus) Spectral OCT - Spectralis OCT	167 ± 21 225 ± 17	202 ± 23 271 ± 20
Ooto S et al., 2010	248	Spectral OCT – 3-D OCT-1000	-	222 ± 19

Table 1. Normal retinal thickness measurements for central fixation point (CFP) and fovea, represented in μm (mean ± standard deviation), obtained by different OCT devices.

There is not a commonly accepted opinion about the variation of retinal thickness with age. Several authors have reported a lack of relation between retinal thickness and age (Browning et al., 2008; Chan et al., 2006; Grover et al., 2010; Hee et al., 1995; Massin et al., 2002; Sanchez-Tochino et al., 2002). Others have found negative correlation between retinal thickness and age in all 9 ETDRS regions (Alamouti & Funk, 2003; Erikson & Alm, 2009), and in five of the 9 ETDRS areas not including the fovea (Ooto et al., 2010). There is a well known decrease in thickness of the NFL with age. According to Erikson and Alm the thinning of the macula with age is 20-25% due to thinning of NFL and 75-80%due to thinning of other retinal layers (Erikson & Alm, 2009). Thus the reduction of retinal thickness with age cannot be contributed to thinning of NFL alone.

It has been reported that men have thicker retinas than women (Browning et al., 2008; Guedes et al., 2003; Hee et al., 1995; Kelty et al., 2008; Massin et al., 2002; Ooto et al., 2010). However, Chan and coauthors and Grover and coauthors did not detect significant inter-sex difference in retinal thickness, but their studied groups had uneven sex distribution (Chan et al., 2006; Grover et al., 2010).

There is published evidence of racial differences in retinal thickness. It has been reported that Blacks and Asians have thinner retinas compared with whites in age-matched groups (Asenfzadeh et al., 2007; Guedes et al., 2003; Kelty et al., 2008). Thus, race may be taken into consideration while interpreting OCT thickness measurements.

The relation of macular thickness to axial length and presence of high myopia has also been described. Retinal thickness in highly myopic eyes (>6D) was higher in the fovea, but lower in the inner and outer regions compared to non-myopic eyes in a study with age-matched groups (Wu et al., 2008). Thus it may be an indication for change in retinal contour of highly myopic eyes and care is needed while interpreting macular pathology on OCT scans of such eyes. The studies of Lam and coauthors and Lim and coauthors showed negative correlation of retinal thickness and axial length (Lam et al., 2007; Lim et al., 2005). However, both studies included highly myopic eyes together with non-myopic eyes, and did not perform age-adjusted analysis. In their investigation on 248 eyes, Ooto and associates found no correlation between macular thickness and age-adjusted axial length (Ooto et al, 2010).

We performed a study including 39 healthy eyes, with almost even sex distribution (21 men; 18 women), accepting refractive error of no more than ± 3D, without glaucoma and all subjects being of Caucasian descent (Koleva-Georgieva & Sivkova, 2010). The automated retinal thickness and volume measurements were obtained by Spectral OCT/SLO Combination Imaging System (OPKO/OTI). A negative correlation between age and retinal thickness and volume in all ETDRS regions, except the temporal inner and temporal outer regions was found, and this relation remained after controlling for gender. Men had thicker retinas than women, and this remained so after controlling for age. These results are in consent with some authors and in discrepancy with others. One reason may be the small sample size in many of the studies, or the heterogeneity of retinal thickness in different populations. Additional studies with larger sample sizes are needed to clarify the situation. If quantitative analysis should be meticulous the normative database for retinal thickness probably should be population-based and obtained for each OCT machine type separately. Still our findings, supported by others, indicate that age, sex, and high myopia must be considered while interpreting retinal thickness data.

3. OCT findings in DME

3.1 Retinal thickness

Retinal edema is defined as any detectable retinal thickening due to fluid accumulation (ETDRS Report Number 10, 1991). Stereoscopic examination of the fundus is the standard method, as defined by the ETDRS, for evaluating macular thickening. However, it is subjective and seems to be insensitive for small changes in retinal thickness (Hee et al, 1995;

Shahidi et al, 1991). The particular value of OCT is the possibility for objective, reliable and repeatable retinal thickness measurements. Since the introduction of OCT several authors have studied the possibility of OCT for early diagnosis of macular edema, and have suggested criteria to detect the so called subclinical diabetic macular edema (Hee et al., 1995, 1998; Massin et al., 2002). There are studies reporting significant differences in retinal thickness between controls and eyes with diabetic retinopathy (without clinically detectable DME) in the fovea (Sanchez-Tochino et al., 2002; Schaudig et al., 2000), superior and nasal quadrants (Schaudig et al., 2000). Difference was also found between healthy eyes and diabetics without diabetic retinopathy in the fovea (Sanchez-Tochino et al., 2002), the paramacular ring (Schaudig et al., 2000) and the superior zone (Sugimoto et al., 2005). When comparing eyes of diabetics with and without retinopathy (and no clinical evidence of macular edema) Sanchez-Tochino and coauthors did not find any significant difference (Sanchez-Tochino et al., 2002), but Schaudig and associates found statistically significant difference in the superior nasal quadrant (Schaudig et al., 2000).

In a clinical study we compared retinal thickness between diabetic patients without clinical evidence of DME (1st group - 57 eyes of 29 patients without diabetic retinopathy; 2nd group - 63 eyes of 32 patients with diabetic retinopathy) and a control group (39 healthy eyes), (Koleva-Georgieva & Sivkova, 2010). All groups were age-matched and with nearly even sex distribution. The tendency of men having thicker retinas than women, and decrease of thickness with age were noted also for diabetic patients from both groups, although not reaching significance for all macular areas. We found significant differences in retinal thickness between controls and diabetics with diabetic retinopathy (group 2) in all macular regions, and also between controls and diabetics without retinopathy (group 1) in all regions except superior inner, inferior inner and nasal inner. It was present also after controlling for age and gender. The differences were present in more macular regions than detected by other authors. It might be due to the greater resolution and precision of the SD OCT that we used. So, OCT could detect early and subtle increase in retinal thickness in eyes with or even without retinopathy in comparison to healthy eyes. When comparing eyes of diabetics without retinopathy (group1) to those with diabetic retinopathy (group 2) we found significant difference in the central fixation point, fovea, superior inner, temporal inner, nasal inner regions and total retinal thickness. This indicated that SD OCT could further distinguish early macular damage in eyes with diabetic retinopathy compared to eyes without retinopathy. These early changes were more likely to develop in the central region and superior macular hemisphere (Koleva-Georgieva & Sivkova, 2010; Schaudig et al., 2000; Sugimoto et al., 2005). This evidence, published by many authors, suggests the possibility of OCT for the early detection of macular edema in diabetic patients.

If we need to know whether a given diabetic patient has early macular damage, detectable by OCT, we have to apply some criteria. Ever since the pioneers of OCT have examined this possibility they have given several criteria: retinal thickness exceeding mean+3SDs (standard deviations) from normal subjects (Hee et al., 1995), retinal thickness exceeding the maximal thickness in normal eyes, difference between the right and left eyes exceeding mean difference in healthy eyes+2SDs, comparison with the database from normal population, and comparison with previous measurements (Hee et al., 1995, 1998). Hee and associates found 3 eyes (from 55 eyes) of diabetics without retinopathy with evidence of early damage according to their criterion on difference between right and left eyes (Hee et al., 1998). Massin and coauthors suggested early macular edema to be present if retinal thickness of an area was greater than the mean +2SDs in the corresponding area of normal subjects (Massin et al., 2002). This will exceed the variation in 95% of the normal population. They detected early macular thickening in 12 eyes (from 70 eyes) of diabetic patients without edema on ophthalmoscopy. In our study we did not apply the criterion of difference between right and left eyes, because Spectral OCT/SLO does not give this information automatically as Stratus TD OCT does. We applied the criterion of retinal thickness exceeding mean+2SDs from normal values for both the central fixation point and the fovea (both being in the clinically significant zone) to distinguish eyes with early subclinical DME (Koleva-Georgieva & Sivkova, 2010). Thirteen eyes were detected with retinal thickness exceeding both 209.6 μm for the central fixation point (176 μm+2x16.8 μm) and 241.1 μm for the fovea (198.3 μm +2x21.4 μm). All 13 eyes had retinopathy - 12 eyes with mild non-proliferative diabetic retinopathy and 1 eye with moderate non-proliferative diabetic retinopathy. In contrast to the finding of Browning and coauthors that only eyes with late stages of retinopathy (severe non-proliferative or proliferative) with no clinically detectable edema had thicker retinas than healthy eyes (Browning et al, 2008), we detected early subclinical macular damage also in eyes with mild and moderate non-proliferative diabetic retinopathy. That's why we believe that OCT examination could be useful in patients with any severity of diabetic retinopathy, even in the earliest stages, and this would be at least for two reasons: first - to screen for early DME and eventually consider a closer follow-up, and second - to have a baseline measurement of retinal thickness for future comparison. This evidence confirms that SD OCT can possibly detect early subclinical macular edema in eyes with diabetic retinopathy. In the clinical setting, it is not advisable to use the above reported values of normal retinal thickness due to differences in population characteristics. However, the preset criteria defining early macular damage may be used, and attention should be paid to age, gender, ethnicity and presence of high myopia.

OCT is also a valuable method for quantifying treatment effects after laser photocoagulation, vitrectomy, or intravitreal application of steroid and anti-VEGF injections. The assessment of the effect of each treatment has to be judged both by the improvement of visual acuity and by the observation of structural changes induced. OCT has proved to be beyond comparison for the latter, and has the value of objectively quantifying even subtle changes in retinal thickness. The high reproducibility of retinal thickness measurements allows OCT to be used for longitudinal objective monitoring of the treatment efficacy. A change in macular thickness of more than 10% of the baseline measurement has been considered as significant and not due to the variability of the method (Massin et al., 2001; Polito et al., 2005). It is worth noting here that fluorescein angiography also has its value in verifying macular ischemia. Several studies have stated that macular ischemia is a possible explanation for the lack of functional improvement in patients with good structural outcome after conservative or surgical treatment (Massin et al., 2003; Otani & Kishi, 2000). However, OCT is becoming the mainstay of objective treatment monitoring and follow-up of patients with macular edema. It is widely accepted in trials and studies (DRCRN, 2010; Estabrook et al., 2007; Otani & Kishi, 2000; Ozdemir et al., 2005; Patel et al., 2006), as well as in clinical settings.

3.2 Retinal microstructure

The main characteristic OCT features of macular edema are: increased retinal thickness, reduced intraretinal reflectivity, irregularity of the layered structure, and flattening of the foveal depression (fig. 2). If edema persists, cystoid cavities may appear (Brancato & Lumbroso, 2004; Saxena & Meredith, 2006; Schumann et al., 2004). In macular edema serous fluid may be present under a detached neurosensory retina as a serous macular detachment (SMD). Hard exudates, hemorrhages and cotton-wool spots may also be present in macular tissue and their characteristics have been described (2.2.2.OCT interpretation - qualitative analysis).

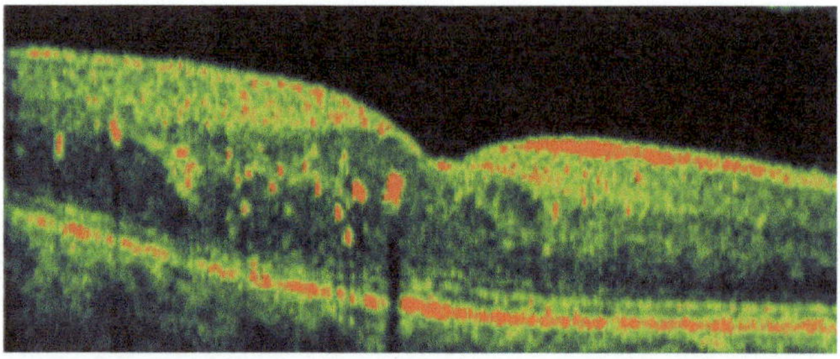

Fig. 2. Simple non-cystoid diabetic macular edema: increased retinal thickness, flattening of the foveal depression, irregularity of the layered structure, hard exudates (multiple red spots with shadowing of underlying tissue), without cystoid spaces.

The accumulation of intraretinal fluid leads to increase in retinal thickness and reduction of optical reflectivity. The layered macular structure becomes irregular. In our studies (Koleva-Georgieva & Sivkova, 2008; 2009), and also in others (Kim et al., 2006; Otani et al, 1999) it was described that areas with reduced reflectivity were located mainly in the outer retinal layers and the inner layers were displaced anteriorly. This was noted especially for simple macular edema, which is the beginning of retinal disruption. According to histopathologic studies of eyes with macular edema, fluid accumulation starts with intracytoplasmic swelling of Müller cells in the outer plexiform layer of Henle (Yanoff et al., 1984). Areas with reduced reflectivity on OCT images probably represent the swollen Müller cells. If macular edema persists, necrosis of Müller cells and the adjacent neurons occurs (Yanoff et al., 1984). This leads to cystoid cavity formation in the retina.

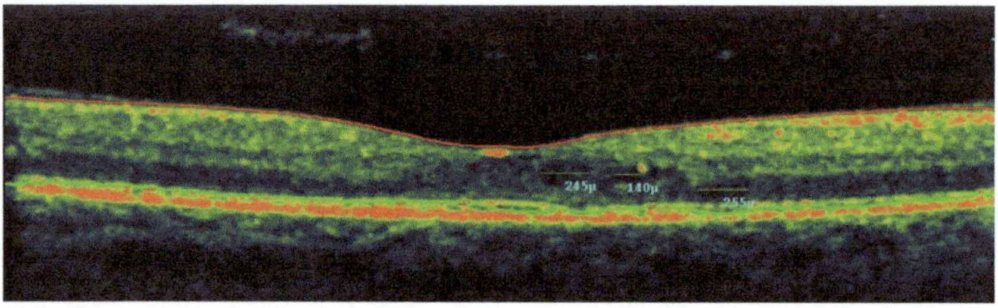

Fig. 3. Mild cystoid diabetic macular edema: intraretinal cystoid spaces with horizontal diameter < 300µm.

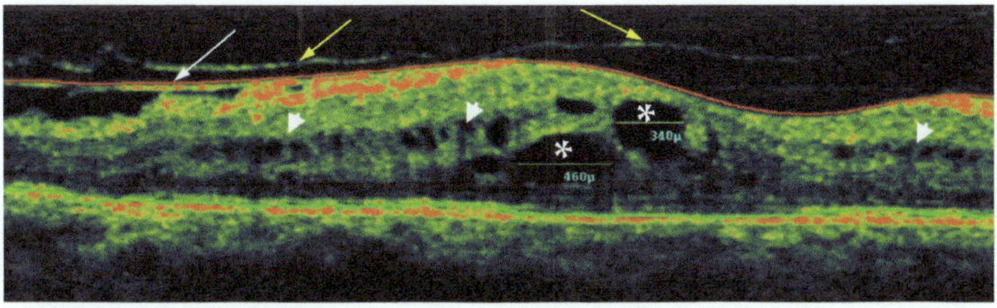

Fig. 4. Intermediate cystoid diabetic macular edema: intraretinal cystoid spaces with horizontal diameter ≥ 300μm < 600μm (star), note smaller cystoid spaces located in the inner layers (white arrowheads), epiretinal membrane with focal adhesions and distortion of retinal contour (white arrow), and posterior hyaloid detached from retinal surface (yellow arrows) with peripapillary adhesion (not shown on this scan).

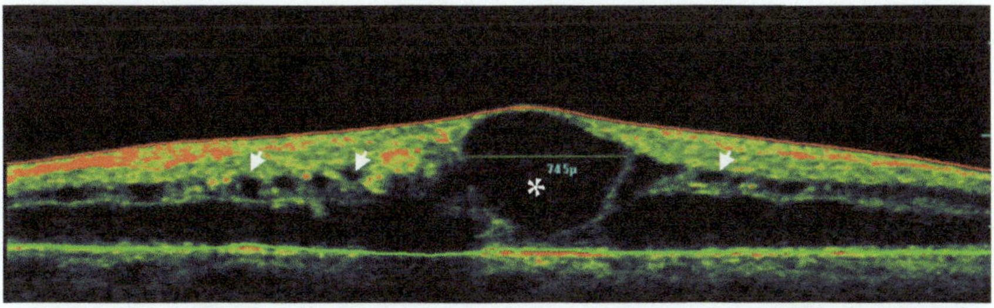

Fig. 5. Severe cystoid diabetic macular edema: intraretinal cystoid spaces with horizontal diameter ≥ 600μm (star), note smaller cystoid spaces located in the inner layers (white arrowheads).

On OCT images cystoid cavities appear as black non-reflective spaces, surrounded by medium-to-low reflective septa (fig. 3, 4 and 5). On en face OCT images cystoid spaces have well defined septae and, since this scan lies in the coronal plane, we may draw out additional information about the extent and location of the cystoid spaces. The cystoid cavities were observed to be located in the outer layers in newly developed edema, and to engage the inner layers in well-established edema forming large confluent cystoid cavities (Otani et al., 1999). In our study we found correlation between the size of cystoid spaces and retinal thickness and visual acuity (Koleva-Georgieva & Sivkova, 2008). We decided to subdivide cystoid DME into mild, moderate, and severe according to the size of cystoid spaces (fig. 3, 4 and 5). The mild cystoid DME presents with small cysts mainly in the outer retinal layers. The cystoid spaces in eyes with intermediate and severe cystoid DME were mainly located in the outer layers, predominantly in the fovea. Still, some of these eyes also had small cysts in the inner layers. We assume that fluid accumulation in cystoid spaces in the inner retinal layers could be a result of the progression of macular edema. With progression, disruption of cystic septae may ensue. Large confluent cystoid cavities may form to involve almost the entire thickness of the retina and give a retinoschisis appearance. In these cases a thin layer of atrophic retinal tissue remains over the retinoschisis spaces, and the eyes have profound visual loss. This probably represents the last stage of retinal disruption. The lower visual acuity in eyes with severe cystoid DME and the statistically significant difference when comparing with the milder cystoid DME types show that the subtypes of cystoid DME could be consecutive stages of macular edema progression with worsening of visual function. We recommend that the size of cystoid spaces should be analyzed when evaluating patients with DME.

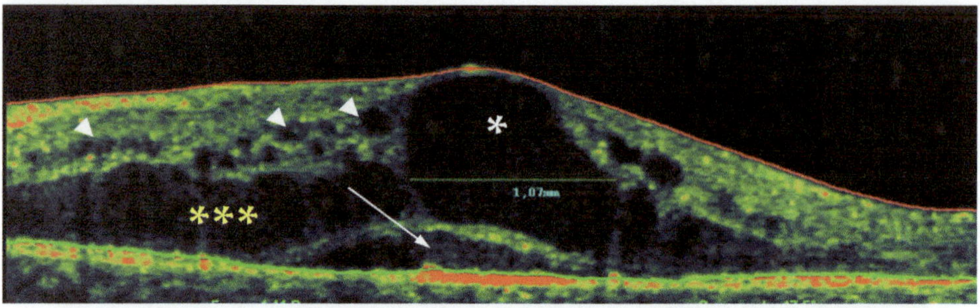

Fig. 6. Serous macular detachment: a dome-shaped hypo-reflective area under the detached neurosensory retina and over the hyper-reflective layer of the pigment epithelium (white arrow), note the association with severe cystoid space (white star), confluent cystoid spaces with retinoschisis appearance (yellow stars), and the small cystoid spaces in the inner layers (arrowheads).

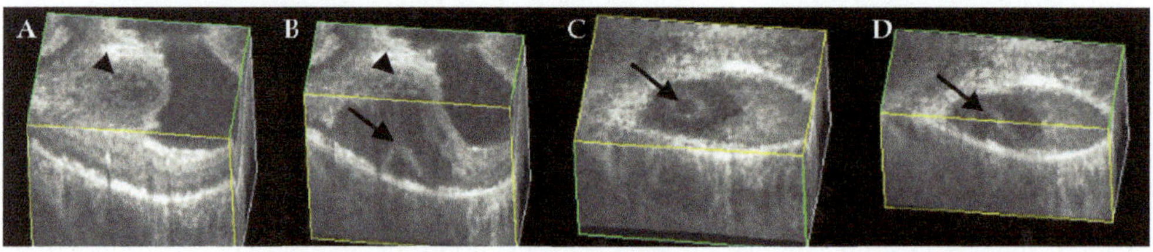

Fig. 7. 3D OCT image reconstruction with consequent coronal and longitudinal slicing: represents serous macular detachment (black arrow) and cystoid spaces (black arrowhead), note that the reflectivity of the serous macular detachment border (representing photoreceptor IS/OS) is more reflective than the cystoid septae.

In eyes with macular edema the pattern of SMD may also be found (Alkuraya et al., 2005; Catier et al., 2005; Kaiser et al., 2001; Kim et al., 2006; Koleva-Georgieva & Sivkova, 2009; Otani et al., 1999; Panozzo et al. 2004). This feature can be detected "in vivo" only by means of OCT, as it does not show on ophthalmoscopy or fluorescein angiography. However, it has been well documented by Wolter in a histopathology study on eyes with DME (Wolter, 1981). The pathogenesis of SMD is not completely understood, and its significance still remains unknown. The most debatable factor is macular traction. Some authors point out traction as a leading cause (Kaiser et al., 2001), while others completely reject this hypothesis (Catier et al., 2005). There are statements that SMD is innocuous and transient (Ozdemir et al., 2005), while others state it is the last stage of chronic edema (Brancato & Lumbroso, 2004).

On OCT scans SMD appears as a low-reflective area under the detached neurosensory retina and over the hyper-reflective line of the pigment epithelium. It is usually confined to the foveal area (fig. 6). On en face OCT scans SMD appears as round area of low reflectivity, surrounded by a medium reflectivity line (fig. 7). In our study on 79 eyes with DME, we found SMD in 9 eyes (11.4%), (Koleva-Georgieva & Sivkova, 2009). This prevalence is comparable to other studies (Alkuraya et al., 2005; Kang et al., 2004; Kim et al., 2006; Otani et al., 1999). In our cohort of studied eyes, SMD was combined predominantly with cystoid edema pattern (intermediate cystoid in 5 eyes, severe cystoid in 3 eyes), and was combined with simple edema pattern only in 1 eye. The cystoid spaces were located in the outer retinal layers and the largest ones leaned to the center of fovea. In 6 eyes we also observed smaller cystoid spaces in the inner retinal layers that tended to be outside the fovea. Hard exudates were seen in 5 eyes. On fluorescein angiography the eyes with SMD presented with diffuse leakage in one eye and cystoid edema pattern in 8 eyes. Macular ischemia was found in 6 eyes. There was similarity in the distribution of macular traction types among eyes with SMD (no traction - 3 eyes, questionable - 3 eyes, and definite - 3 eyes). So, our findings may be in support of the statement that macular ischemia plays important role in the development in SMD, and that macular traction is of equivocal significance (Catier et al., 2005). The height of SMD did not correlate with retinal thickness or with best corrected visual acuity. Eyes with SMD had lower visual acuity than eyes with simple and mild cystoid DME type, and thicker retinas than eyes with simple, mild cystoid and intermediate cystoid DME. The difference was not significant between eyes with SMD and eyes with severe cystoid DME. Some authors state that SMD may be just a transient edema and leaves no functional consequences (Ozdemir et al., 2005). Our findings differ from this statement. In our cohort, SMD was predominantly accompanied by intermediate and severe cystoid edema pattern, there was macular ischemia in 6 of 9 eyes, and visual acuity was worse than that in eyes with simple non-cystoid and mild cystoid DME. On one hand it seemed that the SMD presence did not determine visual function and the low visual acuity could be due to the association of the SMD with large cystoid spaces and presence of macular ischemia. On the other hand we still observed SMD predominantly in eyes with intermediate and severe cystoid edema, which are meant to be advanced and graver types of edema and this association may be meaningful. The number of eyes with SMD in our study was too small and the published data from other studies are controversial. Further larger studies are needed to elucidate the pathogenesis and reveal the functional consequences of SMD. Nevertheless, SD OCT proved to be useful in detecting SMD and accompanying changes in retinal morphology and vitreoretinal interface.

In the past few years, since the introduction of SD OCT, it became possible to accurately visualize the outer retinal layers. The integrity of these layers has has been reported to correlate with with retinal function and discussion in literature is still ongoing about its prognostic value. Several authors have found out that visual acuity has a positive correlation with the survival rate of ELM and IS/OS (Otani et al., 2010), and that the postoperative status of the photoreceptors is related to the final visual function after resolution of normal retinal morphology morphology following surgery surgery for persistent DME (Sakamoto et al., 2009) or epiretinal membrane (ERM), (Mitamura et al., 2009; Oster et al., 2010). The percentage disruption of the photoreceptor IS/OS junction layer is a significant predictor of visual acuity (Maheshwary et al, 2010). Analysis of the integrity of IS/OS and ELM on SD OCT scans should be a part of macular edema evaluation (fig. 8).

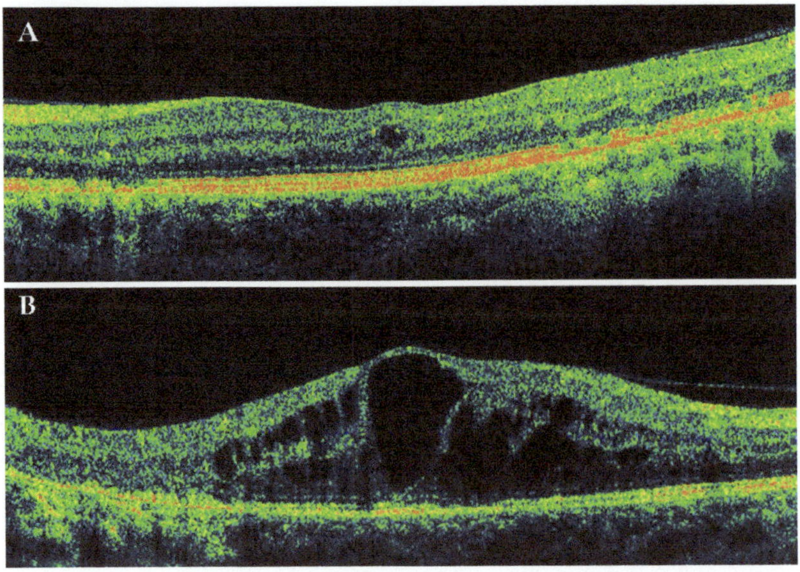

Fig. 8. Outer retinal layers inner segment (IS)/outer segment (OS) and external limiting membrane (ELM): A - intact IS/OS and ELM in eye with mild cystoid diabetic macular edema, B - disturbed integrity in eye with severe cystoid diabetic macular edema.

3.3 Vitreoretinal interface and macular traction

Macular traction is a factor implemented in the pathogenesis of macular edema and there is increasing evidence that releasing it via vitrectomy may be beneficial (DRCRN, 2010; Patel et al., 2006; Yanyali et al., 2007). Macular traction may be induced by vitreoretinal interface abnormalities such as incomplete posterior vitreous detachment (PVD) or ERM. In 1984 Shepens and coauthors postulate the role of incomplete PVD in the formation or progression of macular edema in susceptible eyes, such as of diabetics. Before the introduction of OCT, Hikichi and associates and Nasrallah and associates have evaluated the presence and characteristics of PVD in eyes with DME by ophthalmoscopy. They found relatively small prevalence of complete PVD (27% and 20%) and great number of eyes lacking PVD (64.6% and 77%) in diabetic eyes (Hikichi et al, 1997; Nasrallah et al., 1988). They observed incomplete PVD in 8.4% and 3% of cases and it was ophthalmoscopically detected by a thickened and taut posterior hyaloid. Such cases of thick taut and attached to the top of the raised macular surface posterior hyaloid are easily recognizable on ophthalmoscopy and indicate obvious vitreomacular traction. In other cases, when the posterior hyaloid is thin and slightly detached from the macular surface, it is not visible on ophthalmoscopy, but can be demonstrated on OCT. This type of incomplete PVD is quite common and it resembles the early stages of PVD in normal eyes (Uchino et al., 2001; Gaucher et al., 2005). The role of this type of incomplete PVD in the pathogenesis of macular edema is not fully understood. Several studies have classified the incomplete PVD in order to define its relation with macular edema (Gaucher et al., 2005; Koizumi et al, 2008; Panozzo et al., 2004).

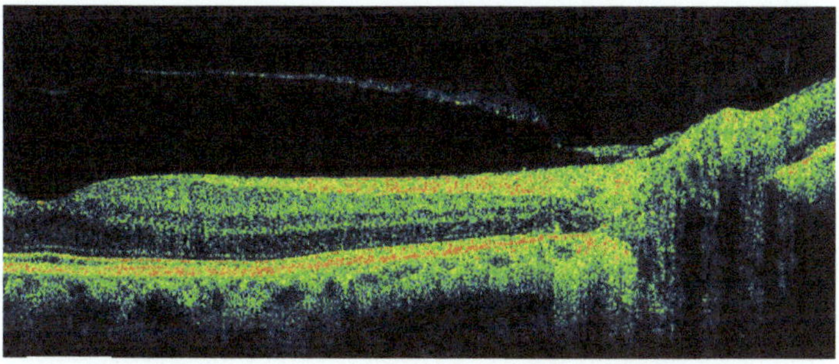

Fig. 9. Questionable macular traction: incomplete posterior vitreous detachment with peripapillary adhesion, without signs of distortion of retinal contour.

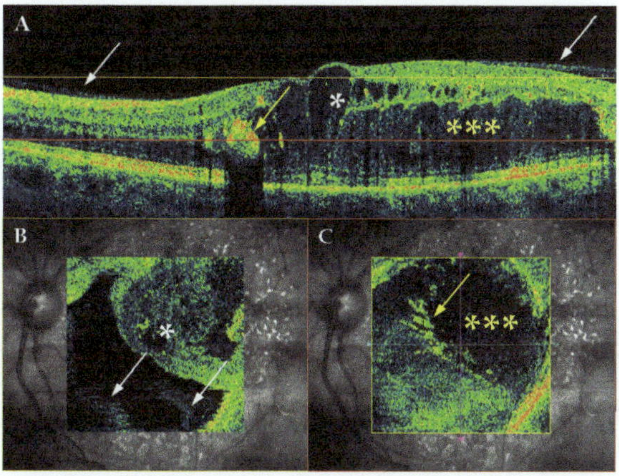

Fig. 10. Questionable macular traction: incomplete posterior vitreous detachment (PVD) in severe cystoid macular edema (A - OCT B-scan, B and C - OCT en face C-scan images with fundus overlay), broad based incomplete PVD without distortion of retinal contour at points of adhesion (white arrow), cystoid space (white star), retinoschisis space (yellow stars), hard exudates (yellow arrow), note that on the en face OCT image the extent and location of the hard exudates, cystoid spaces and the retinoschisis space can be visualized.

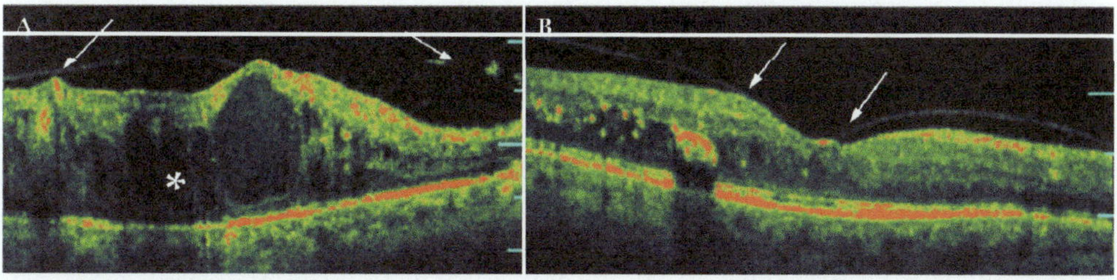

Fig. 11. Definite macular traction caused by incomplete posterior vitreous detachment with distortion of retinal contour at points of adhesion (white arrows), A - accompanying severe cystoid macular edema, note the presence of large confluent cystoid cavity with retinoschisis appearance (star), B - accompanying mild cystoid macular edema.

On OCT scans the posterior hyaloid appears as thin hyper-to-medium reflective line in the non-reflective vitreous cavity at a distance from the retinal surface (fig. 4, yellow arrows, fig. 9, 10 and 11, white arrows). In case of incomplete PVD it may have adhesions to foveal (fig. 10 and 11) or peripapillary (fig. 9) retinal tissue (Gaucher et al., 2005). The vitreomacular adhesion may be broad-based (broad) or narrow-based (focal), (Forte et al., 2007; Koizumi et al. 2008). Panozzo and coauthors have described 3 types of epimacular traction: (1) flat hyper-reflective line, adherent to the retina without significant retinal distortion, (2) continuous hyper-reflective line with multiple points of adhesion, with significant retinal distortion, and (3) antero-posterior traction with "gull wings" configuration. Types (1) and (2) resemble ERM and tangential epiretinal traction, and type (3) represents incomplete PVD with antero-posterior traction and retinal distortion. They do not speculate the cause of traction (ERM or incomplete PVD), but just stress on the presence of distortion of the retinal surface. According to this statement and our clinical findings (Koleva-Georgieva & Sivkova, 2008, 2009), we presume that it is worth to examine retinal surface on OCT scans and differentiate the presence of distortion of the retinal contour at the points of adhesion as this may indicate definite mechanical traction.

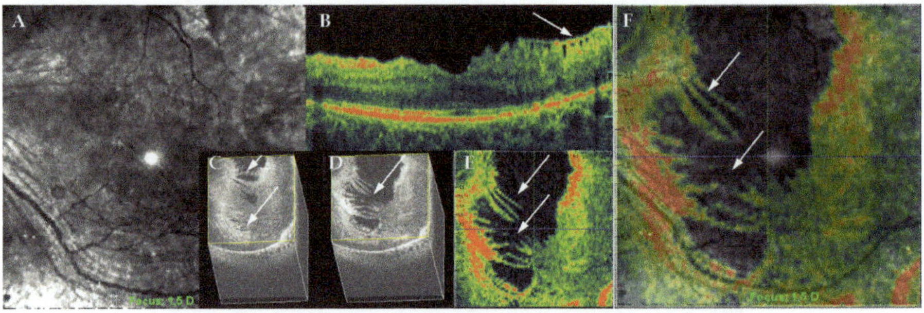

Fig. 12. Definite macular traction: epiretinal membrane (ERM) with distortion of retinal surface contour (white arrows), A - fundus image, B - OCT B-scan, C and D - 3D OCT reconstruction, E - en face C-scan, F - OCT C-scan/fundus image overlay, note the characteristic "brush-like" appearance of the ERM on en face scans.

In patients with diabetic retinopathy secondary ERM may develop and cause tangential macular traction. On OCT scans ERM appears as hyper-reflective line lying on retinal surface (fig. 4, white arrow, fig. 12 B). On en face coronal OCT scan ERM has a characteristic "star-like" or "brush-like" appearance (fig. 12 C, D, E and F). It may lead to loss of foveal depression, increase in macular thickness, and formation of cystoid spaces or pseudoholes. ERMs may have global or focal adherence. Mori and coauthors have described that cases of globally adherent ERMs represent earlier stages of ERM development and are associated with less morphologic changes. ERMs with focal adhesions represent a more advanced stage with significant macular thickening, loss of foveal depression and formation of cystoid spaces (Mori et al., 2004). Secondary ERMs were more likely to have focal adhesions, whereas primary ERMs tended to be globally adherent (Mori et al., 2004). ERM with multiple points of adhesion usually cause distortion of retinal contour which is detectable on SD OCT (Koleva-Georgieva & Sivkova, 2008, 2009) and may indicate more obvious mechanical traction on retina. OCT is helpful in the detection of incomplete PVD and ERM. Since macular traction is one of the causes for the development and persistence of DME, the evaluation of its presence is a substantial part in OCT macular edema assessment. OCT proves to be very useful in diagnosing these vitreoretinal interface abnormalities and follow the postoperative morphological outcome.

4. OCT classification of DME

The first OCT-classification of DME (Otani et al., 1999) is based on retinal morphological changes: "sponge-like swelling", cystoid edema, and serous retinal detachment. Other published classifications are presented by several authors (Kang et al., 2004; Kim et al., 2006; Panozzo et al., 2004). We propose and use in our clinical practice a classification, which summarizes several quantitative and qualitative OCT data: retinal thickness, retinal morphology, retinal topography, macular traction and foveal photoreceptor status. It is based on published data by previous authors and our clinical observations and studies.

I. Retinal thickness:

1. No macular edema - normal macular morphology and thickness not reaching the criteria for subclinical DME;
2. Early subclinical macular edema - no clinically detected retinal thickening on ophthalmoscopy, OCT measured retinal thickness exceeding normal +2SDs for central fixation point and fovea;
3. Established macular edema - retinal thickening and evident morphological characteristics of edema.

II. Retinal morphology:

1. Simple non-cystoid macular edema - increased retinal thickness, reduced intraretinal reflectivity, irregularity of the layered structure, flattening of the foveal depression, without presence of cystoid spaces (fig. 2);
2. Cystoid macular edema - the above criteria, associated with presence of well defined intraretinal cystoid spaces
   - 2.a mild cystoid macular edema - cystoid spaces with horizontal diameter < 300μm (fig.3)
   - 2.b intermediate cystoid macular edema - cystoid spaces with horizontal diameter ≥ 300μm < 600μm (fig. 4)
   - 2.c severe cystoid macular edema - cystoid spaces with horizontal diameter ≥ 600μm, or large confluent cavities with retinoschisis appearance (fig. 5, 10, and 11 A);
3. Serous macular detachment - any of the above, associated with serous macular detachment (hypo-reflective area under the detached neurosensory retina and over the hyper-reflective line of the pigment epithelium), (fig. 6 and 7).

III. Retinal topography:

1. Non-significant macular edema;
2. Clinically significant macular edema, as defined by ETDRS and evaluated on the OCT retinal topography map.

IV. Presence and severity of macular traction (incomplete PVD and/or ERM):

1. No macular traction - presence of complete PVD (Weiss ring detected on ophthalmoscopy), or no PVD (no visible posterior hyaloid line on SD OCT), and no ERM (fig. 2, 5, and 6);

2. Questionable macular traction - incomplete PVD with perifoveal or peripapillary adhesion and/or globally adherent ERM without detectable distortion of retinal surface contour at the points of adhesion (fig. 9 and 10);
3. Definite macular traction - incomplete PVD with perifoveal adhesion and/or focal ERM with detectable distortion of retinal contour at the points of adhesion (fig. 4, white arrow, 11, and 12).

V. Retinal outer layers integrity (IS/OS and ELM):

1. IS/OS and ELM intact (fig. 8 A);
2. IS/OS and ELM with disrupted integrity (fig. 8 B).

5. Future developments in OCT

In 2001, Drexler and associates introduced Ultrahigh Resolution OCT (Drexler et al., 2001). The technology is similar to standard resolution OCT, but the light source is replaced by a broadband Ti:Sapphire short pulse laser. It generates axial resolution of 3 µm in the eye. The advantage of Ultrahigh Resolution OCT is the improved delineation of all retinal layers, more detailed structure imaging and more precise measurements.

In 1997 Podoleanu and associates pioneered the development of a different OCT imaging approach - en face OCT, or scanning the coronal plane (Podoleanu et al., 1997). En face OCT is possible with TD OCT or SD OCT, but the scanning regime has changed from fast scanning in the Z-axis to fast scanning in the XY plane. The axial resolution of en face OCT is similar to conventional OCT, but the transverse resolution is better, leading to a subjectively higher image resolution. En face OCT is combined with confocal Scanning Laser Ophthalmoscopy (SLO), using a single light source. The images in the confocal and the OCT channels are produced simultaneously using the same light source and are therefore in strict pixel-to-pixel correspondence. The SLO provides a high quality fundus image. The exact correspondence allows obtaining of an OCT - SLO fundus image overlay (fig. 10 B and C; fig. 11 F). Analyzing C-scan OCT images is more difficult than B-scan retinal images, but it offers complementary information. The en face plane is the conventional plane of ophthalmoscopy, so analyzing retinal pathology on en face C-scans and on OCT C-scan/SLO fundus image overlays provides additional information about the size, extent and location of pathological features. OCT C-scans may be overlaid with other en face imaging or functional diagnostic methods (fluorescein angiography, ICG angiography, microperimetry, and multifocal electroretinography) thus offering a complex approach to the diagnostic evaluation of macular pathology.

In 2002, Dubois and coworkers reported the development of the ultrahigh resolution full-field en face OCT, which achieves 0.8 µm axial and 1.8 µm transverse resolution (Dubois et al., 2002). It has been used for ex vivo microscopic imaging of subcellular details of animal ocular tissues. In the recent years much research progress has been done in developing adaptive optics to OCT machines. Conventional OCT has good axial resolution (5µm for SD OCT), but low transverse resolution (15-20 µm). It is because of the numerous aberrations of the optics of the system and the eye itself. Adaptive optics corrects these aberrations by wavefront detection and modulation (van Velthoven et al., 2007). Functional OCT methods are also under development, such as polarization-sensitive OCT (combines OCT with tissue birefringence analysis for precise examination of NFL), color Doppler OCT (for supplementary evaluation of retinal blood flow), retinal optophysiology on Ultrahigh Resolution OCT scans (detects changes in the optical properties during a provoked action potential), molecular contrast OCT and nanoparticle based molecular contrast OCT (analyzing tissue or cell structures by use of specific targeted molecules or nanoparticles).

6. Conclusion

OCT is a novel imaging modality that has made significant impact in the diagnostic evaluation of patients with DME. It was a complementary device to stereo-ophthalmoscopy and fluorescein angiography, and now it has become a new imaging standard in retinal diagnostics. The major contribution of OCT is the possibility of obtaining objective and reliable retinal thickness measurements along with "in vivo" visualization of retinal and vitreo-retinal microstructure. The early diagnosis of DME, precise estimation of the different morphologic patterns and presence of macular traction are of uppermost significance in determining the therapeutic approach and prognosis. OCT has proved to achieve these requirements and to ensure objective monitoring of treatment results.

7. References

Alamouti, B. & Funk, J. (2003) Retinal thickness decreases with age: an OCT study. *Br J Ophthalmol*, Vol. 87, No. 7 (July 2003), pp. 899-901

Alkuraya, H., Kanagave, D. & Abu El-Asrar, A.M. (2005). The correlation between optical coherence tomography features and severity of retinopathy, macular thickness, and visual acuity in diabetic macular edema. *Int Ophthalmol*, Vol. 26, No. 3 (June 2005), pp.93-99

Asefzadeh, B., Cavallerano, A.A. & Fisch, B.M. (2007). Racial differences in macular thickness in healthy eyes. *Optom Vis Sci*, Vol. 84, No. 10 (Oct. 2007), pp. E941-E945

Brancato, R. & Lumbroso, B. (1st ed.). (2004). *Guide to optical coherence tomography interpretation*, I.N.C., Roma, Italy

Browning, D.J., Fraser, C.M. & Clark, S. (2008). The relationship of macular thickness to clinically graded diabetic retinopathy severity in eyes without clinically detected diabetic macular edema. *Ophthalmology*, Vol. 115, No. 3 (March 2008), pp. 533-539

Catier, A., Tadayoni, R., Paques, M., Erginay, A., Haouchine, B., Gaudric, A. & Massin, P. (2005). Characterisation of macular edema from various etiologies by optical coherence tomography. *Am J Ophthalmol*, Vol. 140, No. 2 (August 2005), pp. 200-206

Chan, A., Duker, J.S., Ko, T.H., Fujimoto, J.G. & Schuman, J.S. (2006) Normal macular thickness measurements in healthy eyes using Stratus optical coherence tomography. *Arch Ophthalmol*, Vol. 124, No. (February 2006), pp. 193-198

Choma, M., Sarunic, M., Yang, C. & Izatt, J. (2003). Sensitivity advantage of swept sourse and Fourier domain optical coherence tomography. *Opt Express*, Vol. 11, No. 18 (September 2003), pp. 2183-2189

Diabetic Retinopathy Clinical Research Network. (2007). Reproducibility of macular thickness and volume using Zeiss optical coherence tomography in patients with diabetic macular edema. *Ophthalmology*, Vol. 114, No. 8 (August 2007),pp.1520-1525

Diabetic Retinopathy Clinical Research Network. (2008). Retinal thickness on Stratus optical coherence tomography™ in people with diabetes and minimal or no diabetic retinopathy. *Am J Ophthalmol*, Vol. 145, No. 5 (May 2008), pp. 894-901

Diabetic Retinopathy Clinical Research Network Writing Committee. (2010). Vitrectomy outcomes in eyes with diabetic macular edema and vitreomacular traction. *Ophthalmology*, Vol. 117, No. 6 (June 2010), pp. 1087-1093

Domalpally, A., Danis, R.P., Zhang, B., Myers, D. & Kruse, C.N. (2009) Quality issues in interpretation of optical coherence tomograms in macular diseases. *Retina*, Vol. 29, No. 6 (July 2009), pp.775-781

Drexler, W., Morgner, U., Ghanta, R.K., Kaertner, F.X., Schuman, J.S. & Fujimoto,J.G. (2001). Ultrahigh-resolution ophthalmic optical coherence tomography. *Nat Med*, Vol. 7, No. 4 (April 2001), pp. 502-507

Dubois, A., Vabre, L., Boccara, A.C. & Beaurepaire, E. (2002). High-resolution full-field optical coherence tomography with a Linnik microscope. *Appl Opt*, Vol. 41, No. 4 (February 2002), pp. 805-812

Early Treatment Diabetic Retinopathy Study Research Group. (1991). Grading diabetic retinopathy from stereoscopic color fundus photographs - an extension of the modified Airlie house classification. ETDRS report number 10. *Ophthalmology*, Vol. 98, No. 5 Suppl (May 1991), pp. 786-806

El-Ahsry, M., Hedge, V., James, P. & Pagliarini, S. (2008). Analysis of macular thickness in British population using optical coherence tomography (OCT): an emphasis on interocular symmetry. *Curr Eye Res*, Vol. 33, No. 8 (August 2008), pp. 693-699

Eriksson, U. & Alm, A. (2009). Macular thickness decreases with age in normal eyes. A study on the macular thickness map protocol in the Stratus OST. *Br J Ophthalmol*, Vol. 93, No. 11 (November 2009), pp. 1448-1452

Estabrook, E.J., Madhusudhana, K.C., Hannan, S.R. & Newsom, R.S.B. (2007). Can optical coherence tomography predict the outcome of laser photocoagulation for diabetic macular edema? *Ophthalmic Surg Lasers Imaging*, Vol. 38, No. 6 (November/ December 2007), pp. 478-483

Gaucher, D., Tadayoni, R., Erginay, A., Haouchine, B., Gaudrich, A. & Massin, P. (2005). Optical coherence tomography assessment of the vitreoretinal relationship in diabetic macular edema. *Am J Ophthalmol*, Vol. 139, No. 5 (May 2005), pp. 807-813

Grover, S., Murthy, R.K., Brar, V.S. & Chalam, K.V. (2010). Comparison of retinal thickness in normal eyes using Stratus and Spectralis Optical Coherence Tomography. *Invest Ophthalmol Vis Sci*, Vol. 51, No. 5 (May 2010), pp. 2644-2647

Guedes, V., Schuman, J.S., Hertzmark, E., Wollstein, G., Correnti, A., Mancini, R., Lederer, D., Voskanian, S., Velazquez, L., Pakter, H.M., Pedut-Kloizman, T., Fujimoto, J.G. & Mattox, C. (2003). Optical coherence tomography measurement of macular and nerve fiber thickness in normal and glaucomatous human eyes. Ophthalmology, Vol. 110, No. 1 (January 2003), pp. 177-189

Han, I.C. & Jaffe G.J. (2009). Comparison of spectral- and time-domain optical coherence tomography for retinal thickness measurements in healthy and diseased Vol. 147, No. 5 (May 2009), pp. 847-858

Hee, M.R., Puliafito, C.A., Wong, C., Duker, J.S., Reichel, E., Rutledge, B., Schuman, J.S., Swanson, E.A. & Fujimoto, J.G. (1995). Quantitative assessment of macular edema with optical coherence tomography. *Arch Ophthalmol*, Vol. 113, No. 8 (August 2008), pp. 1019-1029

Hee, M.R., Puliafito, C.A., Duker, J.S., Reichel, E., Coker, J.G., Wilkins, J.R., Schuman, J.S., Swanson, E.A. & Fujimoto, J.G. (1998). Topography of diabetic macular edema with optical coherence tomography. *Ophthalmology*,Vol.105, No.2 (Febr 1998), pp.360-370

Hikichi, T., Fujio, N., Akiba, J., Azuma, Y., Takahashi, M. & Yoshida, A. (1997). Association betweeen the short-term natural history of diabetic macular edema and vitreomacular relationship in type II diabetes mellitus. *Ophthalmology*, Vol. 104, No. 3 (March 1997), pp.473-478

Ho, J., Sull, A.C., Vuong, L.N., Chen, Y., Liu, J., Fujimoto, J.G., Schumann, J.S. & Duker, J.S. (2009) Assessment of artifacts and reproducibility across spectral- and time-domain optical coherence tomography. *Ophthalmology*, Vol. 116, No. 10 (October 2009), pp. 1960-1970

Huang, D., Swanson, E.A., Lin, C.P., Schuman, J.S., Stinson, W.G., Chang, W., Hee, M.R., Flotte, T., Gregory, K., Puliafito, C.A. (1991) Optical coherence tomography. *Science*, Vol. 254, No. 5035, pp. 1178-1181

Izatt, J.A., Kulkarni, M.D., Yazdanfar, S., Barton, J.K. & Welch, A.J. (1997). In vivo bidirectional color Doppler flow imaging of picoliter blood volumes using optical coherence tomography. *Opt Lett*, Vol. 22, No. 18 (September 1997), pp. 1439-1441

Kaiser, P.K., Riemann, C.D., Sears, J.E. & Lewis, H. (2001). Macular traction detachment and diabetic macular edema associated with posterior hyaloidal traction *Am J Ophthalmol*, Vol. 131, No. 1 (January 2001), pp. 44-49

Kang, S.W., Park, C.Y. & Ham, D.I. (2004). The correlation between fluorescein angiographic and optical coherent tomographic features in clinically significant diabetic macular edema. *Am J Ophthalmol*, Vol. 137, No. 2 (February 2004), pp. 313-322

Kelty, P.J., Payne, J.F., Trivedi, R.H., Kelty, J., Bowie, E.M. & Burger, B.M. (2008). Macular thickness assessment in healthy eyes based on ethnicity using Stratus OCT optical coherence tomography. *Invest Ophthlamol Vis Sci*, Vol. 49, No. 6 (June 2008), pp. 2668-72

Kim, B.Y., Smith, S.D. & Kaiser, P.K. (2006). Optical coherence tomographic patterns of diabetic macular edema. *Am J Ophthalmol*, Vol. 142, No. 3 (Sept. 2006), pp. 405-412

Koizumi, H., Spaide, R.F., Fisher, Y.L., Freund, K.B., Klancnik, J.M.Jr. & Yanuzzi, L.A. (2008). Three-dimensional evaluation of vitreomacular traction and epiretinal membrane using spectral-domain optical coherence tomography. *Am J Ophthalmol*, Vol. 145, No. 3 (March 2008), pp. 509-517

Koleva-Georgieva, D.N. & Sivkova, N.P. (2008). Types of diabetic macular edema assessed by optical coherence tomography. *Folia Med (Plovdiv)*, Vol. 50, No. 3, (July-September 2008), pp. 30-38

Koleva-Georgieva, D. & Sivkova, N. (2009). Assessment of serous macular detachment in eyes with diabetic macular edema by use of spectral-domain optical coherence tomography. *Graefes Arch Clin Exp Ophthalmol*, Vol. 247, No. 11 (November 2009), pp. 1461-1469

Koleva-Georgieva, D.N. & Sivkova, N.P. (2010) Optical coherence tomography for the detection of early macular edema in diabetic patients with retinopathy. *Foia Med (Plovdiv)*, Vol. 52, No. 1 (January-March 2010), pp. 40-48

Krebs, I., Falkner-Radler, C., Hagen, S., Haas, P., Brannath, W., Lie, S., Ansari-Shahrezaei, S. & Binder, S. (2009) Quality of the threshold algorithm in age-related macular degeneration: Stratus versus Cirrus OCT. *Invest Ophthalmol Vis Sci*, Vol. 50, No. 3 (May 2009), pp. 995-1000

Lam, D.S., Leung, K.S., Mohamed, S., Chan, W.M., Palanivelu, M.S., Cheung, C.Y., Li, E.Y., Lai, R.Y. & Leung, C.K. (2007). Regional variations in the relationship between macular thickness measurements and myopia. *Invest Ophthalmol Vis Sci*, Vol. 48, No. 1 (January 2007), pp. 376-382

Lim, M.C., Hoh, S.T., Foster, P.J., Lim, T.H., Chew, S.J., Seah, S.K. & Aung, T. (2005). Use of optical coherence tomography to assess variations in macular retinal thickness in myopia. *Invest Ophthalmol Vis Sci*, Vol. 46, No. 3 (March 2005), pp. 974-978

Leung, C.K., Cheung, C.Y., Weinreb, RN.., Lee, G., Lin, D., Pang, C.P. & Lam, D.S.C. (2008). Comparison of macular thickness measurements between time domain and spectral domain optical coherence tomography. *Invest Ophthalmol Vis Sci*, Vol. 49, No. 11 (November 2008), pp. 4893-4897

Maheshwary, A.S., Oster, S.F., Yuson, R.M.S., Cheng, L., Mojana, F. & Freeman, W.R. (2010). The association between percent disruption of the photoreceptor inner segment/outer segment and visual acuity in diabetic macular edema. *Am J Ophthalmol* Vol. 150, No. 1 (May 2010), pp. 63-67

Massin, P., Erginay, A., Haouchine, B., Mehidi, A.B., Paques, M. & Gaudrich, A. (2002). Retinal thickness in healthy and diabetic subjects measured using optical coherence tomography mapping software. Eur J Ophtlamol, Vol.12, No. 2 (March-April 2002), pp.102-108

Massin, P., Duguid, G., Erginay, A., Haouchine, B. & Gaudric, A. (2003). Optical coherence tomography for evaluating diabetic macular edema before and after vitrectomy. *Am J Ophthalmol*, Vol. 135, No. 2 (February 2003), pp. 169-177

Mitamura, Y., Hirano, K., Baba, T. & Yamamoto S. (2009). Correlation of visual recovery to presence of photoreceptor inner/outer segment junction in optical coherence images after epiretinal membrane surgery. *Br J Ophthalmol*, Vol. 93, No. 2 (February 2009), pp. 171-175

Mori, K., Gelbach, P.L., Sano, A., Deguchi, T. & Yoneye, S. (2004) Comparison of epiretnal membranes of differing pathologies using optical coherence tomography. *Retina*, Vol. 24, No. 1 (January 2004), pp. 57-62

Nasrallah, F.P., Jalkh, A.E., Van Coppenolle, F., Kado, M., Trempe, C.L., McMeel, J.W. & Schepens, C.L. (1998). The role of the viteous in diabetic macular edema. *Ophthalmology*, Vol. 95, No. 10 (October 1988), pp.1335-1339

Ooto, S., Hangai, M., Sakamoto, A., Tomidokoro, A., Araie, M., Otani, T., Kishi, S., Matsushita, K., Maeda, N., Shirakashi, M., Abe, H., Takeda, H., Sugiyama, K., Saito,H., Iwase, A. & Yoshimura, N. (2010). Three-dimensional profile of macular retinal thickness in normal Japanese eyes. *Invest Ophthalmol Vis Sci*, Vol. 51, No. 1 (January 2010), pp. 465-473

Oster, S.F., Mojana, F., Brar, M., Yuson, R.M., Cheng, L. & Freeman, W.R. (2010). Disruption of the photoreceptor inner segment/outer segment layer on spectral domain-optical coherence tomography is a predictor of poor visual acuity in patients with epiretinal membranes. *Retina*, Vol. 30, No. 5 (May 2010), pp. 713-718

Otani, T., Kishi, S. & Maruyama, Y. (1999). Patterns of diabetic macular edema with optical coherence tomography. *Am J Ophthalmol* Vol. 127, No. 6 (June 1999), pp. 688-693

Otani, T. & Kishi, S. (2000). Tomographic assessment of viteous surgery for diabetic macular edema. *Am J Ophthalmol*, Vol. 129, No. 4 (April 2000), pp.487-494

Otani, T., Yamaguchi, Y & Kishi, S. (2010). Correlation between visual acuity and foveal microstructural changes in diabetic macular edema. *Retina*, Vol. 30, No. 5 (May 2010), pp. 774-780

Ozdemir, H., Karacorlu, M. & Karacorlu, S.A. (2005). Regression of serous macular detachment after intravitreal triamcinolone acetonide in patients with diabetic macular edema. *Am J Ophthalmol*, Vol. 140, No. 2 (August 2005), pp. 251-255

Ozdemir, H., Karacorlu, M. & Karacorlu. S. (2005). Serous macular detachment in cystoid diabetic macular edema. *Acta Ophthalmol Scand*, Vol. 83, No.1 (Feb. 2005), pp.63-66

Panozzo, G., Parolini, B., Gusson, E., Mercanti, A., Pinackatt, S., Bertoldo, G. & Pignatto, S. (2004). Diabetic macular edema: an OCT-based classification. *Semin Ophthalmol*, Vol. 19, No. 1-2 (March-June 2004), pp. 13-20

Patel, J.I., Hykin, P.G., Schadt, M., Luong, V., Fitzke, F. & Gregor, Z.J. (2006). Pars plana vitrectomy for diabetic macular oedema: OCT and functional correlations. *Eye*, Vol. 20, No. 6 (June 2006), pp. 674-680

Paunescu, L.A., Schuman, J.S., Price, L.L., Stark, P.C., Beaton, S., Ishikawa, H., Wollstein, G. & Fujimoto, J.G. (2004) Reproducibility of nerve fiber thickness, macular thickness, and optic nerve head measurements using Stratus OCT. *Invest Ophthalmol Vis Sci*, Vol. 45, No. 6, (June 2004), pp. 1716-1724

Podoleanu, A.G., Dobre, G.M., Webb, D.J. & Jackson, D.A. (1997). Simultaneous en-face imaging of two layers in the human retina by low-coherence reflectometry. *Opt Lett*, Vol. 22, No. 13 (July 1997), pp. 1039-1041

Podoleanu, A. G. (2005) Optical coherence tomography. *Br J Radiology*, Vol. 78, pp. 976-988

Polito, A., Del Borrello, M., Isola, M., Zemella, N. & Bandello, F. (2005). Repeatability and reproducibility of fast macular thickness mapping using Stratus optical coherence tomography. *Arch Ophthalmol*, Vol 123, No. 10 (October 2005), pp.1330-1337

Puliafito, C.A., Hee, M.R., Lin, C.P., Reichel, E., Schuman, J.S, Duker, J.S., Izatt, J.A., Swanson, E.A. & Fujimoto, J.G. (1995). Imaging of macular diseases with optical coherence tomography. *Ophthalmology*, Vol. 102, No.2 (February 1995), pp.217-229

Ray, R., Stinnett, S.S. & Jaffe, G.J. (2005) Evaluation of image artifacts produced by optical coherence tomography of retinal pathology. *Am J Ophthalmol*, Vol. 139, No. 1 (January 2005), pp. 18-29

Sadda, R.S., Wu, Z., Walsh, A.C., Richine, L., Dougall, J., Cortez, R. & LaBree, L.D. (2006) Errors in retinal thickness measurements obtained by optical coherence tomography. *Ophthalmology*, Vol. 113, No. 2 (February 2006), pp. 285-293

Sakamoto, A., Nishijima, K., Kita, M., Oh, H., Tsujikawa, A. & Yoshimura, N. (2009). Association between foveal photoreceptor status and visual acuity after resolution of diabetic macular edema by pars plana vitrectomy. *Graefes Arch Clin Exp Ophthalmol*, Vol. 247, No. 10 (October 2009), pp. 1325-1330

Saxena, S. & Meredith, T.A. (1st ed). (2006). *Optical coherence tomography in retinal diseases.* Jaypee Brothers Medical Publishers (P) Ltd., New Delhi, India

Schaudig, U.H., Glaefke, C., Scholz, F. & Richard G. (2000). Optical coherence tomography for retinal thickness measurement in diabetic patients without clinically significant macular edema. Ophthalmic Surg Lasers, Vol. 31, No. 3 (May-June), pp. 182-186

Schepens, C.L., Avila, M.P., Jalkh, A.E. & Trempe, C.L. (1984). Role of the vitreous in cystoid macular edema. *Surv Ophthalmol* Vol. 28, Suppl (May 1984), pp. 499-504

Schuman, J.S., Puliafito, C.A., Fujimoto, J.G. (2nd ed.). (2004). *Optical coherence tomography of ocular diseases*. SLACK Inc., Thorofare, NJ, USA

Shahidi, M., Ogura, Y., Blair, N.P., Rusin, M.M. & Zeimer, R. (1991). Retinal thickness analysis for quantitative assessment of diabetic macular edema. *Arch Ophthalmol*, Vol. 109, No. 8 (August 1991), pp. 1115-1119

Srinivasan, V.J., Wojtkowski, M., Witkin, A.J., Duker, J.S., Ko, T.H., Carvalho, M., Schuman, J.S., Kowalczyk, A. & Fujimoto, J.G. (2006). High-definition and 3-dimensional imaging of macular pathologies with high-speed ultrahigh-resolution optical coherence tomography. *Ophthalmology*, Vol. 113, No. 11 (November 2006), pp. 2054.e1-2054.14

Toth, C.A., Narayan, D.G., Boppart, S.A., Hee, M.R., Fujimoto, J.G., Birngruber, R., Cain, C.P., DiCarlo, C.D. & Roach, W.P. (1997). A comparison of retinal morphology viewed by optical coherence tomography and by light microscopy. *Arch Ophthalmol*, Vol.115, No. 11 (November), pp. 1425-1428

Uchino, E., Uemura, A. & Ohba, N. (2001). Initial stages of posterior viteous detachment in healthy eyes of older persons evaluated by optical coherence tomography. *Arch Ophthalmol*, Vol. 119, No. 10 (October 2001), pp. 1475-1479

van Velthoven, M.E.J., Faber, D.J., Verbraak, F.D., van Leeuwen, T.G & de Smet, M.D. (2007). Recent developments in optical coherence tomography for imaging the retina. *Prog Retin Eye Res*, Vol. 26, No. 1 (January 2007), pp. 57-77

Williams, R., Airey, M., Baxter, H., Forrester, J., Kennedy-Martin, T. & Girach, A. (2004). Epidemiology of diabetic retinopathy and macular edema: a systematic review. *Eye*, Vol. 18, No. 10 (October 2004), pp. 963-983

Wolf-Schnurrbusch, U.E.K., Cekic, L., Brinkmann, C.K., Iliev, M.E., Frey, M., Rothenbuehler, S.P., Enzmann, V. & Wolf, S. (2009). Macular thickness measurements in healthy eyes using six different optical coherence tomography instruments. *Invest Ophthalmol Vis Sci*, Vol. 50, No. 7 (July 2009), pp. 3432-3437

Wolter, J.R. (1981). The histopathology of cystoid macular edema. *Albrecht Von Graefes Arch Klin Exp Ophthalmol*, Vol. 216, No. 2, pp. 85-101

Wu, P.C., Chen, Y.J., Chen, C.H., Shin, S.J., Yang, H.J. & Kuo, H.K. (2008). Assessment of macular retinal thickness and volume in normal eyes and highly myopic eyes with third generation optical coherence tomography. *Eye*, Vol. 22, No. 4 (April 2008), pp. 551-555

Yanoff, M., Fine, B.S., Brucker, A.Y. & Eagle, R.C.Jr. (1984). Pathology of human cystiod macular edema. *Surv Ophthalmol*, Vol. 28, No. Suppl (May 1984), pp.505-511

Yanyali, A., Horozoglu, F., Celik, E. & Nohutcu, A.F. (2007). Long-term outcomes of pars plana vitrectomy with internal limiting membrane removal in diabetic macular edema. *Retina*, Vol. 27, No. 5 (June 2007), pp.557-566

12

The Effect of Diabetes Mellitus on Retinal Function

Zvia Burgansky-Eliash
Department of Ophthalmology, The Edith Wolfson Medical Center, Holon, Sackler Faculty of Medicine, Tel-Aviv University, Israel

1. Introduction

Diabetic retinopathy (DR) is the leading cause of blindness in adults less than 70 years of age in the western world (Kempen, et al., 2004). It is estimated that 1 in 29 Americans 40 years and older has diabetic retinopathy (4.1 million persons) and 1 in 132 persons has vision-threatening DR (Kempen et al., 2004). Diabetic retinopathy is characterized by microvascular changes. Despite the fact that DR is a common complication of diabetes, many cases are detected only at a late phase where visual acuity is impaired and some irreversible retinal damage has occurred (Aiello, 2003).

Structural changes in the microvasculature during the progression of diabetic retinopathy are well characterized. The earliest detectable changes in diabetic retinopathy are the morphological appearance of microaneurisms and capillary occlusions (Apple DJ, 1985). At an early stage the diabetic eye loses pericytes and undergoes structural alteration in smooth muscle cells, as well as proliferation of endothelial cells (Ansari, et al., 1998, Paget, et al., 1998). The loss of pericytes causes microaneurysm formation, while basement membrane thickening and endothelial cell proliferation lead to vascular occlusion (Dodge & D'Amore, 1992). The challenge in ophthalmologic management of diabetic patients is to detect abnormalities in microvascular hemodynamics before gross morphological changes appear, allowing the physician to intervene in the progress of disease before the damage becomes irreversible

Abnormalities detected in the retina can also provide an indication of the effect of systemic diseases. Standard ophthalmoscopy, however, is observer dependent, and too imprecise to use as a risk indicator of increased cardiovascular morbidity and mortality, either in diabetic (van Hecke, et al., 2006) or in hypertensive patients (van den Born, et al., 2005). A device that automatically assesses functional changes in the retinal microvasculature by detecting and quantifying subtle alterations in flow velocity might serve to overcome the limits of standard morphological evaluation. The functional results obtained by such a method can also help to differentiate between diseases whose structural effects, albeit pronounced, may be open to ambivalent interpretation. Therefore, it appears that development of additional devices based on new principles to measure blood flow and or flow velocity is warranted.

Functional optical imaging of the eye represents a novel non-invasive diagnostic approach for the measurement of retinal blood flow-velocities, mapping of vascular network structure, and for obtaining information about the oximetric (Abramoff, et al., 2006, Grinvald, et al., 2004, Hanazono, et al., 2007) and metabolic status of the retina (Grinvald, et al., 1986, Nelson, et al., 2005).

2. Blood flow velocity measurement in patients with diabetes mellitus

The diabetic pathological processes, which initially are subtle, affect retinal hemodynamics. In the normal retina, autoregulated vascular responses keep the blood flow constant over a range of systemic blood pressures and intraocular pressures (Riva, et al., 1981, Robinson, et al., 1986). Vessels are controlled through local factors, (Haefliger & Anderson, 1997, Matsugi, et al., 1997a, atsugi, et al., 1997b, Riva et al., 1981, Shepro & Morel, 1993) which primarily target smooth muscle cells in arterioles and capillary pericytes (Shepro & Morel, 1993, Sims, 1986). In patients with diabetes, however, there are changes in local vasoactive factors as well as in the response of pericytes to these factors (Bursell, et al., 1997, de la Rubia, et al., 1992, Gillies & Su, 1993, Joussen, et al., 2002, King, et al., 1994, Riva et al., 1981).

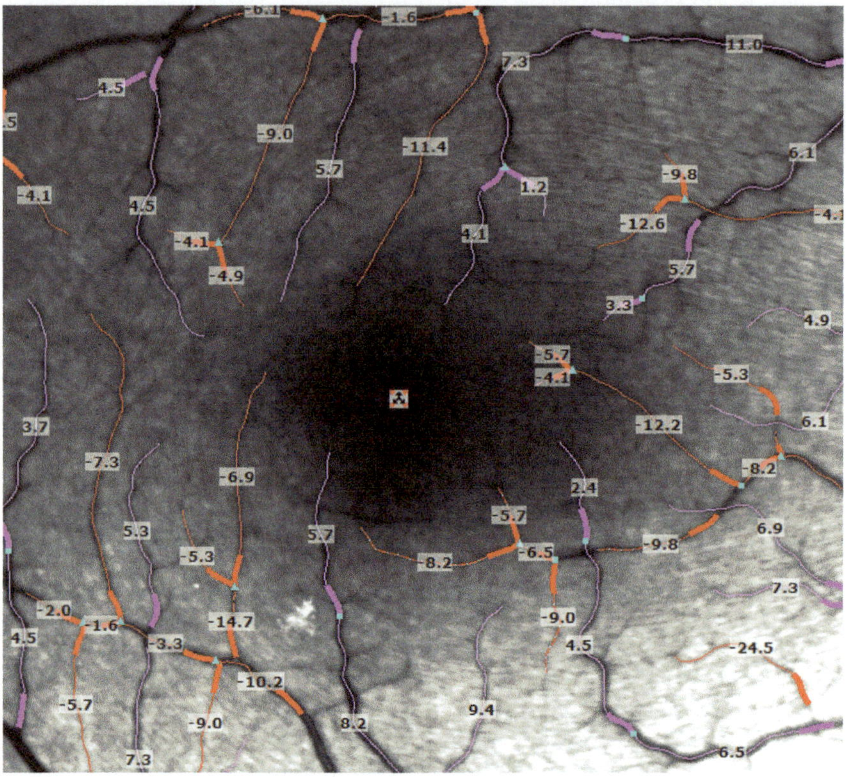

Fig. 1. Blood-flow velocity imaged by Retinal Function Imager in a healthy subject, the velocity (mm/sec) in secondary and tertiary branches of arteries (red) and veins (purple) is shown.

The flow-velocity modality of the Retinal Function Imager (RFI) identifies the motion of red blood cells in retinal vessels by comparing images in a short movie (8- 24 frames) of the retina taken under green light. Each series of 8 frames is acquired within a single short interval of less than 200 msec. To avoid heart-beat pulsation bias of the measured velocities, the timing of a series capture is always triggered on the ECG. The distance traveled by red blood cells in a known time is calculated for each of several retinal blood vessel segments, using a cross-correlation algorithm (Grinvald et al., 2004) and thus directly measuring their average simultaneous velocities. The measured velocity in secondary and tertiary branches of arterioles and venules is recorded by superimposing it on the fundus image (mm/sec; Figure 1).

2.1 Blood flow velocity in patients with Diabetic retinopathy (DR)

To study the effect of DR on the retinal blood flow velocity 42 diabetic patients (58 eyes) and 32 healthy subjects (51 eyes) were recruited (Burgansky-Eliash, et al., 2010). All of the patients in that study group were suffering from adult-onset diabetic mellitus with moderate to severe NPDR in the study eye(s) (ETDRS categories D or E). All subjects were scanned using the RFI resulting in simultaneous measurement of blood-flow velocities in multiple macular vascular segments. In addition, information about medical history and smoking habits were recorded, systemic blood pressure and intraocular pressure were measured and heart rate recording from the RFI was obtained.

The retinal blood flow velocity in the DR patients was significantly slower than in the healthy subjects. The average flow velocities (in mm/sec) of all arterial segments in an eye was 3.74 ± 1.09 for the diabetic patients and 4.19 ± 0.99 for the controls. The difference was significant ($p<0.001$) using model considering parameters variable between the groups (gender, age, systolic blood pressure, heart rate, hypertension and smoking status). The average velocity of all venous segments in an eye was lower than the average arterial velocities: 2.61 ± 0.65 in the diabetic group and 3.03 ± 0.59 in the healthy group. This difference was statistically different ($p=0.004$, table 1).

	NPDR Patients *N* = 58 (eyes)	Healthy Subjects *N* = 51 (eyes)	*P**
Arteries (mm/sec, mean ± SD)	3.74 ± 1.09	4.19 ± 0.99	<0.001
Veins (mm/sec, mean ± SD)	2.61 ± 0.65	3.03 ± 0.59	0.004

* Mixed effect model adjusted for gender, age, systolic blood pressure, heart rate, hypertension and smoking status, NPDR= nonproliferative diabetic retinopathy.

Table 1. Blood-Flow Velocity in Arteries and Veins of Diabetic Patients and Healthy Subjects

The retinal blood-flow velocity and volume in patients with NPDR was compared to controls using multiple measuring devices indicating that blood-flow velocity in general is decreased in patients with NPDR (Arend, et al., 1995, Grunwald, et al., 1986, Hudson, et al., 2005), whereas blood-flow volume measured at or near the level of the whole retina is not decreased (Grunwald et al., 1986, Hudson et al., 2005) and may even be increased (Yoshida, et al., 1983). With the progression of retinopathy, there is evidence showing further reduction in blood flow velocity (Arend, et al., 1991, Blair, et al., 1982, Grunwald et al., 1986, Yoshida et al., 1983) though conflicting data exist (Hudson et al., 2005).

Of the 58 diabetic eyes, 33 (57%) had clinically significant macular edema according to the ETDRS criteria (1991), and 36 (62%) had previously undergone focal laser treatment of the macula. When the diabetic patients were sub grouped according to the presence or absence of macular edema and prior macular laser treatment, differences between subgroups were not significant (P = 0.22 in venules 0.52 in arterioles; in the mixed-effect model, blood-flow velocity is compared between the subgroups taking into account the repeated measures of velocities in the two eyes, gender and age; table 2). These results are consistent with previous findings from examination of arteriole diameters (Jeppesen & Bek, 2006), from laser Doppler flowmetry (Guan, et al., 2006), and from SLO FA videos (Arend et al., 1995) but not in a more recent SLO FA study (Sakata, et al., 2006). Landa et al. found a correlation between RFI average blood flow velocity in retinal veins and the degree of retinal edema represent by OCT central retinal volume(Landa, et al., 2009).

		Diabetic Macular Edema	
		No (*n* = 25)	**Yes (n = 33)**
Macular laser treatment	**No (*n* = 22)**	(*n* = 13) A*: 4.16 ± 1.22 V**: 2.73 ± 0.42	(*n* = 9) A: 3.27 ± 1.0 V: 2.3 ± 0.49
	Yes (*n* = 36)	(*n* = 12) A: 3.8 ± 0.8 V: 2.8 ± 0.71	(*n* = 24) A: 3.65 ± 1.1 V: 2.56 ± 0.71

*A = arteries; **V = veins

Table 2. Effects of Macular Edema and Prior Laser Treatment on Retinal Blood Flow Velocity

2.2 Blood flow velocity in patients with pre-retinopathy diabetes mellitus

After confirming blood flow velocity alternation in the patients with existing DR, a study was performed utilizing the RFI in order to discover hemodynamic changes in patients with diabetes mellitus before morphological changes occur in the retina. This study compared the blood-flow velocity in the retinal vasculature of adult-onset diabetic mellitus patients with no evidence of diabetic retinopathy (23 eyes of DM patients) to that of aged-matched healthy controls (51 eyes of 31). Retinal blood flow velocity was measured using the RFI. Measurement of systemic blood pressure, intraocular pressure, blood glucose level, glycosylated haemoglobin (HbA1C) and body mass index (BMI) were recorded, and heart rate recording from the RFI was obtained.

The average blood-flow velocity in the arteries was 4.7±1.7 mm/sec in the DM group. This was significantly higher than in the healthy subjects (4.1±0.9 mm/sec, $p=0.03$, table 2). As expected, in both groups venous velocity was slower than in the arteries. The DM group had significantly increased venous velocity compared to healthy controls (3.8±1.2 mm/sec vs. 2.9±0.5 mm/sec, respectively; $p<0.0001$). In the DM group, the velocity values of either arteries or veins were not correlated to the duration of diabetes or the levels of glucose, HbA1C or BMI.

	Early DM (N=23)	Healthy (N=51)	*P**
Arteries (mm/sec, mean ± SD)	4.7 ± 1.7	4.1 ± 0.9	0.03
Veins (mm/sec, mean ± SD)	3.8 ± 1.2	2.9 ± 0.5	< 0.001

* Mixed effect model adjusted for gender, age and repeated measures of velocity for both eyes of some patients, DM=diabetes mellitus

Table 3. Blood-Flow Velocity in Arteries and Veins of Diabetic Patients and Healthy Subjects

The increased velocity found in pre-retinopathy patients compared to healthy has the opposite direction to the findings in NPDR patients (Burgansky-Eliash et al., 2010). Thus, the patient/healthy blood-flow velocity relationship reverses during the development of morphological alterations in the retina, as arteries reach the end of their compensating range, or capillary resistance assumes dominance in determining flow volume. In longitudinal studies(Konno, et al., 1996, Rimmer, et al., 1989) decreasing blood-flow velocity over time was found in some but not all diabetic patients.

Considering other causes, the increased velocity found in the DM group might reflect counteracted perfusion abnormalities in diabetic patient retina, stimulated, for example, by changes in blood rheological properties or increased vascular resistance. In diabetic patients there is increased aggregation and reduced deformability of red blood cells, with increased plasma viscosity (Burgansky-Eliash et al., 2010, McMillan, 1975, McMillan, 1978), translating to increased capillary resistance. Vascular resistance can result also from multiple molecular changes associated with long term hyperglycemia as well as endothelial dysfunction. Many of these pathways are interrelated and may be simultaneously activated in retinal cells (Schmetterer & Wolzt, 1999). Some known vasoconstrictor effectors are related to diabetic changes like increased expression of endothelin-1 (ET-1)(Takagi, et al., 1996), and over activation of protein kinase C (PKC)(Grunwald, 1996). Other vasodilatory mechanisms were identified as well, like ET-1 resistance, inhibition of calcium-influx channel in smooth muscle cells, tissue hypoxia(Gardiner, et al., 2007), and increased activity of Nitric oxide syntase(do Carmo, et al., 1998). In addition, in diabetes there is increased leukocytes adhesion to endothelium which is caused by increased expression of adhesion molecules (Miyamoto, et al., 1998) and is associated with endothelial dysfunction(Abiko, et al., 2003). Indeed, in vivo studies found elevated levels of markers of endothelial dysfunction in patients with diabetic retinopathy (soluble intercellular adhesion molecule-1 (sICAM-1) and soluble vascular cell adhesion molecule-1(sVCAM)(van Hecke, et al., 2005). However, studies mimicking retinal capillary obstruction by leukocytes did not detect an effect on retinal blood flow(Abiko et al., 2003). The most physiologically plausible scenario consistent with the findings reported here is that arteries widen in response to impaired capillary perfusion, while venous diameter remains relatively constant. An increase in the arterial/venous diameter ratio is implied by the finding of a greater relative increase in venous velocity (31%) compared to arterial velocity (15%). Excluding an increase in blood pressure, this also implies increased flow volume. Either excessive vasodilatation as a feedback to local ischemia or inhomogeneity in capillary resistance where some capillaries close while other dilate, could produce this over-compensation and increased flow volume. These changes could join a vicious cycle, according to the hemodynamic hypothesis(Parving, et al., 1983, Zatz & Brenner, 1986) that increased blood flow in diabetes patients induces further endothelial damage due to increased shear stress(Kohner, et al., 1995). The decreased vessel density in early diabetes that was found here, was reported previously(Arend et al., 1991).

2.3 The correlation of blood flow velocity to physiological parameters

2.3.1 Correlation to blood pressure

In the healthy group the flow velocity in the arterioles, but not in the venules, was found to be positively correlated with the mean arterial pressure ($r = 0.29$, $p = 0.006$; Figure 2, systolic BP: $r=0.3$, $p=0.04$, diastolic BP: $r=0.4$, $p=0.009$).

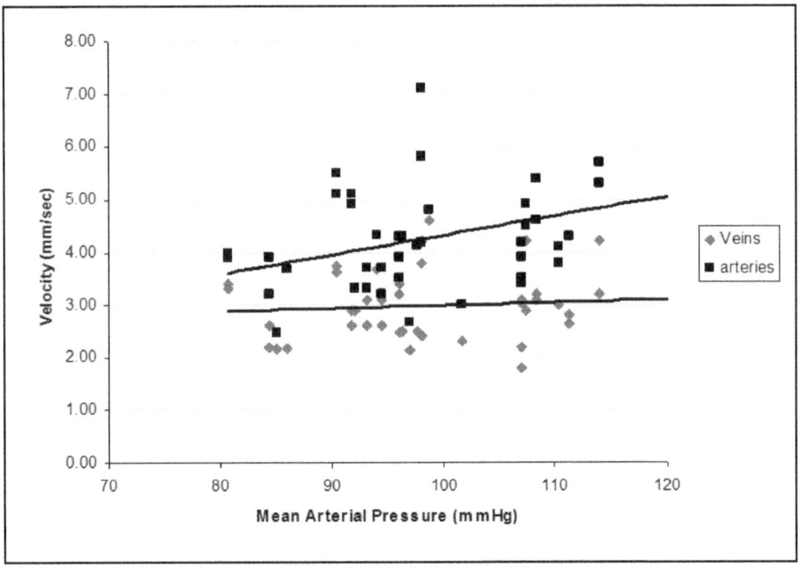

Fig. 2. Correlation between the blood-flow velocity imaged by the Retinal Function Imager and the mean arterial pressure in healthy subjects.

However, there was no significant correlation between flow velocity and mean arterial pressure in the diabetic retinopathy or the pre-retinopathy cohorts. This reduced correlation in the diabetic group compared to the healthy group does not necessary implies that a fundamental dependency is lost. One possibility is that the dependency relationship itself changes as diabetes develops, so that statistical significance is obscured by uncontrolled factors between patients, such as the progress of the disease.

2.3.2 Correlation to heart rate

The average heart rate did not correlate with average velocity of either the healthy, the DM or DR groups. The relationship between retinal blood-flow-velocity and heart rate in individual participants was assessed by correlating the heart rate recorded by the instrument in parallel with each velocity measurement. For each participant we obtained a series of three separate paired measurements of heart rate and flow-velocity. Each value was normalized by the corresponding subject's average. In healthy subjects there is a positive correlation between the heart rate and both arterial and venous velocity ($r=0.4$, $p<0.0001$ for both arteries and veins, figure 3A). In the DM patients a small correlation exists only with the arterial velocity and not with the venous velocity ($r=0.4$, $p=0.0008$ for arteries, $r=0.06$ $p=0.6$ for veins, figure 3B). In the diabetic group, points showed a tendency to cluster around a normalized heart-rate value of 1, because in some members of this group the heart rate over the series was relatively stable. These patients apparently did not differ clinically from the rest of the diabetic retinopathy population. Overall, our diabetic patients demonstrated a correlation between blood-flow velocity and heart rate, although the relationship was less pronounced than in the healthy subjects, possibly because normalized heart rates in the latter group were distributed more widely.

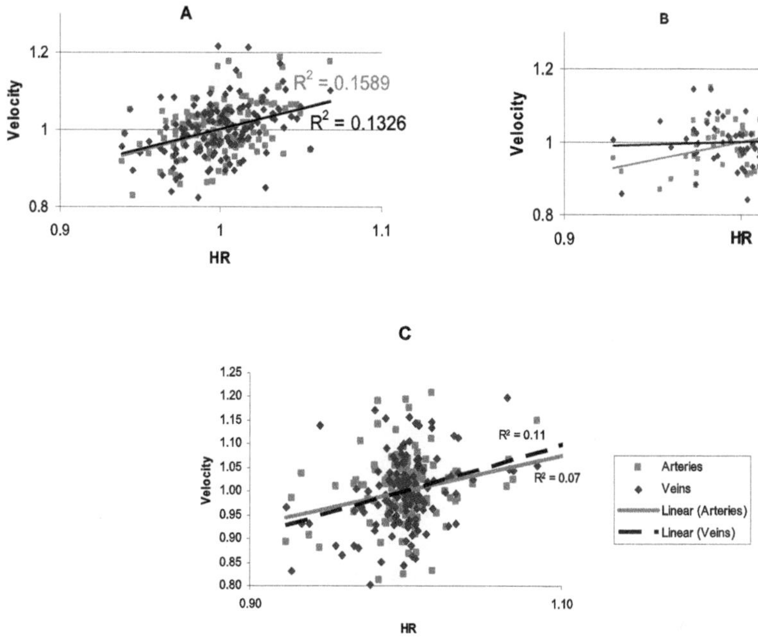

Fig. 3. Correlation between retinal blood flow-velocity and heart rate of all individual series data normalized by the corresponding subject average. A. Healthy group , B. Diabetes mellitus group, C. Diabetic retinopathy group

These findings are consistent with derangement of autoregulatory control mechanisms in diabetic patients (Frederiksen, et al., 2006, Sinclair, et al., 1982), and might be an important characteristic of diabetic retinopathy that warrants future research.

3. Non-invasive Capillary-Perfusion Maps (nCPM)

The retinal function imager (RFI) incorporates a noninvasive method of imaging and mapping the capillaries using the intrinsic contrast chromophore, hemoglobin. Fast acquisition of images at a wavelength strongly absorbed by hemoglobin enables the motion of RBCs to be detected, and by tracing the paths of this perfusing motion, the capillaries can be visualized to create non-invasive capillary-perfusion maps (nCPMs, figure 4). Fifty-eight eyes of 47 patients with diabetes were scanned (average age, 60.3 ± 11.5); 38 had non-proliferative DR (NPDR) and 20 had proliferative diabetic retinopathy (PDR).

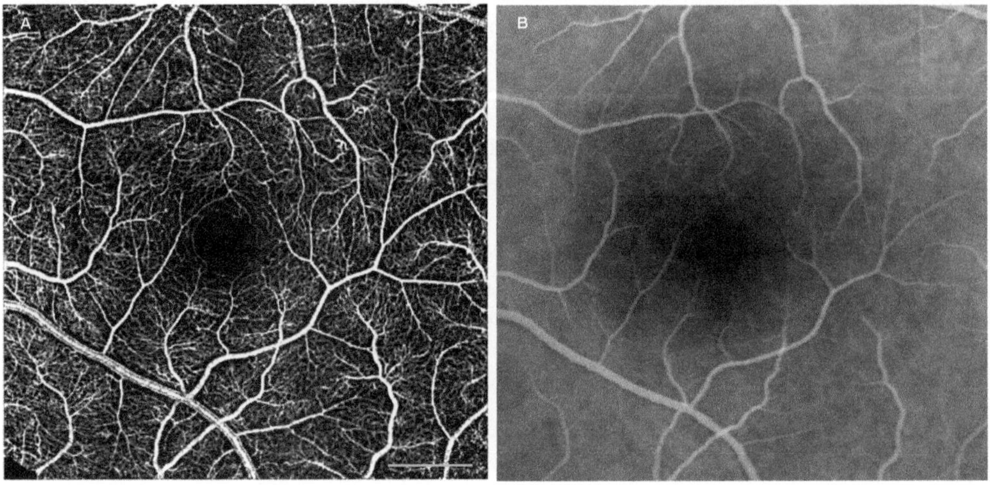

Fig. 4. A. Non-invasive capillary perfusion map in a healthy subject B. corresponding fluorescein angiography (FA) image Scale bar, 500 µm.

Vascular abnormalities seen in the nCPMs of patients with NPDR demonstrate details such as vascular loops and arteriovenous shunts (Figures 5A, 5B). Images of patients with NPDR also demonstrate areas of capillary non-perfusion (Figures. 5C, 5D).

The nCPM images obtained by RFI scanning from eyes with PDR display neovascularization at the optic disc and elsewhere (Figure 6). These coarse, tortuous vessels can be seen protruding from the retina or optic disc surface .

The nCPM provided good capillary perfusion maps that were comparable to the images acquired with an extrinsic contrast agent. Acquisition of nCPM images is non-invasive, comfortable and fast and can be repeated as often as clinically required.

In 14 eyes with DR, a clear image of the fovea was available (in 2 with PDR and in 12 with NPDR). The mean foveal avascular zone (FAZ) diameter and area in these patients were 641.5 ± 82.3 µm and 0.201 ± 0.07 mm^2, respectively (Figure 7b). This was significantly larger than the corresponding values recorded above for healthy subjects (n = 37, Figure 7a; $P < 0.001$ for both diameter and area). Patients with DR were older (average age, 59.2 ± 10.6) than the healthy subjects (average age, 34.8 ± 10.1; $P < 0.001$). However, the correlation between age and FAZ size was not significant. Good correlation was found between FAZ diameter and visual acuity in these patients ($R^2 = 0.34$, $P < 0.05$); thus, poorer visual acuity was associated with larger FAZ diameter.

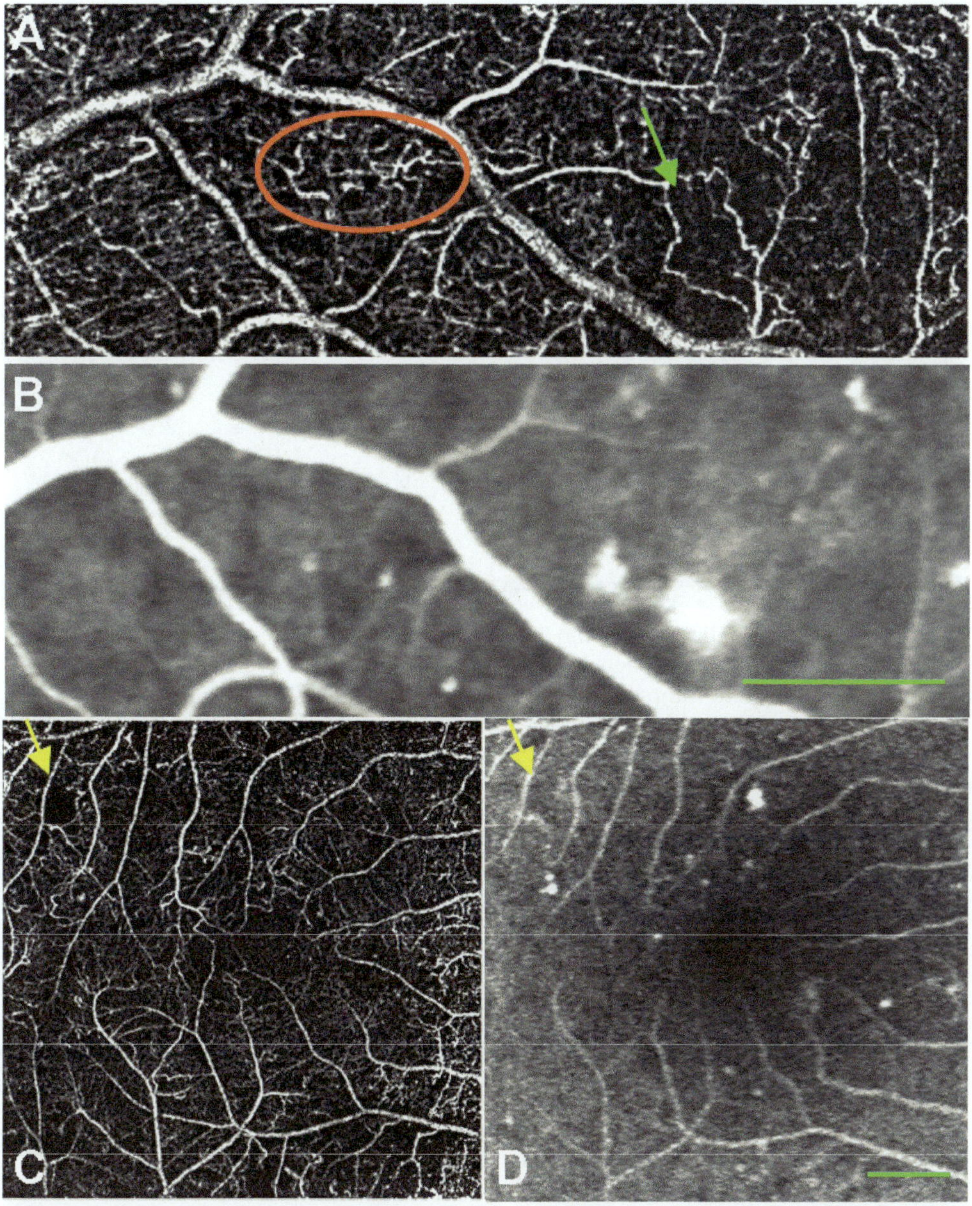

Fig. 5. Non-invasive capillary perfusion map and fluorescein angiographic (FA) images from patients with non-proliferative diabetic retinopathy. A. nCPM of a patient with NPDR. B. Corresponding FA scanning. The nCPM demonstrates vascular loops (red ellipse) and vascular shunts (green arrow). C. nCPM a patient with NPDR. D. Corresponding FA image; yellow arrows demonstrate non-perfusion.

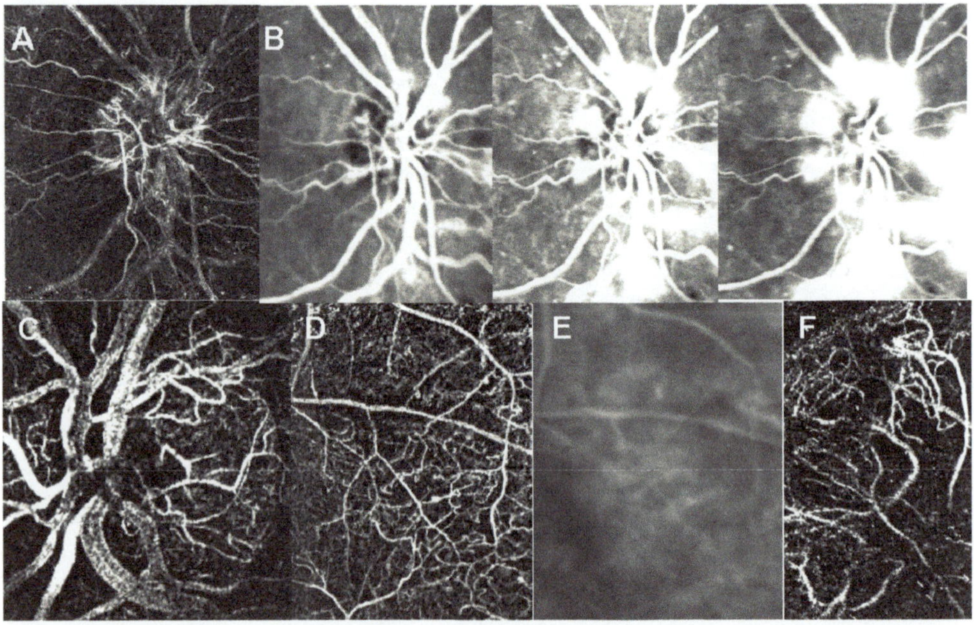

Fig. 6. Non-invasive capillary perfusion imaging of patients with proliferative diabetic retinopathy (PDR). A. nCPM image demonstrating neovascularization of the optic disc (NVD), and B. equivalent fluorescein angiography (FA) images at different stages after fluorescein injection. C. Another example of an nCPM image demonstrating NVD. D. nCPM images showing abnormal vasculature E. Corresponding FA and. F. nCPM image of neovascularization elsewhere (NVE).

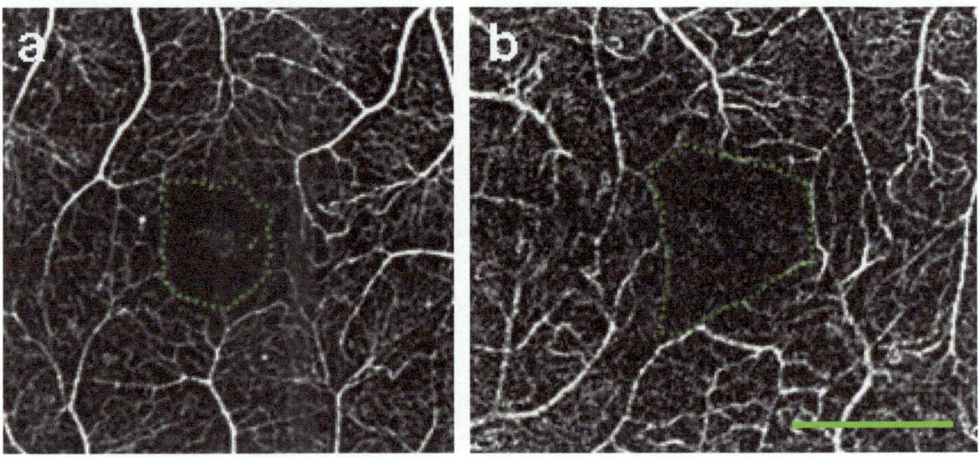

Fig. 7. Foveal avascular zone (FAZ) measurements. A) healthy subject, B) DR patient. Area and diameter, respectively, of FAZ: a) 0.114 mm2, 464 μm; b) 0.225 mm2, 672 μm. The green dotted line encircles the FAZ. Scale bar, 500 μm.

The size of the FAZ reflects the condition of the capillary circulation surrounding the foveal area, and can be a valuable staging tool as it increases under pathological conditions (Conrath, et al., 2005, Yap, et al., 1987). FAZ was measured noninvasively as long as 20 years ago by the entoptic method (Bradley, et al., 1992), revealing an increase in FAZ size in DR patients (Applegate, et al., 1997). That method, however, is subjective and depends on patient training and compliance. Our measurements revealed a significant increase in FAZ size in patients with DR relative to the healthy group. The FAZ measurement obtained by nCPMs in healthy subjects was within the documented range of the FAZ diameter (350–750 μm) (Tyrberg, et al., 2008). Loss of capillaries in the fovea is common in patients with ischemic retinopathies, and FAZ size has been shown to correlate with the visual prognosis in these cases (Mintz-Hittner, et al., 1999, Tyrberg et al., 2008). As previously reported (Applegate et al., 1997), we found a correlation between poorer visual acuity and larger FAZ diameter. Thus, the use of nCPM images should make it possible to measure FAZ easily, and provide a convenient and safe way to monitor this zone for an increase in size and other related changes during follow-up. Measurement of FAZ size can also help to assess suitability for treatment, given that different treatments are needed for a highly ischemic fovea and one that is well perfused (Chung, et al., 2008).

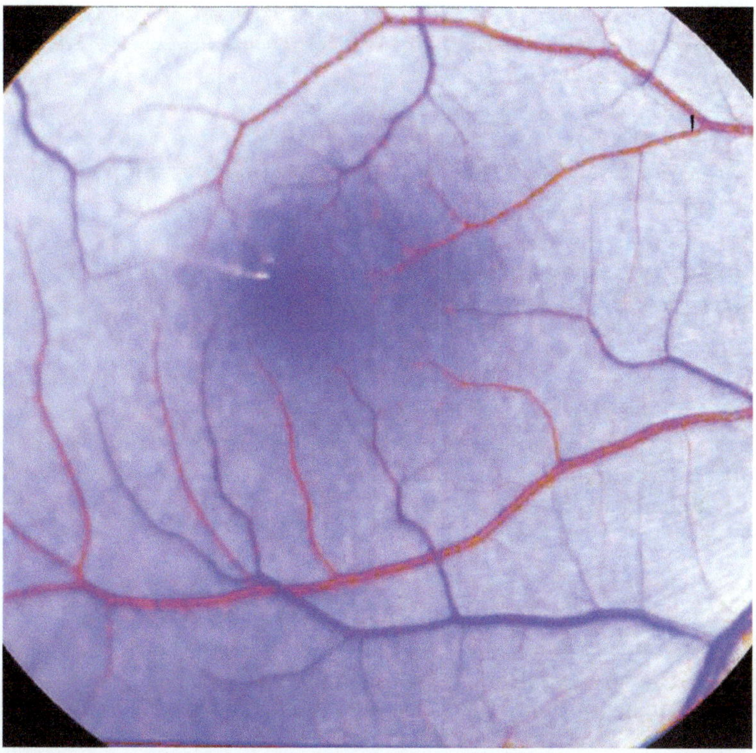

Fig. 8. Qualitative oximetric image obtained with the RFI from the retina of a healthy volunteer. Arteries, veins, and capillaries appear in different colors because of the different oxygen saturation levels of blood.

3. Oxymetry

The balance of oxygen supply and demand in the retina is closely regulated to maintain the processes of visual perception. Alterations in either oxygen supply or consumption might directly indicate the early onset of retinal abnormalities. The difference between the absorption spectra of oxyhemoglobin and deoxyhemoglobin can be used to determine the oxygenation of blood with multispectral imaging methods. Evaluation of retinal oxygen utilization may provide essential information about metabolic state of the retina, and assist in early detection of retinovascular diseases.

In multispectral imaging mode, the RFI can perform spectroscopic decomposition to qualitatively assess the oximetric state of the retina (Izhaky, et al., 2009). A qualitative oximetry map of a healthy volunteer was obtained by acquiring retinal images at two wavelengths (oximetric, 575 ± 5 nm, and isosbestic, 569 ± 5 nm). Differential decomposition analysis was used to generate the oximetry image (Figure 8).

Quantitative retinal oximetry was studied previously in healthy subjects revealing reproducible results that were sensitive to changes in oxygen concentration (Hardarson, et al., 2006). In patients with central retinal vein occlusion, oxygen saturation in veins of the affected eye was lower than in the fellow eye (Hardarson & Stefansson, 2010). Retinal oxymetric evaluation using imaging oximeter (oxygen module by Imedos,GmbH, Jena) of diabetic patients revealed an increase in venous oxygen saturation in patients with diabetic retinopathy, which was in correlation with the severity of the retinopathy (Hammer, et al., 2009). This implies reduced oxygen release to the tissue and tissue hypoxia which was attributed to either capillary closure and formation of arterio-venous shunt vessels or disturbance of vascular auto-regulation.

4. Functional assessment of visual tests and ERG

Retinal reflectance changes in response to photic stimulation carry information about metabolic processes underlying light responses in the retina. High-resolution, contrast agent-free optical imaging based on intrinsic signals in vivo has significantly contributed to understanding of the functional architecture of the neocortex (Grinvald et al., 1986). It reveals activity dependent changes in light reflectance, recorded using a digital camera with high spatial and temporal resolution. Such functional signals are usually small, originating from activity-dependent metabolic, hemodynamic, and fast and slow light-scattering changes (Frostig, et al., 1990, Malonek & Grinvald, 1996).

The RFI is capable of imaging outside the absorption range of photoreceptors under near-infrared light (750–840 nm), and can be used to optically monitor retinal activity in response to a well-defined visual stimulus (562 ±20 nm). The difference between the poststimulated and prestimulated images is used to determine the metabolic state of the retinal compartments. Change in light reflectance in response to a visual stimulus flashing were recorded in the cat retina (Izhaky et al., 2009). Similar experiments conducted on cats, monkeys, and humans have provided functional maps resulting from photic pattern activation(Abramoff et al., 2006, Hanazono, et al., 2008, Hanazono et al., 2007, Srinivasan, et al., 2009).

Electrophysiological studies of visual function in patients with diabetes mellitus demonstrate that functional alterations in the middle and inner retinal layers are present even prior to the development of clinical retinopathy (Bresnick & Palta, 1987, Tzekov & Arden, 1999, Zaharia, et al., 1987). Therefore, the diabetes induces changes in vision function may be not only secondary to vascular damage but also to neurosensory abmormality (Shirao & Kawasaki, 1998). Once diabetic retinopathy develops, additional electroretinogram (ERG) parameters are altered suggesting that photoreceptor abnormalities also occur. The changes are more pronounced compared to preretinopathy stage and there is a significant correlation between retinopathy severity and the magnitude of the functional loss (Holopigian, et al., 1992, van der Torren & Mulder, 1993, Weiner, et al., 1997). Multifocal ERG (mfERG), which maps local function, are abnormal in eyes of diabetic subjects without retinopathy and, to a greater degree, in eyes with mild or moderate NPDR. Moreover, abnormal mfERG implicit times are predictive of the development of new diabetic retinopathy over one and two years and are spatially associated with the retinopathy (Bearse, et al., 2006).

5. Conclusions

This chapter discuss the functional effect of diabetes mellitus on the retina. Retinal blood flow velocity measurements using the retinal function imager (RFI), discovered abnormal results in patients with various stages of diabetic-related ophthalmic condition. The result shows a significant decrease in arterial and venous velocity of patients with diabetic retinopathy and increase in diabetic patients with apparently normal retina compared to normals. The velocity correlation to blood pressure and heart rate was partially lost in the diabetic population either with or without retinopathy. The same technology was used to visualize capillary details without injecting contrast agents. Various vascular abnormalities like shunts and vascular loops were shown. In addition, examples of enlarged avascular zones in the fovea and ischemic retinal areas were presented. Multi-spectral imaging with the RFI was used to create qualitative oxymetry maps. Oxymetry measurement discovered increase in venous oxygen saturation. Imaging and analysis of changes in retinal reflectance in response to photic stimulation provides important information about retinal functionality. Electrophysiological alternations are present in early diabetes prior to the appearance of overt diabetic retinopathy.

6. References

(1991). Grading diabetic retinopathy from stereoscopic color fundus photographs--an extension of the modified Airlie House classification. ETDRS report number 10. Early Treatment Diabetic Retinopathy Study Research Group. *Ophthalmology, 98* (5 Suppl), 786-806.

Abiko, T., Abiko, A., Clermont, A.C., Shoelson, B., Horio, N., Takahashi, J., Adamis, A.P., King, G.L., & Bursell, S.E. (2003). Characterization of retinal leukostasis and hemodynamics in insulin resistance and diabetes: role of oxidants and protein kinase-C activation. *Diabetes, 52* (3), 829-837.

Abramoff, M.D., Kwon, Y.H., Ts'o, D., Soliz, P., Zimmerman, B., Pokorny, J., & Kardon, R. (2006). Visual stimulus-induced changes in human near-infrared fundus reflectance. *Invest Ophthalmol Vis Sci, 47* (2), 715-721.

Aiello, L.M. (2003). Perspectives on diabetic retinopathy. *Am J Ophthalmol, 136* (1), 122-135.

Ansari, N.H., Zhang, W., Fulep, E., & Mansour, A. (1998). Prevention of pericyte loss by trolox in diabetic rat retina. *J Toxicol Environ Health A, 54* (6), 467-475.

Apple DJ, R.M. (1985). Ocular Pathology. Clinical applications and self-assessment. . (St Louis, Toronto, Princeton: Mosby.

Applegate, R.A., Bradley, A., van Heuven, W.A., Lee, B.L., & Garcia, C.A. (1997). Entoptic evaluation of diabetic retinopathy. *Invest Ophthalmol Vis Sci, 38* (5), 783-791.

Arend, O., Remky, A., Harris, A., Bertram, B., Reim, M., & Wolf, S. (1995). Macular microcirculation in cystoid maculopathy of diabetic patients. *Br J Ophthalmol, 79* (7), 628-632.

Arend, O., Wolf, S., Jung, F., Bertram, B., Postgens, H., Toonen, H., & Reim, M. (1991). Retinal microcirculation in patients with diabetes mellitus: dynamic and morphological analysis of perifoveal capillary network. *Br J Ophthalmol, 75* (9), 514-518.

Bearse, M.A., Jr., Adams, A.J., Han, Y., Schneck, M.E., Ng, J., Bronson-Castain, K., & Barez, S. (2006). A multifocal electroretinogram model predicting the development of diabetic retinopathy. *Prog Retin Eye Res, 25* (5), 425-448.

Blair, N.P., Feke, G.T., Morales-Stoppello, J., Riva, C.E., Goger, D.G., Collas, G., & McMeel, J.W. (1982). Prolongation of the retinal mean circulation time in diabetes. *Arch Ophthalmol, 100* (5), 764-768.

Bradley, A., Applegate, R.A., Zeffren, B.S., & van Heuven, W.A. (1992). Psychophysical measurement of the size and shape of the human foveal avascular zone. *Ophthalmic Physiol Opt, 12* (1), 18-23.

Bresnick, G.H., & Palta, M. (1987). Oscillatory potential amplitudes. Relation to severity of diabetic retinopathy. *Arch Ophthalmol, 105* (7), 929-933.

Burgansky-Eliash, Z., Nelson, D.A., Bar-Tal, O.P., Lowenstein, A., Grinvald, A., & Barak, A. (2010). Reduced retinal blood flow velocity in diabetic retinopathy. *Retina, 30* (5), 765-773.

Bursell, S.E., Takagi, C., Clermont, A.C., Takagi, H., Mori, F., Ishii, H., & King, G.L. (1997). Specific retinal diacylglycerol and protein kinase C beta isoform modulation mimics abnormal retinal hemodynamics in diabetic rats. *Invest Ophthalmol Vis Sci, 38* (13), 2711-2720.

Chung, E.J., Roh, M.I., Kwon, O.W., & Koh, H.J. (2008). Effects of macular ischemia on the outcome of intravitreal bevacizumab therapy for diabetic macular edema. *Retina, 28* (7), 957-963.

Conrath, J., Giorgi, R., Raccah, D., & Ridings, B. (2005). Foveal avascular zone in diabetic retinopathy: quantitative vs qualitative assessment. *Eye, 19* (3), 322-326.

de la Rubia, G., Oliver, F.J., Inoguchi, T., & King, G.L. (1992). Induction of resistance to endothelin-1's biochemical actions by elevated glucose levels in retinal pericytes. *Diabetes, 41* (12), 1533-1539.

do Carmo, A., Lopes, C., Santos, M., Proenca, R., Cunha-Vaz, J., & Carvalho, A.P. (1998). Nitric oxide synthase activity and L-arginine metabolism in the retinas from streptozotocin-induced diabetic rats. *Gen Pharmacol, 30* (3), 319-324.

Dodge, A.B., & D'Amore, P.A. (1992). Cell-cell interactions in diabetic angiopathy. *Diabetes Care, 15* (9), 1168-1180.

Frederiksen, C.A., Jeppesen, P., Knudsen, S.T., Poulsen, P.L., Mogensen, C.E., & Bek, T. (2006). The blood pressure-induced diameter response of retinal arterioles decreases with increasing diabetic maculopathy. *Graefes Arch Clin Exp Ophthalmol, 244* (10), 1255-1261.

Frostig, R.D., Lieke, E.E., Ts'o, D.Y., & Grinvald, A. (1990). Cortical functional architecture and local coupling between neuronal activity and the microcirculation revealed by in vivo high-resolution optical imaging of intrinsic signals. *Proc Natl Acad Sci U S A, 87* (16), 6082-6086.

Gardiner, T.A., Archer, D.B., Curtis, T.M., & Stitt, A.W. (2007). Arteriolar involvement in the microvascular lesions of diabetic retinopathy: implications for pathogenesis. *Microcirculation, 14* (1), 25-38.

Gillies, M.C., & Su, T. (1993). High glucose inhibits retinal capillary pericyte contractility in vitro. *Invest Ophthalmol Vis Sci, 34* (12), 3396-3401.

Grinvald, A., Bonhoeffer, T., Vanzetta, I., Pollack, A., Aloni, E., Ofri, R., & Nelson, D. (2004). High-resolution functional optical imaging: from the neocortex to the eye. *Ophthalmol Clin North Am, 17* (1), 53-67.

Grinvald, A., Lieke, E., Frostig, R.D., Gilbert, C.D., & Wiesel, T.N. (1986). Functional architecture of cortex revealed by optical imaging of intrinsic signals. *Nature, 324* (6095), 361-364.

Grunwald, J.E., Bursell, S.E. (1996). Hemodynamic changes as early markers of diabetic retinopathy. *Current Opinion in Endocrinology and Diabetes, 3*, 298-306.

Grunwald, J.E., Riva, C.E., Sinclair, S.H., Brucker, A.J., & Petrig, B.L. (1986). Laser Doppler velocimetry study of retinal circulation in diabetes mellitus. *Arch Ophthalmol, 104* (7), 991-996.

Guan, K., Hudson, C., Wong, T., Kisilevsky, M., Nrusimhadevara, R.K., Lam, W.C., Mandelcorn, M., Devenyi, R.G., & Flanagan, J.G. (2006). Retinal hemodynamics in early diabetic macular edema. *Diabetes, 55* (3), 813-818.

Haefliger, I.O., & Anderson, D.R. (1997). Oxygen modulation of guanylate cyclase-mediated retinal pericyte relaxations with 3-morpholino-sydnonimine and atrial natriuretic peptide. *Invest Ophthalmol Vis Sci, 38* (8), 1563-1568.

Hammer, M., Vilser, W., Riemer, T., Mandecka, A., Schweitzer, D., Kuhn, U., Dawczynski, J., Liemt, F., & Strobel, J. (2009). Diabetic patients with retinopathy show increased retinal venous oxygen saturation. *Graefes Arch Clin Exp Ophthalmol, 247* (8), 1025-1030.

Hanazono, G., Tsunoda, K., Kazato, Y., Tsubota, K., & Tanifuji, M. (2008). Evaluating neural activity of retinal ganglion cells by flash-evoked intrinsic signal imaging in macaque retina. *Invest Ophthalmol Vis Sci, 49* (10), 4655-4663.

Hanazono, G., Tsunoda, K., Shinoda, K., Tsubota, K., Miyake, Y., & Tanifuji, M. (2007). Intrinsic signal imaging in macaque retina reveals different types of flash-induced light reflectance changes of different origins. *Invest Ophthalmol Vis Sci, 48* (6), 2903-2912.

Hardarson, S.H., Harris, A., Karlsson, R.A., Halldorsson, G.H., Kagemann, L., Rechtman, E., Zoega, G.M., Eysteinsson, T., Benediktsson, J.A., Thorsteinsson, A., Jensen, P.K., Beach, J., & Stefansson, E. (2006). Automatic retinal oximetry. *Invest Ophthalmol Vis Sci, 47* (11), 5011-5016.

Hardarson, S.H., & Stefansson, E. (2010). Oxygen saturation in central retinal vein occlusion. *Am J Ophthalmol, 150* (6), 871-875.

Hersh, P.S., Green, W.R., & Thomas, J.V. (1981). Tractional venous loops in diabetic retinopathy. *Am J Ophthalmol, 92* (5), 661-671.

Holopigian, K., Seiple, W., Lorenzo, M., & Carr, R. (1992). A comparison of photopic and scotopic electroretinographic changes in early diabetic retinopathy. *Invest Ophthalmol Vis Sci, 33* (10), 2773-2780.

Hudson, C., Flanagan, J.G., Turner, G.S., Chen, H.C., Rawji, M.H., & McLeod, D. (2005). Exaggerated relative nasal-temporal asymmetry of macular capillary blood flow in patients with clinically significant diabetic macular oedema. *Br J Ophthalmol, 89* (2), 142-146.

Izhaky, D., Nelson, D.A., Burgansky-Eliash, Z., & Grinvald, A. (2009). Functional imaging using the retinal function imager: direct imaging of blood velocity, achieving fluorescein angiography-like images without any contrast agent, qualitative oximetry, and functional metabolic signals. *Jpn J Ophthalmol, 53* (4), 345-351.

Jeppesen, P., & Bek, T. (2006). Impaired retinal autoregulation in small retinal arterioles before and after focal laser treatment for diabetic maculopathy. *Br J Ophthalmol, 90* (2), 198-201.

Joussen, A.M., Poulaki, V., Tsujikawa, A., Qin, W., Qaum, T., Xu, Q., Moromizato, Y., Bursell, S.E., Wiegand, S.J., Rudge, J., Ioffe, E., Yancopoulos, G.D., & Adamis, A.P. (2002). Suppression of diabetic retinopathy with angiopoietin-1. *Am J Pathol, 160* (5), 1683-1693.

Kempen, J.H., O'Colmain, B.J., Leske, M.C., Haffner, S.M., Klein, R., Moss, S.E., Taylor, H.R., & Hamman, R.F. (2004). The prevalence of diabetic retinopathy among adults in the United States. *Arch Ophthalmol, 122* (4), 552-563.

King, G.L., Shiba, T., Oliver, J., Inoguchi, T., & Bursell, S.E. (1994). Cellular and molecular abnormalities in the vascular endothelium of diabetes mellitus. *Annu Rev Med, 45,* 179-188.

Kohner, E.M., & Dollery, C.T. (1970). Fluorescein angiography of the fundus in diabetic retinopathy. *Br Med Bull, 26* (2), 166-170.

Kohner, E.M., Patel, V., & Rassam, S.M. (1995). Role of blood flow and impaired autoregulation in the pathogenesis of diabetic retinopathy. *Diabetes, 44* (6), 603-607.

Konno, S., Feke, G.T., Yoshida, A., Fujio, N., Goger, D.G., & Buzney, S.M. (1996). Retinal blood flow changes in type I diabetes. A long-term follow-up study. *Invest Ophthalmol Vis Sci, 37* (6), 1140-1148.

Landa, G., Garcia, P.M., & Rosen, R.B. (2009). Correlation between retina blood flow velocity assessed by retinal function imager and retina thickness estimated by scanning laser ophthalmoscopy/optical coherence tomography. *Ophthalmologica, 223* (3), 155-161.

Malonek, D., & Grinvald, A. (1996). Interactions between electrical activity and cortical microcirculation revealed by imaging spectroscopy: implications for functional brain mapping. *Science, 272* (5261), 551-554.

Matsugi, T., Chen, Q., & Anderson, D.R. (1997a). Adenosine-induced relaxation of cultured bovine retinal pericytes. *Invest Ophthalmol Vis Sci, 38* (13), 2695-2701.

Matsugi, T., Chen, Q., & Anderson, D.R. (1997b). Suppression of CO2-induced relaxation of bovine retinal pericytes by angiotensin II. *Invest Ophthalmol Vis Sci, 38* (3), 652-657.

McMillan, D.E. (1975). Deterioration of the microcirculation in diabetes. *Diabetes, 24* (10), 944-957.

McMillan, D.E. (1978). Rheological and related factors in diabetic retinopathy. *Int Ophthalmol Clin, 18* (4), 35-53.

Mintz-Hittner, H.A., Knight-Nanan, D.M., Satriano, D.R., & Kretzer, F.L. (1999). A small foveal avascular zone may be an historic mark of prematurity. *Ophthalmology, 106* (7), 1409-1413.

Miyamoto, K., Hiroshiba, N., Tsujikawa, A., & Ogura, Y. (1998). In vivo demonstration of increased leukocyte entrapment in retinal microcirculation of diabetic rats. *Invest Ophthalmol Vis Sci, 39* (11), 2190-2194.

Nelson, D.A., Krupsky, S., Pollack, A., Aloni, E., Belkin, M., Vanzetta, I., Rosner, M., & Grinvald, A. (2005). Special report: Noninvasive multi-parameter functional optical imaging of the eye. *Ophthalmic Surg Lasers Imaging, 36* (1), 57-66.

Paget, C., Lecomte, M., Ruggiero, D., Wiernsperger, N., & Lagarde, M. (1998). Modification of enzymatic antioxidants in retinal microvascular cells by glucose or advanced glycation end products. *Free Radic Biol Med, 25* (1), 121-129.

Parving, H.H., Viberti, G.C., Keen, H., Christiansen, J.S., & Lassen, N.A. (1983). Hemodynamic factors in the genesis of diabetic microangiopathy. *Metabolism, 32* (9), 943-949.

Rimmer, T., Fallon, T.J., & Kohner, E.M. (1989). Long-term follow-up of retinal blood flow in diabetes using the blue light entoptic phenomenon. *Br J Ophthalmol, 73* (1), 1-5.

Riva, C.E., Sinclair, S.H., & Grunwald, J.E. (1981). Autoregulation of retinal circulation in response to decrease of perfusion pressure. *Invest Ophthalmol Vis Sci, 21* (1 Pt 1), 34-38.

Robinson, F., Riva, C.E., Grunwald, J.E., Petrig, B.L., & Sinclair, S.H. (1986). Retinal blood flow autoregulation in response to an acute increase in blood pressure. *Invest Ophthalmol Vis Sci, 27* (5), 722-726.

Sakata, K., Funatsu, H., Harino, S., Noma, H., & Hori, S. (2006). Relationship between macular microcirculation and progression of diabetic macular edema. *Ophthalmology, 113* (8), 1385-1391.

Schmetterer, L., & Wolzt, M. (1999). Ocular blood flow and associated functional deviations in diabetic retinopathy. *Diabetologia, 42* (4), 387-405.

Shepro, D., & Morel, N.M. (1993). Pericyte physiology. *Faseb J, 7* (11), 1031-1038.

Shirao, Y., & Kawasaki, K. (1998). Electrical responses from diabetic retina. *Prog Retin Eye Res, 17* (1), 59-76.

Sims, D.E. (1986). The pericyte--a review. *Tissue Cell, 18* (2), 153-174.

Sinclair, S.H., Grunwald, J.E., Riva, C.E., Braunstein, S.N., Nichols, C.W., & Schwartz, S.S. (1982). Retinal vascular autoregulation in diabetes mellitus. *Ophthalmology, 89* (7), 748-750.

Srinivasan, V.J., Chen, Y., Duker, J.S., & Fujimoto, J.G. (2009). In vivo functional imaging of intrinsic scattering changes in the human retina with high-speed ultrahigh resolution OCT. *Opt Express, 17* (5), 3861-3877.

Takagi, C., Bursell, S.E., Lin, Y.W., Takagi, H., Duh, E., Jiang, Z., Clermont, A.C., & King, G.L. (1996). Regulation of retinal hemodynamics in diabetic rats by increased expression and action of endothelin-1. *Invest Ophthalmol Vis Sci, 37* (12), 2504-2518.

Tyrberg, M., Ponjavic, V., & Lovestam-Adrian, M. (2008). Multifocal electroretinogram (mfERG) in patients with diabetes mellitus and an enlarged foveal avascular zone (FAZ). *Doc Ophthalmol, 117* (3), 185-189.

Tzekov, R., & Arden, G.B. (1999). The electroretinogram in diabetic retinopathy. *Surv Ophthalmol, 44* (1), 53-60.

van den Born, B.J., Hulsman, C.A., Hoekstra, J.B., Schlingemann, R.O., & van Montfrans, G.A. (2005). Value of routine funduscopy in patients with hypertension: systematic review. *Bmj, 331* (7508), 73.

van der Torren, K., & Mulder, P. (1993). Comparison of the second and third oscillatory potentials with oscillatory potential power in early diabetic retinopathy. *Doc Ophthalmol, 83* (2), 111-118.

van Hecke, M.V., Dekker, J.M., Nijpels, G., Moll, A.C., Heine, R.J., Bouter, L.M., Polak, B.C., & Stehouwer, C.D. (2005). Inflammation and endothelial dysfunction are associated with retinopathy: the Hoorn Study. *Diabetologia, 48* (7), 1300-1306.

van Hecke, M.V., Dekker, J.M., Nijpels, G., Stolk, R.P., Henry, R.M., Heine, R.J., Bouter, L.M., Stehouwer, C.D., & Polak, B.C. (2006). Are retinal microvascular abnormalities associated with large artery endothelial dysfunction and intima-media thickness? The Hoorn Study. *Clin Sci (Lond), 110* (5), 597-604.

Weiner, A., Christopoulos, V.A., Gussler, C.H., Adams, D.H., Kaufman, S.R., Kohn, H.D., & Weidenthal, D.T. (1997). Foveal cone function in nonproliferative diabetic retinopathy and macular edema. *Invest Ophthalmol Vis Sci, 38* (7), 1443-1449.

Yap, M., Gilchrist, J., & Weatherill, J. (1987). Psychophysical measurement of the foveal avascular zone. *Ophthalmic Physiol Opt, 7* (4), 405-410.

Yoshida, A., Feke, G.T., Morales-Stoppello, J., Collas, G.D., Goger, D.G., & McMeel, J.W. (1983). Retinal blood flow alterations during progression of diabetic retinopathy. *Arch Ophthalmol, 101* (2), 225-227.

Zaharia, M., Olivier, P., Lafond, G., Blondeau, P., & Brunette, J.R. (1987). Lobular delayed choroidal perfusion as an early angiographic sign of diabetic retinopathy: a preliminary report. *Can J Ophthalmol, 22* (5), 257-261.

Zatz, R., & Brenner, B.M. (1986). Pathogenesis of diabetic microangiopathy. The hemodynamic view. *Am J Med, 80* (3), 443-453.

13

Preventing Diabetic Retinopathy: Red Lesions Detection in Early Stages

C. Mariño, J. Novo, N. Barreira and M.G. Penedo
University of A Coruña
Spain

1. Introduction

Diabetic retinopathy is the most common diabetic eye disease and a leading cause of blindness in industrialized countries. For example, several studies have provided data of its prevalence in several countries like Spain (values between 44.7% and 26.11% depending on the area and the type of diabetes) Fernandez-Vigo et al. (1993); RA et al. (2010), Australia (overall 15.3% of patients with diabetes had retinopathy) Tapp et al. (2003) or USA (40.3% crude prevalence among diabetic patients) Kempen et al. (2004). Moreover, several worlwide programs like the *Aravind Eye Care System* (`http://www.aravind.org/Default.aspx`) promote the sharing of knowlege and resources to avoid blindness, like the caused by diabetic retinopathy.

Diabetic retinopathy is caused by changes in the blood vessels of the retina. For the most of the cases its detection in an early stage would allow for a treatment with a high healing rate. This is why the screening processes are a very valuable method for prevention of this pathology. Typically, a large amount of fundus images (photo of the back of the inside of the eye) have to be analyzed as diabetic patients have both their eyes examined at least once a year. These photos are then examined by an ophthalmologist (eye-doctor) who can determine if there are any visible signs of the disease present. To effectively manage all this information and the workload it produces, automatic techniques for analyzing the images would represent a major improvement, since manual analysis of this amount of information is a very complex and error prone process. These techniques must be robust, sensitive and specific to be implemented in real-life screening applications.

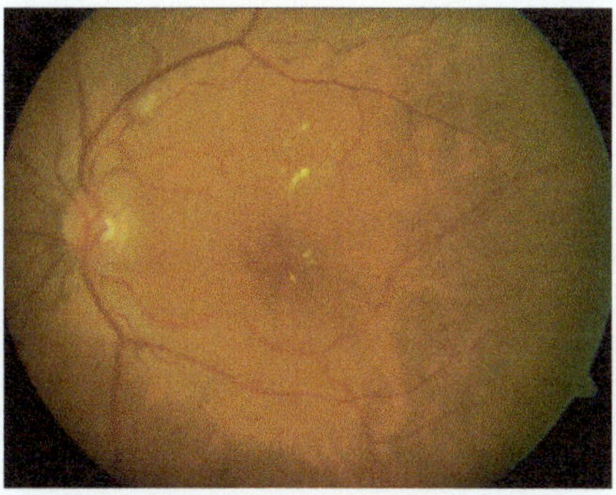

Fig. 1. Digital color retinal image used as input for the diagnosis.

One important symptom of diabetic retinopathy is the development of red lesions such as microaneurysm and white lesions such us exudates and cottonwool spots. Here only red lesions will be located, since they are among the first absolute sign of diabetic retinopathy.

Several studies have been presented to deal with the problem of hard exudates detection. (Leistritz & Schweitzer, 1994) showed that using size, shape, texture, etc. in isolation is insufficient to detect hard exudates accurately. This fact is used in this work too. Several other attempts have been made to detect hard exudates using histogram segmentation. If the background color of a retinal image is sufficiently uniform, a simple and effective method to separate exudates from the background is to select proper thresholds (Leistritz & Schweitzer, 1994; Philips et al., 1993; Ward et al., 1989). In (Goldbaum et al., 1990) Mahalanobis distance is used as the classifier criteria, but results were inconclusive. Many other approximations can be found in literature, like mathematical morphology based (Cree et al., 1997; Spencer et al., 1996) or neural network based (Gardner et al., 1996), with results ranging in sensitivity from 85% and specificity of 76%(Hipwell et al., 2000), sensitivity of 77.5% and specificity of 88.7% in (Sinthanayothin et al., 2002) or sensitivity 93.1% and specificity of 71.4%(Larsen et al., 2003), this last obtained using a commercially available automatic red lesion detection system. More recently, García et al. (García et al., 2009) developed several techniques to deal with the problem of feature detection for the diabetic retinopathy diagnosis and screening, using neural nets like the multilayer perceptron classifier (García et al., 2008) or a radial basis function fed with the output of a logistic regression process, and obtained values ranging in sensitivity from 86.1% to 92.1% and from 71.4% to 86.4% in positive predicted results.

In our work an algorithm for the detection of red lesions in digital color fundus photographs is proposed. The method performs in three stages: in the first stage points candidates to be red lesions are obtained by using a set of correlation filters working in different resolutions, allowing that way the detection of a wider set of points. Then, in the second stage, a region growing segmentation process rejects the points from the prior stage whose size does not fit in the red lesion pattern. Finally, in the third stage three test are applied to the output of the second stage: a shape test to remove non-circular areas, an intensity test to remove that areas belonging to the fundus of the retina and finally a test to remove the points which fall inside the vessels (only lesions outside the vessels are considered). Evaluation was performed on a test composed on images representative of those normally found in a screening set. Moreover, comparison with manually-obtained results from clinical experts are performed, to set the accuracy and reliability of the method.

2. Red lesion detection algorithm

In this work an algorithm for the detection of red lesions in digital color fundus photographs is proposed. The method performs in three stages, as depicted in Fig. 2. In the first stage, working on the green channel of the input (color) image, several correlation filters are applied, each with a different resolution, detecting this way a wider spectrum of features and getting the initial set of candidate lesions. The output of this stage serves as input for the second stage, where a region growing process is used to preprocess the red lesion candidates set obtaining a more accurate set. Finally, in the third stage the previous set of candidates is filtered by means of four filtering processes: a shape (circularity) filter, which rejects regions with "low circularity", an intensity filter, which removes from the set the candidates which does not fulfill the intensity criteria, a correlation mean filter, which removes the candidate areas which represent an outliers in the correlation filter response and finally a last filter which, using the creases of the digital angiography López et al. (2000); Mariño et al. (2006), removes that areas inside or next to vessels. In the following sections each of these stages will be described.

In section 3 description of the correlation filters of the first stage is included. Section 4 provides details on the region growing algorithm. Once the regions have been obtained, the filtering process to discard false positives is described in section 5. Experiments and results are given in section 6 for the different stages of the algorithm, and finally section 7 provides discussion and conclusions.

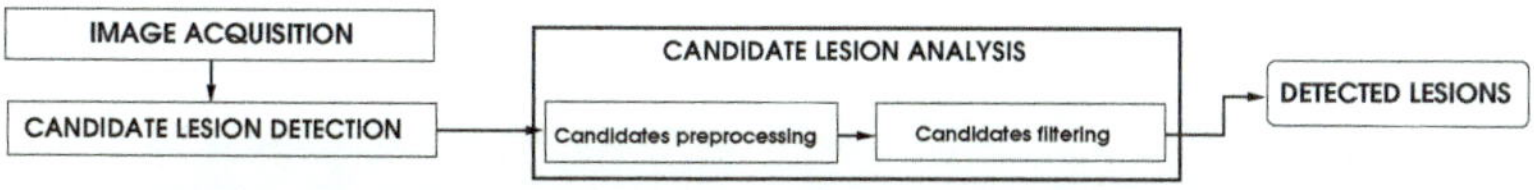

Fig. 2. General schema of the proposed methodology. Once the image is acquired, the correlation filters are applied to get an initial set of candidate lesions.These candidates are analyzed, first preprocessing them using a growing regions algorithm and then applying several filters in order to obtain the final lesions set.

3. Correlation filters set

The goal in this stage is to get the set of candidate red lesions. Since the regions corresponding to lesions have a wide variety of sizes, three correlation filters with different resolutions, F_1, F_2 and F_3, are applied to the image. As proposed in Niemeijer et al. (2005), since red lesions have the highest contrast in the green plane Hoover & Goldbaum (2000), in place of applying the correlation to the gray-level version of the image, green plane I_g is used as the input. In Figure 3 the histogram of the three RGB channels is shown. As depicted, red channel pixels distribution is very scattered, with low frequencies except the very high frequencies. Blue channel is biased to low values with a very short range. Finally, red channel shows a wide range of values within an acceptable frequency range.

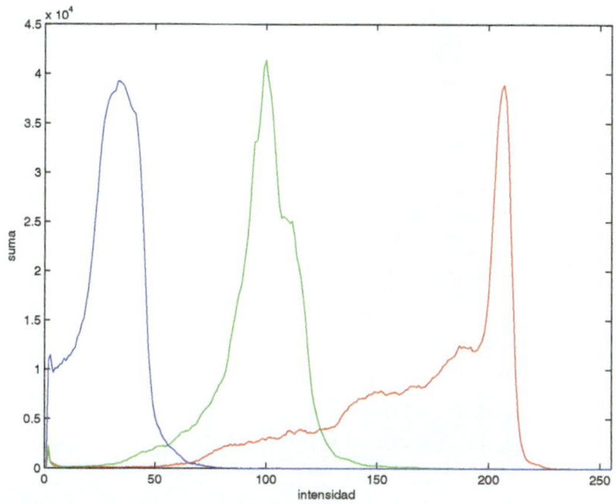

Fig. 3. Histogram of the different RGB channels.

Figure 4 shows an example of the results obtained by an expert clinician working in each of the RGB channels.

Red lesions present three common characteristics:

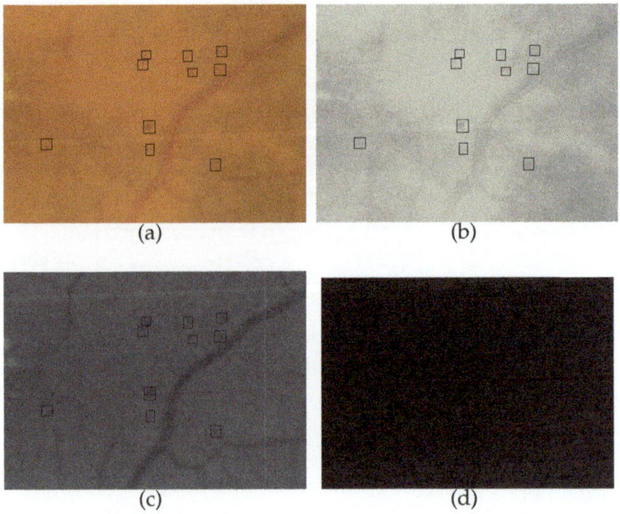

Fig. 4. Result of manual analysis obtained by an expert clinician working on the different RGB channels of a digital retinography. Squares mark the lesions detected by the specialist. 4(a): original retinography, 4(b): results on the red channel, 4(c): results on the green channel and 4(d): results on the blue channel.

Area: red dots are small regions in the image. Figure 5 depicts an histogram of 157 lesions detected by a clinician in the set of available images, showing that the size of the red lesions is never above 200 pixels (a very small size in the 1024×768 pixels sized images used in our work, being in fact $0'0153\%$ of the image).

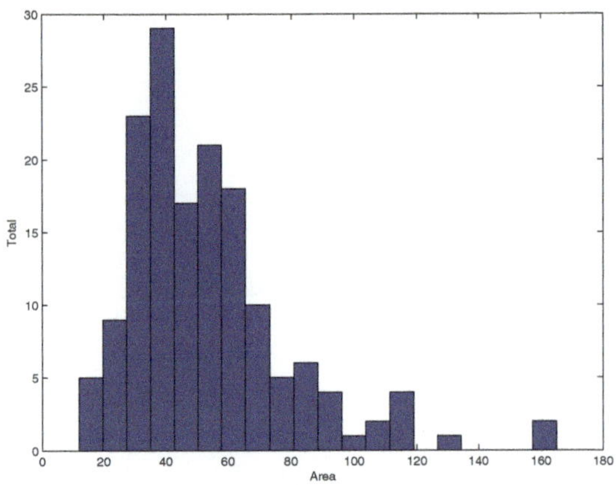

Fig. 5. Histogram of the areas of the red dots. Size of the red lesions is never higher than 200 pixels.

Shape: red dots have an approximately circled shape, although their borders are very irregular. In Figure 6 histogram of the radii of the red lesions is depicted, assuming a perfect circled shape.

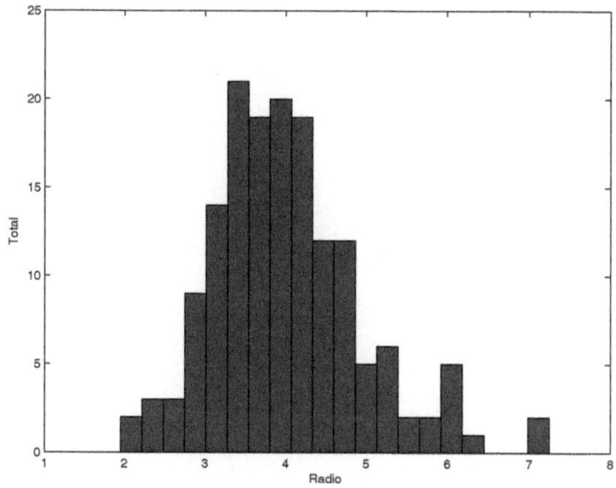

Fig. 6. Histogram of the radii of the red lesions. Radius is always between 2 and 7 pixels long.

Color and intensity: as their name points out, red lesions are mainly red colored, with a color similar to the blood vessels, and are much darker than the surrounding retinal tissues.

Figure 7(a) shows the aspect of a typical red lesion in the green channel of the original image, with the profile in the center of the lesion depicted in 7(b).

In order to design the shapes and sizes of the filter's kernels, red lesions from the images in the test set are isolated and analyzed. As it can be observed in Figure 7(b), a red lesion template can be forged using a Gaussian pattern.

Assuming symmetry in the red lesion, the Gaussian pattern can be described as a one-dimensional function, being the variable the distance (or radius) to the center of the lesion as showed in Equation 1.

$$f(r) = ae^{-br^2} \tag{1}$$

where parameters a and b control the shape of the generated Gaussian curve. In Figure 8 a two-dimensional Gaussian template is depicted.

But, since the red lesions have a circular shape, a second, more "ideal", template was tried to correlate with the red lesions, and results from both templates compared. The kernels of these second filters were designed to be again square-shaped, this time with a circle inside simulating the red lesion. Figure 9 shows one of the kernels used with this approximation.

Our first results were obtained by correlating one filter with the images. This filter was designed with following parameters: 4 pixels of radius, size of 19×19 pixels, depth (b in the equation which models the Gaussian shape) of 30 units (taken from the maximum depth obtained from the red dots marked by clinician in the test images) and for the intensity the mean green channel value of the analyzed image. But with this approximation poor results were obtained, with a high level of false positives (230). Analyzing the results, we concluded that the variability in size of the red lesions lead to these poor results.

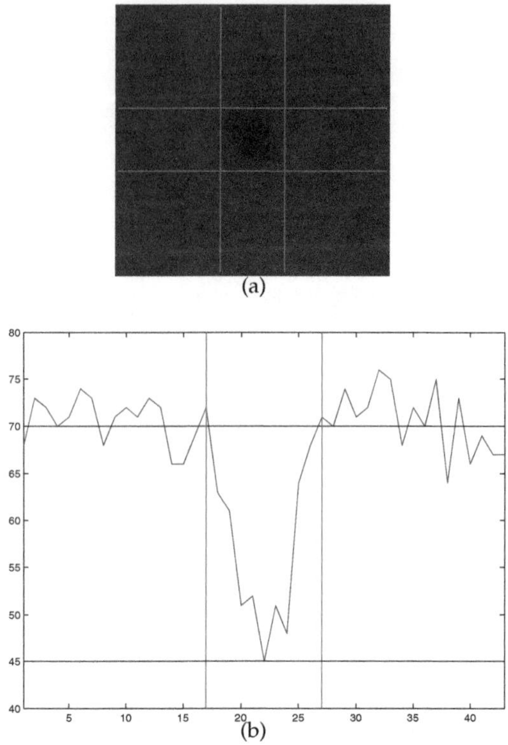

Fig. 7. Green channel view of a red lesion. The pixels belonging to the lesion are darker than the background. Top: lines mark borders of the lesion, located in the centered square. Bottom: profile of the center of a red lesion.

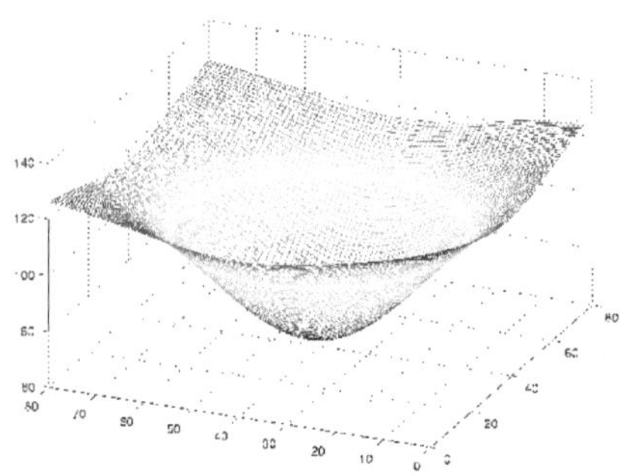

Fig. 8. Example of one of the three Gaussian kernels which the image is correlated with.

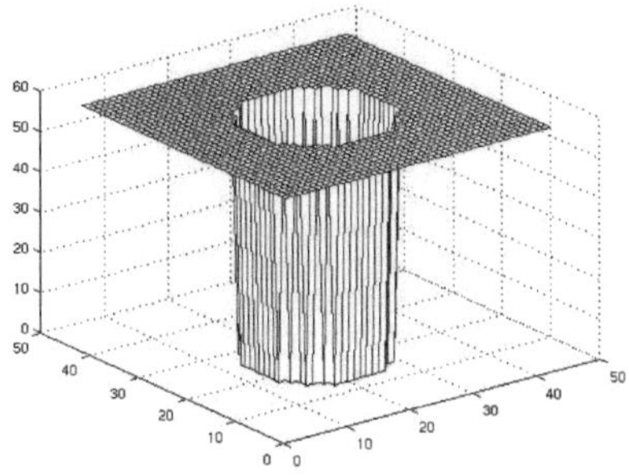

Fig. 9. Example of one of the three kernels which the image is correlated with.

To deal with the problem of the size variability of the lesions to detect, a multiscale solution was designed. In our case, after testing several filter configurations, best results were obtained using three filters with the following parameters:

Radius: 3, 5 and 10 were the selected sizes for the radius of the filters to cover a wide spectrum of red dots radii.

Size: 15×15, 21×21 y 43×43, to cover the more of the red dots sizes detected by the clinician.

Depth: 30 units.

Intensity: the mean green channel value of the analyzed image.

The three images resulting from the correlation with the three filters, C_1, C_2 and C_3, each of size $M \times N$, are combined using equation 2, so that output from this stage R' is an image where each pixel corresponds to the maximum output value from the correlations in its location. Then, a threshold τ is applied to the output, to discard low value correlation pixels, and finally connected regions are built with the values over that threshold. The result from this process will be the candidate red lesion regions.

$$R' = \max\{C_1(x,y), C_2(x,y), C_3(x,y), \\ \forall x, y | 1 \leq x \leq M, 1 \leq y \leq N\} \tag{2}$$

The threshold τ was set to 0.43, the lower value obtained from the profile of the red lesions, as showed in Figure 7(b).

Also, Figure 7(b) shows the profile in the center of the lesion. As it can be observed in that figure, a red lesion template can be forged using a Gaussian pattern.

Assuming symmetry in the red lesion, the Gaussian pattern can be described as a one-dimensional function, being the variable the distance (or radius) to the center of the lesion as showed in Equation 1.

Figure 10 shows the forged red dot template.

Both the correlation kernels were tested with the images test set, and results are included in Table 1. Table 1 shows the early results obtained for images from patients with red lesions

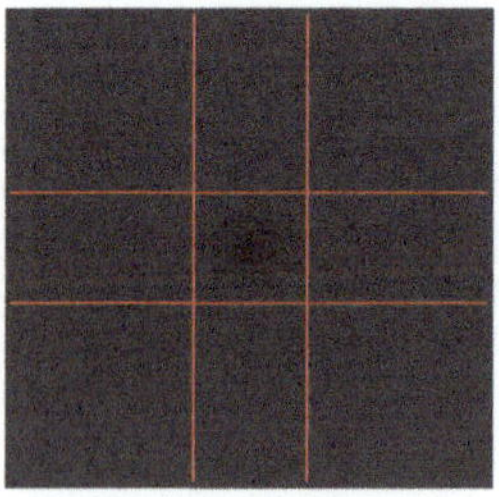

Fig. 10. Example of an artificial red lesion created using a Gaussian template.

and images from healthy patients (no Red Lesions). These results showed an extremely good sensibility but a relatively high average of false positives per image. Although this phase is meant to detect of all the true lesions while successive ones aim to identify them as true or false, an improvement was made in order to lower the false positive rate. But using the same test images images, the results obtained with the circular kernel template allowed to increase the correlation value threshold to 0.5 thus reducing the false positive cases

		Red Lesions	no Red Lesions
Gaussian	Sensibility	95%	N/A
	False positives	186	72
Circular	Sensibility	95%	N/A
	False positives	137	49

Table 1. Red lesions candidates detection sensibility and average false positives per image obtained using three Gaussian templates (first and second rows) and using three circular kernel templates (third and fourth rows).

Despite the meaningful reduction of false positives many areas not belonging to red lesions are obtained in this stage (Figure 11). These areas must, of course, be discarded from the result. This will be the objective of the second stage of the algorithm.

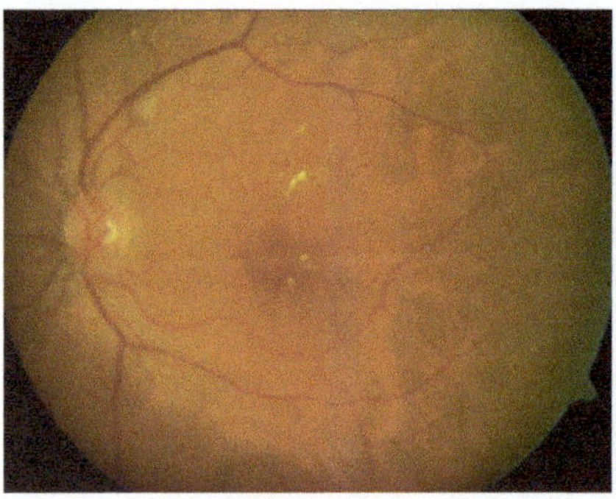

(a)

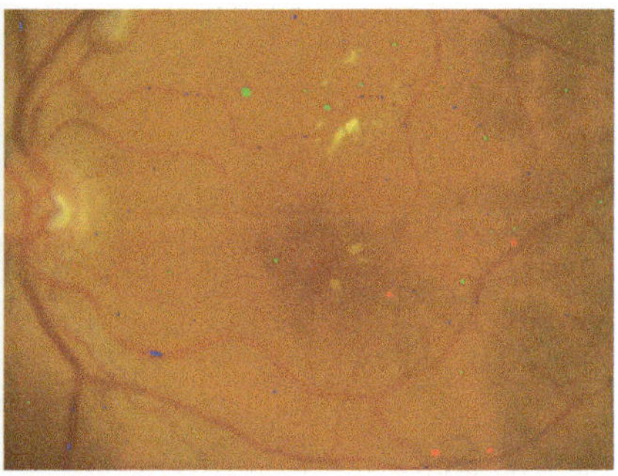

(b)

Fig. 11. 11(a)Digital color retinal image used as input for the diagnosis. 11(b)Cropped region from the output image after applying the correlation filters, equation 2 and threshold to image from Figure 11(a). Candidate red lesions are marked in red, green and blue.

4. Region growing algorithm

To remove false positives from the output of the stage 1, a growing region algorithm is used. The regions which contain less than a given threshold will be removed, since they correspond to noise and false features detected as lesions. In a growing region algorithm, first step consists on finding the seeds for the growing regions. Here the point with the higher correlation value from each region output from stage one will be considered as seed (which will be the center of the lesion, if the region comes from a lesion). Once the seed has been found, the threshold t for the growing process is determined following equation 3Niemeijer et al. (2005).

$$t = i_{seed} - \alpha(i_{seed} - i_{bg}) \tag{3}$$

where i_{seed} is the intensity at the starting seed position, i_{bg} is the intensity of the same pixel in an image resulting from applying a median filter with kernel size 41×41 to I_g and $\alpha \in [0, 1]$. Here $\alpha = 0.5$, as proposed in Niemeijer et al. (2005). Since the illumination in the retina is not uniform along all its area, using I_g provides our algorithm a more robust behaviour against these photometric changes.

Figure 12 depicts the different results obtained by using a simple median filter and by using the estimated values obtained using eq. 3, which clearly improve the results.

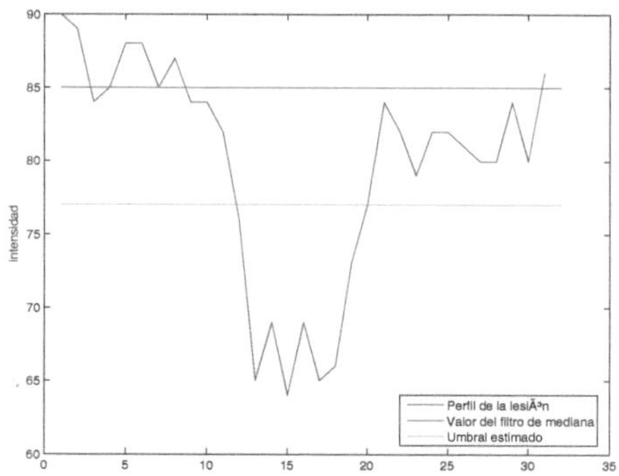

(a)

(b)

Fig. 12. Results obtained using equation 3. 12(a) Profile of a lesion and several growing thresholds (median filter and filter from eq. 3). 12(b) Results from the different growing thresholds: pixels below estimated threshold (eq. 3) are depicted in green and the pixels between this one and the median filter are depicted in red.

Growing starts in the seed pixel and stops when no more connected pixels below the threshold can be found. An illustration of the region growing algorithm is shown in Figure 13.

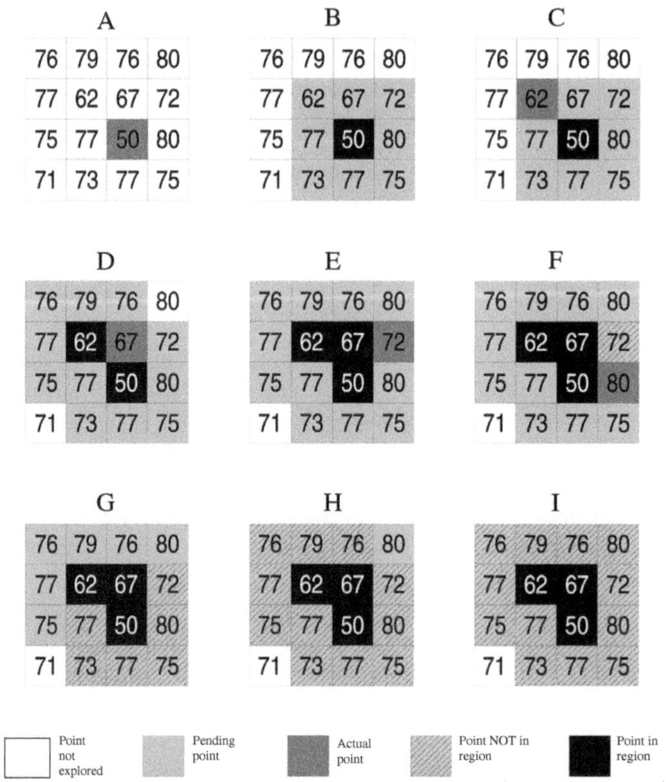

Fig. 13. Illustration of the region growing algorithm. Starting at point (3,3), the algorithm evolves until no new pixels can be added to the region.

And Figure 14 shows the evolution of several regions after region growing algorithm is performed.

The grown objects together form the final candidate object set. If the region size is above $200px$ it will be discarded, since it will be considered as a background area or vessel area. This threshold value has been set empirically, analyzing the sizes of the red lesions in the test set of images, composed by 100 images. Figure 15 depicts the result from this stage applied to image from Figure 11.

Table 2 describes the quality improvement achieved in this stage comparing the false positive average obtained in section 3.

Images type	Red Lesions	no R. Lesions
Sensibility	95%	N/A
False positives	66	18

Table 2. Results obtained applying the growing region algorithm.

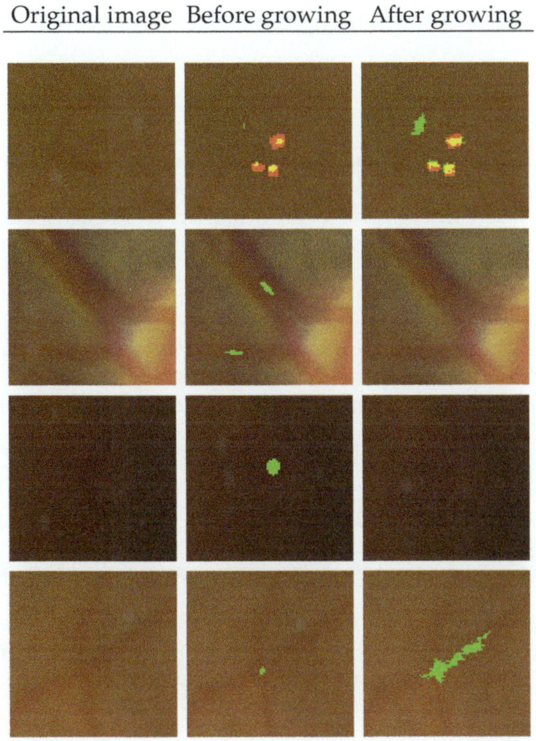

Fig. 14. Region growing examples. In red clinician red lesions marked by clinician is shown, in green output from candidate regions detection is depicted, and in yellow output regions overlaped between both this stages.

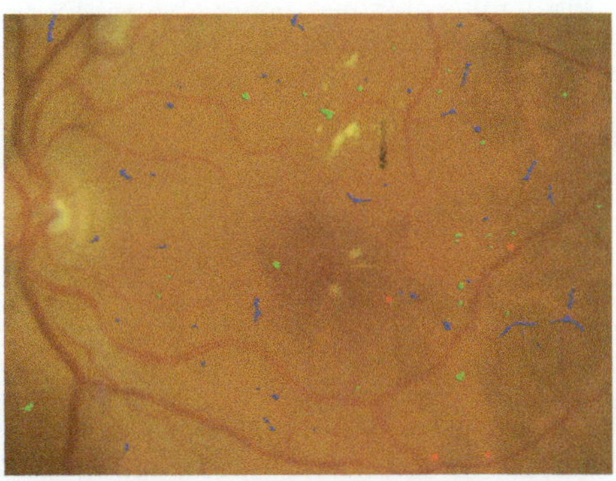

Fig. 15. Cropped region from the output image after applying the growing region process to image (Figure 11). Regions are marked as green and blue areas.

Image in Figure 15 shows some regions that are not red lesions, and should still be removed from results. This goal will be fulfilled by stage three of the algorithm, commented in the next section.

5. Feature based filtering process

After candidate regions are detected and region growing algorithm performed, in the last stage, candidates less adjusted to red lesion profile will be removed. To do so, several high-level knowledge based filters have been designed to improve detection results. This improvement is acquired by removing false positives and not doing so with the true positives.

5.1 Shape filtering

The first applied filtering process consists on removing the regions which does not fit in the regular shape of the red lesions, which are circular shapes. In this step, the degree of circularity for each region is measured, and using a threshold, non-circular shapes are delete from the set of candidate regions. Circularity $\mathcal{C}$ is computed by means of equation 4.

$$\mathcal{C} = \frac{p^2}{4\pi a} \quad (4)$$

where p represents the perimeter of the candidate region and a represents its area.

To deal with the irregular shapes of the candidate region, which makes computation of perimeter and area more difficult, firstly a closing morphological operator Jähne (2005) is applied to the images. This way, inner holes and small irregularities resulting from the region growing stage are removed.

To obtain the perimeter values chaincodes algorithms Russ (1995) were discarded, and a simpler method, counting the pixels of the region which are neighbors of a pixel outside the region, was employed, although this method trends to overestimate perimeter values of figures, which does not represent an important problem for our algorithm, since false positives and red lesions are equally affected by this overestimation. To prove this statement, perimeter values were obtained using chaincodes and using our method, with results depicted in Figure 16. In this graphic circularity values obtained using chaincodes to get the perimeters ($c1$) are shown in the horizontal axe, and values obtained using the method of frontier pixels are shown in vertical axe ($c2$). Although $c2 > c1$ for every values, this does not affect to the filtering process (whatever axe is considered, the more of the false positives is clearly below a threshold).

Once circularity degree has been computed, equation 5 is applied, in order to choose only circular-like regions.

$$Threshold(\mathcal{C}) = \begin{cases} \geq U_t, \text{region accepted} \\ < U_t, \text{ region rejected} \end{cases} \quad (5)$$

The value $U_t = 0.375$ was determined empirically by evaluating the set of test images (Figure 18). Figure 17 shows several examples of candidate regions removed by this filter.

In Figure 19 the result obtained from this filter is depicted, showing the regions accepted marked as blue and green areas.

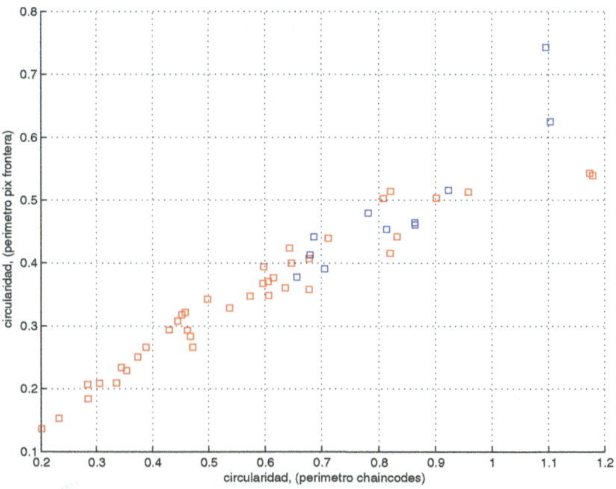

Fig. 16. Circularity values compared. Red squares represent false positives, and blue squares represent true red dots.

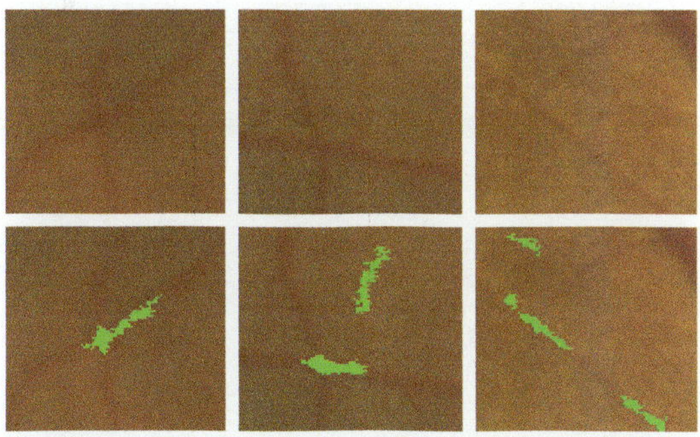

Fig. 17. Regions removed by the circularity filter. Upper row shows the area in the retina and the bottom row removed candidate regions are shown.

Table 3 shows the results obtained applying the circularity filtering to the output of the growing-region algorithm stage.

Images type	Red Lesions	no R. Lesions
Sensibility	85%	N/A
False positives	36	7

Table 3. Results obtained applying the shape filter to the output from stage one described in section 3.

5.2 Intensity filtering

The second filtering process performed in this third stage is an intensity-based filtering. Since red lesions are dark structures, lighter structures can be removed from the set of candidate regions. Since illumination is not constant among images, a robust threshold is needed, and it can not be a constant. From the set of test images, a functional threshold was designed, so that it depends only on the mean value of the green plane image.

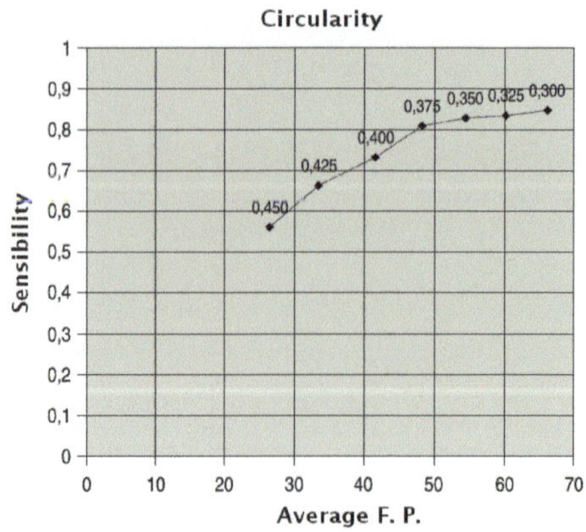

Fig. 18. Sensibility and false positives values depending on the circularity threshold used.

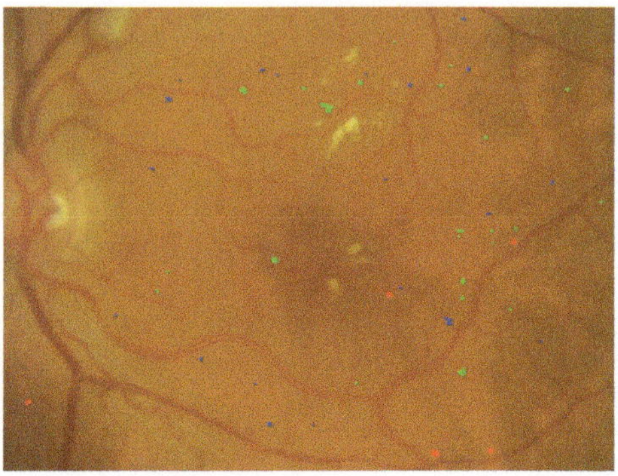

Fig. 19. Cropped region from the output image after applying the shape filtering process. Regions are marked as green and blue areas.

In each of the images, an expert clinician set the right threshold so that minimum of false positives was zero, minimizing the number of false negatives. Equation 6, the intensity threshold, $\mathcal{I}$, was obtained by a minimum square error fitting of a straight line to the set of values obtained from this manual validation.

$$Threshold(\mathcal{I}) = 0.8054\bar{I}_g + 27.3723 \tag{6}$$

where $\bar{I}_g$ represents the mean value of the green plane of the image. Candidate regions above the threshold will be removed, as depicted in Figure 20.

In Figure 21 the result from this process is shown, with candidate regions marked as green and blue areas.

Table 4 shows the obtained intensity filtering results.

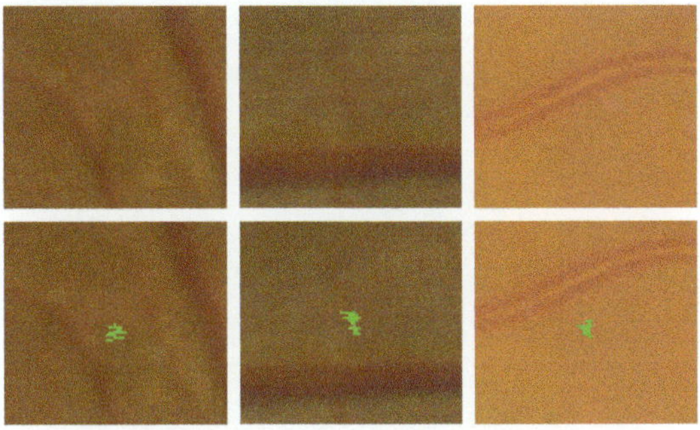

Fig. 20. Regions removed by the intensity filter. Upper row shows the area in the retina and the bottom row removed candidate regions are shown.

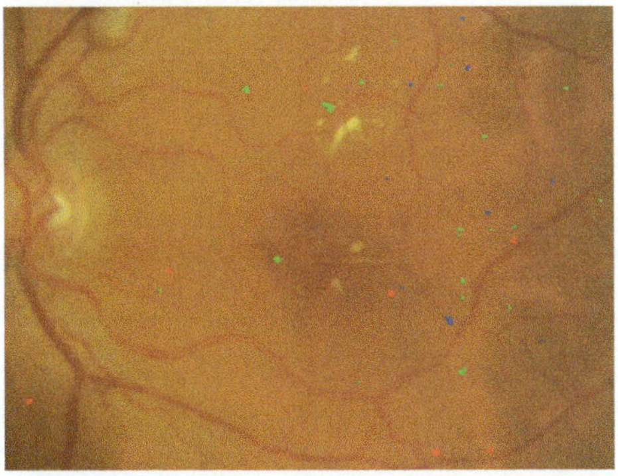

Fig. 21. Cropped region from the output image after applying the intensity filtering process. Regions are marked as green and blue areas.

Images type	Red Lesions	no R. Lesions
Sensibility	87%	N/A
False positives	35	9

Table 4. Results obtained applying the intensity filter to the output from stage one described in section 3.

5.3 Correlation filtering

The third of the filters consists on a correlation-based filter. Taking as basis the correlation image R' from first stage, this filter remove every region whose mean value for this correlation image is not above a given threshold. After testing a set of values in the test images, this threshold was empirically set to the value 0.4 (Figure 22).

In Figure 23 examples of a candidate lesion removed 23(a), and a candidate region preserved 23(b) by the mean correlation filter are depicted. In 23(a), first row shows the original area in the retina (left) and the candidate lesion (right). In second row values of correlation are shown. In 23(b) the same figures are presented with the same interpretation, but in this case values of correlation lead to the preservation of the candidate region.

In Figure 24 the results of the accepted and rejected regions are depicted.

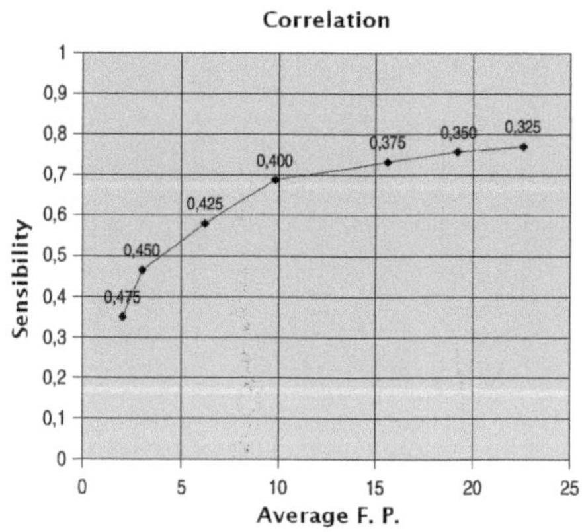

Fig. 22. Sensibility and False Positives values depending on the correlation threshold used.

In Table 5 the performance of the correlation filtering is showed.

Images type	Red Lesions	no R. Lesions
Sensibility	81%	N/A
False positives	22	4

Table 5. Results obtained applying the correlation filtering to the output from stage one described in section 3.

5.4 Creases-based filtering

Finally, in the last of the filtering processes the creases computed from the original digital retinal image are used as landmarks (in Figure 25 the cropped creases image of the Figure 11(a) is shown).

Regions intersected by creases will be removed if its mean value is over 0.25. This filter removes the regions near inside the vascular tree, which must be discarded in the analysis of red lesions. Figure 26 shows an example of a candidate region removed by the creases filter.

Figure 27 represents the variation of false positives and sensibility rate as the mean value set for removal of regions in this filter varies.

Figure 28 depicts the output result from this filter, which is also the final result of the algorithm. Again, red lesions are marked as green and blue areas.

The effectiveness of the crease-based filtering is described in Table 6.

Images type	Red Lesions	no R. Lesions
Sensibility	85%	N/A
False positives	36	7

Table 6. Crease-based filtering results.

Finally, the complete algorithm with all its stages is depicted in Figure 29.

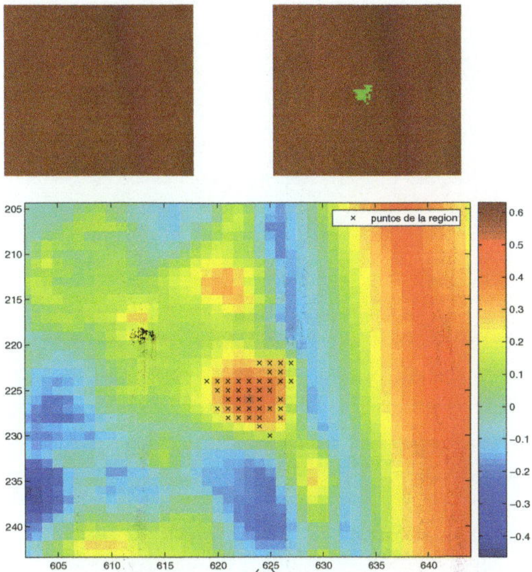

(a)

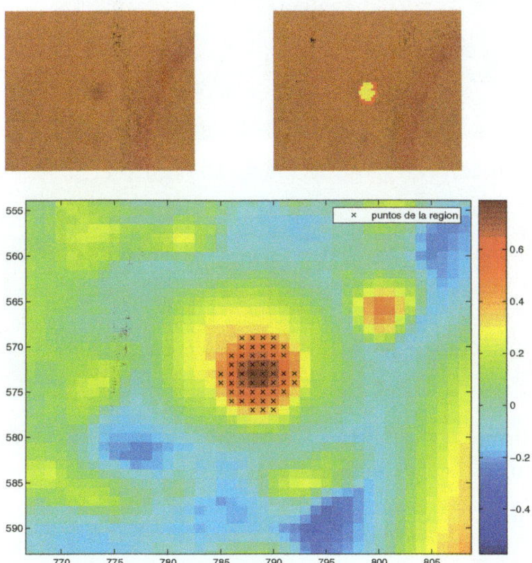

(b)

Fig. 23. Example of a candidate lesion removed 23(a), and a candidate region preserved 23(b) by the mean correlation filter. In 23(a), first row shows the original area in the retina (left) and the candidate lesion (right). In second row values of correlation are shown. In 23(b) the same figures are presented with the same interpretation, but in this case values of correlation lead to the preservation of the candidate region.

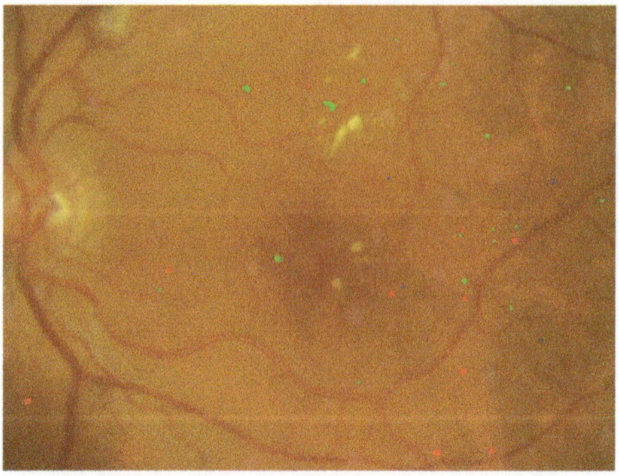

Fig. 24. Cropped region from the output image after applying the correlation filtering process. Regions are marked as green and blue areas.

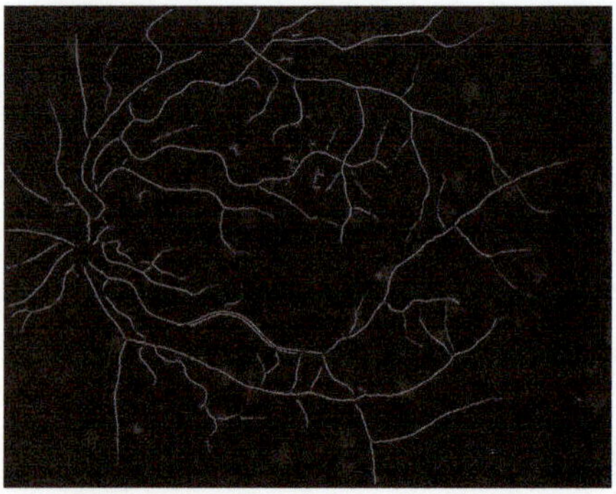

Fig. 25. Creases of the cropped region of the image in Figure 11(a), used to remove regions inside or near vessels.

Fig. 26. Sample of a candidate region removed by the creases filter. From left to right, original image, candidate region and creases image.

6. Validation and results

To validate the algorithm described in previous sections, an experiment was designed in collaboration with the oculists of the Complejo Hospitalario Universitario de Santiago (CHUS) and Instituto Tecnológico de Oftalmología de Santiago (ITO). From the set of 75 images, captured using a Canon CR5 nonmydriatic 3CCD camera at 45° field of view, the clinician manually marked the red lesions detected in 50 of the images. Then, the same images were input to the system, and obtained results were compared. 25 images without lesions were also input to the system, in order to evaluate its response to healthy people images, and to count the number of false positives. Figure 30 shows an image analyzed by the clinician, with the red

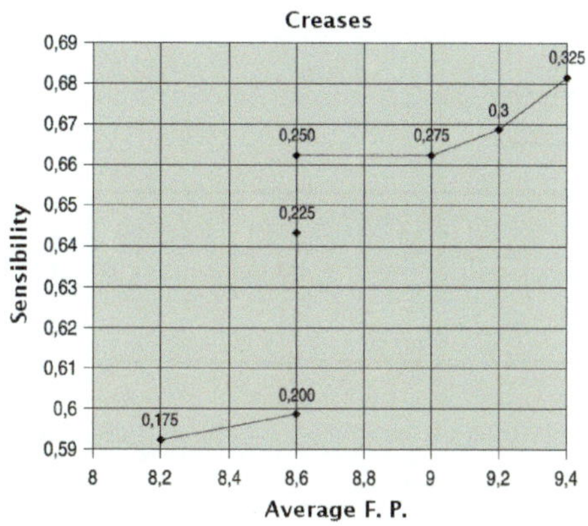

Fig. 27. Sensibility and False Positives values depending on the creases threshold used.

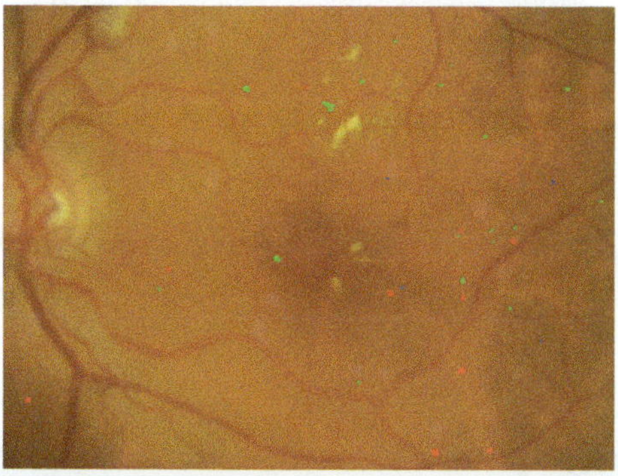

Fig. 28. Cropped region from the output image after applying the creases-based filtering process. Regions are marked as green and blue areas.

lesions marked as yellow areas. To visually compare the results obtained with the algorithm described, the red lesions also detected by the system (true positives) are also rounded by a blue circle, the false positives are marked as green circles, and false negatives are marked as red circles.

Results obtained with the whole test set of 75 images reported the numbers in Table 7, for the images with (first column) and without (second column) red lesions. First and second row show the total number of features detected (not applicable in the case of images without lesions for the manual process) for the manual segmentation and using the algorithm, respectively. In the third row the number of false positives is shown (N.A. in the case of images without red lesions). Fourth row contains the number of successfully recovered lesions, and finally fifth row display the number of false negatives (N.A. in the case of images without red lesions).

From the results in Table 7, it can be seen that 70.7% of the detected lesions are correctly detected, with a sensitivity of 0.785%, which compared with the results from the introduction

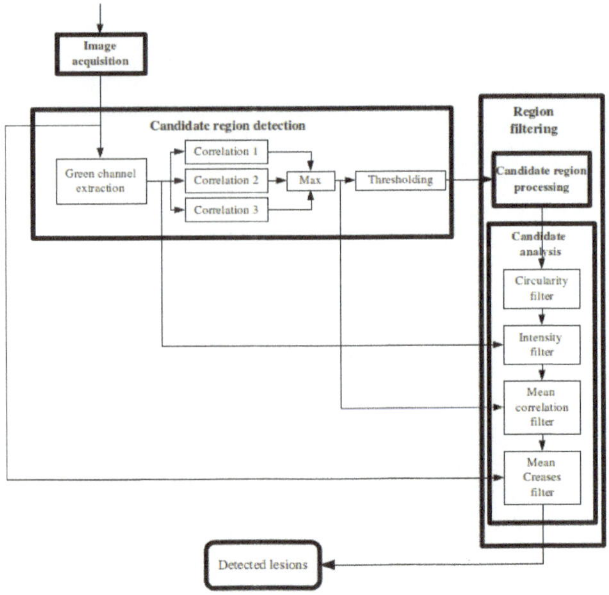

Fig. 29. Representation of the whole algorithm with the different stages where the images are processed.

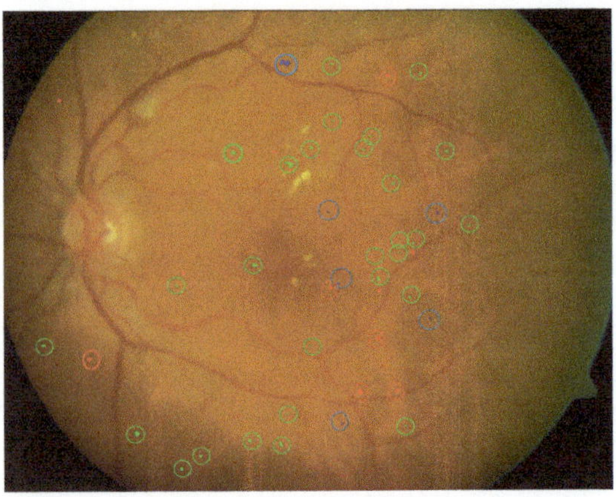

Fig. 30. Comparison of the manual and automatic red lesions detection in image from Figure 11(a). True positives are rounded by a green circle, the false positives are marked as blue circles, and false negatives are marked as red circles.

	Images with red lesions	Images without red lesions
# candidates (manual)	1570.0	N.A.
# candidates (automatic)	1470.0	220.0
# T.P.	1040.0	N.A.
# F.P.	430.0	220.0
# F.N.	530.0	N.A.

Table 7. Numbers obtained in the evaluation of the system for the images with (first column) and without (second column) red lesions. First and second rows show the total number of features detected (not applicable, N.A., in the case of images without lesions for the manual process) for the manual segmentation and using the algorithm, respectively. In the third row the number of false positives is shown (again, N.A. in the case of images without red lesions). Fourth row contains the number of successfully recovered lesions, and finally fifth row display the number of false negatives (N.A. in the case of images without red lesions).

indicates that our system could be a really helpful tool in a real screening system, reducing workload of expert clinicians by pre-filtering patients which present some kind of lesion.

7. Conclusions

In this work a system to assist in the detection of red lesions on digital retinal angiographies have been presented and validated through the whole process. The system performs in three stages: in the first stage candidate areas to be red lesions are detected by means of a set of correlation filters, adapted to different resolutions. This way features of different sizes can be detected. Then, in the second stage, a growing region algorithm together with a matched threshold allows the rejection of candidates which does not fit in the size of the red lesions. Finally, in a third stage, false positives are remove by filtering the output with four matched filters, which analyze several high level knowledge of the candidate regions: shape (searching for circularity), intensity (searching for dark areas), size (with a correlation filter) and finally discarding regions inside the vascular tree by means of the crease lines.

The whole algorithm has proven to be robust and accurate, with a sensitivity of 0.785%, although a bigger set of images and further validation is needed.

8. References

Cree, M., Olson, J., McHardy, K., Sharp, P. & Forrester, J. (1997). A fully automated comparative microaneurysm digital detection system, *Eye* 11: 622–628.

Fernandez-Vigo, J., Macho, J. S., Rey, A. D., Barros, J., Tome, M. & Bueno, J. (1993). The prevalence of diabetic retinopathy in northwest spain.an epidemiological study of diabetic retinopathy in galicia., *Acta Ophthalmologica* Vol. 71(1): 22–26.

García, M., Sanchez, C., López, M., Diez, A. & Hornero, R. (2008). Automatic detection of red lesions in retinal images using a multilayer perceptron neural network, *Proceedings of Conference in Engineering in Medicine and Biology Society*, pp. 5425–5428.

García, M., Sanchez, C., López, M., Poza, J. & Hornero, R. (2009). Detection of hard exudates in retinal images using a radial basis function classifier, *Annals of biomedical engineering* Vol. 37(7): 1448–1463.

Gardner, G., Keating, D., Williamson, T. & Elliot, E. (1996). Detection of diabetic retinopathy using neural network analysis of fundus images, *Br. J. Ophthalmol.* 80(11): 937–948.

Goldbaum, M., Katz, N. & Nelson, M. (1990). The discrimination of similarly colored objects in computer images of the ocular fundus, *Investigat. Ophthalmol.* 31: 617–623.

Hipwell, J., Strachant, F., Olson, J., McHardy, K., Sharp, P. & Forrester, J. (2000). Automated detection of mycroaneurisms in digital red-free photographs: a diabetic retinopathy screening tool, *Diabetic Med.* 19: 588–594.

Hoover, A. & Goldbaum, M. (2000). Locating the optic nerve in a retinal image using the fuzzy convergence of the blood vessels, *IEEE Trans. Med. Imag.* 22(8): 951–958.

Jähne, B. (2005). *Digital image processing*, sexta edn, Springer, Berlín, Alemania.

Kempen, J., O'Colmain, B., Leske, M., Haffner, S., Klein, R., Moss, S., Taylor, H. & Hamman, R. (2004). The prevalence of diabetic retinopathy among adults in the united states, *Arch Ophthalmol.* Vol. 122(4): 552–563.

Larsen, M., Godt, J., Larsen, N., Lund-Andersen, H., Sjølie, A., Agardh, E., Kalm, H., Grunkin, M. & Owens, D. (2003). Automated detection of fundus photographic red lesions in diabetic retinopathy, *Investigat. Ophthalmol. Vis. Sci.* 44(2): 761–766.

Leistritz, L. & Schweitzer, D. (1994). Automated detection and quantification of exudates in retinal images, *SPIE* 2298: 690–696.

López, A., Lloret, D., Serrat, J. & Villanueva, J. (2000). Multilocal creaseness based on the level-set extrinsic curvature, *Computer Vision and Image Understanding* 77(1): 111–144.

Mariño, C., Penedo, M. G., Penas, M., Carreira, M. J. & González, F. (2006). Personal authentication using digital retinal images, *Pattern Analysis and Applications* 9(1): 21–33.

Niemeijer, M., van Ginneken, B., Stall, J., Suttorp-Schulten, M. & Abrámoff, M. (2005). Automatic detection of red lesions in digital color fundus photographs, *IEEE Trans. Med. Imag.* 24(5): 584–592.

Philips, R., Spencer, T., Ross, P., Sharp, P. & Forrester, J. (1993). Quantification of diabetic maculopathy by digital imaging of the fundus, *Eye* 5: 130–137.

RA, P., SA, R., BB, M., FB, J. & MM., I. (2010). Prevalence and relationship between diabetic retinopathy and nephropathy, and its risk factors in the north-east of spain, a population-based study, *Ophthalmic Epidemiology* Vol. 17(4): 251–265.

Russ, J. C. (1995). *The image processing handbook*, third edn, Springer-Verlag and CRC Press and IEEE Press, Nueva York, EE.UU.

Sinthanayothin, C., Boyce, J., Williamson, T., Cook, H., Mensah, E., Lal, S. & Usher, D. (2002). Automated detection of diabetic retinopathy on digital fundus images, *Diabetic Med.* 19: 105–112.

Spencer, T., Olson, J., McHardy, K., Sharp, P. & Forrester, J. (1996). An image processing strategy for the segmentation and quantification in fluorescein angiograms of the ocular fundus, *Computing Biomedical Research* 29: 284–302.

Tapp, R. J., Shaw, J. E., Harper, C. A., de Courten, M. P., Balkau, B., Taylor, D. J. M. H. R., Welborn, T. A. & Zimmet, P. Z. (2003). The prevalence of and factors associated with diabetic retinopathy in the australian population, *Diabetes Care* Vol. 26(6): 1731–1737.

Ward, N., Tomlinson, S. & Taylor, C. (1989). Image analysis of fundus photographs. the detection and measurement of exudates associated with diabetic retinopathy, *Ophthalmology* 96(1): 80–86.

Part 4

Emerging Treatments and Concepts in Diabetic Retinopathy

14

Prophylactic Medical Treatment of Diabetic Retinopathy

Akihiro Kakehashi et al.*
Department of Ophthalmology, Jichi Medical University, Saitama Medical Center, Saitama Japan

1. Introduction

Diabetic retinopathy (DR) is a leading cause of visual loss and blindness in adults in developed and developing countries (Friedman et al., 2011). Clinical trials have shown that intensive glycemic control reduces the incidence and progression of DR (Reichard et al., 1993; Stratton et al., 2001; DCCT, 2002). Other metabolic factors also affect the progression and development of DR. The UK Prospective Diabetes Study Group reported that tight blood pressure control is effective for reducing the incidence of DR (UK Prospective Diabetes Study Group, 1998a, 1998b). The EUCLID study group reported that inhibitors of angiotensin-converting enzyme drugs decreased the progression of retinopathy in patients without hypertension who had type 1 diabetes with little or no nephropathy (Chaturvedi et al., 1998). Lipid-lowering therapy with fenofibrate also might reduce the progression of DR (Chew et al., 2010; Keech et al., 2007). Among the metabolic factors, although glycemic control seems to be the most important, achieving acceptable glucose homeostasis is difficult, even when patients are highly compliant. Furthermore, DR continues to develop and progress even in patients who are treated intensively to achieve better glycemic control. Therefore, it is important to find medical options other than glycemic control to prevent diabetic ocular complications. The metabolic changes that accompany hyperglycemia, such as activation of the polyol pathway (Gabbay, 1973; Lorenzi, 2007; Robison et al., 1988; 1989), activation of protein kinase C (PKC) (Frank, 2002; Liang et al., 2005; Shiba et al., 1993), increased oxidative stress (Gurler et al., 2000; Jennings et al., 1991; Pan et al., 2008; Pinto et al., 2007), leukocyte adhesion to the endothelial cells (McLeod et al., 1995; Miyamoto et al., 1996; Schroder et al., 1991), and accumulation of advanced glycation end products (AGEs)

---

*Ayumi Ota[1], Fumihiko Toyoda[1], Nozomi Kinoshita[1], Hiroko Yamagami[1], Hiroto Obata[1], Takafumi Matsumoto[2], Junichi Tsuji[2], Yoh Dobashi,[3] Wilfred Y. Fujimoto[3,4], Masanobu Kawakami[3] and Yasunori Kanazawa[3]
[1]*Department of Ophthalmology, Jichi Medical University, Saitama Medical Center,*
[2]*Pharmacology Research Laboratories, Dainippon Sumitomo Pharma Co., Ltd.*
[3]*Department of Integrated Medicine I, Jichi Medical University, Saitama Medical Center,*
[4]*Division of Metabolism, Endocrinology and Nutrition,*
University of Washington School of Medicine, Seattle, WA,
[1,2,3]*Japan*
[4]*USA*

(Chibber et al., 1997; Hirata et al., 1997; Kakehashi et al., 2008), are related to the development and progression of diabetic ocular complications. In particular, the polyol pathway is correlated strongly with oxidative stress, activation of PKC, and accumulation of AGEs that lead to induction of vascular endothelial growth factor (VEGF). A key enzyme in the polyol pathway, aldose reductase (AR), is found in the retina and lens (Akagi et al., 1983; Kern & Engerman, 1981). AR inhibitors (ARIs) slowed thickening of the basement membrane of the retinal capillaries and progression of diabetic cataract in experimental studies (Hu et al., 1983; Robison et al., 1983). Thus, the polyol pathway might be the most attractive target for adjunctive treatment to prevent development of diabetic ocular complications. Based on favorable observations from experimental studies using ARIs (Obrosova et al., 2005; Okuda et al., 1985; Robinson et al., 1996; Sun et al., 2006; Yeh et al., 1986), a clinical trial of the ARI, sorbinil, was conducted in 1990, but this drug did not affect the development of DR, and enthusiasm for the clinical application of ARIs waned. To test drugs to treat DR, good animal models of DR would be useful. In this context, the spontaneously diabetic Torii (SDT) rat, a newly established non-obese type 2 diabetes model rat, seems especially appropriate, since it shows advanced DR resembling that in humans (Kakehashi et al., 2006; Kakehashi, 2011a, b; Shinohara et al., 2000). A recent study showed a strong preventative effect of ARIs on the development of DR in this animal model (Kakehashi et al., 2011).

In this chapter, we discuss several studies of medical treatment to prevent DR including our previous and ongoing studies using SDT rats. Among the various medical treatments, we have focused on the ARIs, because we believe that they are the most potent and safest of the potential treatments.

2. ARIs

Many experimental studies of ARIs (Obrosova et al., 2005; Okuda et al., 1985; Robinson et al., 1996; Sun et al., 2006; Yeh et al., 1986) have reported favorable results, with the exception of a clinical trial of sorbinil as mentioned previously.

However, our recent study on the effects of the ARI, fidarestat (SNK-860; Sanwa Kagaku Kenkyusho, Nagoya, Japan), in SDT rats showed that the drug strongly inhibited the development of DR (Kakehashi et al., 2011). We evaluated four rat groups: untreated, low- and high-dose (8 and 32 mg/kg/day) fidarestat-treated SDT rats, and nondiabetic control Sprague-Dawley (SD) rats. We evaluated the DR and measured the retinal sorbitol and reduced glutathione (GSH), VEGF in the ocular fluid, and urinary 8-hydroxy-2'-deoxyguanosine (8-OHdG). Compared with the untreated the incidence of DR was significantly lower in the low- and high-dose fidarestat groups group. Compared with the untreated group, the retinal sorbitol levels were lower in the control and low- and high-dose groups; the retinal GSH levels were higher in the control and the low- and high-dose groups; the VEGF levels were lower in the control and low- and high-dose groups; and the 8-OHdG levels were lower in the control and low- and high-dose groups. The results indicated that fidarestat prevents DR in SDT rats by suppressing oxidative stress and sorbitol production.

Based on these findings, we evaluated the recently developed ARI, ranirestat (AS-3201, Dainippon Sumitomo Pharmaceutical Co., Ltd., Osaka, Japan) for treating DR in SDT rats.

Male SDT rats and SD rats were obtained from CLEA, Inc., Tokyo, Japan. All SDT rats were confirmed to be diabetic based on a non-fasting blood glucose concentration exceeding 19.4 mmol/L. All rats were fed standard rat chow (CRF-1, Oriental Yeast, Inc., Tokyo, Japan) with or without ARI. Epalrestat (Kinedak, Ono Pharmaceutical Co., Ltd., Osaka, Japan), an ARI that is commercially available in Japan, was used as the positive control. The ranirestat-treated rats received the drug once daily; the epalrestat-treated rats were fed chow containing epalrestat at the onset of diabetes; and the SD rats and untreated SDT rats were fed chow without an ARI.

The animals were divided into six groups: normal SD rats (n=8), untreated SDT rats (n=9), ranirestat-treated SDT rats (0.1 mg/kg/day for 40 weeks, n=7; 1.0 mg/kg/day for 40 weeks, n=8; 10.0 mg/kg/day for 40 weeks, n=7), and epalrestat-treated SDT rats (100 mg/kg/day for 40 weeks) (n=8).

The body weight, blood glucose, and glycosylated hemoglobin (HbA1c) were measured once monthly. Blood samples were collected from the tail vein of the non-fasting rats to measure the plasma glucose and glycosylated hemoglobin levels. The body weight was greater in the SD than that in SDT rats with or without treatment ($p<0.01$). The mean plasma glucose levels and HbA1c levels in the SD rats were significantly ($p<0.01$) lower than in the SDT rats with or without treatment. However, there were no significant differences in the blood glucose levels and HbA1c levels between the treated and untreated SDT rats, indicating that an ARI did not affect the glycemic control. Therefore, we did not have to consider any effect of glycemia in interpreting results.

Fluorescein-dextran microscopy was performed after intracardiac injection of fluorescein-dextran (fluorescein isothiocyanate dextran, Sigma, St. Louis, MO, USA), using a modification of the method of D'Amato et al. (1993). With the animals under deep anesthesia induced by intraperitoneal injection of pentobarbital sodium (25 mg/kg body weight, Nembutal, Dainihonseiyaku, Osaka, Japan), 1 ml of phosphate buffered saline containing 50 mg of fluorescein dextran was injected into the left ventricle of each animal. After 5 minutes, the eyes were enucleated for fluorescein microscopy. The retinas were peeled from the eyecups, and the entire retinas were flat-mounted on a slide glass without fixation. A drop of aqueous mounting medium (Crystal/Mount, Biomeda Corp., Foster City, CA, USA) was applied over the retinas and allowed to dry. The flat-mounted retinas were examined by fluorescence microscopy (Nikon SMZ1500 with P-FLA fluorescence attachment, Nikon, Tokyo, Japan). As we reported previously (Kakehashi et al., 2006), DR was diagnosed when extensive fluorescein leakage was seen around the optic disc, and we classified the DR into three stages: no retinopathy (no dye leakage), mild retinopathy (mild dye leakage around the optic disc), and severe retinopathy (extensive dye leakage throughout the entire retina) (Fig. 1).

With the animals under deep anesthesia induced by intraperitoneal injection of pentobarbital sodium, the eyes were enucleated for conventional histopathologic studies and placed in a fixative (Superfix KY-500, Kurabo, Tokyo, Japan) to avoid iatrogenic retinal detachment. The fixed eyes were washed in 0.1% mol/L cacodylate buffer and embedded in paraffin. The paraffin block was cut into 4-μm sections and stained with hematoxylin and eosin for conventional histopathologic examination. As reported previously (Kakehashi et al., 2006), DR was diagnosed when large retinal folds mimicking tractional retinal detachment around the optic disc were observed.

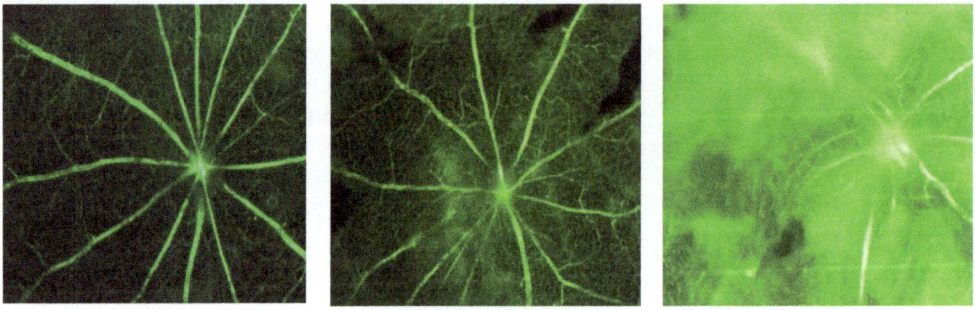

Fig. 1. Classification of diabetic retinopathy. Retinopathy (-), no dye leakage; retinopathy(+), mild dye leakage around the optic disc; retinopathy (++), extensive dye leakage throughout the retina.

Compared with controls (7/9 eyes), DR did not develop in any ranirestat-treated groups (0.1 mg/kg/day; 1.0 mg/kg/day; 10.0 mg/kg/day for 40 weeks) (0/7, 0/8, 0/7 eyes, $p<0.01$, chi-square test). Mild DR developed in the epalrestat-treated group (100 mg/kg/day for 40 weeks) (2/8 eyes; $p=0.09$ by the chi-square test). Epalrestat did not prevent development of DR in SDT rats. The incidence of DR was significantly ($p<0.01$) lower in the ranirestat-treated groups compared with the untreated group.

Immunohistochemical procedures were based on the standard avidin-biotin horseradish peroxidase method using the appropriate antibody and developed with AEC Substrate Chromogen (DakoCytomation, Carpinteria, CA, USA). VEGF was immunostained with a monoclonal antibody for human VEGF (1:25 dilution, Immuno-Biological Laboratories Co., Ltd., Fujioka, Japan). Carboxymethyl-lysine (CML) was immunostained with a monoclonal antibody for human AGEs (1:50 dilution for CML, Trans Genic Inc., Kumamoto, Japan). Bovine serum was used as the primary antibody for the negative control. The immunostaining grades were divided into three groups: minimal (-), moderate (+), and severe (++). Minimal staining was characterized by almost no retinal staining, moderate staining by light red retinal staining, and severe staining by intense dark red retinal staining. Fig. 2 shows immunostaining for CML and VEGF. Immunostaining for CML was very strong in the untreated eye (upper left) compared with minimal staining in the ranirestat-treated (10 mg/kg/day for 40 weeks) eye (lower left). Immunostaining for VEGF was moderate in the untreated eye (upper right) compared with minimal staining in the ranirestat-treated eye (lower right).

Strong immunostaining for CML was seen in eight of nine eyes of the untreated SDT rats. The staining significantly ($p<0.05$) decreased to the moderate level in the eyes treated with 1.0 mg/kg/day and 10.0 mg/kg/day of ranirestat, except for those treated with 0.1 mg/kg/day of ranirestat ($p=0.111$). Epalrestat did not have a significant ($p=0.241$) effect. Moderate immunostaining for VEGF was seen in eight of nine eyes in the untreated SDT rats, and this decreased significantly ($p<0.05$) to minimal staining in the rats treated with 1.0 mg/kg/day and 10.0 mg/kg/day of ranirestat, but not in those treated with the 0.1 mg/kg/day dose of ranirestat ($p=0.117$). Epalrestat did not have a significant effect ($p=0.247$).

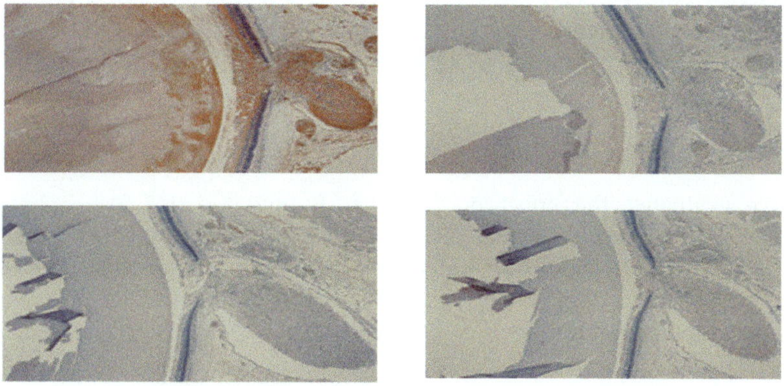

Fig. 2. Immunostaining for CML and VEGF. Immunostaining for CML shows strong staining in the untreated eye (upper left) compared with minimal staining in the ranirestat-treated eye (lower left). Immunostaining for VEGF shows moderate staining in the untreated eye (upper right) compared with minimal staining in the ranirestat-treated eye (lower right).

The retinal sorbitol and fructose levels were measured. ARI activity was determined after the liquid chromatography-tandem mass spectrometry method was performed. Briefly, rats were anesthetized with sodium pentobarbital (50 mg/kg, intra peritoneally; Abbott, Abbott Park, IL, USA), and the retinas were removed, promptly cooled with liquid nitrogen, and stored at −50°C. The samples for the sorbitol and fructose assay were prepared by protein precipitation followed by a solid-phase extraction procedure. The API 4000 Mass Spectrometer (AB SCIEX, Tokyo, Japan) was operated in the selected-reaction monitoring mode under optimized conditions to detect sorbitol- or fructose-negative ions formed by atmospheric pressure chemical ionization. At 15 weeks, the sorbitol levels in the retina of the SDT rats treated with ranirestat (10.0 mg/kg/day) were lower than in the untreated eyes. Eparlestat did not affect the retinal sorbitol levels. However, there were no significant differences in the sorbitol levels among the treated and untreated SDT rats at 40 weeks. Retinal fructose levels were lower at 15 weeks in SDT rats treated with ranirestat (10.0 mg/kg/day) than those that were untreated. Eparlestat did not affect the retinal fructose levels. At 40 weeks, there were no significant differences in the retinal fructose levels among the rat groups.

3. Other options for prophylactic medical treatment of DR

3.1 PKC β inhibitor

Liang and coworkers (2005) reported amelioration of vascular dysfunction in diabetic rats using an oral PKC β inhibitor. Those authors later reported that VEGF increases intraocular vascular permeability through activation of PKC in vivo and suggested that oral pharmacologic therapies involving PKC β-isoform-selective inhibitors might be effective for treating DR (Aiello et al., 1997). Based on their report, the oral PKC β inhibitor, ruboxistaurin (RBX) (LY333531, Eli Lilly and Co., Indianapolis, IN), administered to patients with diabetes with no or mild DR, ameliorated diabetes-induced retinal circulation time abnormalities (Aiello et al., 2006). Another multicenter, double-masked, randomized, placebo-controlled study in patients with diabetes with moderate to very severe nonproliferative diabetic retinopathy showed that RBX was well tolerated and reduced the risk of visual loss but did not prevent DR progression (PKC-DRS Study Group, 2005).

We evaluated the effect of our PKC β inhibitor (JTT-010, Takatsuki, Japan) on the development of diabetic ocular complications in SDT rats. The rats had delayed oscillatory potentials on electroretinography, but DR developed eventually. We concluded that PKC β inhibitors may require concurrent administration of antihyperglycemic drugs to achieve maximal therapeutic effects on DR (Sasase et al., 2009).

3.2 Anti-AGE agents

Previous studies have suggested the concept of "metabolic memory" associated with accumulation of AGEs as DR develops (Chibber et al., 1997; Genuth et al., 2005; Hammes et al., 1999). Another anti-AGE agent, pyridoxamine, also prevented development of DR (Stitt et al., 2002). However, clinical trials of anti-AGE agents for the treatment of DR have not yet been conducted.

Based on those reports, we evaluated the effects of oral aminoguanidine and pyridoxamine on the development of cataract and DR in SDT rats (Toyoda et al., 2011) and reported that aminoguanidine prevented accumulation of CML and resulted in almost complete inhibition of DR, but pyridoxamine did not prevent DR. Aminoguanidine seems to be a stronger inhibitor of DR than pyridoxamine.

3.3 Anti-leukocyte adhesion agents

Leukocyte adhesion to the diabetic retinal vasculature is thought to be the critical early event in the pathogenesis of DR, resulting in breakdown of the blood-retinal barrier and in capillary nonperfusion (Gurler et al., 2000; Hu et al., 1983). Adamis and coworkers (1994) reported that the antileukocyte adhesion agents, anti-intercellular adhesion molecule-1 antibody (Miyamoto et al., 1999) and anti-CD 18 antibody (Barouch et al., 2000), were useful for treating experimental DR. They also showed an antileukocyte adhesion effect using a PKC β inhibitor (Nonaka et al., 2000) and receptor for the AGEs (Kaji et al., 2007). Nagai et al. (2007) reported an inhibitory effect of an angiotensin II type 1 receptor blocker on retinal leukostasis in diabetic mice.

We tested several commercially available antileukocyte adhesion agents in diabetic rats. We first evaluated the effectiveness of the sulphonylurea gliclazide for decreasing the adhesion of neutrophils to endothelial cells and leukocyte entrapment in the retinal microcirculation of streptozotocin (STZ)-induced diabetic rats. We showed that gliclazide attenuated retinal leukostasis irrespective of hyperglycemia in diabetic rats, whereas another sulphonylurea, glibenclamide, did not. This indicated that gliclazide, among the sulphonylurea drugs, might be selectively beneficial for preventing development of DR (Kinoshita et al., 2002). We also evaluated the effectiveness of topical nipradilol, a topical antiglaucoma αβ-blocker and nitric oxide donor, on retinal microvascular leukocyte adhesion in diabetic rats. Topical nipradilol significantly reduced retinal leukostasis in the retinal microcirculation of STZ-induced diabetic rats, and we think that nipradilol may be a prophylactic agent that can inhibit development of early DR through its nitric oxide donor effects on the microcirculation. We believe that most antileukocyte adhesion agents can slow progression of DR but do not inhibit it completely. Good glycemic control or other additional medical treatments are needed to achieve a maximal effect on DR.

3.4 Anti-VEGF agents

Since the VEGF levels increase as DR progresses (Adamis et al., 1994; Aiello et al., 1994; Amin et al., 1997; Lutty et al., 1996), VEGF is very important in the development and progression of DR. VEGF is also a vascular permeability factor and plays an important role in the development of diabetic macular edema (DME) (Mathews et al., 1997). Based on these observations, several anti-VEGF agents such as an anti-VEGF antibody (Adamis et al., 1996), soluble VEGF-receptor chimeric proteins (Aiello et al., 1995), and antisense phosphorothioate oligodeoxynucleotides against VEGF (Robinson et al., 1996) have been tested in an animal model of retinal neovascularization mimicking DR. The results were very promising. Based on these favorable results in animal studies, several clinical studies have been undertaken to evaluate treatment of DME using an anti-VEGF antibody. The RESOLVE Study evaluated the safety and efficacy of intravitreal ranibizumab (Lucentis, Genentech, Inc., South San Francisco, CA) for treating patients with DME (Massin et al., 2010). Ranibizumab is a fully humanized monoclonal antibody fragment, which binds to multiple variants of VEGF-A, and is approved to treat age-related macular degeneration. The results indicated that intravitreal ranibizumab improves visual acuity and reduces macular thickness in DME. The Diabetic Retinopathy Clinical Research Network (DRCR.net) is evaluating and comparing several medical treatments for DME. The DRCR.net is a collaborative network formed in September 2002 that is dedicated to facilitating multicenter clinical studies of DR, DME, and associated conditions. Currently, there are more than 109 participating sites with over 320 physicians throughout the United States (http://drcrnet.jaeb.org/). The DRCR.net reported that intravitreal ranibizumab combined with laser treatment is more effective than laser treatment with or without triamcinolone. The anti-VEGF agents inhibit VEGF and increase capillary permeability. Macular edema is resolved by blocking increased capillary permeability. However, a drawback of the anti-VEGF agents is that they do not have long-term efficacy, so repeated injections are usually required. Moreover, a 2% prevalence of endophthalmitis over 12 months in the RESOLVE Study is worrisome. To minimize the number of intravitreal injections, gene therapy using a safe virus vector, such as an adeno-associated virus (Ideno et al., 2007), may be a future option for treating DME.

4. Comments

Good glycemic control is the most important factor for preventing the development and progression of diabetic ocular complications. However, it is also difficult to obtain good glycemic control in many clinical cases. In this chapter, we discussed several additional medical therapeutic options for diabetic ocular complications. PKC β inhibitors and antileukocyte adhesion agents might help prevent DR, but neither was sufficient without good concurrent glycemic control or other additional medical treatments. Anti-VEGF agents have a strong therapeutic effect in DME; however, they do not have long-term efficacy and the possibility of complications, such as endophthalmitis, associated with injection of anti-VEGF agents into the vitreous is a concern. Thus, anti-VEGF agents do not seem to be safe therapeutic options for preventing diabetic ocular complications. Oral anti-AGE agents seem to be good prophylactic medical treatments for DR in experimental animal studies. Clinical trials of oral anti-AGE agents for treating DR are worthwhile. Among the several prophylactic medical treatments for DR, we focused on the ARIs in this chapter. Epalrestat, which is commercially available in Japan, has been widely used to treat diabetic neuropathy. Although the effect of eparlestat on DR has not been clearly recognized in a clinical trial, the safety and clinical effects of long-term oral administration of the drug for treating diabetic neuropathy have been established. Thus, we believe that our findings suggest the potential therapeutic usefulness of a new ARI, ranirestat, for preventing DR. Importantly, it appears that ranirestat might prevent DR even without strict glycemic control. We look forward to the development and evaluation of new ARIs with minimal side effects for use in future clinical studies to prevent DR.

5. References

Adamis, A. P., Miller, J.W., Bernal, M.T., D'Amico, D.J., Folkman J., Yeo T.K. & K. Yeo T. (1994) Increased vascular endothelial growth factor levels in the vitreous of eyes with proliferative diabetic retinopathy. *Am J Ophthalmol,* Vol. 118, No. 4 (October 1994), pp. 445-450, ISSN 0002-9394

Adamis, A. P., Shima, D.T., Tolentino, M.J., Gragoudas, E.S., Ferrara, N., Folkman J., D'Amore, P.A. & Miller J.W. (1996) Inhibition of vascular endothelial growth factor prevents retinal ischemia-associated iris neovascularization in a nonhuman primate. *Arch Ophthalmol,* Vol. 114, No. 1 (January 1996), pp. 66-71, ISSN 0003-9950

Aiello, L. P., Avery R.L., Arrigg, P.G., Keyt, B.A., Jampel, H.D., Shah, S. T., Pasquale, L.R., Thieme, H., Iwamoto, M.A., Park, J.E. et al. (1994) Vascular endothelial growth factor in ocular fluid of patients with diabetic retinopathy and other retinal disorders. *N Engl J Med,* Vol. 331, No. 22 (December 1994), pp. 1480-1487, ISSN 0028-4793

Aiello, L. P., Pierce, E.A., Foley E.D., Takagi H., Chen H., Riddle L., Ferrara N., King, G.L. & Smith L.E. (1995) Suppression of retinal neovascularization in vivo by inhibition of vascular endothelial growth factor (VEGF) using soluble VEGF-receptor chimeric proteins. *Proc Natl Acad Sci U S A,* Vol. 92, No. 23 (November 1995), pp. 10457-10461, ISSN 0027-8424

Aiello, L. P., Bursell, S. E., Clermont, A., Duh, E., Ishii, H., Takagi, C., Mori, F., Ciulla, T. A., Ways, K., Jirousek, M., Smith, L. E., King, G. L. (1997) Vascular endothelial growth factor-induced retinal permeability is mediated by protein kinase C in vivo and suppressed by an orally effective beta-isoform-selective inhibitor. *Diabetes,* Vol. 46, No. 9 (September 1997), pp.1473-80, ISSN 0012-1797

Aiello, L. P., Clermont A., Arora V., Davis, M.D., Sheetz, M.J. & Bursell, S.E. (2006) Inhibition of PKC beta by oral administration of ruboxistaurin is well tolerated and ameliorates diabetes-induced retinal hemodynamic abnormalities in patients. *Invest Ophthalmol Vis Sci,* Vol. 47, No. 1 (January 2006), pp. 86-92, ISSN 0146-0404

Akagi, Y., Kador, P.F., Kuwabara, T. & Kinoshita, J.H. (1983) Aldose reductase localization in human retinal mural cells. *Invest Ophthalmol Vis Sci,* Vol. 24, No. 11 (November 1983), pp. 1516-1519, ISSN 0146-0404

Amin, R. H., Frank, R. N., Kennedy, A., Eliott, D., Puklin, J. E., Abrams, G. W. (1997) Vascular endothelial growth factor is present in glial cells of the retina and optic nerve of human subjects with nonproliferative diabetic retinopathy. *Invest Ophthalmol Vis Sci,* Vol. 38, No. 1 (January 1997), pp. 36-47, ISSN 0146-0404

Barouch, F. C., Miyamoto, K., Allport J.R., Fujita K., Bursell, S.E., Aiello L.P., Luscinskas, F.W. & Adamis, A.P. (2000) Integrin-mediated neutrophil adhesion and retinal leukostasis in diabetes. *Invest Ophthalmol Vis Sci,* Vol. 41, No. 5 (April 2000), pp. 1153-1158, ISSN 0146-0404

Chaturvedi, N., Sjolie, A.K., Stephenson, J.M., Abrahamian, H., Keipes M., Castellarin, A., Rogulja-Pepeonik, Z. & Fuller, J.H. (1998) Effect of lisinopril on progression of retinopathy in normotensive people with type 1 diabetes. The EUCLID Study Group. EURODIAB Controlled Trial of Lisinopril in Insulin-Dependent Diabetes Mellitus. *Lancet,* Vol. 351, No. 9095 (January 1998), pp. 28-31, ISSN 0140-6736

Chew, E. Y., Ambrosius, W.T., Davis, M.D., Danis, R.P., Gangaputra, S., Greven, C.M., Hubbard, L., Esser, B.A., Lovato, J.F., Perdue, L.H., Goff, D.C., Jr., Cushman, W.C., Ginsberg, H.N., Elam, M.B., Genuth, S., Gerstein, H.C., Schubart, U. & Fine, L.J. (2010) Effects of medical therapies on retinopathy progression in type 2 diabetes. *N Engl J Med,* Vol. 363, No. 3 (July 2010), pp. 233-244, ISSN 1533-4406

Chibber, R., Molinatti, P.A., Rosatto, N., Lambourne, B. & Kohner, E.M. (1997) Toxic action of advanced glycation end products on cultured retinal capillary pericytes and endothelial cells: relevance to diabetic retinopathy. *Diabetologia,* Vol. 40, No. 2 (February 1997), pp. 156-164, ISSN 0012-186X

D'Amato, R., Wesolowski, E., Smith, L. E. (1993) Microscopic visualization of the retina by angiography with high-molecular-weight fluorescein-labeled dextrans in the mouse. *Microvasc Res,* Vol. 46, No. 2 (September 1993), pp. 135-42, ISSN 0026-2862

DCCT (2002) Effect of intensive diabetes treatment on the microvascular complications of type 1 diabetes mellites. The Diabetes Control and Complications Trial. *JAMA,* vol 287, No. 19, (May 2002), pp. 2563-9, ISSN 0098-7484

Frank, R. N. (2002) Potential new medical therapies for diabetic retinopathy: protein kinase C inhibitors. *Am J Ophthalmol,* Vol. 133, No. 5 (May 2002), pp. 693-698, ISSN 0002-9394

Friedman, D. S., Ali, F. & Kourgialis, N. (2011) Diabetic retinopathy in the developing world: how to approach identifying and treating underserved populations. *Am J Ophthalmol,* Vol. 151, No. 2 (February 2011), pp. 192-194 e191, ISSN 1879-1891

Gabbay, K. H. (1973) The sorbitol pathway and the complications of diabetes. *N Engl J Med,* Vol. 288, No. 16 (April 1973), pp. 831-836, ISSN 0028-4793

Genuth, S., Sun, W., Cleary, P., Sell, D.R., Dahms, W., Malone, J., Sivitz, W. & Monnier, V.M. (2005) Glycation and carboxymethyl lysine levels in skin collagen predict the risk of future 10-year progression of diabetic retinopathy and nephropathy in the Diabetes Control and Complications trial and epidemiology of diabetes interventions and complications participants with type 1 diabetes. *Diabetes,* Vol. 54, No. 11 (November 2005), pp. 3103-3111, ISSN 0012-1797

Gurler, B., Vural, H., Yilmaz, N., Oguz, H., Satici, A. & Aksoy, N. (2000) The role of oxidative stress in diabetic retinopathy. *Eye,* Vol. 14, Pt 5 (October 2000), pp. 730-735, ISSN 0950-222X

Hammes, H. P., Alt, A., Niwa, T., Clausen, J.T., Bretzel, R.G., Brownlee, M. & Schleicher, E.D. (1999) Differential accumulation of advanced glycation end products in the course of diabetic retinopathy. *Diabetologia,* Vol. 42, No. 6 (June 1999), pp. 728-736, ISSN 0012-186X

Hirata, C., Nakano, K., Nakamura, N., Kitagawa, Y., Shigeta, H., Hasegawa, G., Ogata, M., Ikeda, T., Sawa, H., Nakamura, K., Ienaga, K., Obayashi, H. & Kondo, M. (1997) Advanced glycation end products induce expression of vascular endothelial growth factor by retinal Muller cells. *Biochemical and Biophysical Research Communications,* Vol. 236, No. 3 (July 1997), pp. 712-715, ISSN 0006-291X

Hu, T. S., Datiles, M. & Kinoshita, J.H. (1983) Reversal of galactose cataract with sorbinil in rats. *Invest Ophthalmol Vis Sci,* Vol. 24, No. 5 (May 1983), pp. 640-644, ISSN 0146-0404

Ideno, J., Mizukami, H., Kakehashi, A., Saito, Y., Okada, T., Urabe, M., Kume, A., Kuroki, M., Kawakami, M., Ishibashi, S. & Ozawa, K. (2007) Prevention of diabetic retinopathy by intraocular soluble flt-1 gene transfer in a spontaneously diabetic rat model. *Int J Mol Med,* Vol. 19, No. 1 (January 2007), pp. 75-79, ISSN 1107-3756

Jennings, P. E., McLaren, M., Scott, N.A., Saniabadi, A.R. & Belch, J.J. (1991) The relationship of oxidative stress to thrombotic tendency in type 1 diabetic patients with retinopathy. *Diabetic Medicine: a Journal of the British Diabetic Association,* Vol. 8, No. 9 (November 1991), pp. 860-865, ISSN 0742-3071

Kaji, Y., Usui, T., Ishida, S., Yamashiro, K., Moore, T. C., Moore, J., Yamamoto, Y., Yamamoto, H., Adamis, A. P. (2007) Inhibition of diabetic leukostasis and blood-retinal barrier breakdown with a soluble form of a receptor for advanced glycation end products. *Invest Ophthalmol Vis Sci,* Vol. 48. No. 2 (February 2007), pp. 858-65, ISSN 0146-0404

Kakehashi, A., Saito, Y., Mori, K., Sugi, N., Ono, R., Yamagami, H., Shinohara, M. Tamemoto, H., Ishikawa, S.E., Kawakami, M. & Kanazawa, Y. (2006) Characteristics of diabetic retinopathy in SDT rats. *Diabetes Metab Res Rev,* Vol. 22, No. 6 (November-December 2006), pp. 455-461, ISSN 1520-7552

Kakehashi, A., Inoda, S., Mameuda, C., Kuroki, M., Jono, T., Nagai, R., Horiuchi, S., Kawakami, M. & Kanazawa, Y. (2008) Relationship among VEGF, VEGF receptor, AGEs, and macrophages in proliferative diabetic retinopathy. *Diabetes Res Clin Pract,* Vol. 79, No. 3 (March 2008), pp. 438-445, ISSN 1872-8227

Kakehashi, A. (2011a) Diabetic ocular complications in the SDT Rat. *The Open Diabetes Journal,* Vol. 4, No. Special issue 2011 (April 2011), pp. 37-40, 1876-5246.

Kakekashi, A. (2011b) Nobel animal model of diabetic complications: SDT rat. *The Open Diabetes Journal,* Vol. 4, No. Special issue 2011(April 2011), p. 14

Kakehashi, A., Takezawa, M., Toyoda, F., Kinoshita, N., Kambara, C., Yamagami, H., Kato, N., Ishikawa, S., Kawakami, M. & Kanazawa, Y. (2011) Aldose reductase inhibitor fidarestat prevents diabetic ocular complications in spontaneously diabetic Torii rats. *The Open Diabetes Journal,* Vol. 4, Special issue 2011 (April 2011), pp. 101-107

Keech, A. C., Mitchell, P., Summanen, P.A., O'Day, J., Davis, T.M., Moffitt, M.S., Taskinen, M.R., Simes, R.J., Tse, D., Williamson, E., Merrifield, A., Laatikainen, L.T., d'Emden, M.C., Crimet, D.C., O'Connell, R.L. & Colman, P.G. (2007) Effect of fenofibrate on the need for laser treatment for diabetic retinopathy (FIELD study): a randomised controlled trial. *Lancet,* Vol. 370, No. 9600 (November 2007), pp. 1687-1697, ISSN 1474-547X

Kern, T. S. & Engerman, R.L. (1981) Distribution of aldose reductase in ocular tissues. *Exp Eye Res,* Vol. 33, No. 2 (August 1981), pp. 175-182, ISSN 0014-4835

Kinoshita, N., Kakehashi, A., Inoda, S., Itou, Y., Kuroki, M., Yasu, T., Kawakami, M. & Kanazawa, Y. (2002) Effective and selective prevention of retinal leukostasis in streptozotocin-induced diabetic rats using gliclazide. *Diabetologia,* Vol. 45, No. 5 (May 2002), pp. 735-739, ISSN 0012-186X

Liang, H. R., Takagaki, T., Foltz, R.L. & Bennett, P. (2005) Quantitative determination of endogenous sorbitol and fructose in human erythrocytes by atmospheric-pressure chemical ionization LC tandem mass spectrometry. *J Chromatogr B Analyt Technol Biomed Life Sci,* Vol. 824, No. 1-2 (September 2005), pp. 36-44, ISSN 1570-0232

Lorenzi, M. (2007) The polyol pathway as a mechanism for diabetic retinopathy: attractive, elusive, and resilient. *Exp Diabetes Res,* Vol. 2007, pp. 61038, ISSN 1687-5303

Lutty, G. A., McLeod, D.S., Merges, C., Diggs, A. & Plouet, J. (1996) Localization of vascular endothelial growth factor in human retina and choroid. *Arch Ophthalmol,* Vol. 114, No. 8 (August 1996), pp. 971-977, ISSN 0003-9950

Massin, P., Bandello, F., Garweg, J.G., Hansen, L.L., Harding, S.P., Larsen, M., Mitchell, P., Sharp, D., Wolf-Schnurrbusch, U.E., Gekkieva, M., Weichselberger, A. & Wolf, S. (2010) Safety and efficacy of ranibizumab in diabetic macular edema (RESOLVE Study): a 12-month, randomized, controlled, double-masked, multicenter phase II study. *Diabetes Care,* Vol. 33, No. 11 (November 2010), pp. 2399-2405, ISSN 1935-5548

Mathews, M. K., Merges, C., McLeod, D.S. & Lutty, G.A. (1997) Vascular endothelial growth factor and vascular permeability changes in human diabetic retinopathy. *Invest Ophthalmol Vis Sci,* Vol. 38, No. 13 (December 1997), pp. 2729-2741, ISSN 0146-0404

McLeod, D. S., Lefer, D.J., Merges, C. & Lutty, G.A. (1995) Enhanced expression of intracellular adhesion molecule-1 and P-selectin in the diabetic human retina and choroid. *Am J Pathol,* Vol. 147, No. 3 (September 1995), pp. 642-653, ISSN 0002-9440

Miyamoto, K., Ogura, Y., Hamada, M., Nishiwaki, H., Hiroshiba, N. & Honda, Y. (1996) In vivo quantification of leukocyte behavior in the retina during endotoxin-induced uveitis. *Invest Ophthalmol Vis Sci,* Vol. 37, No. 13 (December 1996), pp. 2708-2715, ISSN 0146-0404

Miyamoto, K., Khosrof, S., Bursell, S.E. , Rohan, R., Murata, T., Clermont, A.C., Aiello, L.P., Ogura, Y. & Adamis, A.P. (1999) Prevention of leukostasis and vascular leakage in streptozotocin-induced diabetic retinopathy via intercellular adhesion molecule-1 inhibition. *Proc Natl Acad Sci U S A,* Vol. 96, No. 19 (September 1999), pp. 10836-10841, ISSN 0027-8424

Nagai, N., Izumi-Nagai, K., Oike, Y., Koto, T., Satofuka, S., Ozawa, Y., Yamashiro, K., Inoue, M., Tsubota, K., Umezawa, K. & Shida, S. (2007) Suppression of diabetes-induced retinal inflammation by blocking the angiotensin II type 1 receptor or its downstream nuclear factor-kappaB pathway. *Invest Ophthalmol Vis Sci,* Vol. 48, No. 9 (September 2007), pp. 4342-4350, ISSN 0146-0404

Nonaka, A., Kiryu, J., Tsujikawa, A, Yamashiro, K., Miyamoto, K., Nishiwaki, H., Honda, Y. & Ogura, Y. (2000) PKC-beta inhibitor (LY333531) attenuates leukocyte entrapment in retinal microcirculation of diabetic rats. *Invest Ophthalmol Vis Sci,* Vol. 41, No. 9 (August 2000), pp. 2702-2706, ISSN 0146-0404

Obrosova, I. G., Pacher, P., Szabo, C., Zsengeller, Z., Hirooka, H., Stevens, M.J. & Yorek, M.A. (2005) Aldose reductase inhibition counteracts oxidative-nitrosative stress and poly(ADP-ribose) polymerase activation in tissue sites for diabetes complications. *Diabetes,* Vol. 54, No. 1 (January 2005), pp. 234-242, ISSN 0012-1797

Okuda, J., Yashima, K., Inagaki, K. & Miwa, I. (1985) Effects of an aldose reductase inhibitor, 1-[(p-bromophenyl)-sulfonyl]hydantoin, on cataract formation and tissue polyol levels in galactosemic rats. *Chem Pharm Bull,* Vol. 33, No. 7 (July 1985), pp. 2990-2995, ISSN 0009-2363 .

Pan, H. Z., Zhang, H., Chang, D., Li, H. & Sui, H. (2008) The change of oxidative stress products in diabetes mellitus and diabetic retinopathy. *Br J Ophthalmol,* Vol. 92, No. 4 (April 2008), pp. 548-551, ISSN 1468-2079

Pinto, C. C., Silva, K.C., Biswas, S.K., Martins, N., De Faria, J.B. & De Faria, J.M. (2007) Arterial hypertension exacerbates oxidative stress in early diabetic retinopathy. *Free Radic Res,* Vol. 41, No. 10 (October 2007), pp. 1151-1158, ISSN 1071-5762

PKC-DRS Study Group (2005) The effect of ruboxistaurin on visual loss in patients with moderately severe to very severe nonproliferative diabetic retinopathy: initial results of the Protein Kinase C beta Inhibitor Diabetic Retinopathy Study (PKC-DRS) multicenter randomized clinical trial. *Diabetes,* Vol. 54, No. 7 (July 2005), pp. 2188-97, ISSN 0012-1797

Reichard, P., Nilsson, B.Y. & Rosenqvist, U. (1993) The effect of long-term intensified insulin treatment on the development of microvascular complications of diabetes mellitus. *N Engl J Med,* Vol. 329, No. 5 (July 29, 1993), pp. 304-309, ISSN 0028-4793

Robinson, G. S., Pierce, E. A., Rook, S. L., Foley, E., Webb, R., Smith, L. E. (1996) Oligodeoxynucleotides inhibit retinal neovascularization in a murine model of proliferative retinopathy. *Proc Natl Acad Sci U S A,* Vol. 93, No. 10 (May 1996), pp. 4851-6, ISSN 0027-8424

Robison, W. G., Jr., Kador, P.F. & Kinoshita, J.H. (1983) Retinal capillaries: basement membrane thickening by galactosemia prevented with aldose reductase inhibitor. *Science,* Vol. 221, No. 4616 (September 1983), pp. 1177-1179, ISSN 0036-8075

Robison, W. G., Jr., Nagata, M. & Kinoshita, J.H. (1988) Aldose reductase and retinal capillary basement membrane thickening. *Exp Eye Res,* Vol. 46, No. 3 (March 1988), pp. 343-348, ISSN 0014-4835

Robison, W. G., Jr., Nagata, M., Tillis, T.N., Laver, N. & Kinoshita, J.H. (1989) Aldose reductase and pericyte-endothelial cell contacts in retina and optic nerve. *Invest*

Ophthalmol Vis Sci, Vol. 30, No. 11 (November 1989), pp. 2293-2299, ISSN 0146-0404

Robinson, W. G., Jr., Laver, N.M., Jacot, J.L., Glover, J.P., Basso, M.D., Blouin, P. & Hohman, T.C. (1996) Diabetic-like retinopathy ameliorated with the aldose reductase inhibitor WAY-121,509. *Invest Ophthalmol Vis Sci,* Vol. 37, No. 6 (May 1996), pp. 1149-1156, ISSN 0146-0404

Sasase, T., Morinaga, H., Abe, T., Miyajima, K., Ohta, T., Shinohara, M., Matsushita, M., Kakehashi, A. (2009) Protein kinase C beta inhibitor prevents diabetic peripheral neuropathy, but not histopathological abnormalities of retina in Spontaneously Diabetic Torii rat. *Diabetes, Obesity & Metabolism,* Vol. 11, No. 11 (November 2009), pp.1084-7. ISSN 1462-8902

Schroder, S., Palinski, W. & Schmid-Schonbein, G.W. (1991) Activated monocytes and granulocytes, capillary nonperfusion, and neovascularization in diabetic retinopathy. *Am J Pathol,* Vol. 139, No. 1 (July 1991), pp. 81-100, ISSN 0002-9440

Shiba, T., Inoguchi, T., Sportsman, J.R., Heath, W.F., Bursell, S. & King, G.L. (1993) Correlation of diacylglycerol level and protein kinase C activity in rat retina to retinal circulation. *Am J Physiol,* Vol. 265, No. 5, Pt 1 (November 1993), pp. E783-793, ISSN 0002-9513

Shinohara, M., Masuyama, T., Shoda, T, Takahashi, T., Katsuda, Y., Komeda, K., Kuroki, M., Kakehashi, A. & Kanazawa, Y. (2000) A new spontaneously diabetic non-obese Torii rat strain with severe ocular complications. *Int J Exp Diabetes Res,* Vol. 1, No. 2, pp. 89-100, ISSN 1560-4284

Stitt, A., Gardiner, T.A., Alderson, N.L., Canning, P., Frizzell, N., Duffy, N., Boyle, C., Januszewski, A.S., Chachich, M., Baynes, J.W. & Thorpe, S.R. (2002) The AGE inhibitor pyridoxamine inhibits development of retinopathy in experimental diabetes. *Diabetes,* Vol. 51, No. 9 (September 2002), pp. 2826-2832, ISSN 0012-1797

Stratton, I. M., Kohner, E.M., Aldington, S.J., Turner, R.C., Holman, R.R., Manley, S.E. & Matthews, D.R. (2001) UKPDS 50: risk factors for incidence and progression of retinopathy in Type II diabetes over 6 years from diagnosis. *Diabetologia,* Vol. 44, No. 2 (February 2001), pp. 156-163, ISSN 0012-186X

Sun, W., Oates, P.J., Coutcher, J.B., Gerhardinger, C. & Lorenzi, M. (2006) A selective aldose reductase inhibitor of a new structural class prevents or reverses early retinal abnormalities in experimental diabetic retinopathy. *Diabetes,* Vol. 55, No. 10 (October 2006), pp. 2757-2762, ISSN 0012-1797

Toyoda, F., Kakehashi, A., Ota, A., Kinoshita, N., Kambara, C., Yamagami, H., Tamemoto, H., Ueba, H., Dobashi, Y., Ishikawa, S., Kawakami, M. & Kanazawa, Y. (2011) Prevention of proliferative diabetic retinopathy and cataract in SDT rats with aminoguanidine, an anti-advanced glycation end product agent. *The Open Diabetes Journal,* Vol. 4, No. Special issue (April 2011), pp. 108-113

UK Prospective Diabetes Study Group. (1998a) Efficacy of atenolol and captopril in reducing risk of macrovascular and microvascular complications in type 2 diabetes: UKPDS 39. *BMJ,* Vol. 317, No. 7160 (September 1998), pp. 713-720, ISSN 0959-8138

UK Prospective Diabetes Study Group. (1998b) Tight blood pressure control and risk of macrovascular and microvascular complications in type 2 diabetes: UKPDS 38. *BMJ*, Vol. 317, No. 7160 (September 1998), pp. 703-713, ISSN 0959-8138

Yeh, L. A., Rafford, C.E., Beyer, T.A. & Hutson, N.J. (1986) Effects of the aldose reductase inhibitor sorbinil on the isolated cultured rat lens. *Metab Clin Exp*, Vol. 35, No. 4 Suppl 1 (April 1986), pp. 4-9, ISSN 0026-0495

15

Treatment of Diabetic Macular Edema – Latest Therapeutic Developments

Yeon Sung Moon and Na Rae Kim*
Inha University School of Medicine
Korea

1. Introduction

Macular edema is a frequent manifestation of diabetic retinopathy and an important cause of impaired vision in individuals with diabetes (Klein et al., 1984; Moss et al., 1998). The Wisconsin Epidemiologic Study of Diabetic Retinopathy (WESDR), a population-based study in southern Wisconsin, estimated that after 20 years of known diabetes, the prevalence of diabetic macular edema (DME) was approximately 28% in both type 1 and type 2 diabetes (Klein, et al., 1984)

Despite recent attempts at strict glycemic control and optimization of other important systemic parameters such as hypertension and hyperlipidemia, diabetic retinopathy continues to be a leading cause of new onset vision loss worldwide in the working age population (DCCT Group, 1995). Although severe vision loss can occur from proliferative diabetic retinopathy (PDR), DME accounts for the majority of vision loss (Moss, et al., 1998).

Treatment for DME is continuously evolving. While focal laser photocoagulation remains the standard of care, a new wave of studies is emerging that shows the benefits of adjunctive therapy for DME. The goal of this chapter is to briefly summarize recent strategies for the treatment of DME.

2. Treatment of diabetic macular edema

DME has been an area of particular interest for clinical investigators. Although PDR is the cause of severe vision loss, DME is more prevalent and is the leading cause of moderate vision loss in patients with diabetic retinopathy. By disruption of the inner blood–retinal barrier, retinal vessels become permeable, leading to the exudation of fluid and lipids into the macula, which ultimately leads to a decline in vision (Bhagat et al., 2009).

The Early Treatment for Diabetic Retinopathy Study (ETDRS) was the first randomized and controlled trial to examine therapy for DME, and it demonstrated that focal (direct/grid) laser photocoagulation reduces moderate vision loss caused by DME by 50% or more (ETDRS group, 1987a). The ETDRS also indicated that focal laser treatment is not an ideal therapy. Focal laser treatment failed to prevent vision loss in a large number of patients, and it did not improve vision in the majority of patients (ETDRS group, 1985).

---

*Yeon Sung Moon and Na Rae Kim have contributed equally to this chapter.

2.1 Laser treatment

Laser photocoagulation remains the standard of care and the only treatment with proven efficacy in a large-scale clinical trial for this condition. The ETDRS demonstrated the efficacy of focal/grid photocoagulation in reducing the risk of moderate vision loss from DME (ETDRS group, 1991). The beneficial outcomes of focal/grid laser in an era of improved glycemic control were confirmed and expanded in recent clinical trials conducted by the Diabetic Retinopathy Clinical Research Network (DRCR.net) (Aiello et al., 2010; Beck et al., 2009; DRCR net, 2008).

Focal/grid photocoagulation has potential side effects, including laser scar expansion, paracentral scotomata, elevation of central visual field thresholds, and secondary choroidal neovascularization and subretinal fibrosis (Guyer et al., 1992; Han et al., 1992; Schatz et al., 1991). Modifications to the focal/grid photocoagulation technique have been made in response to these potential side effects. A comparison across studies suggests that outcomes with current modified techniques may be similar to those obtained with the original ETDRS technique (DRCR net, 2009).

2.1.1 Focal / grid laser photocoagulation

To characterize the severity of macular edema and for treatment guidelines, the term clinically significant macular edema (CSME) is defined: retinal thickening at or within 500µm of the foveal center, hard exudates at or within 500µm of the foveal center with adjacent retinal thickening, or retinal thickening greater than 1 disc diameter in size, within 1 disc diameter of the foveal center (ETDRS group, 1985, 1987a).

There is good evidence that focal laser treatment preserves vision in eyes with DME. The ETDRS randomized 1490 eyes with DME to receive focal laser treatment or observation (ETDRS group, 1985). Retreatment was applied at 4-month intervals if CSME persisted, one or more treatable lesions were identified, and the investigator believed these lesions were responsible for the edema (ETDRS group, 1987b). At 3 years, treatment significantly reduced moderate visual loss as compared with observations, with the greatest benefits in eyes with CSME (ETDRS group, 1987b)

Although focal laser photocoagulation reduces the risk of moderate visual loss by approximately 50%, approximately 12% of treated eyes still lose vision, many because of persistent DME (ETDRS group, 1985). Kim et al. assessed macular optical coherence tomography (OCT) findings of DME patients to determine whether specific OCT patterns are predictive of visual outcome after focal laser photocoagulation (Kim et al., 2009). DME was classified into four different OCT patterns, which are: diffuse retinal thickening, cystoids macular edema, serous retinal detachment, and vitreomacular interface abnormalities (Figure 1). In this study, eyes with diffuse retinal thickening achieved a greater visual acuity increase than eyes with other patterns.

It is unclear how focal retinal laser exerts its effects. One theory is that it improves oxygenation to the inner retina by eliminating highly oxygen-dependent photoreceptors (Gottfredsdottir et al., 1993; Stefansson, 2001). Another theory is that the laser reduces the retinal capillary area and thereby reduces leakage (Wilson et al., 1988). Other authors postulate that photocoagulation restores the outer blood–retinal barrier (Bresnick, 1983).

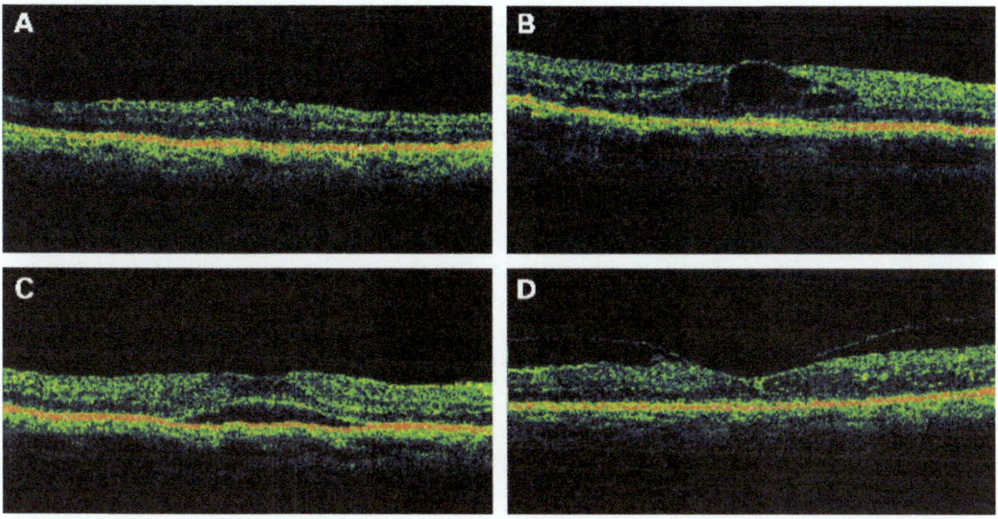

Fig. 1. Different patterns of diabetic macular edema by optical coherence tomography. (A) Diffuse retinal thickening appears as a sponge-like retinal swelling with areas of reduced intraretinal reflectivity. (B) Cystoid macular edema showing intraretinal cystoid spaces. (C) Serous retinal detachment showing shallow elevation of the retina, with an optically clear space between the retina and the retinal pigment epithelium. (D) Vitreomacular interface abnormalities showing a highly reflective band over the inner retinal surface and extending towards the optic nerve or peripherally.

2.1.2 Modified ETDRS direct/grid photocoagulation

Although effective, ETDRS protocol for photocoagulation may require placement of burns close to the center of the macula. Over time, laser burns may develop into areas of progressive retinal pigment epithelium and retinal atrophy that become larger than the original laser spot size and this may encroach upon fixation (Schatz, et al., 1991). In an attempt to reduce these adverse effects, many retinal specialists now treat patients using burns that are lighter and less intense than what was originally specified in the ETDRS, although no clinical trials have been performed to show improved outcomes with this approach (Akduman & Olk, 1999).

These include specifications with maximal spot sizes of 50μm, allowing the use of yellow and green wavelengths, not requiring blanching of large microaneurysms as long as the subjacent retinal pigment epithelium is lightly blanched, and removing the requirement for fluorescein angiography to guide treatment (Abu el Asrar & Morse, 1991; Fong et al., 2007). A modified ETDRS focal/grid photocoagulation protocol including all these changes has been adopted as the standard laser technique for DME used in DRCR Network studies.

2.1.3 Mild Macular Grid (MMG) laser photocoagulation

An alternative approach is the mild macular grid (MMG) technique, the application of mild, widely spaced burns throughout the macula (avoiding the foveal region). By design, some burns could be placed in clinically normal appearing retina if the entire retina was not abnormally thickened, including areas within the macula that are relatively distant from the area of thickening. The lighter burns applied to the macula are theoretically less likely to result in thermal injury to the overlying retina and less likely to break the Bruch membrane. The widespread application also might lead to improved oxygenation, development of healthier retinal pigment epithelium, and overall physiologic improvement of the entire macula.

The DRCR Network trial was designed to compare 2 laser techniques for previously untreated DME. One technique was the most commonly used approach in current clinical practice, the modified ETDRS technique, and the other approach was the MMG technique. At 12 months after treatment, the MMG technique was less effective at reducing OCT–measured retinal thickening than the current modified ETDRS laser photocoagulation approach. The visual acuity outcomes with both approaches were not substantially different. (Fong, et al., 2007).

2.1.4 Subthreshold Micropulse Diode Laser Photocoagulation (SMDLP)

Many laser modalities such as argon blue-green, argon green, krypton and diode have been used to achieve a clinically visible burn (threshold burn) according to the conventional photocoagulation protocol (Akduman & Olk, 1997; Olk, 1990). Subthreshold micropulse diode laser photocoagulation (SMDLP) is designed to target the retinal pigment epithelium while minimizing the negative thermal effects on the neural retina and deeper structures. A micropulse diode laser allows subthreshold therapy without a visible burn end point, and has been shown to be as effective as standard argon laser photocoagulation in reducing DME, while potentially allowing for more frequent re-dosing (Jain et al., 2010).

A study comparing the efficacy and side effects of conventional green laser photocoagulation and SMDLP treatment for diabetic CSME was conducted with prospective, randomized, double-masked manner. There were no statistically significant differences in best-corrected visual acuity (BCVA), contrast sensitivity and retinal thickness between the two laser modalities at 0, 4 and 12 months. It is found that laser scarring was much more apparent with conventional green laser than with the SMDLP (Figueira et al., 2009).

Recently, Lavinsky et al. conducted a prospective, randomized, controlled, double-masked clinical trial comparing modified ETDRS focal/grid laser photocoagulation with normal-density or high-density SMDLP for the treatment DME. In this study, the subthreshold micropulse 810-nm diode laser technique delivered in a high-density manner was superior to the standard mETDRS photocoagulation over at least 1 year of follow-up, with significantly more eyes gaining substantial vision and significantly fewer eyes losing substantial vision. (Lavinsky et al., 2011).

2.2 Steroid treatment

Corticosteroids are potent anti-inflammatory agents that can counteract many of the pathological processes thought to play a role in the development of macular edema. Corticosteroids prevent leukocyte migration, reduce fibrin deposition, stabilize endothelial cell tight junctions, and inhibit synthesis of vascular endothelial growth factor (VEGF), prostaglandins, and proinflammatory cytokines (Joussen et al., 2007; Kern, 2007; Leopold, 1985; Nauck et al., 1998).

The rationale for the use of corticosteroids to treat DME follows from the observation that the increase in retinal capillary permeability that results in edema may be caused by a breakdown of the blood retina barrier mediated in part by VEGF (Aiello et al., 1997; Antonetti et al., 1999; Senger et al., 1983). Corticosteroids have been demonstrated to inhibit the expression of VEGF and the VEGF gene (Nauck, et al., 1998; Nauck et al., 1997).

2.2.1 Intravitreal triamcinolone

In 2001-2002, the first reports were published of the use of intravitreal injection of triamcinolone acetonide for DME (Jonas & Sofker, 2001; Martidis et al., 2002), suggesting that intravitreal triamcinolone was potentially an efficacious treatment for DME. This treatment gained widespread use, most commonly as a dose of 4 mg of Kenalog® (Bristol-Myers Squibb, Princeton NJ), despite the lack of data from a controlled study demonstrating efficacy that exceeded risks.

In light of the short-term results from early reports of intravitreal triamcinolone for DME, the DRCR Network conducted a randomized clinical trial to evaluate the efficacy and safety of two doses of preservative-free intravitreal triamcinolone (1 mg and 4 mg) in comparison with standard focal/grid photocoagulation. At 4 months, both triamcinolone groups had greater improvement in visual acuity and macular thickness than the focal laser; however, by year one, there was no difference between the groups, and by the second year, the laser group demonstrated better visual acuity and more reduced macular thickness results over the corticosteroid groups (DRCR net, 2008). Another study in a subset of randomized subjects who completed the 3-year follow-up do not indicate a long-term benefit of intravitreal triamcinolone relative to focal/grid photocoagulation in patients with DME similar to those studied in this clinical trial (Beck, et al., 2009).

More recently, Gillies et al. reported that treatment with intravitreal triamcinolone acetonide plus laser resulted in a doubling of improvement in vision by 10 letters or more compared with a laser only over 2 years in eyes with DME. However, this treatment was associated with cataracts and a raised intraocular pressure (Gillies et al., 2011)

2.2.2 Peribulbar triamcinolone

Peribulbar injections have been performed using anterior combined sub-Tenon and subconjunctival, posterior sub-Tenon, and retrobulbar approaches. Theoretically, adverse effects may be presumed to be lower than those of intravitreal triamcinolone acetonide. A peribulbar corticosteroid injection is of particular interest for eyes with DME that have good visual acuity where the risks of an intravitreal injection of corticosteroid may not be justified (E. Chew et al., 2007).

The DRCR Network conducted a pilot study evaluating the effects of both anterior and posterior sub-Tenon delivery of peribulbar corticosteroids, with or without focal photocoagulation, in eyes with DME and good visual acuity. In cases of DME with good visual acuity, peribulbar triamcinolone, with or without focal photocoagulation, is unlikely to be of substantial benefit (E. Chew, et al., 2007). The group further reported long-term effects of anterior and posterior peribulbar injections of triamcinolone acetonide. The results suggested that the risk of intraocular pressure elevation and cataract development is increased with anterior peribulbar triamcinolone acetonide injections while ptosis development is increased with the posterior peribulbar injections (E. Y. Chew et al., 2011).

2.2.3 Dexamethasone implant

The treatment of macular edema is considerably limited by the difficulty in delivering effective doses of therapeutic agents into the vitreous cavity. In recent years, the development of a sustained-release intravitreal dexamethasone implant (Ozurdex® , Allergan Inc, Irvine, CA) enabled more controlled delivery of the drug, with a potentially lower rate of adverse events (Herrero-Vanrell et al., 2011).

In a previous study to evaluate the safety and efficacy of dexamethasone implant vs. observation in eyes with persistent DME, treatment with a 700µg intravitreal dexamethasone drug delivery system is well tolerated and produces significant improvements in BCVA, central retinal thickness, and fluorescein leakage, compared with observation (Haller, Kuppermann, et al., 2010).

2.2.4 Fluocinolone acetonide

Extended release intravitreal inserts of fluocinolone acetonide have also been evaluated for the treatment of DME. As fluocinolone acetonide has been in use for many years as a dermal product, its pharmacology, systemic metabolism and elimination are well established.

A nonbiodegradable fluocinolone acetonide, Retisert® (Bausch & Lomb, Rochester, NY) is FDA-approved for the treatment of uveitis. Surgical implantation of this polymer device initially showed evidence of benefit in reducing macular thickness in DME; however 20% of patients required filtering surgery for high intraocular pressures within 24 months (Pearson et al., 2005).

Iluvien® (Alimera Sciences, Alpharetta, GA) is another reservoir implant currently being studied in phase III trials for the treatment of DME. It was hypothesized that fluocinolone acetonide inserts may cause fewer problems with glaucoma than the surgically implanted device because of lower in vitro release rates of fluocinolone acetonide (0.2 and 0.5µg/day) and also because of a more posterior location in the eye, which may decrease exposure to the trabecular meshwork in the anterior chamber while still delivering adequate levels of fluocinolone acetonide to the retina. In a small phase II trial in patients with persistent DME despite focal laser, both 0.2- and 0.5-µg/day fluocinolone acetonide inserts significantly improved visual acuity in patients with DME over 2 years. Significantly fewer incisional glaucoma procedures were needed in the low-dose insert group (Campochiaro et al., 2010).

2.3 Anti-Vascular Endothelial Growth Factor (Anti-VEGF) injection

An alternative treatment approach, and to now, available for less than a decade, is the use of intravitreal therapies targeting VEGF (Nicholson & Schachat, 2010), the most potent known promoter of vascular permeability (Senger et al., 1990). Clinical studies have established that VEGF concentrations are elevated in eyes with DME (Funatsu et al., 2003; Funatsu et al., 2005), and preclinical studies have demonstrated that VEGF levels increased after its onset in a manner temporally correlated with the breakdown of the blood–retinal barrier (Qaum et al., 2001). Several mechanisms are believed to underlie these actions; in addition to the direct action of VEGF on the permeability of intact blood vessels, it also promotes an influx of inflammatory cells that produces endothelial cell apoptosis in the retinal vasculature (Adamis & Berman, 2008).

2.3.1 Pegaptanib

Pegaptanib (Macugen®; Eyetech Pharmaceuticals, Inc. and Pfizer Inc, New York) is a ribonucleic acid aptamer that targets the VEGF165 isoform that is currently approved in a number of countries worldwide for the treatment of neovascular age-related macular degeneration.

Cunningham et al. assessed the efficacy of pegaptanib for the treatment of DME. In a phase II trial, subjects treated with pegaptanib had better visual acuity outcomes, were more likely to show a reduction in central retinal thickness, and were deemed less likely to need additional therapy with photocoagulation at follow-up than those assigned to sham injection (Cunningham et al., 2005).

A phase 2/3, randomized, double-masked, 2-year trial has been performed to assess the safety and efficacy of intravitreal pegaptanib sodium 0.3 mg compared with sham injections in subjects with DME, with focal/grid photocoagulation being permitted as needed after week 18. In this study, intravitreal pegaptanib sodium 0.3 mg was well tolerated and demonstrated superior efficacy over the sham in the treatment of patients with DME. The proportion of patients with ≥10 letters (or 2 lines) of visual acuity improvement at week 54 was statistically significantly greater in the pegaptanib group versus those in the sham treatment arm ($P = 0.0047$; primary efficacy endpoint) (Sultan et al., 2011).

2.3.2 Ranibizumab

Ranibizumab (Lucentis®; Genentech, South San Francisco, California) is a humanized antibody fragment directed at all isoforms of VEGF-A and is fabricated specifically for intravitreal use. Ranibizumab is now FDA-approved for the treatment of age-related macular degeneration as well as macular edema associated with retinal vein occlusion.

For diabetic macular edema, an initial small pilot study showed efficacy of intravitreal injections of ranibizumab in reducing macular thickness and improving visual acuity (Nguyen et al., 2006).

Acting upon the favorable results of their pilot study, a 6-month, phase II, multicenter, randomized controlled trial, the Ranibizumab for Edema of the mAcula in Diabetes-2 (READ-2) study was designed. Patients with DME were randomized to three groups. Group 1 received four injections of ranibizumab, group 2 received focal laser at baseline and again at 3 months if needed; and group 3 had combination of laser treatment and injections of ranibizumab. The ranibizumab only group gained a mean of 7.24 ETDRS letters, the laser-only group lost 0.43 letters, and the combination group had gained 3.80 letters (Nguyen et al., 2009).

Data at twenty-four-months were also reported for the READ-2 study. After the initial 6 months, all patients were followed up every 2 months. Patients in group 1 could be re-injected if they had persistent or recurrent DME, patients in group 2 could receive ranibizumab alone or laser only, and patients in group 3 could receive ranibizumab alone or in combination with laser. After 24 months, patients gained 7.7, 5.1, and 6.8 letters in the three groups, respectively, and the percentage of patients who gained three or more lines of visual acuity was 24, 18 and 26%, respectively (Nguyen et al., 2010).

One-year safety and efficacy results from the Ranibizumab in Diabetic Macular Edema Study (RESOLVE) have also been reported. This was a phase II, randomized clinical trial comparing 0.3 and 0.5mg ranibizumab with sham injections for the treatment of DME in 151 eyes. Patients received three monthly injections initially, followed by continuation of monthly injections on an as-needed basis with the opportunity for rescue focal laser treatment. In addition, after the first month, dose doubling (0.05 to 0.10 ml) was allowed based on pre-specified criteria. At the end of the 12-month assessment period, ranibizumab led to a mean gain of 10.3 letters from the baseline compared with a decline of 1.4 letters in the sham patients. Macular thickness reduction was also greater in the ranibizumab group vs. the sham group (Massin et al., 2010).

The DRCR Network group has reported 1-year results of a phase III, randomized controlled trial comparing four groups: sham injection plus prompt laser, ranibizumab plus prompt laser, ranibizumab plus deferred laser, and triamcinolone plus prompt laser. A total of 854 eyes of 691 patients were enrolled. In the ranibizumab groups, patients received at least four initial injections, after which retreatment was based on specific retreatment criteria. Change in mean visual acuity was greater in both ranibizumab groups (both +9 letters) vs. the laser only (+3 letters) and the triamcinolone group (+4 letters). Reduction in macular thickness was similar in all three injection groups and was greater than that in the laser only group (Elman et al., 2010).

The expanded 2-year results reported are similar to the results published previously and reinforce the conclusions originally reported. At the 2-year visit, compared with the sham plus prompt laser group, the mean change in the visual acuity letter score from the baseline was 3.7 letters greater in the ranibizumab plus prompt laser group, 5.8 letters greater in the ranibizumab plus deferred laser group, and 1.5 letters worse in the triamcinolone plus prompt laser group (Elman et al., 2011).

The 12-month, phase III, randomized, double-masked, multicenter, laser-controlled RESTORE study was designed to assess whether ranibizumab monotherapy or combined with laser was superior to laser alone in patients with visual impairment due to DME. The results from the RESTORE study demonstrated that treatment with ranibizumab as a monotherapy and combined with laser treatment is superior to laser treatment in rapidly improving and sustaining visual acuity in patients with visual impairment due to DME. There were no efficacy differences detected between the ranibizumab and ranibizumab combined with laser treatment arms (Mitchell et al., 2011).

2.3.3 Bevacizumab

Bevacizumab (Avastin®; Genentech, South San Francisco, California) inactivates all VEGF isoforms and is indicated for systemic use as an adjunct cancer chemotherapeutic agent (Van Meter & Kim, 2010). Bevacizumab, which is a full-length humanized monoclonal G1 antibody, has emerged as a therapeutic agent for retinal diseases (Arevalo et al., 2009), and has been used as an off-label agent in a number of ocular diseases, including diabetic retinopathy (Gunther & Altaweel, 2009).

The DRCR Network group conducted a phase II study over 3 months in 121 eyes, comparing five treatment arms: focal photocoagulation, two intravitreal injections of 1.25mg bevacizumab, two intravitreal injections of 2.5mg bevacizumab, one 1.25mg bevacizumab followed by a sham injection at week 6, and two 1.25mg bevacizumab injections combined with focal photocoagulation. Compared with laser alone, eyes in groups 2 and 3 had an improvement in visual acuity after 3 months (-1 letter vs. +5 and +7 letters, respectively). There was a greater initial reduction in macular thickness after 3 weeks in groups 2 (-35µm) and 3 (-86µm) compared with laser (+21µm); however, this difference did not persist by week 12 (Scott et al., 2007).

A subsequent 3-arm randomized clinical trial demonstrated the superiority of intravitreal bevacizumab injection either alone or in combination with triamcinolone acetonide over macular laser photocoagulation in visual acuity improvement up to 24 weeks in primary treatment of DME. This improving effect persisted longer in the intravitreal bevacizumab group (up to 36 weeks) than in the intravitreal bevacizumab/intravitreal triamcinolone acetonide group (up to 12 weeks). In the macular laser photocoagulation group, no improvement in visual acuity was observed at all follow-up visits. In regard to central macular thickness reduction, there was no meaningful superiority of the intravitreal bevacizumab and intravitreal bevacizumab/intravitreal triamcinolone groups over the macular laser photocoagulation group (Soheilian et al., 2009).

The intravitreal Bevacizumab or Laser Therapy in the management of diabetic macular edema study (BOLT) was designed to compare bevacizumab therapy to laser for DME. This study was a randomized controlled trial comparing intravitreal bevacizumab 1.25mg with laser therapy in 80 patients who had previously received focal laser for DME. Patients in the bevacizumab arm received injections every 6 weeks for the first 3 months and every 6 weeks as needed thereafter, while those in the laser group received as needed laser every 4 months. The bevacizumab arm had superior visual acuity results at 12 months (+8 vs. -0.5 letters), a 5.1 times greater odds of gaining at least 10 letters, and a trend toward greater decrease in macular thickness (130 vs. 68µm) (Michaelides et al., 2010).

2.3.4 VEGF-Trap

VEGF Trap-Eye® (Regeneron Pharmaceuticals., Tarrytown, New York, NY, and Bayer Healthcare Pharmaceuticals, Berlin, Germany) is a 115-kDA recombinant fusion protein consisting of the VEGF binding domains of human VEGF receptors 1 and 2 fused to the Fc domain of human immunoglobulin-G1 (Holash et al., 2002). Animal studies have demonstrated that intravitreal VEGF Trap-Eye has theoretic advantages over ranibizumab and bevacizumab, including a longer half life in the eye and a higher binding affinity to VEGF-A (Gaudreault et al., 2005). In addition, the fusion protein binds placental growth factors 1 and 2, which have been shown to contribute to excessive vascular permeability and retinal neovascularization (Rakic et al., 2003).

A phase I study showed that a single intravitreal injection of VEGF Trap-Eye effected biological activity by improving visual acuity and reducing excess retinal thickness in 5 eyes with DME (Do et al., 2009).

On the basis of a sound biological rationale and encouraging phase I results, a phase II multicenter, randomized clinical trial, the DME and VEGF Trap-Eye: INvestigation of Clinical Impact (DA VINCI) study was designed to compare intravitreal VEGF Trap-Eye with standard macular laser treatment after the modified ETDRS protocol. In this phase II randomized clinical trial, intravitreal VEGF Trap-Eye was superior to macular laser treatment by the modified ETDRS protocol for the treatment of DME over a 24-week period. VEGF Trap-Eye resulted in significantly better mean visual acuity outcomes (+8.5 to +11.4

vs. +2.5 letters gained) and greater mean reductions in retinal thickness (-127.3 to -194.5μm vs. -67.9μm) compared with laser alone (Do et al., 2011).

2.4 Vitrectomy

The vitreous has been implicated as a cause of macular edema in people with diabetes via several mechanical and physiologic mechanisms, all of which are postulated to lead to increased vascular permeability. Widespread or diffuse DME that is unresponsive to focal laser treatment may benefit from a vitrectomy. The presence of vitreous traction and macular edema, now readily documented with OCT, in association with visual impairment is also a common indication for the need of a vitrectomy. Complications of vitrectomy include recurrent vitreous hemorrhage, retinal tears and detachment, cataract formation and glaucoma (Figueroa et al., 2008; Harbour et al., 1996; Hartley et al., 2008; Ikeda et al., 1999; Lewis et al., 1992; Pendergast et al., 2000; Tachi & Ogino, 1996; Yamamoto et al., 2001).

In a prospective study of 87 eyes undergoing vitrectomy for DME associated with at least moderate visual loss and vitreomacular traction, the median change in visual acuity at 6 months was an improvement of 3 letters, with visual acuity improving by ≥ 10 letters from the baseline to 6 months in 38% and worsening by ≥ 10 letters in 22%. Reduction in OCT central subfield thickness to < 250μm occurred in almost half, and most eyes had a reduction of thickening of ≥ 50% (Haller, Qin, et al., 2010).

2.5 Protein kinase C inhibitor

An increased understanding of the pathophysiology of diabetic microangiopathy and the mechanisms of glycaemic vascular damage might facilitate the development of new therapeutic agents that ameliorate microvascular complications, even or especially when tight glycaemic control is unattainable. Hyperglycaemia-induced *de novo* synthesis of diacylglycerol in vascular cells leads to preferential activation of the PKC-β isoform, which is strongly implicated in the pathogenic processes involved in diabetic microangiopathy such as ischemia, leakage, neovascularization and abnormal vasodilator function (Idris & Donnelly, 2006).

2.5.1 Protein kinase C *β* inhibitor (Ruboxistaurin)

The Protein Kinase C β inhibitor Diabetic Retinopathy Study (PKC-DRS) was designed to test the primary hypothesis that ruboxistaurin, a β-isoform–selective protein kinase C inhibitor, would delay the progression of diabetic retinopathy. Ruboxistaurin was well tolerated without significant adverse effects. Compared with a placebo, 32 mg/day ruboxistaurin was associated with a delayed occurrence of moderate visual loss. However, in patients with moderately severe to very severe nonproliferative diabetic retinopathy at the baseline, ruboxistaurin did not prevent retinopathy progression to the proliferative disease state (PKC-DRS group, 2005).

2.5.2 PKC412

Orally administered PKC412 at doses of 100mg/day or higher may significantly reduce macular edema and improve visual acuity in diabetic subjects. However, concern regarding liver toxicity with systemic therapy makes local delivery an appealing approach (Campochiaro, 2004).

2.6 Others

2.6.1 HMG-CoA reductase inhibitor (Atorvastin)

Lipids have a definite role in the pathogenesis of diabetic retinopathy. Because of the increased permeability and leakage of the retinal capillaries, extravascular deposition of less soluble plasma lipoprotein occurs. The mass of lipid-filled macrophages is visible on funduscopy as hard exudates (Watanabe et al., 1988).

Statins act by competitively inhibiting 3-hydroxy-3-methylglutaryl-coenzyme A (HMG-CoA) reductase, the first committed enzyme of the HMG-CoA reductase pathway. Sen et al. found that statins retard the progression of retinopathy in patients with diabetes mellitus and hypercholesterolemia (Sen et al., 2002), whereas other studies have reported that statins limit the severity of hard exudates and subfoveal lipid migration in CSME (Gordon et al., 1991; Gupta et al., 2004).

A recent study evaluated the efficacy and safety of atorvastatin and described its effect on hard exudates and macular edema in patients with diabetes mellitus and dyslipidemia. In this study, aggressive treatment of hyperlipidemia resulted in significant improvement in hard exudates and fluorescein leakage. The lipid-lowering drug atorvastatin was safe when administered to patients with diabetes mellitus and useful in the management of DME in patients with an abnormal lipid profile (Panagiotoglou et al., 2010).

3. Conclusion

Although, focal laser photocoagulation is the standard-of-care treatment for DME, it is not a cure. During the last decade, a number of additional treatments for DME have been proposed. Such treatments include intravitreal injection of corticosteroids such as triamcinolone acetonide, intravitreal injection of aptamers or antibodies targeted at VEGF, vitrectomy, and pharmacologic therapy with oral protein kinase C beta inhibitors.

In particular, anti-VEGF therapies, in conjunction with laser or as standalone treatments, have shown promise in not only maintaining but also improving visual acuity. Intravitreal triamcinolone also has a role in treating patients with DME refractory to laser and anti-VEGF therapy, and it remains to be seen whether extended-release corticosteroid devices might play a role in the management of DME. Diabetic patients with macular edema who have a taut posterior hyaloid membrane may benefit from pars plana vitrectomy and removal of the posterior hyaloids

The pathogenesis of DME is complex, and a variety of factors and biochemical pathways are involved, which provides an opportunity for the development of a number of therapeutic modalities to treat the condition.

4. Acknowledgements

This work was supported by Inha university Research grant.

5. References

Abu el Asrar, A. M., & Morse, P. H. (1991). Laser photocoagulation control of diabetic macular oedema without fluorescein angiography. *Br J Ophthalmol, 75*(2), 97-99, ISSN 0007-1161 (Print)

Adamis, A. P., & Berman, A. J. (2008). Immunological mechanisms in the pathogenesis of diabetic retinopathy. *Semin Immunopathol, 30*(2), 65-84, ISSN 1863-2297 (Print)

Aiello, L. P., Bursell, S. E., Clermont, A., Duh, E., Ishii, H., Takagi, C., Mori, F., Ciulla, T. A., Ways, K., Jirousek, M., Smith, L. E., & King, G. L. (1997). Vascular endothelial growth factor-induced retinal permeability is mediated by protein kinase C in vivo and suppressed by an orally effective beta-isoform-selective inhibitor. *Diabetes, 46*(9), 1473-1480, ISSN 0012-1797 (Print)

Aiello, L. P., Edwards, A. R., Beck, R. W., Bressler, N. M., Davis, M. D., Ferris, F., Glassman, A. R., Ip, M. S., & Miller, K. M. (2010). Factors associated with improvement and worsening of visual acuity 2 years after focal/grid photocoagulation for diabetic macular edema. *Ophthalmology, 117*(5), 946-953, ISSN 1549-4713 (Electronic)

Akduman, L., & Olk, R. J. (1997). Diode laser (810 nm) versus argon green (514 nm) modified grid photocoagulation for diffuse diabetic macular edema. *Ophthalmology, 104*(9), 1433-1441, ISSN 0161-6420 (Print)

Akduman, L., & Olk, R. J. (1999). Subthreshold (invisible) modified grid diode laser photocoagulation in diffuse diabetic macular edema (DDME). *Ophthalmic Surg Lasers, 30*(9), 706-714, ISSN 1082-3069 (Print)

Antonetti, D. A., Barber, A. J., Hollinger, L. A., Wolpert, E. B., & Gardner, T. W. (1999). Vascular endothelial growth factor induces rapid phosphorylation of tight junction proteins occludin and zonula occluden 1. A potential mechanism for vascular permeability in diabetic retinopathy and tumors. *J Biol Chem, 274*(33), 23463-23467, ISSN 0021-9258 (Print)

Arevalo, J. F., Sanchez, J. G., Wu, L., Maia, M., Alezzandrini, A. A., Brito, M., Bonafonte, S., Lujan, S., Diaz-Llopis, M., Restrepo, N., Rodriguez, F. J., & Udaondo-Mirete, P. (2009). Primary intravitreal bevacizumab for diffuse diabetic macular edema: the Pan-American Collaborative Retina Study Group at 24 months. *Ophthalmology, 116*(8), 1488-1497, 1497 e1481, ISSN 1549-4713 (Electronic)

Beck, R. W., Edwards, A. R., Aiello, L. P., Bressler, N. M., Ferris, F., Glassman, A. R., Hartnett, E., Ip, M. S., Kim, J. E., & Kollman, C. (2009). Three-year follow-up of a randomized trial comparing focal/grid photocoagulation and intravitreal triamcinolone for diabetic macular edema. *Arch Ophthalmol, 127*(3), 245-251, ISSN 1538-3601 (Electronic)

Bhagat, N., Grigorian, R. A., Tutela, A., & Zarbin, M. A. (2009). Diabetic macular edema: pathogenesis and treatment. *Surv Ophthalmol, 54*(1), 1-32, ISSN 0039-6257 (Print)

Bresnick, G. H. (1983). Diabetic maculopathy. A critical review highlighting diffuse macular edema. *Ophthalmology, 90*(11), 1301-1317, ISSN 0161-6420 (Print)

Campochiaro, P. A. (2004). Reduction of diabetic macular edema by oral administration of the kinase inhibitor PKC412. *Invest Ophthalmol Vis Sci, 45*(3), 922-931, ISSN 0146-0404 (Print)

Campochiaro, P. A., Hafiz, G., Shah, S. M., Bloom, S., Brown, D. M., Busquets, M., Ciulla, T., Feiner, L., Sabates, N., Billman, K., Kapik, B., Green, K., & Kane, F. (2010).

Sustained ocular delivery of fluocinolone acetonide by an intravitreal insert. *Ophthalmology, 117*(7), 1393-1399 e1393, ISSN 1549-4713 (Electronic)

Chew, E., Strauber, S., Beck, R., Aiello, L. P., Antoszyk, A., Bressler, N., Browning, D., Danis, R., Fan, J., Flaxel, C., Friedman, S., Glassman, A., Kollman, C., & Lazarus, H. (2007). Randomized trial of peribulbar triamcinolone acetonide with and without focal photocoagulation for mild diabetic macular edema: a pilot study. *Ophthalmology, 114*(6), 1190-1196, ISSN 1549-4713 (Electronic)

Chew, E. Y., Glassman, A. R., Beck, R. W., Bressler, N. M., Fish, G. E., Ferris, F. L., & Kinyoun, J. L. (2011). Ocular side effects associated with peribulbar injections of triamcinolone acetonide for diabetic macular edema. *Retina, 31*(2), 284-289, ISSN 1539-2864 (Electronic)

Cunningham, E. T., Jr., Adamis, A. P., Altaweel, M., Aiello, L. P., Bressler, N. M., D'Amico, D. J., Goldbaum, M., Guyer, D. R., Katz, B., Patel, M., & Schwartz, S. D. (2005). A phase II randomized double-masked trial of pegaptanib, an anti-vascular endothelial growth factor aptamer, for diabetic macular edema. *Ophthalmology, 112*(10), 1747-1757, ISSN 1549-4713 (Electronic)

DCCT Group. (1995). The effect of intensive diabetes treatment on the progression of diabetic retinopathy in insulin-dependent diabetes mellitus. The Diabetes Control and Complications Trial. *Arch Ophthalmol, 113*(1), 36-51, ISSN 0003-9950 (Print)

Do, D. V., Nguyen, Q. D., Shah, S. M., Browning, D. J., Haller, J. A., Chu, K., Yang, K., Cedarbaum, J. M., Vitti, R. L., Ingerman, A., & Campochiaro, P. A. (2009). An exploratory study of the safety, tolerability and bioactivity of a single intravitreal injection of vascular endothelial growth factor Trap-Eye in patients with diabetic macular oedema. *Br J Ophthalmol, 93*(2), 144-149, ISSN 1468-2079 (Electronic)

Do, D. V., Schmidt-Erfurth, U., Gonzalez, V. H., Gordon, C. M., Tolentino, M., Berliner, A. J., Vitti, R., Ruckert, R., Sandbrink, R., Stein, D., Yang, K., Beckmann, K., & Heier, J. S. (2011). The DA VINCI Study: Phase 2 Primary Results of VEGF Trap-Eye in Patients with Diabetic Macular Edema. *Ophthalmology*, ISSN 1549-4713 (Electronic)

DRCR net. (2008). A randomized trial comparing intravitreal triamcinolone acetonide and focal/grid photocoagulation for diabetic macular edema. *Ophthalmology, 115*(9), 1447-1449, 1449 e1441-1410, ISSN 1549-4713 (Electronic)

DRCR net. (2009). The course of response to focal/grid photocoagulation for diabetic macular edema. *Retina, 29*(10), 1436-1443, ISSN 1539-2864 (Electronic)

Elman, M. J., Aiello, L. P., Beck, R. W., Bressler, N. M., Bressler, S. B., Edwards, A. R., Ferris, F. L., 3rd, Friedman, S. M., Glassman, A. R., Miller, K. M., Scott, I. U., Stockdale, C. R., & Sun, J. K. (2010). Randomized trial evaluating ranibizumab plus prompt or deferred laser or triamcinolone plus prompt laser for diabetic macular edema. *Ophthalmology, 117*(6), 1064-1077 e1035, ISSN 1549-4713 (Electronic)

Elman, M. J., Bressler, N. M., Qin, H., Beck, R. W., Ferris, F. L., 3rd, Friedman, S. M., Glassman, A. R., Scott, I. U., Stockdale, C. R., & Sun, J. K. (2011). Expanded 2-year follow-up of ranibizumab plus prompt or deferred laser or triamcinolone plus prompt laser for diabetic macular edema. *Ophthalmology, 118*(4), 609-614, ISSN 1549-4713 (Electronic)

ETDRS group. (1985). Photocoagulation for diabetic macular edema. Early Treatment Diabetic Retinopathy Study report number 1. Early Treatment Diabetic

Retinopathy Study research group. *Arch Ophthalmol, 103*(12), 1796-1806, ISSN 0003-9950 (Print)

ETDRS group. (1987a). Photocoagulation for diabetic macular edema: Early Treatment Diabetic Retinopathy Study Report no. 4. The Early Treatment Diabetic Retinopathy Study Research Group. *Int Ophthalmol Clin, 27*(4), 265-272, ISSN 0020-8167 (Print)

ETDRS group. (1987b). Treatment techniques and clinical guidelines for photocoagulation of diabetic macular edema. Early Treatment Diabetic Retinopathy Study Report Number 2. Early Treatment Diabetic Retinopathy Study Research Group. *Ophthalmology, 94*(7), 761-774, ISSN 0161-6420 (Print)

ETDRS group. (1991). Early photocoagulation for diabetic retinopathy. ETDRS report number 9. Early Treatment Diabetic Retinopathy Study Research Group. *Ophthalmology, 98*(5 Suppl), 766-785, ISSN 0161-6420 (Print)

Figueira, J., Khan, J., Nunes, S., Sivaprasad, S., Rosa, A., de Abreu, J. F., Cunha-Vaz, J. G., & Chong, N. V. (2009). Prospective randomised controlled trial comparing sub-threshold micropulse diode laser photocoagulation and conventional green laser for clinically significant diabetic macular oedema. *Br J Ophthalmol, 93*(10), 1341-1344, ISSN 1468-2079 (Electronic)

Figueroa, M. S., Contreras, I., & Noval, S. (2008). Surgical and anatomical outcomes of pars plana vitrectomy for diffuse nontractional diabetic macular edema. *Retina, 28*(3), 420-426, ISSN 0275-004X (Print)

Fong, D. S., Strauber, S. F., Aiello, L. P., Beck, R. W., Callanan, D. G., Danis, R. P., Davis, M. D., Feman, S. S., Ferris, F., Friedman, S. M., Garcia, C. A., Glassman, A. R., Han, D. P., Le, D., Kollman, C., Lauer, A. K., Recchia, F. M., & Solomon, S. D. (2007). Comparison of the modified Early Treatment Diabetic Retinopathy Study and mild macular grid laser photocoagulation strategies for diabetic macular edema. *Arch Ophthalmol, 125*(4), 469-480, ISSN 0003-9950 (Print)

Funatsu, H., Yamashita, H., Ikeda, T., Mimura, T., Eguchi, S., & Hori, S. (2003). Vitreous levels of interleukin-6 and vascular endothelial growth factor are related to diabetic macular edema. *Ophthalmology, 110*(9), 1690-1696, ISSN 0161-6420 (Print)

Funatsu, H., Yamashita, H., Sakata, K., Noma, H., Mimura, T., Suzuki, M., Eguchi, S., & Hori, S. (2005). Vitreous levels of vascular endothelial growth factor and intercellular adhesion molecule 1 are related to diabetic macular edema. *Ophthalmology, 112*(5), 806-816, ISSN 1549-4713 (Electronic)

Gaudreault, J., Fei, D., Rusit, J., Suboc, P., & Shiu, V. (2005). Preclinical pharmacokinetics of Ranibizumab (rhuFabV2) after a single intravitreal administration. *Invest Ophthalmol Vis Sci, 46*(2), 726-733, ISSN 0146-0404 (Print)

Gillies, M. C., McAllister, I. L., Zhu, M., Wong, W., Louis, D., Arnold, J. J., & Wong, T. Y. (2011). Intravitreal triamcinolone prior to laser treatment of diabetic macular edema: 24-month results of a randomized controlled trial. *Ophthalmology, 118*(5), 866-872, ISSN 1549-4713 (Electronic)

Gordon, B., Chang, S., Kavanagh, M., Berrocal, M., Yannuzzi, L., Robertson, C., & Drexler, A. (1991). The effects of lipid lowering on diabetic retinopathy. *Am J Ophthalmol, 112*(4), 385-391, ISSN 0002-9394 (Print)

Gottfredsdottir, M. S., Stefansson, E., Jonasson, F., & Gislason, I. (1993). Retinal vasoconstriction after laser treatment for diabetic macular edema. *Am J Ophthalmol, 115*(1), 64-67, ISSN 0002-9394 (Print)

Gunther, J. B., & Altaweel, M. M. (2009). Bevacizumab (Avastin) for the treatment of ocular disease. *Surv Ophthalmol, 54*(3), 372-400, ISSN 0039-6257 (Print)

Gupta, A., Gupta, V., Thapar, S., & Bhansali, A. (2004). Lipid-lowering drug atorvastatin as an adjunct in the management of diabetic macular edema. *Am J Ophthalmol, 137*(4), 675-682, ISSN 0002-9394 (Print)

Guyer, D. R., D'Amico, D. J., & Smith, C. W. (1992). Subretinal fibrosis after laser photocoagulation for diabetic macular edema. *Am J Ophthalmol, 113*(6), 652-656, ISSN 0002-9394 (Print)

Haller, J. A., Kuppermann, B. D., Blumenkranz, M. S., Williams, G. A., Weinberg, D. V., Chou, C., & Whitcup, S. M. (2010). Randomized controlled trial of an intravitreous dexamethasone drug delivery system in patients with diabetic macular edema. *Arch Ophthalmol, 128*(3), 289-296, ISSN 1538-3601 (Electronic)

Haller, J. A., Qin, H., Apte, R. S., Beck, R. R., Bressler, N. M., Browning, D. J., Danis, R. P., Glassman, A. R., Googe, J. M., Kollman, C., Lauer, A. K., Peters, M. A., & Stockman, M. E. (2010). Vitrectomy outcomes in eyes with diabetic macular edema and vitreomacular traction. *Ophthalmology, 117*(6), 1087-1093 e1083, ISSN 1549-4713 (Electronic)

Han, D. P., Mieler, W. F., & Burton, T. C. (1992). Submacular fibrosis after photocoagulation for diabetic macular edema. *Am J Ophthalmol, 113*(5), 513-521, ISSN 0002-9394 (Print)

Harbour, J. W., Smiddy, W. E., Flynn, H. W., Jr., & Rubsamen, P. E. (1996). Vitrectomy for diabetic macular edema associated with a thickened and taut posterior hyaloid membrane. *Am J Ophthalmol, 121*(4), 405-413, ISSN 0002-9394 (Print)

Hartley, K. L., Smiddy, W. E., Flynn, H. W., Jr., & Murray, T. G. (2008). Pars plana vitrectomy with internal limiting membrane peeling for diabetic macular edema. *Retina, 28*(3), 410-419, ISSN 0275-004X (Print)

Herrero-Vanrell, R., Cardillo, J. A., & Kuppermann, B. D. (2011). Clinical applications of the sustained-release dexamethasone implant for treatment of macular edema. *Clin Ophthalmol, 5*, 139-146, ISSN 1177-5483 (Electronic)

Holash, J., Davis, S., Papadopoulos, N., Croll, S. D., Ho, L., Russell, M., Boland, P., Leidich, R., Hylton, D., Burova, E., Ioffe, E., Huang, T., Radziejewski, C., Bailey, K., Fandl, J. P., Daly, T., Wiegand, S. J., Yancopoulos, G. D., & Rudge, J. S. (2002). VEGF-Trap: a VEGF blocker with potent antitumor effects. *Proc Natl Acad Sci U S A, 99*(17), 11393-11398, ISSN 0027-8424 (Print)

Idris, I., & Donnelly, R. (2006). Protein kinase C beta inhibition: A novel therapeutic strategy for diabetic microangiopathy. *Diab Vasc Dis Res, 3*(3), 172-178, ISSN 1479-1641 (Print)

Ikeda, T., Sato, K., Katano, T., & Hayashi, Y. (1999). Vitrectomy for cystoid macular oedema with attached posterior hyaloid membrane in patients with diabetes. *Br J Ophthalmol, 83*(1), 12-14, ISSN 0007-1161 (Print)

Jain, A., Collen, J., Kaines, A., Hubschman, J. P., & Schwartz, S. (2010). Short-duration focal pattern grid macular photocoagulation for diabetic macular edema: four-month outcomes. *Retina, 30*(10), 1622-1626, ISSN 1539-2864 (Electronic)

Jonas, J. B., & Sofker, A. (2001). Intraocular injection of crystalline cortisone as adjunctive treatment of diabetic macular edema. *Am J Ophthalmol, 132*(3), 425-427, ISSN 0002-9394 (Print)

Joussen, A. M., Smyth, N., & Niessen, C. (2007). Pathophysiology of diabetic macular edema. *Dev Ophthalmol, 39*, 1-12, ISSN 0250-3751 (Print)

Kern, T. S. (2007). Contributions of inflammatory processes to the development of the early stages of diabetic retinopathy. *Exp Diabetes Res, 2007*, 95103, ISSN 1687-5303 (Electronic)

Kim, N. R., Kim, Y. J., Chin, H. S., & Moon, Y. S. (2009). Optical coherence tomographic patterns in diabetic macular oedema: prediction of visual outcome after focal laser photocoagulation. *Br J Ophthalmol, 93*(7), 901-905, ISSN 1468-2079 (Electronic)

Klein, R., Klein, B. E., Moss, S. E., Davis, M. D., & DeMets, D. L. (1984). The Wisconsin epidemiologic study of diabetic retinopathy. IV. Diabetic macular edema. *Ophthalmology, 91*(12), 1464-1474, ISSN 0161-6420 (Print)

Lavinsky, D., Cardillo, J. A., Melo, L. A., Jr., Dare, A., Farah, M. E., & Belfort, R., Jr. (2011). Randomized Clinical Trial Evaluating mETDRS versus Normal or High-Density Micropulse Photocoagulation for Diabetic Macular Edema. *Invest Ophthalmol Vis Sci, 52*(7), 4314-4323, ISSN 1552-5783 (Electronic)

Leopold, I. H. (1985). Nonsteroidal and steroidal anti-inflammatory agents. In M. L. Sears & A. Tarkkanen (Eds.), *Surgical Pharmacology of the Eye*. ISBN 0881670472 9780881670479, New York: Raven Press.

Lewis, H., Abrams, G. W., Blumenkranz, M. S., & Campo, R. V. (1992). Vitrectomy for diabetic macular traction and edema associated with posterior hyaloidal traction. *Ophthalmology, 99*(5), 753-759, ISSN 0161-6420 (Print)

Martidis, A., Duker, J. S., Greenberg, P. B., Rogers, A. H., Puliafito, C. A., Reichel, E., & Baumal, C. (2002). Intravitreal triamcinolone for refractory diabetic macular edema. *Ophthalmology, 109*(5), 920-927, ISSN 0161-6420 (Print)

Massin, P., Bandello, F., Garweg, J. G., Hansen, L. L., Harding, S. P., Larsen, M., Mitchell, P., Sharp, D., Wolf-Schnurrbusch, U. E., Gekkieva, M., Weichselberger, A., & Wolf, S. (2010). Safety and efficacy of ranibizumab in diabetic macular edema (RESOLVE Study): a 12-month, randomized, controlled, double-masked, multicenter phase II study. *Diabetes Care, 33*(11), 2399-2405, ISSN 1935-5548 (Electronic)

Michaelides, M., Kaines, A., Hamilton, R. D., Fraser-Bell, S., Rajendram, R., Quhill, F., Boos, C. J., Xing, W., Egan, C., Peto, T., Bunce, C., Leslie, R. D., & Hykin, P. G. (2010). A prospective randomized trial of intravitreal bevacizumab or laser therapy in the management of diabetic macular edema (BOLT study) 12-month data: report 2. *Ophthalmology, 117*(6), 1078-1086 e1072, ISSN 1549-4713 (Electronic)

Mitchell, P., Bandello, F., Schmidt-Erfurth, U., Lang, G. E., Massin, P., Schlingemann, R. O., Sutter, F., Simader, C., Burian, G., Gerstner, O., & Weichselberger, A. (2011). The RESTORE study: ranibizumab monotherapy or combined with laser versus laser monotherapy for diabetic macular edema. *Ophthalmology, 118*(4), 615-625, ISSN 1549-4713 (Electronic)

Moss, S. E., Klein, R., & Klein, B. E. (1998). The 14-year incidence of visual loss in a diabetic population. *Ophthalmology, 105*(6), 998-1003, ISSN 0161-6420 (Print)

Nauck, M., Karakiulakis, G., Perruchoud, A. P., Papakonstantinou, E., & Roth, M. (1998). Corticosteroids inhibit the expression of the vascular endothelial growth factor gene in human vascular smooth muscle cells. *Eur J Pharmacol, 341*(2-3), 309-315, ISSN 0014-2999 (Print)

Nauck, M., Roth, M., Tamm, M., Eickelberg, O., Wieland, H., Stulz, P., & Perruchoud, A. P. (1997). Induction of vascular endothelial growth factor by platelet-activating factor and platelet-derived growth factor is downregulated by corticosteroids. *Am J Respir Cell Mol Biol, 16*(4), 398-406, ISSN 1044-1549 (Print)

Nguyen, Q. D., Shah, S. M., Heier, J. S., Do, D. V., Lim, J., Boyer, D., Abraham, P., & Campochiaro, P. A. (2009). Primary End Point (Six Months) Results of the Ranibizumab for Edema of the mAcula in diabetes (READ-2) study. *Ophthalmology, 116*(11), 2175-2181 e2171, ISSN 1549-4713 (Electronic)

Nguyen, Q. D., Shah, S. M., Khwaja, A. A., Channa, R., Hatef, E., Do, D. V., Boyer, D., Heier, J. S., Abraham, P., Thach, A. B., Lit, E. S., Foster, B. S., Kruger, E., Dugel, P., Chang, T., Das, A., Ciulla, T. A., Pollack, J. S., Lim, J. I., Eliot, D., & Campochiaro, P. A. (2010). Two-year outcomes of the ranibizumab for edema of the mAcula in diabetes (READ-2) study. *Ophthalmology, 117*(11), 2146-2151, ISSN 1549-4713 (Electronic)

Nguyen, Q. D., Tatlipinar, S., Shah, S. M., Haller, J. A., Quinlan, E., Sung, J., Zimmer-Galler, I., Do, D. V., & Campochiaro, P. A. (2006). Vascular endothelial growth factor is a critical stimulus for diabetic macular edema. *Am J Ophthalmol, 142*(6), 961-969, ISSN 0002-9394 (Print)

Nicholson, B. P., & Schachat, A. P. (2010). A review of clinical trials of anti-VEGF agents for diabetic retinopathy. *Graefes Arch Clin Exp Ophthalmol, 248*(7), 915-930, ISSN 1435-702X (Electronic)

Olk, R. J. (1990). Argon green (514 nm) versus krypton red (647 nm) modified grid laser photocoagulation for diffuse diabetic macular edema. *Ophthalmology, 97*(9), 1101-1112; discussion 1112-1103, ISSN 0161-6420 (Print)

Panagiotoglou, T. D., Ganotakis, E. S., Kymionis, G. D., Moschandreas, J. A., Fanti, G. N., Charisis, S. K., Malliaraki, N. E., & Tsilimbaris, M. K. (2010). Atorvastatin for diabetic macular edema in patients with diabetes mellitus and elevated serum cholesterol. *Ophthalmic Surg Lasers Imaging, 41*(3), 316-322, ISSN 1542-8877 (Print)

Pearson, A., Levy, B., & Group., F. A. I. S. (2005). Fluocinolone Acetonide Intravitreal Implant to Treat Diabetic Macular Edema: 2–year Results of a Multi–Center Clinical Trial. *Invest Ophthalmol Vis Sci, 46*, E-Abstract P4673.

Pendergast, S. D., Hassan, T. S., Williams, G. A., Cox, M. S., Margherio, R. R., Ferrone, P. J., Garretson, B. R., & Trese, M. T. (2000). Vitrectomy for diffuse diabetic macular edema associated with a taut premacular posterior hyaloid. *Am J Ophthalmol, 130*(2), 178-186, ISSN 0002-9394 (Print)

PKC-DRS group. (2005). The effect of ruboxistaurin on visual loss in patients with moderately severe to very severe nonproliferative diabetic retinopathy: initial results of the Protein Kinase C beta Inhibitor Diabetic Retinopathy Study (PKC-DRS) multicenter randomized clinical trial. *Diabetes, 54*(7), 2188-2197, ISSN 0012-1797 (Print)

Qaum, T., Xu, Q., Joussen, A. M., Clemens, M. W., Qin, W., Miyamoto, K., Hassessian, H., Wiegand, S. J., Rudge, J., Yancopoulos, G. D., & Adamis, A. P. (2001). VEGF-initiated blood-retinal barrier breakdown in early diabetes. *Invest Ophthalmol Vis Sci, 42*(10), 2408-2413, ISSN 0146-0404 (Print)

Rakic, J. M., Lambert, V., Devy, L., Luttun, A., Carmeliet, P., Claes, C., Nguyen, L., Foidart, J. M., Noel, A., & Munaut, C. (2003). Placental growth factor, a member of the VEGF family, contributes to the development of choroidal neovascularization. *Invest Ophthalmol Vis Sci, 44*(7), 3186-3193, ISSN 0146-0404 (Print)

Schatz, H., Madeira, D., McDonald, H. R., & Johnson, R. N. (1991). Progressive enlargement of laser scars following grid laser photocoagulation for diffuse diabetic macular edema. *Arch Ophthalmol, 109*(11), 1549-1551, ISSN 0003-9950 (Print)

Scott, I. U., Edwards, A. R., Beck, R. W., Bressler, N. M., Chan, C. K., Elman, M. J., Friedman, S. M., Greven, C. M., Maturi, R. K., Pieramici, D. J., Shami, M., Singerman, L. J., & Stockdale, C. R. (2007). A phase II randomized clinical trial of intravitreal bevacizumab for diabetic macular edema. *Ophthalmology, 114*(10), 1860-1867, ISSN 1549-4713 (Electronic)

Sen, K., Misra, A., Kumar, A., & Pandey, R. M. (2002). Simvastatin retards progression of retinopathy in diabetic patients with hypercholesterolemia. *Diabetes Res Clin Pract, 56*(1), 1-11, ISSN 0168-8227 (Print)

Senger, D. R., Connolly, D. T., Van de Water, L., Feder, J., & Dvorak, H. F. (1990). Purification and NH2-terminal amino acid sequence of guinea pig tumor-secreted vascular permeability factor. *Cancer Res, 50*(6), 1774-1778, ISSN 0008-5472 (Print)

Senger, D. R., Galli, S. J., Dvorak, A. M., Perruzzi, C. A., Harvey, V. S., & Dvorak, H. F. (1983). Tumor cells secrete a vascular permeability factor that promotes accumulation of ascites fluid. *Science, 219*(4587), 983-985, ISSN 0036-8075 (Print)

Soheilian, M., Ramezani, A., Obudi, A., Bijanzadeh, B., Salehipour, M., Yaseri, M., Ahmadieh, H., Dehghan, M. H., Azarmina, M., Moradian, S., & Peyman, G. A. (2009). Randomized trial of intravitreal bevacizumab alone or combined with triamcinolone versus macular photocoagulation in diabetic macular edema. *Ophthalmology, 116*(6), 1142-1150, ISSN 1549-4713 (Electronic)

Stefansson, E. (2001). The therapeutic effects of retinal laser treatment and vitrectomy. A theory based on oxygen and vascular physiology. *Acta Ophthalmol Scand, 79*(5), 435-440, ISSN 1395-3907 (Print)

Sultan, M. B., Zhou, D., Loftus, J., Dombi, T., & Ice, K. S. (2011). A phase 2/3, multicenter, randomized, double-masked, 2-year trial of pegaptanib sodium for the treatment of diabetic macular edema. *Ophthalmology, 118*(6), 1107-1118, ISSN 1549-4713 (Electronic)

Tachi, N., & Ogino, N. (1996). Vitrectomy for diffuse macular edema in cases of diabetic retinopathy. *Am J Ophthalmol, 122*(2), 258-260, ISSN 0002-9394 (Print)

Van Meter, M. E., & Kim, E. S. (2010). Bevacizumab: current updates in treatment. *Curr Opin Oncol, 22*(6), 586-591, ISSN 1531-703X (Electronic)

Watanabe, J., Wohltmann, H. J., Klein, R. L., Colwell, J. A., & Lopes-Virella, M. F. (1988). Enhancement of platelet aggregation by low-density lipoproteins from IDDM patients. *Diabetes, 37*(12), 1652-1657, ISSN 0012-1797 (Print)

Wilson, D. J., Finkelstein, D., Quigley, H. A., & Green, W. R. (1988). Macular grid photocoagulation. An experimental study on the primate retina. *Arch Ophthalmol, 106*(1), 100-105, ISSN 0003-9950 (Print)

Yamamoto, T., Akabane, N., & Takeuchi, S. (2001). Vitrectomy for diabetic macular edema: the role of posterior vitreous detachment and epimacular membrane. *Am J Ophthalmol, 132*(3), 369-377, ISSN 0002-9394 (Print)

16

Calcium Dobesilate in Prevention and Treatment of Diabetic Retinopathy

Oldřich Farsa
Faculty of Pharmacy, University of Veterinary and Pharmaceutical Sciences Brno
Czech Republic

1. Introduction

Diabetic retinopathy is a leading cause of adult vision loss and blindness. Angioprotective drugs are one of possibilities, which can be used in treatment of diabetic retinopathy. Nearly all of them are very efficient antioxidants or reactive oxygen and nitrogen species (RONS) scavengers. They often contain phenolic groups. Most of them are glycosides of plant origin with aglycones of flavonoid structure, i.e. aglycones are polyhydroxylated derivatives of 2-phenyl-4*H*-chromen-2-one or 2-phenyl-4*H*-1-benzopyran-4-one. Quercetin, which is the aglycone of many glycosides including rutoside, can serve as a typical example. Other glycosides, such as a saponoside escine (Reparil®) isolated from seeds of horse chestnut *Aesculus hippocastaneum*, have triterpenic aglycones. (In fact, escin is a mixture of several related compounds. The particular structure on the Figure I express escin I that is a mixture of two geometric isomers. They differ in *E* or *Z* configuration of 2-methylbut-2-enoyl, which is attached to originally hydroxyl oxygen in position 21β of the triterpenoid scaffold.) (Kim et al., 2004, Carrasco & Vidrio, 2007). Flavonoid glycosides have poor bioavailability that is due to their low lipophilicity. This problem has been solved by etherification of phenolic groups of flavonoid aglycones with hydroxyalkyl such as hydroxyethyl groups (troxerutin) in past (Agolini & Cavallini, 1987, Wadworth & Faulds, 1992) Troxerutin was demonstrated to attenuate neovascularization in retinopathy in streptozocin-induced diabetic rats (Chung et al., 2005). More recently, increased bioavailability of flavonoid glycosides is reached by micronisation without changing their chemical structures. Preparations such as Detralex® or Daflon® contain standardized and micronized flavonoid fraction characterized by its content of diosmin, which is their main active constituent. Their activity in the treatment of diabetic retinopathy was clearly demonstrated (Lacombe et al., 1989). There is nearly only one exception among these quite complex compounds: calcium dobesilate (Danium ®, Doxium ®, Dexium®), which is a very simple synthetic molecule: calcium 2,5-dihydroxybenzenesulfonate (see Figure 1)

Calcium dobesilate is also almost the only one angioprotective drug that recently remains the object of interest in treatment of diabetic retinopathy including clinical studies (Leal et al. 2010, Einarsdottir & Stefansson, 2009, Ribeiro et al., 2006), and even it was used as a standard for determination of the particular activity of a traditional Chinese herbal medicine preparation (Luo et al. 2009).

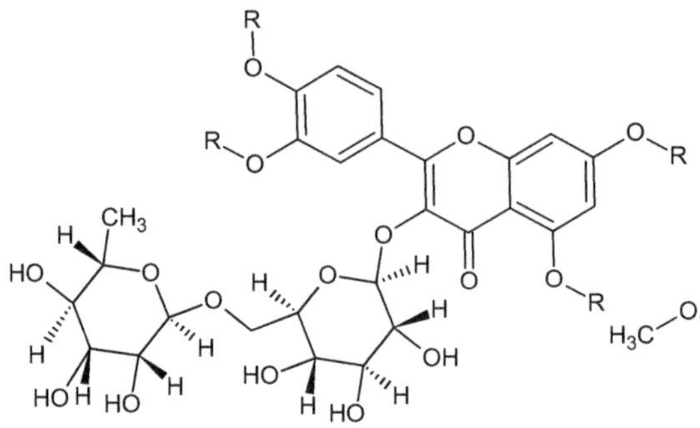

R = -H rutin (rutosid)

R = $-OCH_2CH_2OH$ troxerutin

free aglycone with R = -H and free -OH in pos. 3 = quercetin

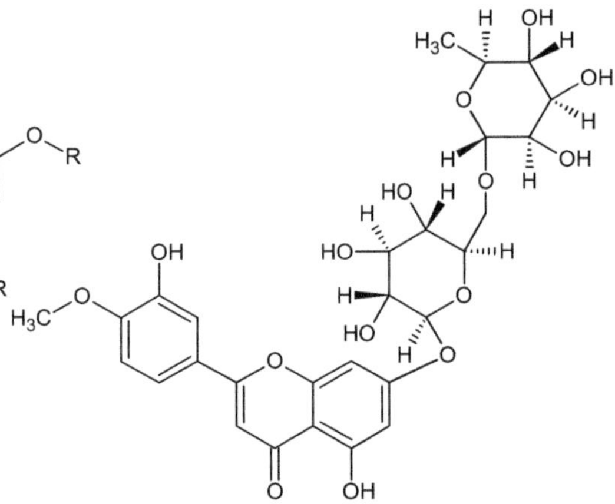

diosmin

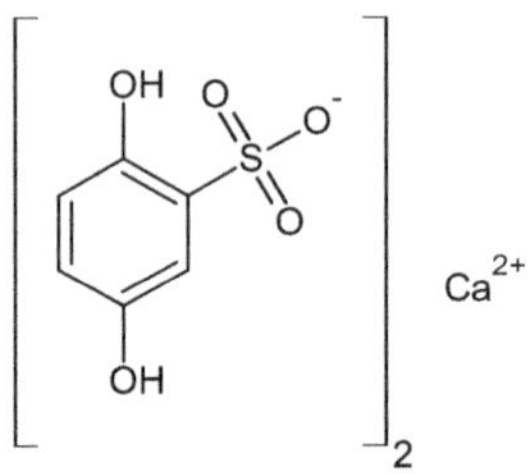

calcium dobesilate

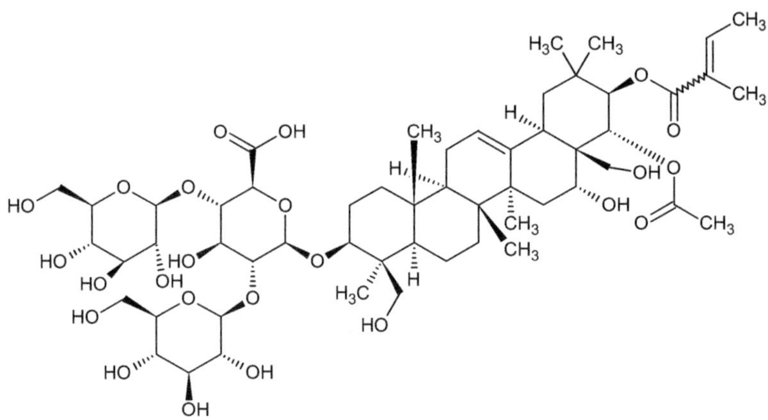

escin I

Fig. 1. Calcium dobesilate as the simplest structure among angioprotective drugs.

2. Calcium dobesilate: Chemical, historical and bibliographical data

2.1 Early syntheses of 2,5-dihydroxybenzenesulfonic acid and its salts

The first synthesis of 2,5-dihydroxybenzenesulfonic acid that can be found is that in the article of Seyda (Seyda, 1883). On principle it was sulfonation of hydroquinone with diluted sulfuric acid in mild conditions, the reaction temperature did not exceed 50°C, for 3 hours. During this period, starting hydroquinone gradually dissolved in diluted sulfuric acid. After cooling of the solution for 24 hours, formed crystals of 2,5-dihydroxybenzenesulfonic acid were filtered off. The filtrate was diluted with water and under boiling saturated with barium carbonate. The excessive barium carbonate was then together with formed barium sulfate filtered off. The filtrate was being concentrated *in vacuo* until a white crystalline syrupy mass was formed. This viscous liquid was then poured on a porous ceramic plate to be dried. Thus barium 2,5-dihydroxybenzenesulfonate was yielded. Potassium 2,5-dihydroxybenzenesulfonate was prepared by adding of potassium carbonate into an aqueous solution of barium 2,5-dihydroxybenzenesulfonate followed by filtering-off of formed barium carbonate and concentration of the filtrate *in vacuo* into a viscous liquid that was then diluted with double volume of absolute ethanol. A brown precipitate, which had been formed was then filtered off and all the ethanol was distilled off from the filtrate with exclusion of air. Crystalline mass formed from the filtrate was then recrystallized from water to give transparent octaedric crystals. Sodium 2,5-dihydroxybenzenesulfonate was prepared similarly by adding of sodium carbonate into a solution of the barium salt. It was formed in the concentrated aqueous solution as a mass consisted from microscopic octaedric crystals. Lead 2,5-dihydroxybenzesulfonate was prepared from the crude 2,5-dihydroxybenzenesulfonic acid and lead carbonate. It precipitated from a concentrated aqueous solution as an amorphous solid that was no more soluble in water. However, it was soluble in concentrated acetic acid. The lead salt gave the free 2,5-dihydroxybenzenesulfonic acid by reaction with sulfane (see Figure 2).

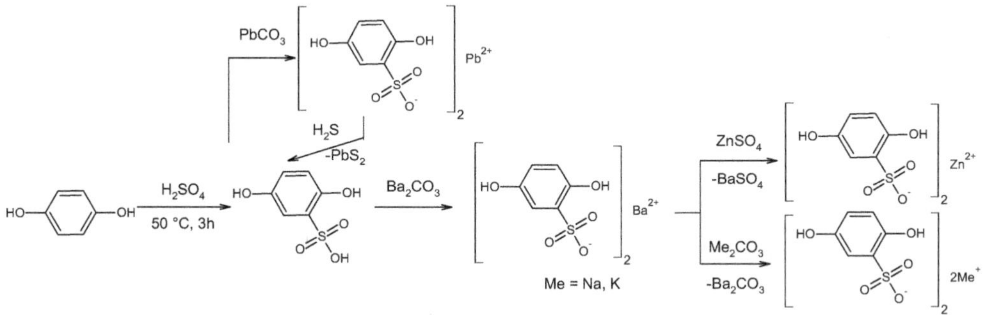

Fig 2. Early syntheses of 2,5-dihydroxybenzenesulfonic acid and some its metallic salts.

2.2 Industrial „redox" one-pot synthesis of calcium dobesilate vs. sulfonation followed by neutralization

Estéve-Subirana (Estéve-Subirana, 1970) has developed a different synthesis of calcium dobesilate, which is also simple and suitable for the industrial production of it. It consists of only one reaction of calcium hydrogensulfite with 1,4-benzoquinone. Such a procedure could be classified as a „redox substitution" due to changes of the oxidation states of both sulfur atom and benzene ring. However, such a synthesis is not suitable for low scale preparations of calcium dobesilate including those that are performed by students in practical classes in subjects such as medicinal or organic chemistry. These practical educations can be met by students of fields such as pharmacy or chemistry at appropriate schools or faculties. The main problem of the Estéve-Subirana's procedure consists in use of calcium hydrogensulfite, which is not commercially available in solid state. Its concentrated aqueous solution is frequently prepared by reaction of gaseous sulfur dioxide with an aqueous suspension of calcium carbonate. This reaction can proceed in a special bubble column reactor typical for industrial processes such as the procedure developed by Rückauf and colleagues (Rückauf et al., 1990).

$$CaCO_3 + SO_2 + H_2O \longrightarrow Ca(HSO_3)_2 + CO_2$$

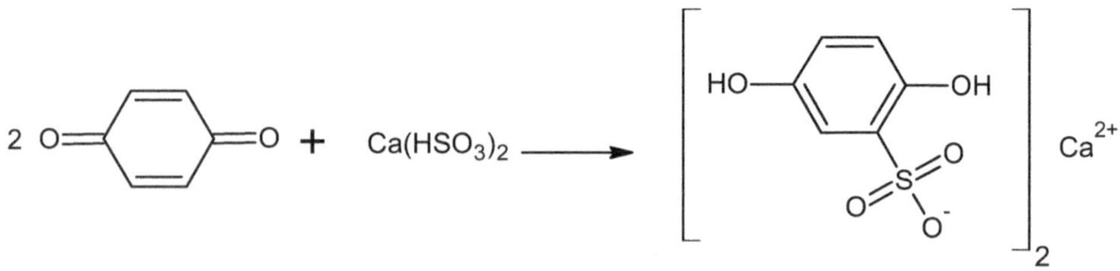

Fig. 3. Preparation of calcium dobesilate according to Estéve-Subirana (Estéve-Subirana, 1970) preceeded with preparation of calcium hydrogensulfite according to Rückauf et al. (Rückauf et al. , 1990).

To develop a simple and effective synthesis of calcium dobesilate that does not require calcium hydrogensulfite, we returned to sulfonation of hydroquinone. After we had tried several procedures using diluted sulfuric acid without significant successes (Šablatura, 2005), we came back to the original preparation of Seyda (Seyda, 1883). We modified his synthesis of barium 2,5-dihydroxybenzenesulfonate for preparation calcium dobesilate in conditions of today. Hydroquinone was sulfonated with concentrated sulfuric acid, a resulted mixture was then neutralized short boiling with calcium carbonate. Poorly soluble calcium sulfate precipitate was then filtered off. The filtrate was evaporated nearly to dryness. The residuum was disperged in concentated ethanol and filtered. The ethanolic filtrate was evaporated to dryness. Recrystallization of the residuum from the mixture butan-1-ol / chloroform gave calcium dobesilate in the form of its monohydrate (see Fig. 4).

Crystallization trials from several with various ratios alcohol / water mixtures led in most to solid solvates, e.g. calcium dobesilate : propan-2-ol 1 : 1.3 (dobesilate : alcohol ratio was estimated from ^{1}H-NMR spectrum). Simple confirmation of identity of the product by determination of its melting point is impossible because of high value of its melting temperature, but it can be identified by simple spectrophotometry in UV region according to Czech Pharmacopoeia 2005 Edition (Czech Pharmacopoeia 2009, 2009) (see also bellow). This procedure was published in a journal devoted to chemical education (Farsa & Šablatura, 2008) and in more detailed and modified form also in an instruction manual for practical courses in medicinal chemistry (Beneš & Farsa, 2007). It is notable that, short time after its publishing, very similar procedures of preparation of calcium dobesilate appeared in Chinese patents (Yao 2010, Yang et al. 2010).

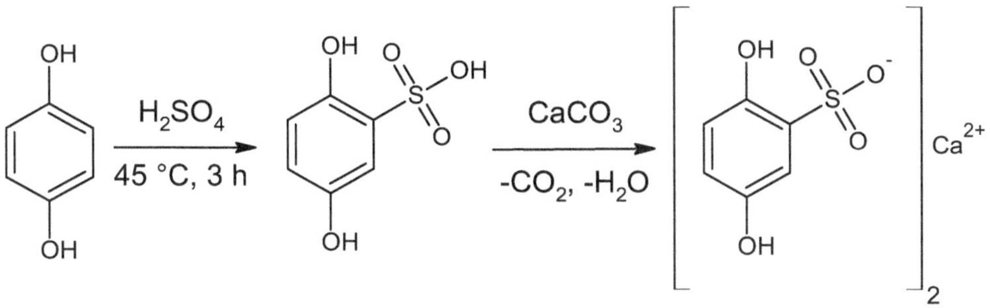

Fig. 4. Preparation of calcium dobesilate proposed for practical courses in chemical disciplines

2.3 Spectral data and other important physico-chemical properties of calcium dobesilate

Infrared spectra of calcium dobesilate measured in a potassium bromide tablet contained significant absorption bands at wawenumbers 3410, 1500, 1470, 1220, 1080, 880, 815 and 640 cm^{-1} (Estéve-Soler, 1977) A ^{1}H nuclear magnetic resonance spectrum (^{1}H-NMR) of calcium dobesilate recorded in deuterium oxide contained following signals (values of chemical shifts δ are in ppm): 7.13 (bs, 3H, aromatic hydrogens), 6.70 (s, 2H, 2 OH) and 4.75 (s, 2H, H_2O). The least signal served also as the reference one. There was evident from the ratio of integral areas that the investigated sample was calcium dobesilate monohydrate (Estéve-Soler, 1977). ^{1}H-NMR measured by the author in deuterated dimethyl sulfoxide (DMSO-D_6) was a little different. It contained the following signals (chemical shifts δ are in ppm, coupling constants J in Hz): 9.78 (s, 1H, OH), 8.84 (s, 1H, OH), 6.80 (d, 1H, J=2.4, arom. H), 6.57 (m, 2H, arom. H), 3.37 (s, 4H, 2 H_2O). The integral area of the signal assigned to water hydrogens corresponded to 4 hydrogen atoms per one dobesilate anion so that this sample was calcium dobesilate tetrahydrate (see Fig. 5). A ^{13}C nuclear magnetic resonance spectrum (^{13}C-NMR) of the same sample of calcium dobesilate was recorded by the author also in DMSO-D_6 in attached proton test (APT) mode. This type of carbon NMR spectrum enables to differ between carbon atoms with odd and even number of hydrogen atoms attached to every particular carbon atom so that in our case to distinguish between aromatic carbons with one hydrogen and those with no hydrogen. It contained the following signals (the values of chemical shift in ppm): 148.8 (CH), 145.8 (CH), 130.6 (CH), 117.9 (CSO_3^-), 116, 5 (COH), 112.8 (COH) (see Fig. 5).

Also ultraviolet spectra, which are advantageous namely for purity determination, have been known for decades. They have been recorded from various solvents such as water, methanol or aqueous hydrochloric acid. (Negritescu et al., 1979, Kračmár et al., 1988, Chen & Xiao, 2008). These electronic spectra are relatively easy to obtain because of low prices of needed UV spectrophotometers in comparison with NMR or IR spectrometers. This is probably one of the reasons for which some pharmacopoeias use this method for confirmation of identity of calcium dobesilate monohydrate, which is official as a drug substance (Czech Pharmacopoeia 2009, 2009, European Pharmacopoeia Edition 7.2, 2011). In accordance with both pharmacopoeias, the UV spectrum of calcium dobesilate measured in water can have absorption maxima at 221 and 301 nm and the specific absorbance at 301 nm in the range 174 to 181 (see Fig. 6).

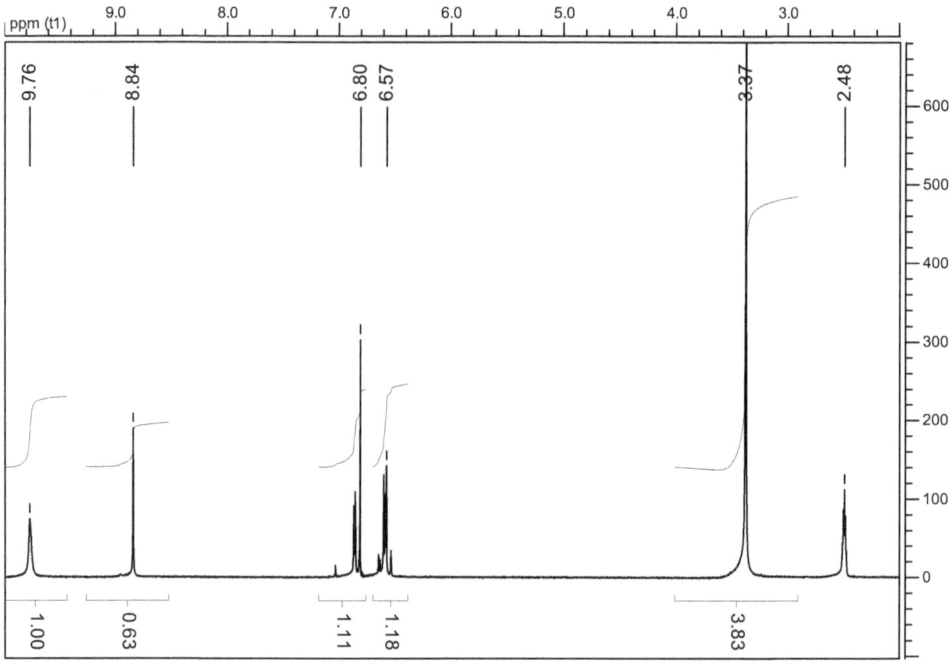

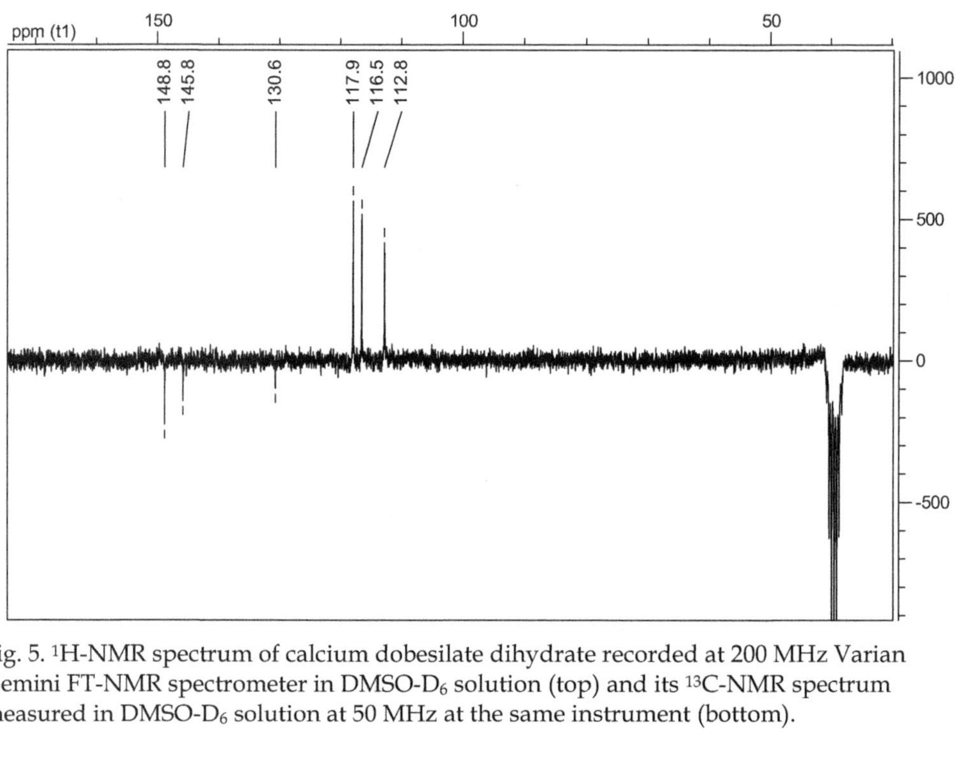

Fig. 5. ^{1}H-NMR spectrum of calcium dobesilate dihydrate recorded at 200 MHz Varian Gemini FT-NMR spectrometer in DMSO-D_6 solution (top) and its ^{13}C-NMR spectrum measured in DMSO-D_6 solution at 50 MHz at the same instrument (bottom).

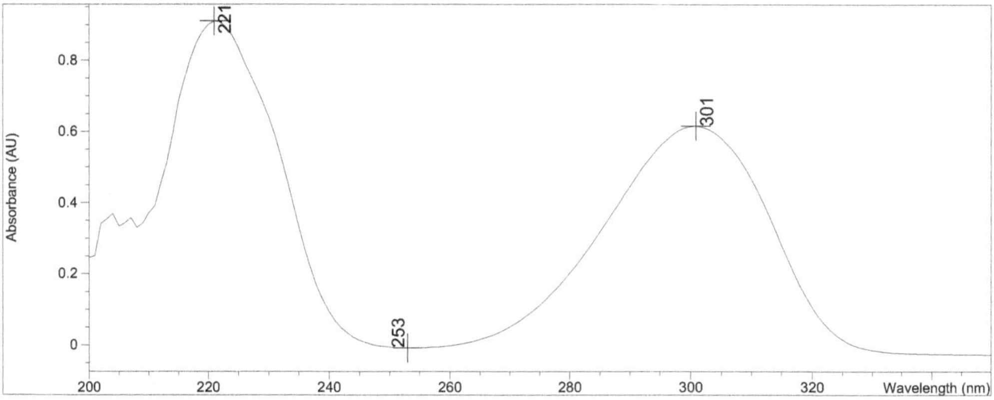

Fig. 6. Ultraviolet spectrum of calcium dobesilate measured in an aqueous solution at Agilent 8453 diode array UV-VIS spectrophotometer in accordance with requirements of the European Pharmacopoeia (European Pharmacopoeia Edition 7.2, 2011).

As it was mentioned above, melting point of calcium dobesilate monohydrate is out of range of measurement of common melting point apparatuses and thus it is not suitable for identification of calcium dobesilate monohydrate as a substance. Milne states that anhydrous calcium dobesilate melts above 300°C under decomposition (Milne, 2002).

The pharmacopoeias state that calcium dobesilate monohydrate is very soluble in water, freely soluble in anhydrous ethanol, very slightly soluble in propan-2-ol and practically insoluble in dichloromethane (Czech Pharmacopoeia 2009, 2009, European Pharmacopoeia Edition 7.2, 2011). In fact, it is extremely soluble in water: three weight parts of calcium dobesilate monohydrate dissolve in one part of boiling water. This ratio of the compound and the solvent can be used for purifying of the drug by recrystallization (Nováček et al., 1987).

Since calcium dobesilate is a hydroquinone derivative it can be easily oxidized into calcium 3,6-dioxocyclohexa-1,4-diene-1-sulfonate (see Fig. 7).

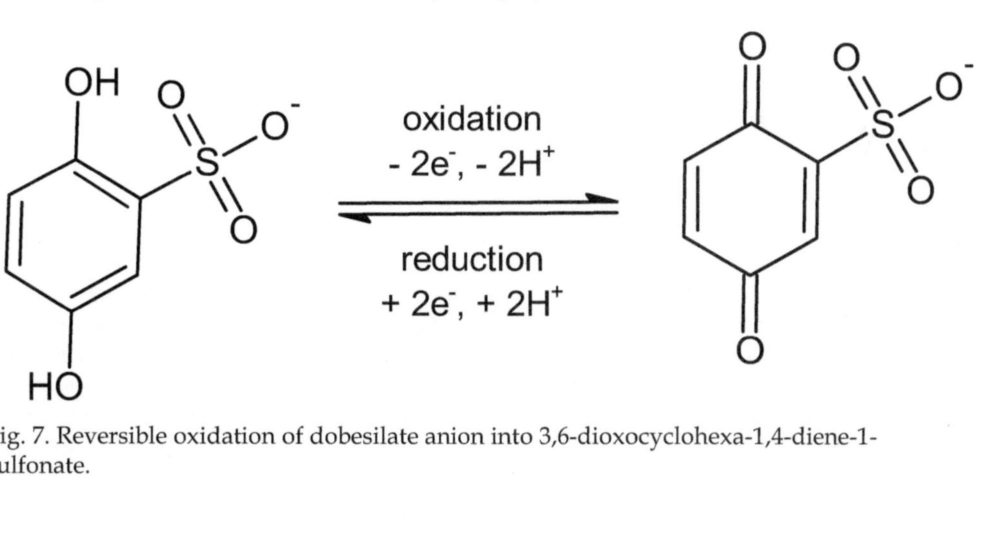

Fig. 7. Reversible oxidation of dobesilate anion into 3,6-dioxocyclohexa-1,4-diene-1-sulfonate.

Reversibility of this reaction has been repeatedly demonstrated by cyclic voltammetry with various types of electrodes. (Zheng et al., 2007, Zhang & Zhang, 2009, Zhang et al., 2011). Such methods have reached very low detection limit for calcium dobesilate up to 4.0×10^{-8} mol L^{-1} and have been resistant to interference with other reducing compounds occurring in body liquids such as uric acid, serotonin, and ascorbic acid (Hu et al., 2009). That is why they have been successfully used not only for identification and assay of calcium dobesilate in substance samples and drug formulations (Guangzhi et al., 2009) but also in biological samples (Zheng et al., 2007). The influence of bovine serum albumin (BSA) on the electrochemical behavior of calcium dobesilate was also investigated. The stoichiometric coefficient and the association constant of calcium dobesilate with BSA were obtained by this technique in addition to those obtained by UV-spectrophotometry. It was found that the peak currents in cyclic voltammetry diagrams decreased and the peak potentials stayed almost unchanged in the presence of BSA, indicating that there might exist an interaction between calcium dobesilate and BSA (Xu et al., 2009). Oxidation of calcium dobesilate is also used for its titrimetric assay by means of cerimetry with potentiometric end-point determination required by some pharmacopoeias (European Pharmacopoeia 7.2, 2011, Czech Pharmacopoeia 2009, 2009). This method gives more accurate results than chelatometric titrimetry using N,N'-ethylenediaminetetraacetic acid (EDTA) for complexation of calcium ion of calcium dobesilate (Zhang & Xu, 1999). The activity of calcium dobesilate as a reduction agent is also reason of its radical-scavenging activity, which plays an important role in its mechanism of action as a drug of diabetic retinopathy (see further).

The chromatographic behaviour of calcium dobesilate is determined by its extremely low lipophilicity as it is an ionic salt. Thin-layer chromatography (TLC) on a silica gel normal phase was being used for identification of hydroquinone as an impurity in calcium dobesilate substance. While hydroquinone migrates in the required mobile phase dichloromethane : methyl acetate : ethyl acetate 20 : 30 : 50, calcium dobesilate remains at the start (Czech Pharmacopoeia 2002, 2002, Šablatura, 2006). Reversed phase high performance liquid chromatography (reversed phase-high performance liquid chromatography) methods for identification and content assay of calcium dobesilate namely in various samples have been reported. Assays of calcium dobesilate in dog blood plasma for pharmacokinetic purposes after its single (Plessas et al., 1986a) and repeated (Plessas et al., 1986b) administration were performed using a C18 column. A similar method using a Hypersil® octadecylsilyl silica gel (ODS) column and UV detection in absorption maximum of calcium dobesilate at 301 nm with mobile phase methanol : water 7 : 3 and flow rate 1.0 mL min^{-1} has been developed for determination of calcium dobesilate in pharmaceuticals (Zhu & Chen, 2005). Slightly different conditions, mobile phase acetonitrile : water buffer pH 2.5 1 : 1, flow rate 1.0 mL min^{-1} and detection wavelength 290 nm, were used in a procedure suitable for simultaneous determination of calcium dobesilate and lidocaine hydrochloride, dexamethasone acetate, butylhydroxyanisol and hydroquinone as a degradation product of calcium dobesilate in suppositories and an ointment. The retention times ranged between 2.4 min for the most hydrophilic calcium dobesilate to 17.1 min for the most hydrophilic BHA (Zivanovic et al., 2005). Also recent pharmacopoeias utilize reversed phase-high performance liquid chromatography using a spherical end-capped ODS column, mobile phase acetonitrile : aqueous buffer solution 1 : 9, flow rate 0.8 mL min^{-1} and detection wavelength 220 nm for the test for presence of impurities, namely hydroquinone. calcium dobesilate could have the retention time about 6 min in this system (European Pharmacopoeia 7.2, 2011, Czech Pharmacopoeia 2009, 2009). Finally, Rona and Ary reported a reversed phase-high performance liquid chromatography procedure suitable for determination of calcium dobesilate in human plasma for purposes of bioequivalence studies. They used a C16 reverse phase modified with inserted amide moiety. Such phases have been recommended as suitable for separation of polar compounds (Sigma-Aldrich, 2011). The mixture phosphate buffer pH 2.5 : acetonitrile 3 : 1 was used as a mobile phase, the detection wavelength was 305 nm (Rona & Ary, 2001). It is interesting that no high performance liquid chromatography procedure using electrochemical detection has been reported although redox properties of calcium dobesilate offer this possibility of sensitive detection.

2.4 Polymorphism, solvate complexes and co-crystals of calcium dobesilate

Calcium dobesilate monohydrate is the most common crystalline form of calcium dobesilate and is also official in many pharmacopoeias. It is also a subject of a mild misunderstanding between some pharmacopoeias and Chemical Abstracts or their electronic version, the data base SciFinder, because the Chemical Abstracts Service reference number (CAS RN) 20123-80-2 is in the pharmacopoeias (European Pharmacopoeia 7.2, 2011, Czech Pharmacopoeia 2009, 2009) assigned to this monohydrate while in SciFinder to anhydrous calcium dobesilate. Calcium dobesilate monohydrate is then referred in SciFinder under CAS RN 117552-79-1 (SciFinder, 2011). Calcium dobesilate monohydrate has been characterized by powder X-ray diffraction spectrum (Lu, 2005) and by two methods of differential thermal analysis (DTA); thermogravimetric analysis (TGA) a differential scanning calorimetry (DSC). Caproiu and colleagues reported based on DTA that calcium dobesilate monohydrate showed dehydration starting at 115°C and ending at 180°C (Caproiu et al., 1988) while Lu stated the dehydration interval between 134°C and 180°C (Lu, 2005). Calcium dobesilate dihydrate, sesquihydrate, i.e. hydrate containing 1.5 mol water per 1 mol calcium dobesilate, and non-stoichiometric hydrates containing 5/7, 5/4, 1.6 and 2.6 mol water per 1 mol calcium dobesilate respectively have been patented (Huang, 2007).

Calcium dobesilate has been patented as an active ingredient of its mixed-phase co-crystaline form. Such co-crystals are based on a theory that the additive(s), which are also known as co-crystal formers, are co-crystallized as minor non-stoichiometric components in the active agent's crystalline matrix. This co-crystalline phase has then semi-crystalline nature and contains a high incidence of crystal defects. Any excess additive that is not co-crystallized with the active agent forms a separate phase (Additive Phase) apart from the active agent, which results in the mixed phase co-crystal composition. The Additive Phase and the active agent crystals containing co-crystallized additive can be tightly agglomerated forming a mixed phase co-crystal particle. The unique physical properties obtained by this process of preparation can include changes in apparent solubility, crystallinity, water wetability, dissolution rates, physical powder properties (e.g., bulk density, absolute density, refractive index, x-ray diffraction, spectral, flowability, hygroscopicity, adsorption, and compaction), bioavailability, apparent permeability, apparent taste, and/or stability (Goldman, 2005). Calcium dobesilate is believed to form co-crystals with co-crystal former, which has at least one functional group selected from amine, amide, pyridine, imidazole, indole, pyrrolidine, carbonyl, carboxyl, hydroxyl, phenol, sulfone, sulfonyl, mercapto and methylsulfanyl, such that calcium dobesilate and co-crystal former are capable of co-crystallizing from a solution phase under crystallization conditions (Almarsson et al., 2011). Calcium dobesilate has also been patented as a component of an ionic liquid (Rogers et al., 2010) that can be used for overcoming of influence polymorphism in drug substances (Rogers et al., 2007). calcium dobesilate can also form solvates with propylene glycol, which could be more stable than hydrates (Tawa et al, 2010). However, none of these patents contains a particular example of processing of calcium dobesilate.

3. Activities found in *In Vitro* and animal models

3.1 Antioxidant and antiradical activity

Antioxidant or reduction activity of calcium dobesilate is a result of its hydroquinone structure. This was mentioned above in section 2.3 in relationship to its analytical behaviour (compare Fig. 8) but this type of reactivity has also an important impact to its biological activity. The ability of 2,5-dihydroxybenzenesulfonic acid salts to reduce mercurous and silver nitrates to metallic mercury and silver respectively was first observed by Seyda (Seyda, 1883). Calcium dobesilate was shown to actively interact with toxic superoxide anion radical $O_2^{\circ -}$.This reactive oxygen species (ROS) was generated either by UV irradiation of an aqueous solution of glycyltryptohphan at 280 nm, or by irradiation of a mixture of glycyltryptophan with riboflavine with visible light. Thus calcium dobesilate showed the activity similar to that of superoxide dismutase (Lozovskaia et al., 1990). This result was confirmed in the experiment in which superoxide radicals were generated in the system xanthine/xanthine oxidase/ferrous chloride, but potency of calcium dobesilate to scavenge superoxide radicals was 23 times less than that of rutin that was used for comparison. However, calcium dobesilate was as potent as rutin in scavenging hydroxyl radicals generated *in vitro* via the iron-catalyzed Haber-Weiss reaction from superoxide anion (IC_{50} = 1.1 vs 0.7 μM, respectively). In human erythrocytes, calcium dobesilate reduced phenazine methosulfate dependent lipid peroxydation, although the effect was observed at high concentration (Brunet et al., 1998a). Oral treatment with calcium dobesilate significantly protected diabetic rat retina against a free radicals mediated injury induced by ischemia/reperfusion. This was observed in an *in vivo* experiment with streptozotocin-induced diabetic rats (Szabo et al., 2001). The results of these experiments support the hypothesis that the antioxidant properties of calcium dobesilate could play a role in its angioprotective properties *in vivo*. The antioxidant effects of calcium dobesilate were further investigated in relation to the oxidative status, apoptosis and in vitro proliferation of human peripheral blood mononuclear cells (PBMC) isolated from healthy donors. Calcium dobesilate alone did not modify cell growth in vitro until 10 μM. This molecule counteracted oxidative damages generated by the high reducing aldose 2-deoxy-D-ribose (dR). PBMC incubated with the reducing sugars D(-)-ribose and 2-deoxy-D-ribose (dR) exhibited characteristic patterns of apoptosis, such as DNA fragmentation and morphological changes, which can be prevented by exogenous antioxidants such as N-acetyl-L-cysteine (Barbieri et al., 1994) and/or other agents (Anderson et al., 1994). Calcium dobesilate was shown to reduce apoptosis by delaying both membrane permeability changes and DNA fragmentation. Calcium dobesilate 10 μM affected in a time-dependent dynamics several parameters representative of the cellular oxidative status. In particular, calcium dobesilate significantly increased the activity of glutathione S-transferase (GST) after three days of treatment and also, but to a lower extent, the activity of γ-glutamyltransferase (γ-GT). Both enzymes are known to be involved in the glutathione (GSH) metabolic cycle. This enzymatic behaviour was reversed at seven days of treatment, with a significant GST decrease and a γ-GT activation. After seven days of calcium dobesilate exposure, the intracellular GSH content was enhanced and this resulted in a dramatic decrease in lipid peroxidation, underlining the powerful antioxidant properties of calcium dobesilate in human PBMC. (Graber et al., 1998). These results indicate that *in vitro* antioxidant effects of calcium dobesilate manifest *in vivo* by reduced lipid peroxidation and contribute to the prevention of apoptosis.

3.2 Angioprotective action of calcium dobesilate against reactive oxygen species-induced capillary permeability

Microvascular permeability seems to be strongly increased by ROS generated *in situ*. In an *in vivo* experiment in rats, calcium dobesilate administered intraperitoneally (i.p.), intravenously (i.v.) and orally (p.o.) significantly reduced microvascular permeabilization induced by ROS in the rat peritoneal cavity. ROS were generated again either with the system xanthine / xanthine oxidase or with PMS/NADH. Microvascular permeabilization was quantified by Evans blue extravasation. The activity of calcium dobesilate was comparable to that of rutin (Brunet et al., 1998b).

3.3 Enhancement of nitric oxide synthase activity in endothelial cells

The term endothelium-derived relaxing factor was originally proposed by Robert Furchgott for a then unknown factor leading to relaxation of the smooth muscle of large arteries in response to acetylcholine. Nitric oxide NO, which is in fact a free radical, was later found to be the mediator of this response. Most of NO in the body is synthesized by the endothelial isoform of NO synthase (NOS) from its precursor L-arginine (Palmer et al., 1988a), which is inhibited by false substrates of NOS, e.g., L-N^G-monomethyl arginine (L-NMMA) (Palmer et al., 1988b). NOS is a highly regulated protein and the endothelial form (eNOS) is predominantly found in endothelial cells. In them, two different isoenzymes can be expressed, depending on the activation state of these cells. In resting, non-activated endothelial cells a constitutive enzyme (ecNOS) is expressed (Moncada & Higgs, 1993) and after challenge with proinflammatory cytokines and/or bacterial endotoxin a cytokine-inducible enzyme (iNOS) is expressed in addition (Suschek et al., 1993). The constitutive, calcium-dependent isoenzyme produces low amounts of NO for short periods of time (Palacios et al., 1989). This endothelium-derived NO plays a crucial role in blood pressure regulation (Rees et al., 1989), in inhibition of platelet aggregation and platelet adhesion (Radomski et al., 1987a, b), and in modulating leukocyte adhesion, an essential step early in tissue inflammation (Kubes et al., 1991, Zimmerman et al., 1992). The inducible, cytosolic, calcium-independent NO synthase is expressed only after cell activation and releases large amounts of NO for longer periods of time that functions as cytotoxic and immune regulatory effector molecule (Kröncke et al., 1995). Diabetes-induced vascular function abnormalities are besides other biochemical and morphological changes also reflected by decreased synthesis of NO (Durante et al., 1988, McVeigh et al., 1992). Magnesium 2,5-dihydroxybenzenesulfonate or magnesium dobesilate was used instead of calcium dobesilate in an experiment concerned with investigation of influence of dobesilate on NOS activities. The reason of usage of this compound was to eliminate a direct activation of the constitutive calcium-dependent NOS by calcium ions. In search for an effect on endothelial NO production, macrovascular endothelial cells from rat aorta, microvascular endothelial cells from rat exocrine pancreatic tissue, and capillary endothelial cells from rat islets, werecultured in the presence or absence of magnesium dobesilate. The activity of ecNOS in resident cells as well as of iNOS in cytokine-activated cells was measured indirectly by recording the citrulline concentrations in culture supernatants. In each of the different endothelial cells magnesium dobesilate incubation (0.25 ± 1 mM) for 24 h led to a significant and concentration-dependent increase in ecNOS-activities. With cytokine-activated endothelial cell cultures only moderate effects were observed with little or no concentration-dependency. Addition of the NOS-inhibitor L-NMMA led to a significant suppression of citrulline formation in all cultures as an evidence for the enzyme specificity of these effects. Both iNOS- and ecNOS-specific reverse transcription and semi-quantitative polymerase chain reaction (RT-PCR) with RNA from resident or cytokine-activated endothelial cells gave no evidence for an increase in NOS-specific mRNA after MgD-treatment. Furthermore, dobesilate-mediated enhancement of NO synthesis in resting endothelial cells was not due to iNOS induction in these cells, as no iNOS-specific signal was found by RT-PCR (Suschek et al., 1997). Results of these experiments were supported by an additional study in which calcium dobesilate was found to enhance the endothelium-dependent relaxation induced by acetylcholine in rabbit isolated aorta artery. This effect was clearly endothelium dependent because, after the endothelium had been removed, the effect disappeared. The experiments were carried out on approximately 2 - 3 wide rings prepared by cutting of the arteries. The effect of calcium dobesilate was inhibited when the rings were incubated with increasing concentration of another known NOS inhibitor N^G-nitro-L-arginine methyl ester (L-NAME), and this effect was reversed wit L-arginine, the substrate in NO synthesis (Ruiz et al., 1997).

3.4 Influence of calcium dobesilate on apoptosis in vessel and other tissues

Since apoptosis is closely linked with oxidation stress some aspects of anti-apoptic effects of calcium dobesilate were mentioned above in section 3.1. In a clinical study, the influence of calcium dobesilate to apoptosis of varicose veins in comparison with diosmin-hesperidin combination was investigated. Patients were treated either with calcium dobesilate or with diosmin-hesperidin six weeks prior to the surgical removal of the particular varicose vein. Tissue samples obtained from such veins of 56 patients were immunohistochemically stained with antibodies of anti-bcl-2 and anti-bax thus aimed at anti-apoptic (bcl-2) and pro-apoptic (bax) proteins. Significant differences in the presence of bcl-2 protein expression between the untreated patient group and the group treated with calcium dobesilate suggest that calcium dobesilate could be of benefit in treatment of vascular disorders by down-regulating apoptosis (Iriz et al., 2008). On the other hand, calcium dobesilate is capable to elicit growth arrest of some types of cancer, in particular glioma (Cuevas et al., 2005) and basal cell carcinoma (Cuevas & Arrazola, 2005), and induce apoptosis of their cells.

3.5 Effects of calcium dobesilate on expression of adhesion molecules ICAM-1 and VCAM-1

Diabetes causes metabolic and physiologic abnormalities in the retina, and inflammation seems to play a critical role in the development of diabetic retinopathy. Those changes include the upregulation of inducible NOS, cyclooxygenase-2, intercellular adhesion molecule-1 (ICAM-1), caspase-1, vascular endothelial growth factor (VEGF), and nuclear factor kappa B (NF-κB), which leads to increased production of NO, prostaglandin E2, and cytokines (Adamis & Berman, 2008, Kern, 2007). It has also been demonstrated that the adhesion of leukocytes to retinal vessels is increased in the retinas of diabetic animals, and this increase is correlated with changes in tight junction proteins and increased blood–retinal barrier (BRB) permeability (Barber et al., 2000, Klaassen et al., 2009). The increase in leukostasis is also associated with an increase in the expression of ICAM-1 by retinal endothelial cells (Miyamoto et al., 1999). NF-κB regulates the expression of adhesion molecules, such as ICAM-1, and NF-κB activation has been correlated with the increase in leukostasis and BRB breakdown in diabetic rat retinas (Joussen et al., 2002). In a study on streptozotocin-induced diabetic rats, diabetes increased the BRB permeability and retinal thickness. These changes were inhibited by Calcium dobesilate treatment. Calcium dobesilate also inhibited the increase in leukocyte adhesion to retinal vessels or endothelial cells and in ICAM-1 levels, induced by diabetes or elevated glucose. Moreover, CaD decreased oxidative stress and p38 mitogen-activated protein kinase (p38 MAPK) and NF-κB activation caused by diabetes. Thus, calcium dobesilate can prevent the BRB breakdown induced by diabetes, by restoring tight junction protein levels and organization and decreasing leukocyte adhesion to retinal vessels. The protective effects of calcium dobesilate probably involves the inhibition of p38 MAPK and NF-κB activation, possibly through the inhibition of oxidative/nitrosative stress (Leal et al., 2011).

Vascular cell adhesion molecule-1 (VCAM-1) is also an important marker of the endothelial function. Similarly to ICAM-1, the concentration of its soluble form (sVCAM-1) is elevated in diabetes and diabetic retinopathy (Nowak et al., 2008, Clausen et al., 2000). The influence of calcium dobesilate on the levels of sVCAM-1 and sICAM-1 was investigated in a clinical trial in mildly obese male smokers. Endothelial dysfunction in these subjects was confirmed by means of increased levels of sVCAM-1, sICAM-1 and related parameters, but no effect of calcium dobesilate on levels of cell adhesion molecules was observed after 3 months of treatment with with 1000 mg calcium dobesilate dobesilate daily(Schram et al., 2003).

3.6 Angiogenesis inhibition

Calcium dobesilate was investigated for its ability to interfere with the process of angiogenesis in a mouse gelatine sponge assay using acidic fibroblast growth factor (aFGF) as an inducer of neovascularization. According to the reported results, calcium dobesilate remarkably reduced vessel ingrowth in aFGF-containing subcutaneous sponges in mice. These findings suggest that calcium dobesilate could be an effective agent in the treatment of angiogenesis-dependent diseases involving FGFs (Cuevas et al., 2005). This knowledge was successfully used in the treatment of erythematotelangiestatic rosacea, which is characterized by uncontrolled angiogenesis (Cuevas & Arrazola, 2005). Angiogenesis is, however, recently considered to be a main contributor to the pathogenesis of diabetic retinopathy (Aiello, 2003,Campochiaro, 2000; Campochiaro and Hackett, 2003). The anti-angiogenic effect of calcium dobesilate can also be mediated by aminopeptidases inhibition, namely by inhibition of aminopeptidase N (Yang et al., 2007).

3.7 Reduction of retinal albumin leakage by calcium dobesilate

The action of calcium dobesilate on retinal albumin leakage in streptozotocin-diabetic rats was investigated together with relevant in vivo retinal antioxidant and permeability markers, i.e., carboxymethyl-lysine-advanced glycation end product (CML-AGE) formation and vascular endothelial cell growth factor (VEGF) overexpression. Twenty days after streptozotocin administration, diabetic rats were treated for 10 days with calcium dobesilate (100 mg/kg/day per os) or vehicle. Retinal albumin leakage, CML-AGE formation, and VEGF overexpression were evaluated by immunohistochemistry of frozen eye sections. Diabetic rats exhibited dramatic increases in retinal albumin leakage (31% of positive vessels vs. 0.2% in nondiabetic rats, CML-AGE retinal occurrence (40±3% vs. undetectable positive vessels), and retinal VEGF protein expression (14.6±1.1 vs. 3.5±0.5 VEGF-positive spots/field). Calcium dobesilate significantly reduced retinal albumin leakage (by 70%), retinal CML-AGEs contents (by 62%), and retinal VEGF expression (by 69.4%). In conclusion, calcium dobesilate orally given to diabetic rats markedly reduced retinal hyperpermeability, CML-AGE contents, and VEGF overexpression. These results strongly suggest that calcium dobesilate stabilizes blood–retinal barrier in diabetic retinopathy (Rota et al., 2004).

3.8 Influence of calcium dobesilate on platelets and blood viscosity

Platelet-active drugs are in general of potential benefit in the prevention of diabetic microangiopathy. Calcium dobesilate was shown to reduce aggregation and the release reaction induced by thrombin and collagen in rabbit platelets (Michal & Gotti, 1988). Calcium dobesilate also increased platelet cAMP concentrations *in vitro* and *ex vivo* probably through activation of adenylate cyclase (Michal and Gotti, 1988). In addition, this drug reduced platelet electrophoretic mobility (Heidrich et al., 1983), and it inhibited, in a time- and concentration-dependent manner, platelet-activating factor (PAF) production by the EA926 endothelial cell line stimulated by thrombin (Bussolino et al., 1986). The effects of PAF on the microvasculature bed of glomerular or pulmonary microcirculation suggest that PAF might play a role in microcirculation disease. The rheological properties of blood in diabetes mellitus have received increasing attention since Skovborg and colleagues demonstrated elevation of whole-blood viscosity in diabetics (Skovborg et al., 1966). In particular, evidence has accumulated that abnormal blood viscosity plays a role in the pathogenesis of diabetic retinopathy. Increased blood viscosity in diabetes mellitus has been attributed to changes in plasma protein composition (Barnes et al., 1977, Hoare et al., 1976, Hudomel et al., 1977, Skovborg et al., 1966); and to increased aggregation of red blood cells (McMillan, 1976). The mechanism by which hyperviscosity contributes to the deterioration of the microcirculation in the retina and other organs in diabetics is that, by increasing the resistance to blood flow, it causes blood stasis, especially in the capillaries and postcapillary venules, which are the sites where the very early lesions of diabetes microangiopathy characteristically appear. In some studies, calcium dobesilate has been demonstrated to decrease hyperviscosity in blood (Barras & Graf, 1980, Vojnikovic, 1991), perhaps through a fibrinogen-lowering effect (Barras & Graf, 1980, Vinnazzer & Hachen, 1987).

3.9 Influence of calcium dobesilate on plasma levels of endothelin

Endothelin-1 (ET-1) was discovered by Yanagisawa and colleagues in 1988 (Yanagisava et al., 1988) in the supernatant of aortic endothelial cells. ET-1 is a potentand prolonged vasoconstrictor and mitogenic endothelium derived peptide, and has been considered as a marker for endothelial damage and potential contributor to the developmentof the atherogenic process. Increased circulating ET-1 levels was found in patients with atherosclerosis, as well as in patients with Type 2 diabetes mellitus suggesting arole in the pathogenesis of these disorders (Ak et al., 2001). Plasma ET-1 plays also an important role in the whole patho-physiological process of diabetic retinopathy. Its plasma concentrations correlate to the severity of the disease, measures of their plasma concentrations can help to predict the severity of the disease. They also enable to distinguish between proliferative and non-proliferative diabetic retinopathy (Cao et al., 2009). In a clinical study, the plasma ET-1 concentrations were determined in 45 diabetes mellitus patients. The changes of ET-1 in 20 diabetic retinopathy patients before and after treatment with calcium dobesilate and 30 normal controls were observed. The level of plasma endothelin was higher in diabetes mellitus patients than that of the controls, which was even higher in diabetic retinopathy. After treatment with calcium dobesilate, the plasma ET-1 level decreased significantly (Zhong & Guo, 1997).

4. Pharmacokinetics and metabolism of calcium dobesilate

Studies on the metabolism and pharmacokinetics of calcium dobesilate were carried out by Benakis and colleagues (Benakis et al., 1974). They reported the results of blood levels of calcium dobesilate labeled with ^{35}S isotope, protein binding and urinary excretion in humans. The studies in humans were performed by the administration of the drug *p.o.* or *i.v.* After *i.v.* medication, 500 mg, the maximum value is obtained 5 min after administration and is about 65 mg/ml. This value of dicreases rapidly, the plasma half-life being 1 hr. After administration by the oral route, 500 mg in a capsule, the maximum value was obtained at the 6th hour after medication and is about 8mg/ml, and a plateau was obtained between the 3rd and the 10th hour. Levels decreased slowly and were undetectable 24 hours after administration. Intestinal absorption was 15% per hour during the first 7 hours and then decreased to 5% per hour. More than 80% of the drug is absorbed in the first 8 hours. The drug is 20–25% protein bound. The specific affinity of the drug to aggregated and nonaggregated platelets has been demonstrated. Calcium dobesilate does not cross the blood-brain barrier. Urinary elimination in the first 24 hours reaches 75% after *i.v.* medication and 50% after oral medication.

5. Clinical findings and usage of calcium dobesilate in prevention and treatment of diabetic retinopathy

5.1 Results of clinical studies

While the results of various *in vitro* experiments suggest that calcium dobesilate would have to be effective in the treatment of diabetic retinopathy, the results of clinical trials are ambiguous. One of the first clinical studies was a double-blind, randomized trial, which lasted for 2 years. The authors investigated the efficacy of calcium dobesilate on diabetic retinopathy in 51 patients, 17 were on placebo. The statistical analysis of the results indicated that calcium dobesilate acts as a potent angioprotector, capable of preventing both intra. and extraretinal hemorrhages. The drug also lowered the incidence of exudate formation and improved visual acuity (Salama Benarroch et al., 1977). A double-blind cross-over clinical trial performed on 18 diabetics, the results of which were published in the same year, investigated the effect of calcium dobesilate on capillary resistance and background retinopathy in comparison with placebo. Each treatment lasted 8 months. The study gave no evidence of a significant beneficial effect of calcium dobesilate on the capillary resistance in diabetics or on the course of the diabetic retinopathy (Larsen et al., 1977). The additional two independent, double-blind, controlled studies were performed to evaluate the efficacy of calcium dobesilate for the treatment of nonproliferative diabetic retinopathy. In the first suty, forty-two patients underwent a six-month crossover evaluation while receiving calcium dobesilate (750 mg per day) and placebo in random order. In the second ome, thirty-six patients received calcium dobesilate (1,000 mg per day) or placebo for one year. Evaluation by clinical examination, fluorescein angiography, angiography, and fundus photography failed to demonstrate any beneficial effect of calcium dobesilate (Stamper et al., 1978). On the other hand, the study with 50 patients who had diabetic retinopathy open-angle glaucoma, raised intraocular pressure, and hyperviscosity of whole blood, plasma, and aqueous humor and received 1,500 mg of calcium dobesilate daily for 3 months or pacebo exhibited the significant improvement of the state of the retina, the visual acuity, the intraocular pressure and the 3 viscosity values in the calcium dobesilate group (Vojnikovic, 1984). In a retrospective controlled study, 54 patients with diabetic retinopathy received calcium dobesilate (mean 650 mg/day) for 6-30 months (mean 18 months) and were compared to a correspondingly selected control group. The patients were divided into three subgroups (mild, moderate, and severe diabetic retinopathy). Microaneurysms, blot hemorrhages, striate hemorrhages, and hard exudates were assessed semiquantitatively from panorama fundus photographs, using a scoring system. The effect of calcium dobesilate was statistically significant for cases with moderate diabetic retinopathy on summing up the scores of the various retinal lesions. No effect on diabetic maculopathy or visual acuity was observed (Adank & Koerner, 1985). A more recent study, however, carried out in 197 patients, showed that 2 g of calcium dobesilate daily for 2 years had exhibited a significantly better activity than placebo on prevention of BRB disruption, independently of diabetes control. Tolerance was very good (Ribeiro et al., 2006). One of the most recent studies was concerned with the infuence of calcium dobesilate on development of clinically significant macular oedema (CSME) within a follow-up period of 5 years. It was performed on 635 patients from 40 centers in 11 countries. They were treated with 1500 mg of calcium dobesilate per day in three divided doses of 500 mg or with placebo for period up to 5 years. Unfortunately, this trial showed that calcium dobesilate did not reduce the risk of development of CSME (Haritoglou et al., 2009).

6. Safety and important adverse effects of calcium dobesilate

Adverse events with calcium dobesilate do not occur very frequently and have the following distribution in terms of frequency: fever (26%), gastrointestinal disorders (12.5%), skin reactions (8.2%), arthralgia (4.3%), and agranulocytosis (4.3%). No deaths have been attributed to calcium dobesilate. Most adverse events are rare and unrelated to the pharmacological properties of calcium dobesilate. (Allain et al., 2004). Agranulocytosis, which was first reported in 1992 (Kulessa et al., 1992), is probably the most serious adverse effect of calcium dobesilate. The estimated prevalence of agranulocytosis is 0.32 cases/million treated patients, i.e. ten times less than the calculated prevalence of agranulocytosis in the general population (Allain et al., 2004). Moreover, there is no case report that would attribute agranulocytosis clearly to calcium dobesilate during a simple treatment of diabetic retinopathy.

7. Dosage and aplication forms of calcium dobesilate

Calcium dobesilate is predominantly administered *p.o.* in uncoated tablets. Initial dosage in early stages of microangiopathies, namely diabetic retinopathy, is 250 mg calcium dobesilate three times a day (three tablets per day). After 2-3 weeks it is possible to decrease dosage to the keeping level 250-500 mg calcium dobesilate per day. Diminished performance of liver or kideys has no impact to dosage of calcium dobesilate (Medicinal products database of the State institute for Drug Control, 2011).

7.1 Intraocular preparations of calcium dobesilate

Except of usually administerd oral tablets, some topic preparations of calcium dobesilate have also been reported. Ocular preparations for a local treatment of diabetic retinopathy and related disorders like glaucoma are the matter of the patent application of Velpandian (Velpandian, 2006). The simpliest eye solution, which is the Composition I of the Example 1 of this patent, contain 1 % weight-volume (w/v) calcium dobesilate, 0.76 % w/v sodium chloride for isotonisation and 0.1 % w/v sodium metabisulfite as an antioxidant. The Composition II is similar but contains only 0.70 % w/v sodium chloride and furtherly 0.4 % w/v hydroxypropylmethylcellulose as an viscosity-increasing agent. The Compositions III a IV are water insoluble and water soluble eye oitments respectively. The micronized form of calcium dobesilate in concentration 1 % w/v is used for preparation of both. The vehicle for water insoluble oitment is the white petrolatum mixed with a mineral oil, for the water soluble one it is a mixture of polyethylene glycols. Both oitments contain suitable antimicrobial preservatives in concentration 0.01 % w/v and 0.001 % w/v respectively. The composition V is a controlled-release gel based on a suitable gel-forming polymer and contain also 1 % w/v calcium dobesilate.

8. Conclusion

Calcium dobesilate is one of the oldest drugs used in the treatment of diabetic retinopathy. The first reports concerning its usage appeared in the late 1960th (Sevin & Cuendet, 1969a, b). Its mechanisms of action have been gradually elucidated. Many of them are related to its reactivity as a reducing agent. Now it is known that they include lowering of reactive oxygen species-induced capillary permeability, enhancement of nitric oxide synthase activity in endothelial cells, influence of calcium dobesilate on apoptosis in vessel and other tissues, effects of calcium dobesilate on expression of cellular adhesion molecules, angiogenesis inhibition, reduction of retinal albumin leakage, influence of calcium dobesilate on platelets and blood viscosity, influence of calcium dobesilate on plasma levels of endothelin and others. Despite certain doubts of its efficiency originating from results of some clinical trials calcium dobesilate still remains the only angioprotective agent that reduces the progression of diabetic retinopathy (Garay et al., 2005).

9. Acknowledgements

The author is grateful to the Internal grant agency of the University of Veterinary and Pharmaceutical Sciences Brno for the financial support by the grant No. 26/2010/FaF.

10. References

Adamis, A. P. & Berman, A. J. (2008). Immunological mechanisms in the pathogenesis of diabetic retinopathy. Semin Immunopathol, Vol. 30, No. 2, (April 2008), pp.(65–84), ISSN 1863-2297

Adank, C. & Koerner, F. (1985). Calcium dobesilate in diabetic retinopathy. A retrospective controlled study. *Ophthalmologica,* Vol. 190, No. 2, (February 1985), pp. (102-111), ISSN 0030-3755

Aiello, L.M.. (2003). Perspectives on diabetic retinopathy. *American journal of ophthalmology,* Vol. 136, No. 1, (July 2003), pp. (122-135), ISSN 0002-9394

Agolini, G. & Cavallini, G. M. (1987). Long-term therapy of retinal vasculopathies with oral administration of high doses of O-(beta-hydroxyethyl)-rutoside. *La Clinica terapeutica,* Vol. 120, No. 2, (January 1987), pp. (101-110), ISSN 0009-9074

Ak, G., Buyukberber, S., Sevinc., A, Turk, H. M., Ates, M., Sari, R., Savli, H. & Cigli, A. (2001). The relation between plasma endothelin-1 levels and metabolic control, risk factors, treatment modalities, and diabetic microangiopathy in patients with Type 2 diabetes mellitus. *Journal of diabetes and its complications,* Vol. 15, No. 3, (May-June 2001), pp. (150-157), ISSN 1056-8727

Allain, H., Ramelet, A. A., Polard, E. & Bentué-Ferrer, D. (2004). Safety of calcium dobesilate in chronic venous disease, diabetic retinopathy and haemorrhoids. *Drug Safety,* Vol. 27, No. 9, (August 2004), pp. (649-660), ISSN 0114-5916

Almarsson, O., Bourghol Hickey, M., Peterson, M. L., Zaworotko, M. J., Moulton, B. & Rodriguez-Hornedo, N. (2011). *US 7927613* (19.04.2011)

Anderson, D., Yu,T. W., Phillips, B. J. & Schmezer, P. (1994). The effect of various antioxidants and other modifying agents on oxygen-radical-generated DNA damage in human lymphocytes in the COMET assay. *Mutation Research - Fundamental and Molecular Mechanisms of Mutagenesis,* Vol. 307, No. 1, (May 1994), pp. (261–270), ISSN 1386-1964

Barbieri, D., Grassilli, E., Monti, D., Salvioli, S., Franceschini, M. G., Franchini, A., Bellesia, E., Salomoni, P., Negro, P., Capri, M., Troiano, L., Cossarizza, A. & Franceschi, C. (1994). D-ribose and 2-deoxy-D-ribose induce apoptosis in human quiescent peripheral blood mononuclear cells. *Biochemical and Biophysical Research Communications,* Vol. 201, No. 3, (June 1994), pp. (1109-1116), ISSN 1090-2104

Barras, J. & Graf, C. (1980) Hyperviscosity in diabetic retinopathy treated with Doxium (calcium dobesilate). *Vasa,* Vol. 9, No. 2, (April-June 1980), pp. (161–164), ISSN0301-1526

Barber, A. J., Antonetti, D.A. & Gardner, T. W. (2000). Altered expression of retinal occludin and glial fibrillary acidic protein in experimental diabetes. *Investigative Ophthalmology and Visual Science,* Vol. 41, No. 11, (October 2000), pp. (3561–3568), ISSN 1552-5783

Barnes, A.J., Locke, P., Scudder, P.R., Dormandy, T. L., Dormandy, J. A. & Slack, J. (1977). Is hyperviscosity a treatable component of diabetic microcirculatory disease? *Lancet,* Vol. 2, No. 8042, (October 1977), pp. (789-791), ISSN: 0140-6736

Benakis, A., Glasson, B., Bouvier, C. A., Ritschard, J., Krahenbuhl, B., Jung, A. & Hachen, H. J. (1974). Metabolism and pharmacokinetics of calcium dobesilate in humans. *Therapie,* Vol. 29, No. 2, (March-April 1974), pp. (211-219), ISSN 0040-5957

Beneš, L. & Farsa, O. (2007). Medicinal Chemistry. An instruction manual for practical courses. University of Veterinary and Pharmaceutical Sciences, ISBN 978-80-7305-003-0, Brno, Czech Republic

Brunet, J., Farine, J. C., Garay, R. P. & Hannaert, P. (1998a). In vitro antioxidant properties of calcium dobesilate. *Fundamental & clinical pharmacology,* Vol. 12, No. 2, (February 1998), pp. (205-212), ISSN 0767-3981

Brunet, J., Farine, J. C., Garay, R. P. & Hannaert, P. (1998b). Angioprotective action of calcium dobesilate against reactive oxygen species-induced capillary permeability in the rat. *European Journal of Pharmacology,*Vol. 358, No. 3, (October 1998), pp. (213-220), ISSN 0014-2999

Bussolino, F., Biffignandi, P. & Arese, P. (1986). Platelet-activating factor: a powerful lipid autacoid possibly involved in microangiopathy. *Acta Haematologica,*Vol. 75, No. 3, (March 1986), pp. (129-140), ISSN 0001-5792

Campochiaro, P. A. (2000). Retinal and choroidal neovascularization. *Journal of Cellular Physiology,* Vol. 184, No. 3, (September 2000), pp. (301–310), ISSN 0021-9541

Campochiaro, P. A. & Hackett, S. F. (2003). Ocular neovascularization: a valuable model system. *Oncogene.* Vol. 22, No.429, (Septebmer 2003), pp. (6537-6548). ISSN . 0950-9232

Cao, W., Jiang, Y. & Chen, Y. (2009). Clinical significance of changes of ET-1/CGRP contents in patients with diabetic retinopathy. *Guoji Yanke Zazhi,*Vol. 9, No. 2, (February 2009), pp. (309-310), ISSN 1672-5123

Caproiu, R., Praisler-Stoica, M., Tanase, A. & Georgescu, D. (1988). Characterization of calcium 2,5-dihydroxybenzenesulfonate (calcium dobesilate) by thermal analysis. *Revistade Chimie,* Vol. 39, No. 6, (June 1988), pp. (528-530), ISSN 0034-7752

Carrasco, O. F. & Vidrio, H. (2007). Endothelium protectant and contractile effects of the antivaricose principle escin in rat aorta. *Vascular pharmacology,*Vol. 47, No. 1, (July 2007), pp. (68-73), ISSN 1537-1891

Chen, Y. & Xiao, Y. (2008). Detection of calcium dobesilate in calcium dobesilate capsules: a comparison of HPLC and UV spectrophotometry. *Guangdong Yaoxueyuan Xuebao,* Vol. 24, No. 5, (May 2008), pp. (480-483), ISSN 1006-8783

Chung, H. K., Choi, S. M., Ahn, B. O., Kwak, H. H., Kim, J. H. & Kim, W. B. (2005). *Arzneimittelforschung,* Vol. 55, No. 10, (November 2005), pp.(573-80), ISSN 0004-4172

Clausen, P., Jacobsen, P., Rossing, K., Jensen, J. S., Parving, H. H. & Feldt-Rasmussen, B. (2000). Plasma concentrations of VCAM-1 and ICAM-1 are elevated in patients with Type 1 diabetes mellitus with microalbuminuria and overt nephropathy. *Diabetic medicine : a journal of the British Diabetic Association,* Vol. 17, No. 9, (September 2000), pp.(644-649), ISSN 0742-3071

Cuevas, P. & Arrazola, J. M. (2005). Treatment of basal cell carcinoma with dobesilate. *Journal of the American Academy of Dermatology,* Vol. 53, No. 3, (September 2005), pp. (525-526), ISSN 1368-5031

Cuevas, P., Díaz-González, D., Sánchez, I., Lozano, R, M., Giménez-Gallego, G. & Dujovny, M. (2006). Dobesilate inhibits the activation of signal transducer and activator of transcription 3, and the expression of cyclin D1 and bcl-XL in glioma cells. *Neurological Research,* Vol.28, No. 2, (March 2006), pp. (127-130, ISSN 0161-6412

Cuevas, P., Sanchez, I., Lozano, R. M. & Gimenez-Gallego, G.. (2005). Dobesilate is an angiogenesis inhibitor. *European Journal of Medical Research,*.Vol. 10, No. 9, (September 2005), pp. (369-372), ISSN 0949-2321

Czech Pharmacopoeia 2002. (2002). Grada, ISBN 80-247-0464-1, Prague, Czech Republic

Czech Pharmacopoeia 2009. (2009). Grada, ISBN 80-247-2994-7, Prague, Czech Republic

Durante, W., Sen, A. K., Sunahara & F. A. (1988). Impairment of endothelium-dependent relaxation in aortae from spontaneously diabetic rats. *British Journal of Pharmacology,*Vol. 94, No. 2, (June 1988), pp. (463-468), ISSN 0007-1188

Einarsdottir, A. B. & Stefansson, E. (2009). Prevention of diabetic retinopathy. *Lancet,* Vol. 373, No. 9672, (April 2009), pp. (1316-1318), ISSN 0140-6736

Estéve-Soler, J. (1977). Verfahren zur Herstellung des Kalziumsalzes der 2,5-dihydroxybenzolsulfonsäure. *DD 125668* (11.5.1977)

Estéve-Subirana, A. (1970): Therapeutically active derivatives of p-dihydroxybenzene. *US 3509207* (28.4.1970)

European Pharmacopoeia 7.2. (2011). European Directorate for the Quality of Medicines & Health Care, ISBN 978-92-871-6704-0, Strasbourg Cedex, France

Farsa O., Šablatura M. (2008). An alternative synthesis of calcium dobesilate, a simple venous insufficiency drug, suitable for use in medicinal or organic Chemistry practical courses. *Khimyia/Chemistry,* Vol. 17, No. 4 (July-August 2008), pp. (281-285), ISSN 0861-9255

García Benayas, E., García Díaz, B. & Pérez, G. (1997). Calcium dobesilate-induced agranulocytosis. *Pharmacy world & science,* Vol. 19, No. 5, (October 1997), pp. (251-252), ISSN 0928-1231

Garay, R.P., Hannaert, P. & Chiavaroli, C. (2005). Calcium dobesilate in the treatment of diabetic retinopathy. *Treatments in Endocrinology,* Vol. 4, No. 4, (July-August 2005), pp. (221-232), ISSN 1175-6349

Goldman, D. (2005). Method of preparation of mixed phase co-crystals with active agents. *CA 2548281* (23.06.2005)

Graber, R., Farine, J. C., Fumagalli, I., Tatti, V. & Losa, G.A. (1998). Calcium Dobesilate protects human peripheral blood mononuclear cells from oxidation and apoptosis. *Apoptosis,* Vol 3, No. 1, (1998), pp. (41-49), ISSN 1360-8185

Guangzhi, H., Long, C., Yong, G., Shijun, S. & Xiaolai, W. (2009). Selective electrochemical sensing of calcium dobesilate based on the nano-Pd/CNTs modified pyrolytic graphite electrode. *Talanta,* Vol. 78, No.3, (March 2009), pp. (1211-1214), ISSN . 0039-9140

Haritoglou, C, Gerss, J., Sauerland, C., Kampik, A. & Ulbig, M. W. (2009). Effect of calcium dobesilate on occurrence of diabetic macular oedema (CALDIRET study): randomised, double-blind, placebo-controlled, multicentre trial. *The Lancet,* Vol. 373, No. 9672, (April 2009), pp. (1364 – 1371), ISSN 0140-6736

Heidrich, H., Gerke, E. & Nekarda, H. (1983). Thrombozytenaggregationshemmung unter Calciumdobesilat. *Arzneimittel-Forschung/Drug Research,*Vol. 33, No. 4, (April 1983), pp. (580-582), ISSN 0004-4172

Hoare, E., Barnes, A. & Normandy, J. (1976) Abnormal blood viscosity in diabetes mellitus and retinopathy. *Biorheology* , Vol. 13, No. 1, (January - February 1976), pp. (21–25), ISSN0006-355X

Hu, G. Ma, Y., Guo, Y. & Shao, S. (2009). Selective electrochemical sensing of calcium dobesilate based on an ordered mesoporous carbon-modified pyrolytic graphite electrode. *Journal of Electroanalytical Chemistry,*Vol. 633, No. 1, (August 2009), pp. (264-267), ISSN 1572-6657

Huang, Z. (2007). New formulations of 2,5-dihydroxybenzenesulfonic acid for improving microcirculation and protecting blood vessel. *CN 101081823* (05.12.2007)

Hudomel, J., Nemeth, B., Palfalvy, M. & Farkas A. (1977). Effect of calcium dobesilate (Doxium) on blood hyperviscosity in cases of diabetic retinopathy. *Ophthalmic Research,* Vol. 9, No. 1, (January - February 1977), pp. (25–30), ISSN 0030-3747

Iriz, E., Vural C., Ereren, E., Poyraz, A., Erer, D., Oktar, L., Golgot, L., Halit, V., Soncul, H. (2008). Effects of calcium dobesilate and diosmin-hesperidin on apoptosis of venous wall in primary varicose veins. *Vasa,* Vol. 37, No. 3, (August 2008), pp. (233-240), ISSN 0301-1526

Joussen, A. M., Poulaki, V., Mitsiades, N., Kirchhof, B., Koizumi, K., Döhmen, S. & Adamis, A. P. (2002). Nonsteroidal anti-inflammatory drugs prevent early diabetic retinopathy via TNF-alpha suppression. *The FASEB Journal,* Vol. 16, No. 3, (March 2002), pp. (438–440), ISSN 0892-6638

Kern, T. S. (2007). Contributions of inflammatory processes to the development of the early stages of diabetic retinopathy. *Experimental Diabetes Research,* Vol. 2007, Article ID 95103, pp. (95-103), ISSN 1687-5214

Kim, M., Park, B.-Y., Moon, C.-H., Park, E.-K. & Kim, K. (2004). Composition containing horse chestnut extract for anti-angiogenic and matrix metalloproteinase inhibitory activity. *EP 1438059* (July 21, 2004)

Klaassen, I., Hughes, J. M., Vogels, I. M., Schalkwijk, C. G., Van Noorden, C. J. & Schlingemann, R. O. (2009). Altered expression of genes related to blood-retina barrier disruption in streptozotocin-induced diabetes. *Experimental eye research,* Vol. 89, No. 1, (June 2009), pp. (4–15), ISSN 0014-4835

Kračmár, J, Kračmárová, J., Kovářová, A. & Stejskal, Z. (1988). UV spectrophotometry in drug control. 37: New active substances containing benzene, pyridine and quinoline chromophores. Part 8: Impact of substitution and solvent. *Pharmazie,* Vol. 43, No. 3, (March 1988), pp.(173-176), ISSN 0031-7144

Kröncke, K.D., Fehsel, K. & Kolb-Bachofen, V. (1995). Inducible nitric oxide synthase and its product nitric oxide, a small molecule with complex biological activities. *Biological Chemistry Hoppe-Seyler,* Vol. 376, No. 6, (June 1995), pp. (327-343), ISSN 0177-3593

Kubes, P., Suzuki, M. & Granger, D.N. (1991). Nitric oxide: An endogenous modulator of leukocyte adhesion. *Proceedings of the National Academy of Sciences of the United States of America,* Vol. 88, No. 11, (June 1991), pp. (4651-4655), ISSN 0027-8424

Kulessa, W., Becker, E. W., Berg, P. A. (1992). Recurrence of agranulocytosis after taking calcium dobesilate. *Deutsche medizinische Wochenschrift,* Vol. 117, No. 10, (March 1992), pp. (372-374), ISSN 0012-0472

Lacombe, C., Lelievre, J. C., Bucherer, C. & Grimaldi, A. (1989). Activity of Daflon 500 mg on the hemorheological disorders in diabetes. *International angiology : a journal of the International Union of Angiology,* Vol. 8, Supl. 4, (October-December 1989), pp. (48-48), ISSN 0392-9590

Larsen, H. W., Sander, E., Hoppe, R. (1977). The value of calcium dobesilate in the treatment of diabetic retinopathy. A controlled clinical trial. *Diabetologia,* Vol. 13, No. 2, (April 1977), pp. (105-109), ISSN 0012-186X

Leal, E. C., Martins, J.,Voabil, P., Liberal, J., Chiavaroli, C., Bauer, J., Cunha-Vaz, J. & Ambrosio, A. F. (2010). Calcium dobesilate inhibits the alterations in tight junction proteins and leukocyte adhesion to retinal endothelial cells induced by diabetes. *Diabetes,* Vol. 59, No. 10, (October 2010), pp. (2637-2645), ISSN 0012-1797

Lozovskaia, E. L., Kaplunskii, G. D., Sapezhinskii, I. I. (1990). Superoxide dismutase activity and photosensitizing properties of 2,5-dihydroxybenzolsulfonate. *Biofizika,* Vol. 35, No. 6, (June 1990), pp. (912-916), ISSN 0006-3029

Lu, J. R. (2005). Synthesis and structural analysis of calcium dobesilate monohydrate. *Zhongguo Xiandai Yingyong Yaoxue,* Vol. 22, No. 2, (February 2005), pp. (124-126), ISSN 1007-7693

Luo, X. X., Duan, J. G., Liao, P. Z., Wu, L., Yu, Y. G., Qiu, B., Wang, Y. L., Li, Y. M., Yin, Z. Q., Liu, X. L. & Yao, K. (2009). Effect of qiming granule on retinal blood circulation of diabetic retinopathy: a multicenter clinical trial. *Chinese journal of integrative medicine,* Vol. 15, No. 5, (October 2009), pp. (384-388), ISSN 1672-0415

McMillan, D. (1976). Plasma protein changes, blood viscosity and diabetic microangiopathy. *Diabetes,* Vol. 25, No. Suppl. 2, (January 1976), pp. (25–33), ISSN 0012-1797

McVeigh, G. E., Brennan, G. M., Johnston, G. D., McDermott, B. J., McGrath, L. T., Henry, W. R., Andrews, J. W. & Hayes, J. R. (1992). Impaired endothelium-dependent and independent vasodilation in patients with type 2 (non-insulin-dependent) diabetes mellitus. *Diabetologia,* Vol. 35, No. 8, (August 1992), pp. (771-776), ISSN 0012-186X

Michal, M. & Gotti, C. (1988). Effect of calcium dobesilate on platelet function. *Thrombosis Research,*Vol. 51, No. 6, (September 1988), pp. (593-605), ISSN 0049-3848

Milne, G. W. A. (Ed.) (2002). *Drugs: Synonyms & Properties.* Ashgate Publ. Co., ISBN: 0-566-08228-4, Brookfield, Vt., USA

Miyamoto, K., Khosrof, S., Bursell, S. E., Rohan, R., Murata, T., Clermont, A. C., Aiello, L. P., Ogura. Y. & Adamis, A. P. (1999). Prevention of leukostasis and vascular leakage in streptozotocin-induced diabetic retinopathy via intercellular adhesion molecule-1 inhibition. *Proceedings of the National Academy of Sciences of the United States of America,* Vol. 96, No. 19, (September 1999), pp. (10836–10841), ISSN 0027-8424

Moncada, S. & Higgs, A. (1993). The L-arginine-nitric oxide pathway. *The New England Journal of Medicine,* Vol. 329, No. 27, (December 1993), pp. (2002-2012), ISSN 0028-4793

Negritescu, S., Belu, D, Dragoi, R., Sisman, E., Cosmin, A., Candidatu, A. & Georgescu, D. (1979). Analytical studies on 2,5-dihydroxybenzenesulfonic acid salts as antihemorrhagic drugs. *Revistade Chimie,* Vol. 30, No. 9, (September 1979), pp. (912-915), ISSN: 0034-7752

Nováček, A., Sedláčková, V., Horáček, L. & Šimek, P. (1987). A method of purification of 2,5-dihydroxybenzenedulfonic acid calcium salt. *CS 8402981,* (15.09.1987)

Nowak, M., Wielkoszyński, T., Marek, B., Kos-Kudła, B., Świętochowska, E., Siemińska, L., Kajdaniuk, D., Głogowska-Szelag, J. & Nowak, K. (2008). Blood serum levels of vascular cell adhesion molecule (sVCAM-1), intercellular adhesion molecule (sICAM-1) and endothelial leucocyte adhesion molecule-1 (ELAM-1) in diabetic retinopathy. *Clinical and experimental medicine,* Vol. 8, No. 3, (September 2008), pp. (159–164), ISSN 1591-8890

Palacios, M., Knowles, R. G. & Palmer, R. M. J. (1989). Nitric oxides from L-arginine stimulates the soluble guanylate cyclase in adrenal glands. *Biochemical and Biophysical Research Communications,* Vol. 165, No. 2, (December 1989), pp. (802-810), ISSN 1090-2104

Palmer, R. M. J., Ashton D. S. & Moncada, S. (1988). Vascular endothelial cells synthesize nitric oxide from L-arginine. *Nature,* Vol. 333, No. 6174, (June 1988), pp. (664–666), ISSN 0028-0836

Palmer, R. M. J., Rees, D. D., Ashton, D. S. & Moncada, S. (1988). L-Arginine is the physiological precursor for the formation of nitric oxide in endothelium-dependent relaxation. *Biochemical and Biophysical Research Communications,* Vol. 153, No. 3 , (June 1988), pp. (1251–1256), ISSN 1090-2104

Plessas, C. T., Karayannakos, P., Plessas, S. T., Costakis, A., Donta, I. & Skalkeas, G. (1986a). Pharmacokinetics of calcium dobesilate in beagle dogs after a single administration. *European journal of drug metabolism and pharmacokinetics,* Vol. 11, No. 4, (April 1986), pp. (303-308), ISSN 0378-7966

Plessas, C. T., Karayannakos, P., Plessas, S. T., Costakis, A., Donta, I. & Skalkeas, G. (1986b). Pharmacokinetics of calcium dobesilate in beagle dogs after repeated administration. *European journal of drug metabolism and pharmacokinetics,* Vol. 11, No. 4, (April 1986), pp. (309-312), ISSN 0378-7966

Radomski, M. W., Palmer, R. M. J. & Moncada, S. (1987a). Comparative pharmacology of endothelium-derived relaxing factor, nitric oxide and prostacyclin in platelets. *British Journal of Pharmacology,* Vol. 92, No. 3, (November 1987), pp. (181-185), ISSN 0007-1188

Radomski, M. W., Palmer, R. M. J. & Moncada, S. (1987b). Endogenous nitric oxide inhibits human platelet adhesion to vascular endothelium. *Lancet,* Vol. 2, No. 8567, (November 1987), pp. (1057-1059), ISSN 0140-6736

Rees, D. D., Palmer, R. M. J. & Moncada, S. (1989). Role of endothelium-derived nitric oxide in the regulation of blood pressure. *Proceedings of the National Academy of Sciences of the United States of America,* Vol. 86, No. 9, (May 1989), pp. (3375-3381), ISSN 0027-8424

Ribeiro, M. L., Seres, A. I., Carneiro, A. M., Stur, M., Zourdani, A., Caillon, P. & Cunha-Vaz, J. G. (2006). Effect of calcium dobesilate on progression of early diabetic retinopathy: a randomised double-blind study. *Graefe's archive for clinical and experimental ophthalmology,* Vol. 244, No. 12, (December 2006), pp. (1591-1600), ISSN 0721-832X

Rogers, R. D., Daly, D. T., Gurau, G., MacFarlane, D., Turanjanin, J., Dean, P. M., Scott, J., Bica, K. & Seddon, K. R. (2010). Dual functioning ionic liquids and salts thereof. *World Patent Application WO 2010/078300* (08.07.2010)

Rogers, R. D., Daly, D. T., Swatloski, R. P., Hough, W. L., Davis, J. H. Jr., Smiglak, M., Pernak, J. & Spear, S. K. (2007). Multi-functional ionic liquid compositions for overcoming polymorphism and imparting improved properties for active pharmaceutical, biological, nutritional, and energetic ingredients. *US Patent Application 20070093462* (26.04.2007)

Róna, K. & Ary, K. (2001). Determination of calcium dobesilate in human plasma using ion-pairing extraction and high-performance liquid chromatography. *Journal of Chromatography B: Biomedical Sciences and Applications,* Vol. 755, No. 1-2, (May 2001), pp. (245-251), ISSN 0378-4347

Rota, R., Chiavaroli, C., Garayc, R. P. & Hannaert, P. (2004). Reduction of retinal albumin leakage by the antioxidant calcium dobesilate in streptozotocin-diabetic rats. *European Journal of Pharmacology,* Vol. 495, No. 2-3, (July 2004), pp.(217– 224), ISSN 0014-2999

Rückauf H., Turek, F. & Dietrich, W. (1990). Verfahren zur Herrstellung von Hydrogensulfitlösungen. *DD 282899* (26.9.1990)

Ruiz, E., Lorente, R. & Tejerina, T. Effects of calcium dobesilate on the synthesis of endothelium-dependent relaxing factors in rabbit isolated aorta. *British Journal of Pharmacology,*Vol. 121, No. 4, (June 1997), p. (711–716), ISSN 0007-1188

Šablatura, M. (2006). *Development and optimization of a novel exercise for practical courses in Medicinal Chemistry I. Master thesis.* University of Veterinary and Pharmaceutical Sciences, Brno, Czech Republic

Salama Benarroch, I., Nano, H., Pérez, H., Elizalde, F., Bisceglia, H. & Salama. A. (1977). Assessment of calcium dobesilate in diabetic retinopathy. A double-blind clinical investigation. *Ophthalmologica,* Vol. 174, No. 1, (January 1977), pp. (47-51), ISSN 0030-3755

Schram, M. T., Stam, F., de Jongh, R. T., de Vries, G., van Dijk, R. A., Serné, E. H., Lampe, D., Nanayakkara, P. W., Tushuizen, M. E., Scheffer, P. G., Schalkwijk, C. G., Kamper A. M., Stehouwer, C. D . (2003). The effect of calcium dobesilate on vascular endothelial function, blood pressure, and markers of oxidation in obese male smokers: a placebo-controlled randomised clinical trial. *Atherosclerosis,* Vol. 170, No. 1, (September 2003), pp. (59-72), ISSN 0021-9150

Sci Finder (July 2011). Substance Detail 20123-80-2. In: *Sci Finder, a Data Base of the American Chemical Society,* 12. 07. 2011, Available from https://scifinder.cas.org/scifinder/view/scifinder/scifinderExplore.jsf

Sevin, R., Cuendet, J. F. (1969a). The action of calcium dobesilate in diabetic retinopathy. *Bulletins et mémoires de la Société française d'ophtalmologie,* Vol. 82, pp. (170-180), ISSN 0081-1092

Sevin, R., Cuendet, J. F. (1969b). Calcium dobesilate in diabetic retinopathy. *Ophthalmologica,* Vol. 159, No. 1, (January–February 1969), pp. (126-135), ISSN 0030-3755

Seyda, A. (1883). Über Sulfonsäuren des Hydrochinons. *Berichte der Deutschen Chemischen Gesellschaft,* Vol.16, No.1, (January-June 1883), pp. (687-694), ISSN 0009-2940

Sigma-Aldrich. (July 2011). SUPELCOSIL™ ABZ+Plus HPLC Column, In: *Sigma-Aldrich online catalog,* 12. 07. 2011, Available from http://www.sigmaaldrich.com/catalog/ProductDetail.do?lang=en&N4=59194C30|SUPELCO&N5=SEARCH_CONCAT_PNO|BRAND_KEY&F=SPEC

Skovborg, F., Nielsen, A.V., Schlichtkrull, J. & Ditzel, J. (1966). Blood-viscosity in diabetic patients. *Lancet,*Vol. 1, No. 7429, (January 1966), pp. (129-131), ISSN 0140-6736

Stamper, R. L., Smith, M. E., Aronson, S. B., Cavender, J. C., Cleasby, G. W., Fung, W. E. & Becker, B. (1978). The effect of calcium dobesilate on nonproliferative diabetic retinopathy: a controlled study. *Ophthalmology,* Vol. 85, No. 6, (June 1978), pp. (594-606), ISSN 0161-6420

State Institute for Drug Control. (August 2011). SPC 98886. Summary of data concerning the preparation Danium ®., In: *Medicinal products database,* 02. 08. 2011, Available from http://www.sukl.eu/modules/medication/search.php?data[search_for]=Danium &data[code]=&data[atc_group]=&data[material]=&data[path]=&data[reg]=&data[radio]=none&data[rc]=&data[with_adv]=0&search=Search&data[listing]=20

Suschek, C., Kolb, H. & Kolb-Bachofen, V. (1997). Dobesilate enhances endothelial nitric oxide synthase-activity in macro- and microvascular endothelial cells. British Journal of Pharmacology.Vol. 122, No. 7, (December 1997), pp. (1502-1508), ISSN 0007-1188

Suschek, C., Rothe, H., Fehsel, K., Enczmann, J. & Kolb-Bachofen, V. (1993). Induction of a macrophage-like nitric oxide synthase in cultured rat aortic endothelial cells. *Journal of Immunology,* Vol. 151, (September 1993), pp. (3283-3291), ISSN 0022-1767

Szabo, M. E., Haines, D., Garay, E., Chiavaroli, C., Farine, J. C., Hannaert, P., Berta, A. & Garay, R. P. (2001). Antioxidant properties of calcium dobesilate in ischemic /reperfused diabetic rat retina. *European Journal of Pharmacology,* Vol. 428, No. 2, (October 2001), pp. (277-286), ISSN 0014-2999

Tawa, M., Almarsson, O. & Remenar, J. (2010) Pharmaceutical propylene glycol solvate compositions. *US 7790905* (07.09.2010)

Velpandian, T. (2006). Pharmacetical compositions of calcium dobesilate. *IN 1327/DEL/2006* (01.06.2006)

Vinazzer, H. & Hachen, H. J. (1987). Influence of calcium dobesilate (Doxium) on blood viscosity and coagulation parameters in diabetic retinopathy. *Vasa,* Vol. 16, No. 2, (March - April 1987), pp. (190-192), ISSN 0301-1526

Vojnikovic, B. (1984). Hyperviscosity in whole blood, plasma, and aqueous humor decreased by doxium (calcium dobesilate) in diabetics with retinopathy and glaucoma: a double-blind controlled study. *Ophthalmic Research,* Vol. 16, No. 3, (May-June 1984), pp. (150-162), ISSN 0030-3747

Vojnikovic, B. (1991). Doxium (calcium dobesilate) reduces blood hyperviscosity and lowers elevated intraocular pressure in patients with diabetic retinopathy and glaucoma. *Ophthalmic Research,* Vol. 23, No. 1, (January-February 1991), pp. (12-20), ISSN 0030-3747

Wadworth, A. N. & Faulds, D. (1992). Hydroxyethylrutosides. A review of its pharmacology, and therapeutic efficacy in venous insufficiency and related disorders. *Drugs,* Vol. 44, No. 6, (June 1992), pp. (1013-1032), ISSN 0012-6667

Xu, H., Li, X., Zhang, J., Zhang, Z. & Liu, K. (2009). *Analytical Letters,* Vol. 42, No. 8, (May 2009), pp. (1094-1110), ISSN 0003-2719

Yanagisawa, M., Kurihara, H., Kimura, S., Tomobe, Y. & Kobayashi, M. (1988). A novel potent vasoconstrictor peptide produced by vascular endothelial cells. *Nature,* Vol. 332, No. 6163, (March 1988), pp. (411-415), ISSN 0028-0836

Yang, E., Shim, J.S., Woo, H.-J., Kim, K.-W. & Kwon, H.J. (2007). Aminopeptidase N/CD13 induces angiogenesis through interaction with a pro-angiogenic protein, galectin-3.

Biochemical and Biophysical Research Communications, Vol. 363, No. 2, (November 2007), pp. (336-341), ISSN 1090-2104

Yang, Y., Ma G. & Long, H. (2010). Process for preparation of calcium dobesilate hydrate. *CN 101880248* (10.11.2010)

Yao, C. (2010). Process for preparation of calcium dobesilate nanopowder. *CN 101898980* (1.12.2010)

Zhang, Y., Du, F. Y. & Wei, L. L. (2011). Electrochemical behavior of calcium dobesilate at a gold nanoparticles modified glassy carbon electrode and its determination. Fenxi Shiyanshi,Vol. 30, No. 3, (March 2011), pp. (50-53), ISSN 1000-0720

Zhang, Y. & Zhang, Z. F. (2009). Lihua Jianyan, Huaxue Fence, Vol. 45, No. 11, (June 2009), pp. (1296-1301), ISSN 1001-4020

Zhang, Z. & Xu, Z. (1999). Comparison of two titration methods of calcium 2,5-dihydroxybenzenesulfonate. Huagong Shikan, Vol. 13, No. 11, (November 1999), pp. (36-38), ISSN 1002-154X

Zheng, J., Zhang, Y. & Yang, P. (2007). An ionic liquid-type carbon paste electrode for electrochemical investigation and determination of calcium dobesilate. *Talanta.* Vol. 73, No. 5, (April 2007), pp.(920–925), ISSN 0039-9140

Zhong, H. & Guo, L. (1997). The plasma levels of endothelin in diabetic retinopathy and their changes after treatment with doxium. *Hunan Yike Daxue Xuebao - Bulletin of Hunan Medical University,* Vol. 22, No. 1, (January 1997), pp. (56-58), ISSN 1000-5625

Zhu, F. & Chen, J. (2005). Determination of calcium dobesilate in drugs by HPLC. Baoji Wenli Xueyuan Xuebao, Ziran Kexueban, Vol. 25, No. 2, (February 2005), pp. (119-121), ISSN 1007-1261

Zimmerman, G.A., Prescott, S.M. & McIntyre, T.M. (1992). Endothelial cell interactions with granulocytes: tethering and signalling molecules. *Immunology Today,*Vol. 13, No. 3, (March 1992), pp. (93-100), ISSN 0167-5699

Zivanovic, L., Zecevic, M., Markovic, S., Petrovic, S. & Ivanovic, I. (2005). Validation of liquid chromatographic method for analysis of lidocaine hydrochloride, dexamethasone acetate, calcium dobesilate, buthylhydroxyanisol and degradation product hydroquinone in suppositories and ointment. *Journal of Chromatography A,*Vol. 1088, No. 1-2, (September 2005), pp. (182-186), ISSN 0021-9673

17

The Role of Sex Hormones in Diabetic Retinopathy

Jeffery G. Grigsby[1], Donald M. Allen[2], Richard B. Culbert[3,4], Gerardo Escobedo[4], Kalpana Parvathaneni[1], Brandi S. Betts[1] and Andrew T.C. Tsin[1]
[1]*Department of Biology, University of Texas at San Antonio, San Antonio, Texas*
[2]*Department of Biology, University of Texas of the Permian Basin, Odessa, Texas*
[3]*Department of Surgery, Texas Tech School of Medicine, Midland, Texas*
[4]*Premier Retina Specialists, Midland, Texas*
[1, 2,3,4]*United States of America*

1. Introduction

The role sex hormones play in the etiologies of human proliferative diseases such as cancers of the breast and the male and female gonads have long been described (Beatson 1896; Lacassagne 1936; Love and Philips 2002). Lacassagne in 1937 suggested that "a therapeutic antagonist to the congestion of oestrone in the breast should be found to prevent breast cancer" (Lacassagne 1936). Finally, in 1962 Jenson et al. suggested an assay to detect the presence of estrogen receptor (ER) and suggested it be used to determine which breast cancers were susceptible to estrogen (Jensen 1962). Other human pathologies such as cardiovascular and autoimmune disease have also been linked to sex hormones (Ansar Ahmed et al. 1985; Mendelsohn and Karas 2005). Even though sex hormone receptors have been identified in the eye, the role that sex hormones play in the development of eye disease, such as that occurring with diabetes, is less described (Gupta et al. 2005). In this chapter, we hope to enlighten the reader about the presence of sex hormone receptors in various eye tissues, present how sex hormones are involved in the mechanisms that control the development of proliferative diabetic retinopathy and offer insight into areas where modulation of these mechanisms could be controlled by blockers of sex hormone receptors.

2. Epidemiology

2.1 Sex differences in the prevalence of retinopathy noted in epidemiological studies

The role of gender as a contributing factor in diabetic retinopathy has long been debated. Numerous and seemingly contradictory studies have shown either a male predisposition, a female predisposition, or no significant difference between the sexes in development or progression of diabetic retinopathy.

Earlier population studies such as the Wisconsin Epidemiological Study of Diabetic Retinopathy (WESDR) were done with predominantly white cohorts (Klein et al. 2008; Klein et al. 2010). The 25 year results of this WESDR showed that being male was an independent risk factor for the progression of diabetic retinopathy, although not a risk factor for the development of proliferative diabetic retinopathy or for visual impairment due to diabetes (Klein et al. 2010). However, many other studies show no correlation between gender and either severity or progression of diabetic retinopathy (Janka et al. 1989; Klein et al. 1994; Lloyd et al. 1995). The possibility that ethnicity or race played a role in gender differences in diabetic retinopathy was evaluated. The Los Angeles Latino Eye Study showed that in Latinos with type 2 diabetes, males were more likely to develop diabetic retinopathy (Varma et al. 2007). A study in India also demonstrated increased risk of diabetic retinopathy for men who develop diabetes over the age of forty (Raman et al. 2011). However, other studies in various ethnic groups show no gender differences. No gender difference was reported in proliferative diabetic retinopathy in Pima Indians (Nelson et al. 1989). Comparing Mexican-Americans in San Antonio to non-hispanic whites in Wisconsin found no gender differences in either group (Haffner et al. 1988). Another study in India found no male predisposition to diabetic retinopathy (Namperumalsamy et al. 2009). Studies of Pacific Islanders have found no gender predisposition in prevalence or progression of diabetic retinopathy (Smith et al. 2007; Tapp et al. 2006). Asians in China and Singapore also demonstrated no gender differences in prevalence of diabetic retinopathy (Wang et al. 2009; Wong et al. 2008). A multi-ethnic study in the United States did not indicate an increased risk for males for retinopathy in white, black, Hispanic or Chinese cohorts (Wong et al. 2006). The Early Treatment of Diabetic Retinopathy Study (ETDRS) trial found increased risk for women to have progression of diabetic retinopathy, but this occurred only in one subgroup (Davis et al. 1998). All other subgroups showed no gender differences in progression of retinopathy or development of proliferative retinopathy, and therefore the differences in that subgroup were thought to be spurious.

This disparity of results indicates that there probably are other confounding factors that have not been considered in these studies. Variations in human leukocyte antigen (HLA) haplotypes may affect risk for diabetes and diabetic retinopathy (Rand et al. 1985). Unaccounted disparity in HLA expression between groups in studies may lead to apparent differences that are not actually present. The fact that most studies that do show an effect indicate a greater risk in men may indicate there is variable expression of a factor present in men, such as androgenic hormones, that may have accounted for the increased risk of progression of diabetic retinopathy.

2.2 Puberty

While the levels of sex hormones increase during puberty, it is important to remember that the levels of growth hormones and secondary growth factors also increase during puberty. In fact Merimee reported a clinical observation that diabetic dwarfs exhibit little retinopathy (Merimee 1990). Another interesting clinical observation reported by Bell in a case study of agonadal (without ovaries) female twins demonstrated a lack of retinopathy after a long duration of very poorly controlled diabetes (A1c's as high as 15.6%) (Bell 1995). When trying to determine how puberty affects the prevalence of retinopathy, one must consider the endocrinological environment of an individual: 1) pre-puberty, 2) during puberty, and 3) after puberty. The search to determine the effect of the attainment of puberty on the development of retinopathy has evolved, but is not without controversy.

There has been much discussion on the presence of a pre-pubertal "grace period" from the development of retinopathy. One obvious consideration is that patients past puberty have had the disease longer. Some studies have suggested that puberty does not offer protection against the development of retinopathy, but that the infrequency of occurrence is related to the short duration of the disease during pre-pubescence (Constable et al. 1984; Knuiman et al. 1986; Porta et al. 2004; Szabo et al. 1967). Porta et al., in a retrospective analysis of 628 patients with diabetes and an onset of <29 years, found that retinopathy (determination of pubertal age was not available) may take longer to develop in patients who develop diabetes before puberty, but that after 20 years duration the prevalence of retinopathy is no longer influenced by the age of onset (Porta et al. 2004). In a previous prospective work, Porta et al. report that onset of diabetes before puberty could be an additional risk factor to the development of proliferative retinopathy (Porta et al. 2001).

Knowles et al. (1965) and Murphy et al. (1990) proposed there was a constant interval from the time of the adolescent growth spurt to the development of retinopathy and the years before this growth spurt were not an important consideration in the development of retinopathy. Further, Klein et al. (1985) found in a southern Wisconsin population-based study that the presence of retinopathy was more strongly associated with the duration of a patient's diabetes after the age of 13 than before it. Kostraba et al. also supported this conclusion, stating the "post-pubertal duration of IDDM may be a more accurate determinant of the development of microvascular complications and diabetes-related mortality than total duration" (Kostraba et al. 1989). Kernell et al. found "that children are at low risk before the age of 13 and before puberty" (Kernell et al. 1997). Using the Tanner scale of sexual maturity, Murphy et al., found no difference in the prevalence of retinopathy, considering pubertal status, in children with diabetes of less than 5 years duration, but did find post-pubescent youth with diabetes of 5 to 10 years duration were more likely to have retinopathy than prepubescent youth with the same duration of diabetes. They also found a higher rate of retinopathy in post-pubescent youth than prepubescent youth in the group of subjects with duration of diabetes greater than 10 years, but the numbers in the group of prepubescent youth were too small for statistical comparison. They determined that post-pubescent youth were 4.8X more likely to have retinopathy than prepubescent or pubescent youth when comparing subjects of the same age and duration of diabetes (Murphy et al. 1990). Many other studies reveal a protective effect of the pre-pubertal period for the development of retinopathy (Krolewski et al. 1986; Olsen et al. 2004; Svensson et al. 2004). Olsen et al. found in a Danish nationwide prospective study in patients followed for 8 years that, while the contribution of the pre-pubertal duration of type 1 diabetes does contribute to the development of retinopathy, it contributes only half as much as the post-pubertal period of time. (Olsen et al. 2004).

2.3 Pregnancy

The devastating effects of diabetic retinopathy during pregnancy have been well documented. Despite tight glycemic control, diabetic retinopathy presents a major problem during child bearing years. In the United States 10% of all pregnancies have complications as a result of diabetes mellitus (Vargas et al. 2010). Previously the prognosis for pregnancy in women who have diabetes with microvascular disease was so poor that many physicians advised such patients to avoid or even terminate their pregnancies (Moloney and Drury 1982). Numerous articles have documented the acceleration of diabetic retinopathy during pregnancy, the pathogenesis of which still remains unclear (Klein et al. 1990; The Diabetes Control and Complications Trial Group 1993).

A myriad of physiologic events occur during pregnancy. Some studies show that the ability of the retina to autoregulate its blood flow is impaired (Ernest et al. 1983; Grunwald et al. 1984; Grunwald et al. 1995; Rassam et al. 1995). Other changes include hormonal, metabolic, immunologic, as well as differences in cardiovascular and hematologic systems (Chen et al. 1994; Rosenn et al. 1992; Schocket et al. 1999). After the first 3-4 weeks of a normal human pregnancy large quantities of estrogens are produced nearly exclusively by the placenta from dehydroepiandrosterone sulfate (DHEA). In the placenta it is desulfurylated, converted to androstenedione, aromatized to estrone and converted to 17-β estradiol (E2) before entering circulation. At full term half of the estradiol precursors are from the fetal circulation and half from the maternal. In addition, progesterone is formed in large amounts in the placenta from steroid precursors. Near full term this amount consumes what would be an equivalent of 1/4 to 1/3 of the daily low density lipoprotein (LDL) turnover of non-pregnant adults (Wilson et al. 1998). In fact, the extreme elevation of estrogen and progesterone is the greatest of the pregnancy associated endocrine alterations (Jovanovic-Peterson and Peterson 1991). Sone et al. found that while E2 levels at physiological concentrations did not increase VEGF concentrations in a human endometrial adenocarcinoma cell line, progesterone (P4) at physiological concentrations did significantly raise VEGF levels in bovine retinal pigment epithelial cells (Sone et al. 1996). Furthermore, Larinkari et al. have demonstrated that those pregnant patients with progressive retinopathy had progesterone and estradiol at the upper limits of the normal pregnancy ranges (Larinkari et al. 1982; Sone et al. 1996). Suzuma et al. found that E2 at normal physiological levels for pregnancy increased VEGFR-2 levels (Suzuma et al. 1999). Advanced glycation end-products (AGE) accumulate at an increased rate in hyperglycemia and have been implicated in the development of diabetic retinopathy. Tanaka et al. using human vascular endothelial cells found that the AGE receptor (RAGE) increases with exposure to E2 at normal pregnancy physiological levels and that this increase was blocked with the selective estrogen receptor modulator (SERM) tamoxifen (Tanaka et al. 2000).

3. Levels of testosterone, estrogen and progesterone

Testosterone is formed from its precursor androstenedione and to a lesser extent from DHEA. In males, testosterone is produced mainly by Leydig cells of the testes. Testosterone can be converted by peripheral tissues to the more active dihydrotestosterone (DHT) by the enzyme 5α-reductase or it can be converted into estradiol (E2) by an "A" ring aromatase. In males, the conversion of testosterone to E2 by aromatase achieves masculinization of brain neurons (Wu et al. 2009). In the female ovary, testosterone secreted by thecal cells of the follicles is aromatized by granulosa cells into estradiol.

In males testosterone levels reach ≈250 ng/L by the second trimester of gestation. 2-3 months after birth, the levels fall to 50ng/L and remain low until puberty (age 12-17), when they rise to adult levels of 500-750ng/L. Levels of testosterone decline slowly after middle age, but inadequate testosterone levels can be augmented by hormone replacement therapy

(Wilson et al. 1998). In females, testosterone levels are normally low: 30-50 ng/L throughout life (Forest 1975). Serum testosterone is converted into inactive metabolites by the liver.

Levels of E2 are low in girls (1.6-2.6 pg/mL) but even lower in boys (0.4 to 1.1 pg/mL (Janfaza et al. 2006). During puberty (age 8-13) estrogen rises to adult levels and varies during the menstrual cycle. Estradiol shows a pre-ovulatory peak (190pg/ml) by day 14 of the cycle and peaks broadly (≈100pg/mL) during the luteal phase from days 18-25 (Levin and Hammes 2011; Thorneycroft et al. 1971). Progesterone is low except for a broad peak at 10 ng/mL during the luteal phase of the menstrual cycle. After menopause, E2 falls, reaching levels similar to those found in adult males (8-40 pg/mL) (Lee et al. 2006). Estrogen replacement can be used to ameliorate the side effects of low estradiol. Contraception employs small doses of an ethinylestradiol and progesterone, but studies have shown no relationship between current and past use of contraceptives and diabetic retinopathy (Klein et al. 1990).

4. Known sex hormone effects on vessel walls

4.1 General concepts

The role sex hormones play in the maintenance of the blood vessel walls has been an area of great interest recently. While much work has been done to elucidate the role of estrogen, the role of androgens has heretofore not received as much attention and consequently is not as well understood (Kaushik et al. 2010; Vitale et al. 2010). DHT has a higher affinity for AR and is converted from testosterone in target cells (Imperato-McGinley and Canovatchel 1992). Androgen receptors (AR) have been identified in vascular endothelial cells, vascular smooth muscle cells (VSM), macrophages and monocytes (Villablanca et al. 2010). Estradiol alone has little effect on the production of androgen receptor (Wynne and Khalil 2003). The concentration of AR is less in females than males and it appears to be regulated by a combination of estradiol and testosterone (Villablanca et al. 2010).

There are two estrogen receptors, ERα and ERβ, with overlapping distribution in body tissues. Each sub-type has several variants (Orshal and Khalil 2004). ERα and ERβ have been identified in the vasculature in endothelial cells, VSM, macrophages and monocytes (Villablanca et al. 2010). ERα is thought to promote protective effects to vascular injury. ERβ is believed to be the dominant form in VSM, especially in women (Mendelsohn 2002).

The two subtypes of progesterone receptor (PR), progesterone receptor A (PRA) and progesterone receptor B (PRB), have been found in vascular endothelial cells, VSM and macrophages (Thompson and Khalil 2003; Vazquez et al. 1999; Villablanca et al. 2010). The PRB subtype seems to have a role in gene transcription and cell proliferation of VSM (Pieber et al. 2001).

Sex hormones have gender-specific effects on cardiovascular risk factors such as lipid metabolism, obesity (central weight gain, i.e. android) and glucose metabolism possibly explaining the differences in cardiovascular disease (CVD) risk between men and women (Carani et al. 1997; Fonseca 2009; Liu et al. 2002; Vitale et al. 2010). All of these risk factors, along with blood pressure, are also risk factors of retinopathy and as such are another link between sex hormones and the development and progression of retinopathy (Cunha-Vaz 2011).

4.2 Vascular tone

For some time a correlation between blood pressure and progression of retinopathy has been noted in epidemiologic studies demonstrating that lower blood pressures result in less diabetic retinopathy. This has now been confirmed by large randomized studies (Epidemiology of Diabetes Interventions and Complications (DCCT/EDIC) Study Research Group 2005; The Diabetes Control and Complications Trial Group 1993; UK Prospective Diabetes Study Group 1998). It is well established that adolescent and premenopausal women have lower blood pressures than age matched males and that blood pressure in women rises after menopause. Systolic and diastolic blood pressures in men less than 60 years old are higher than in women by 6-7 and 3-5 mmHg (Dubey et al. 2002). Also blood pressure in women can be affected by the menstrual cycle, pregnancy and supplementation of estrogens (Mendelsohn and Karas 2005). While ERα and ERβ both mediate important effects on blood vessels animal studies indicate that ERβ controlled genes are the ones involved in arterial tone and blood pressure control (Vitale et al. 2010).

One way in which sex hormones interact with the walls of blood vessels is in the way they control vascular tone. Nitric oxide (NO) is a dilator and relaxant of blood vessels acting through its effects on VSM. It is produced by vessel endothelial cells in a reaction catalyzed by endothelial nitric oxide synthase (eNOS) requiring O_2 and NADPH where arginine is oxidized to citrulline, releasing NO (Berg et al. 2007). NO then diffuses from endothelial cells to VSM where it can activate guanylcyclase, producing cyclic GMP from GTP and triggering events leading to vessel dilation. Estrogen in both genomic and a non-genomic pathways can lead to the production of eNOS thus increasing production of NO. Furthermore, arterial endothelial NO release is greater in females than males (Orshal and Khalil 2004).

Less is known about the effects of androgens on blood pressure than are known about the effects of estrogens on blood pressure. (Dubey et al. 2002). Generally it has been found that androgen levels are inversely related to blood pressure (Kaushik et al. 2010). The Rotterdam population-based prospective study found an association toward higher blood pressure in the lower androgenic group, but this did not reach the predetermined level of significance in their study (Hak et al. 2002). The effect *in vitro* of testosterone on VSM is toward vasodilation and is mediated through the nitric oxide (NO) pathway (Kaushik et al. 2010). However, testosterone has also been linked to pro-hypertensive effects. In male spontaneously hypertensive rats testosterone has been found to increase the activity of tyrosine hydroxylase, the rate limiting enzyme in norepinephrine synthesis (Dubey et al. 2002). Furthermore, testosterone has been linked to increased expression of artery thromboxane A_2 resulting in enhanced coronary constriction (Dubey et al. 2002). In murine models hypertension has been prevented by orchidectomy. This normalization of blood pressure is reversed by supplementation of testosterone. These effects seem to be generated through AR since the AR blocker flutamide has been shown to eliminate the blood pressure difference between male and female mice (Kaushik et al. 2010).

Other research has looked at how the control of the renin-angiotension system is influenced by sex hormones. It has been proposed that testosterone may activate the renin-angiotension system and that E2 inhibits renin release and angiotension converting enzyme (ACE) (Orshal and Khalil 2004). The fact that there are no gender differences in the effectiveness of

ACE inhibitors when they are used to treat hypertension may mean that this male/female difference is insignificant (Kaushik et al. 2010). Normal physiological levels of E2 can result in increased cyclooxygenase (COX-1) expression with resulting prostacyclin synthesis in sheep fetal pulmonary artery and human umbilical vein endothelial cells (HUVEC). Prostacyclin synthesis is linked to vascular relaxation. Although several mechanisms have been proposed, COX inhibitors such as nonsteroidal anti-inflammatory drugs (NSAIDs) have been linked to increased blood pressure (Orshal and Khalil 2004; Qi et al. 2002).

The effects of progesterone on vascular activity are not clear. In some tissues it has no effect while in others it can lead to vascular relaxation. The vasodilator effect of progesterone may be related to non-genomic relaxant effects (Orshal and Khalil 2004).

4.3 Lipids

Brown et al. found a "marked accumulation" of retinal exudate in patients with high triglyceride levels (Brown et al. 1984). Dodson and Gibson in a study on patients with type 2 diabetes found that hypercholesterolemia was a risk factor in the development of diabetic maculopathy (Dodson and Gibson 1991). In epidemiological studies Chew et al., and Klein et al. found that increased blood lipid levels are associated with diabetic retinopathy in that subjects with elevated lipids had a greater risk of developing high-risk PDR and a greater risk of vision loss from DME (Chew et al. 1996; Klein et al. 1991). Chowdhury et al. conclude that a toxic effect of LDL on pericytes could be enhanced by LDL glycation or oxidation (Chowdhury et al. 2002).

Although there has been some variation in study conclusions, epidemiological and observational studies have generally concluded that low endogenous testosterone levels in men are associated with lipid profiles consisting of decreased high-density lipoprotein (HDL) cholesterol levels and increased total cholesterol, triglycerides and LDL levels compared to normal or higher levels. This is referred to as Hypoandrogen Metabolic Syndrome (HAM) and often accompanies the metabolic syndrome of central obesity and insulin resistance (Kaushik et al. 2010). Multiple studies have reached a similar conclusion and found that men with higher levels of testosterone generally have better lipid profiles including high HDLs and lower triglycerides (Kaushik et al. 2010). Supplementation of testosterone in hypoandrogenesis is generally considered to decrease HDLs and only modestly affect LDLs (Mendelsohn and Karas 2005). Lower testosterone levels in men have also been linked to central adiposity, insulin resistance, hyperinsulinemia and type 2 diabetes (Webb and Collins 2010). Testosterone, acting through the adipocyte androgen receptors, increases expression of β-adrenergic receptor, protein kinase A, and lipase (Wu and von Eckardstein 2003).

The actions of estrogens on the blood lipid levels of women have been studied for many years. Lipid levels are affected by the action of endogenous sex steroid hormones and hormone replacement therapy (HRT) on liver lipoprotein metabolism. In an analysis of several studies Mumford et al. found that total cholesterol and LDL levels were highest during the follicular phase of the menstrual cycle and were lower during the luteal phase. They found HDLs to be higher during the follicular and peri-ovulatory phases. In a meta-analysis of sex steroid use by transsexual individuals, Elamin et al. found a reduction in HDL in female to male patients receiving androgens and an increase in HDLs in male to female patients receiving estrogens. They found triglyceride levels increased in both female to male patients receiving androgens and male to female patients receiving estrogens (Elamin et al. 2010).

After menopause it has been found that LDLs and triglyceride levels rise and HDL levels decrease. HRT appears to positively affect lipid levels by lowering total cholesterol, LDLs and raising HDLs, but negatively affects lipid levels by raising triglycerides (Mendelsohn and Karas 2005). Some controversy has arisen over the delivery method of HRT. Nanda et al. found that HRT transdermal therapy (estrogen 50 μg/day) had the advantage of lowering triglyceride levels as opposed to oral (conjugated equine estrogens 0.625mg/day) (Nanda et al. 2003). The Women's Health Initiative (WHI) trial and the Heart and Estrogen/Progestin Replacement Study (HERS) found that a favorable lipid profile developed using exogenous estrogens, but also found using estrogen with progestin was associated with elevated levels of CVD. Progesterone is believed to either have a neutral effect on lipids or to negatively affect estrogen's positive effects (Hulley et al. 1998; Mumford et al. 2011; Rossouw et al. 2002).

5. Sex hormone effects on specific components in the vessel wall

The events leading to the retinal damage associated with hyperglycemia such as the breakdown of the blood retinal barrier, vessel basement membrane thickening, formation of microaneursyms, hemorrhages, cotton-wool spots, capillary obliteration and acellular capillaries can be traced to the damage occurring to micro-vessel endothelial cells, pericytes and their surrounding basement membrane. It has been noted that these sequelae develop as a result of the early loss of capillary endothelial cells and pericytes in the retina (Cunha-Vaz 2011).

5.1 Endothelium

The initial recruitment of leukocytes into vasculature during the development of retinopathy involves a process referred to as rolling - the initial slowing and loose attachment of leukocytes to the vascular endothelium. This attachment is transient and reversible and its essential function is to slow down the leukocytes as they travel through the vessel lumen. The leukocyte integrins VLA-4, $\alpha_4\beta_7$-integrin, Mac-1 and LFA-1 are the principle attachment proteins of leukocytes whose corresponding ligands on endothelial cells are ICAM and VCAM-1. Rolling may be followed by activation of the leukocyte, adhesion to the endothelial cell and subsequent transendothelial migration through the vessel luminal layer of endothelial cells. While macrophages play positive roles in tissue repair they may contribute to diabetic retinopathy as chronic mediators of inflammation (Duh 2009). It is believed that leukocyte recruitment increases under certain conditions such as atherosclerosis, hypercholesteremia and diabetes (Hammes and Porta 2010). Elevated expression of ICAM-1 has been shown in the blood vessels of diabetic patients and animals and soluble VCAM-1 has been detected in the serum of persons with type 1 diabetes (Hammes and Porta 2010; Miyamoto et al. 1999). The results of increased cell adhesion of leukocytes to retinal capillary endothelial cells can be correlated with leukostasis, capillary occlusion, blood-retinal barrier disruption, increased retinal edema, endothelial cell injury and death (Hammes and Porta 2010).

McCrohon et al. using a co-culture of monocytes and HUVEC found that dihydrotesterone (DHT) increases the level of VCAM-1 in HUVEC and that this results in an increase of adhesion of these cells to monocytes. This effect was blocked by the AR blocker hydroxyflutamide (McCrohon et al. 1999). In a similar experiment, Death et al. found that DHT increased expression of VCAM-1 in male human endothelial cells through a mechanism involving NF-κB that was blocked by hydroxyflutamide (Death et al. 2004). Others have shown DHT and testosterone can inhibit VCAM-1 and ICAM-1, but Mukherjee et al. demonstrated that VCAM-1 inhibition in HUVECs can be reversed by an aromatase inhibitor, demonstrating that the apparent VCAM-1 inhibition by testosterone was caused by the aromatase conversion of testosterone to estrogen (Mukherjee et al. 2002; Villablanca et al. 2010).

As one might expect, estrogen inhibits the expression of ICAM-1 and VCAM-1 in the vascular endothelium during inflammation (Cid et al. 1994; Simoncini et al. 1999; Villablanca et al. 2010). Interestingly this inhibition was blocked by the ER antagonist ICI 182,780, but the selective estrogen receptor modulator (SERM) tamoxifen had no inhibitory effects (Simoncini et al. 1999). It is believed VCAM-1 inhibition occurs through ERβ. While progesterone at supra-physiological levels inhibits expression of VCAM-1, another progestin, medroxyprogesterone acetate (MPA) does not. When tested with HUVECs at normal physiological concentrations progesterone has no effect on ICAM-1 or VCAM-1 expression. When estrogen and progesterone are used concurrently progesterone increases the estrogen inhibition of ICAM-1 and VCAM-1 in human iliac artery at supra-physiological levels (Villablanca et al. 2010).

Proliferation of endothelial cells can be viewed as a positive or negative factor. It can be positive as a vessel repair mechanism, or negative as in tube vessel formation such as occurs in proliferative diabetic retinopathy or rheumatoid arthritis. In conditions such as atherosclerosis and diabetic retinopathy an intact endothelium is important due to its role in providing "an antithrombotic and anticoagulant surface" (Vazquez et al. 1999). Gender differences have been found to exist with endothelial cell proliferation. Liu et al. found testosterone, when used at nanomolar concentrations, increased the proliferation of male rat vascular endothelial cells (VEC), but had no effect on the proliferation of female VEC. Nanomolar E2 increased the increased proliferation of both male and female VEC. Vazquez found that progesterone had an inhibitory effect on endothelial cell proliferation acting through PR in WT mice (Vazquez et al. 1999). Espinosa-Heidmann studied 9 month old female mice (middle aged) with either: 1) a sham operation, 2) an ovariectomy with empty pellets, or 3) an ovariectomy with an E2 pellet. After choroidal thermal burns they found that female ovariectomized mice with E2 supplementation had a larger area of neovascularization compared to either sham operated female mice, ovariectomized female mice, or male mice implanted with an estrogen pellet. They hypothesized that the E2 "in the absence of other ovarian hormones, paradoxically increased the severity of choroidal neovascularization (CNV) in middle aged female mice" (Espinosa-Heidmann et al. 2005). Tanemura et al., using the fact that pre-menopausal women are more susceptible to choroidal neovascularization than men, found greater neovascularization using laser-induced photocoagulation in female rats than in male rats. They found that E2 and photocoagulation increased the expression of ERβ and VEGFR-2 and found no change in the expression of ERα mRNA at any time after photocoagulation. Using a culture of HUVEC to measure cell proliferation of transfected endothelial cells they found a significant increase in cell number in those overexpressing ERβ, but no change in cell number in cells overexpressing ERα (Tanemura et al. 2004).

5.2 Basement membrane

New blood vessel growth is complex involving breakdown of a vessel wall, endothelial cell migration, proliferation, tube formation and formation of a new basement membrane (Folkman 1995). Extracellular matrix proteins work as a scaffold whereby cell migration, proliferation and capillary formation can occur. Basic fibroblast growth factor (FGF-2) is a potent extracellular cytokine which functions in these stages of neovascularization. FGF-2 is unique in that it lacks a sequence to allow its release from then endothelial cell where it is manufactured. Albuquerque et al. found that FGF-2 release into the cell media is enhanced when estrogen is present in a cell culture of human coronary artery endothelial cells and that this enhancement can be blocked by the ER blocker ICI 182,780. Furthermore, they found this enhancement was inhibited by inhibition of protein kinase C, indicating that estrogen does not necessarily result directly in the production of more FGF-2, but that it may function with cell matrix proteins to enhance the release of FGF-2 (Albuquerque et al. 1998). Extracellular matrix proteases which are regulated post-translationally also play an important role in basement membrane remodeling. As an example, tPA and uPA are plasminogen activators which are inhibited by the plasminogen activator inhibitor (PAI-1). When endotheliąl cells are quiescent, such as when they are confluent, estrogen functions to increase PAI-1 production and reduces production of tPA and uPA, decreasing protease activity. When cells are activated such as in angiogenesis, estrogen decreases PAI-1 production and consequently increases tPA and uPA production thus accelerating protease activity (Rubanyi and Kauffman 1998).

5.3 Pericytes

Pericytes are derived from the same pluripotent mural precursor cells as vascular smooth muscle cells (Hammes and Porta 2010). They appear to play a role in supporting the microcirculation against hydrostatic pressure and also function to sustain vessel stability through physical and chemical signaling with vessel endothelial cells (Hall 2006). It is believed pericyte loss is the first damage occurring with hyperglycemia (Hammes 2005; Vidro et al. 2008). Brignardello et al. using bovine retinal capillary pericytes found that DHEA, a precursor to both testosterone and estrogen, reduced pericyte loss resulting from high glucose as a result of its antioxidant properties. They report that this effect was not produced through either AR or ER (Brignardello et al. 1998). In a study of rabbits fed a high-fat diet, which has been known to increase oxidative stress, Aragno et al. found that DHEA restored the rabbits oxidative balance. This supports Brignardello's hypothesis that the protective cellular effect of DHEA is through its antioxidant properties (Aragno et al. 2009). Nanomolar concentrations of DHT and E2 had no effect on pericyte loss as a result of high glucose (Brignardello et al. 1998).

6. Hormone receptors in the retina

Sex hormones and sex hormone receptors are present in the retina from an early stage. Many areas of the brain and retina develop in a sexually dimorphic manner during prenatal, perinatal and postnatal development. Salyer et al. using Long-Evans rats found that prenatally and early postnatally in normal rats males had thicker retinas than females. This increased thickness was reduced using flutamide, an androgen inhibitor, but not significantly so compared to normal males or testosterone-treated males, indicating that the process was not entirely mediated through AR. Females at this life-stage had undetectable testosterone levels, but when these females were treated with testosterone their retinal thickness did not differ significantly from normal or testosterone-treated males. To help rule out the conversion of testosterone to estrogen Salyer et al. using immunocytochemistry found no aromatase present in the neuroretina at this stage of development, but they did find quantities of it in the retinal pigment epithelium (RPE) (Salyer et al. 2001). Interestingly, Kobayashi et al. found evidence of 17β-hydroxysteroid dehydrogenase type IV in the RPE of chick embryo eye. 17β-hydroxysteroid dehydrogenase type IV is an enzyme which converts E2 to less reactive estrone (Kobayashi et al. 1997). It has been proposed its function is to protect the embryonic eye against excessive amounts of E2 (Gupta et al. 2005). Messenger RNAs of AR have been found in adult rat retina and uvea, rabbit retina and choroid and human RPE (Rocha et al. 2000; Wickham et al. 2000). In addition, Rocha et al. found the mRNA for 5α reductase, which translates the enzyme which converts testosterone to the more active DHT in the RPE (Rocha et al. 2000). Prabhu et al. found AR protein in all layers of rat retina except the ganglion and outer nuclear layers (Prabhu et al. 2010). However, in an interesting comparison of transformed rat cell lines from brain capillary endothelial cells and retinal capillary endothelial cells, Ohtsuki et al. found dominant expression of AR in the brain capillary cells, but not the retinal capillary cells. DHT acting through AR, in brain capillary endothelial cells (but not the retinal capillary endothelial cells), up-regulated the mRNA for organic anion transporter 3 (OAT3) a protein which is found in blood brain barrier (Ohtsuki et al. 2005).

ERs are nuclear receptors but may be also be located either in the cytoplasm or in the cell plasma membrane (Marquez and Pietras 2001; Simoncini et al. 2000). As discussed, ER has been found in the vascular endothelium of organs other than the gonads including the retina (Gupta et al. 2005; Ogueta et al. 1999; Suzuma et al. 1999). The ligand for either ERα or ERβ can be a form of estrogen or a selective estrogen receptor modulator (SERM). ERα has been mapped to the long arm of chromosome 6 and the ERβ has been mapped to band q22-24 of chromosome 14 (Enmark and Gustafsson 1999). ERα and ERβ are highly conserved with >95% homology for the DNA-binding domain. The two ERs differ functionally in how they are regulated. The β-receptor lacks ligand-independent transcriptional activity as compared to ERα, meaning when the ligand-dependent carboxy area of ERβ is blocked from its ligand, it retains very little activity (Manni and Verderame 2002).

The ligand-independent area of ERα usually displays only weak activity; however in certain cell types it can exhibit strong independent activity (Berry et al. 1990). A pre-requisite for transcriptional activity of the estrogen receptors are their compatibilities with certain co-activators (Shibata et al. 1997); thus, differences in the composition of the highly variable (Enmark and Gustafsson 1999) amino area of ERα and ERβ results in differences in intrinsic activity related to differences in affinity for their co-activators (Webb et al. 1998). It should also be noted there is significant variability between ERα and ERβ in their ligand-binding domains, ≈50% variability(Enmark and Gustafsson 1999). These differences suggest it may be possible to create pharmaceuticals which could activate one but not the other.

Prior to activation with estrogen, ERα and ERβ are held in the nucleus attached to a molecular chaperone such as heat shock protein 90 (HSP90) (Webb et al. 1998). Estrogen combines with estrogen receptors to create either homo- or hetero-dimers (Cowley et al. 1997; Osborne et al. 2000; Pettersson et al. 1997). These dimers combine with appropriate coactivators and bind to estrogen response elements (ERE) on the DNA which consist of an inverted repeat of two half-sites with the consensus motif AGGTCA spaced by 3 base pairs. ERα has been detected in pre-menopausal human female retinas (descending amounts 35 years>49 years>74 years) and in human male retinas. Interestingly, Ogueta et al. found the amount of ERα in males was intermediate between the levels found in 49 to 74 year old females. They localized ERα in the retina to the nuclei of the outer and inner nuclear layers, the outer plexiform layer (horizontal and bipolar cells), the nuclei of the ganglion cell layer and the RPE (Ogueta et al. 1999). ERβ has been localized to the RPE and also to neovascular tissue evolving from the choroid in both males and females in a manner which is dependent on estrogen concentration (Giddabasappa et al. 2010; Gupta et al. 2005; Marin-Castano et al. 2003).

7. Effects of sex hormones on individual steps in retinopathy

Due to prevailing evidences of the roles of sex hormones and sex hormone receptors in the development and maintenance of retina, Gupta et al. commented that "it is likely that sex-based incidences of retinal disorders may be regulated by estrogens (Gupta et al. 2005). We suggest androgens and progesterone also play a role.

7.1 Vascular cell maintenance

It is well established that the incidence and progression of retinopathy is related to the control of systemic factors such as blood pressure and blood glucose management (The Diabetes Control and Complications Trial Group 1993; UK Prospective Diabetes Study Group 1998). Furthermore lipid levels and waist-hip ratio have been correlated with the progression to proliferative retinopathy (Dorchy et al. 2002; Porta et al. 2001). As discussed above, blood pressure, lipid levels and waist-hip ratio have all been linked to the effects of sex hormones.

At the cellular level there are factors in the response of retinal capillary endothelial cells, pericytes and basement membrane that are often at least partially under the control of sex hormones. Leukostasis is positively influenced by the expression of ICAM and VCAM-1 with androgens and estrogens modulating expression of these attachment proteins. The upregulation of these proteins by DHT has been blocked by the androgen receptor blocker hydroxyflutamide (McCrohon et al. 1999). Estrogens inhibited ICAM and VCAM-1 expression (Cid et al. 1994; Simoncini et al. 1999; Villablanca et al. 2010). Progestins seemed to inhibit VCAM-1 expression while medroxyprogesterone did not. Progesterone used concurrently with estrogen further enhances the estrogen inhibition of ICAM-1 and VCAM-1 (Villablanca et al. 2010).

Androgens have been found to increase vascular endothelial cell proliferation in males. E2 has been found to increase endothelial cell proliferation in both males and females and progesterone has a negative effect on this proliferation. Thus sex hormones can play an important role in vascular repair (Liu et al. 2002). However it can also be a negative in conditions such as the progression of proliferative diabetic retinopathy. Remodeling of the basement membrane is an important element in the development of neovascularization. E2 plays a role in the control of the extracellular cytokines FGF-2 and PAI-1 which maintain some control over this process (Albuquerque et al. 1998; Rubanyi and Kauffman 1998). It is well known that pericyte and endothelial cell communication plays an important role in the health of retinal capillaries (Hall 2006). It is also well known that pericyte loss is one of the first damaging effects of hyperglycemia. The fact that sex hormones can work to protect pericytes further links the role of sex hormones to the cell responses to diabetes. Furthermore, as discussed previously, sex hormones and their cognate receptors are well known to populate the retina of humans.

7.2 Angiogenesis

Vascular endothelial growth factor (VEGF) is well known as a controller of angiogenesis (Aiello et al. 1994; Folkman 1971).

Suzuma et al. used bovine retinal microvascular endothelial cells and Mueller et al. used human primary and Ishikawa uterine cells to show an increase in VEGF linked to E2 exposure (Mueller et al. 2000; Suzuma et al. 1999). Kazi et al. have demonstrated in rat uterine luminal cells that E2 required the P13K/AKT pathway to increase VEGF gene expression (Kazi et al. 2009). Grigsby et al. using a primate cell line of rhesus monkey retinal endothelial cells (RhREC) showed a decrease in VEGF levels with E2 exposure, which only partially recovered with the concurrent use of tamoxifen and raloxifene (Grigsby et al. 2011).

Pigment epithelium-derived factor (PEDF) is a 50-kDa glycoprotein secreted by the RPE (Tombran-Tink et al. 1991; Tombran-Tink and Johnson 1989). It has been shown to be the most important inhibitor of angiogenesis in mammalian eyes, strongly suggesting that decreased levels of it play an important role in angiogenic eye diseases such as proliferative diabetic retinopathy (Dawson et al. 1999; Takenaka et al. 2005). Gao et al., using Brown Norway rats, found PEDF levels to be inversely related to VEGF levels. The latter was inversely linked to retinal oxygen concentrations in a balance controlling angiogenesis (Gao et al. 2001). Cheung et al. found in human ovarian and surface epithelial cells that ER is an important upstream regulator of PEDF. They further found that E2 reduced PEDF levels, and that this reduction could be modulated by the introduction of the ER antagonist, ICI 182,780 (Cheung et al. 2006). In normoxic conditions Grigsby et al. found that, in response to E2, PEDF levels were reduced in RhREC cells. Furthermore, this reduction in response to E2 could be mitigated by concurrent exposure to tamoxifen or raloxifene, but the relative change in PEDF and in VEGF did not exactly correspond to cell growth patterns indicating that additional factors are involved in E2-induced proliferation of RhREC (Grigsby et al. 2011).

8. Conclusions

There is ample evidence that sex hormones do play a role in the development and progression of diabetic retinopathy in humans. For clinicians, there is evidence the attainment of puberty and especially pregnancy should raise the level of suspicion of the presence or progression of retinopathy.

Androgens and androgen blockers could possibly have mixed results in treating or preventing retinopathy. Androgens can raise blood pressure, have negative results on blood lipids, and increase levels of ICAM and VCAM-1. Low levels of androgens are linked with metabolic syndrome in males and can negatively affect lipid levels, blood glucose, blood pressure and increase hip-waist ratio. However, DHEA, a testosterone precursor, has been shown to be effective in protecting pericytes against the effects of high glucose (Brignardello et al. 1998).

It is believed high glucose levels can induce oxidative stress through several mechanisms (Brownlee 2001; Cunha-Vaz 2011 Du et al. 2000). Nishikawa et al. found superoxides may be generated in either complex I or complex III of the mitochondria, especially as a result of hyperglycemia (Nishikawa et al. 2000). The toxicity of glucose and consequent vascular damage has been postulated to occur through four supposedly dissimilar mechanisms: 1) activation of protein kinase C, 2) aldose reductase activation, 3) advanced glycation endproduct formation (AGE) and 4) the hexosamine pathway. What has been described as the "unifying hypothesis" is that reactive oxygen species formation is the upstream event that occurs in each of these mechanisms (Brownlee 2001; Cunha-Vaz 2011). Giddabasappa et al. have recently described their work on ARPE-19 cells in which they find that ERβ protects these cells from oxidative damage by protecting the mitochondria and up-regulating ERβ and antioxidant genes (Giddabasappa et al. 2010).

Similar to the "timing hypothesis" of hormone replacement therapy in human females where estrogen replacement is only appropriate during certain peri-menopausal stages, estrogen may play different roles depending on the stage of retinopathy. At an early stage the proliferation of endothelial cells induced by estradiol may be a benefit as a reparative mechanism; however, at a stage where proliferative retinopathy is threatening vision this increased proliferation and could lead to pathological vessel formation (Espinosa-Heidmann et al. 2005; Grigsby et al. 2011; Suzuma et al. 1999).

Since selective estrogen receptor modulators (SERM) can stimulate or depress estrogen effects depending on the type of ER or co-activators present in a particular cell, a SERM, or a co-activator blocker might be designed to suppress only that ER found in the retinal microvascular endothelial cell environment or to reduce leukostasis by inhibiting ICAM or VCAM-1 (Smith and O'Malley 2004). Their actions can be either non-genomic or genomic. Tamoxifen has been approved by the US-FDA for reducing the incidence of breast cancer in women at high risk for developing the disease, and in the treatment of metastatic breast cancer (Tamoxifen 2007). It has been used for over 30 years to treat estrogen-sensitive breast cancer. Raloxifene (Evista©) was originally approved for the treatment and prevention of post-menopausal bone loss and, more recently, for reducing the risk of invasive breast cancer in postmenopausal women with osteoporosis as well as in postmenopausal women at high risk for invasive breast cancer (Tamoxifen 2007). Both tamoxifen and raloxifene inhibit cell proliferation in breast tissue, but only raloxifene inhibits cell proliferation in the uterus; in fact, tamoxifen has been linked to an increase in uterine cancer (Cuzick et al. 2002). The use of tamoxifen has also been linked to cataract formation (Zhang et al. 1994). Grigsby et al. are the first to demonstrate that raloxifene is as effective as tamoxifen in reducing the E2-induced proliferation in a primate retinal endothelial cell line. Results from this cell study on tamoxifen and raloxifene inhibition of E2-induced cell proliferations suggest that tamoxifen and raloxifene have similar potency to block estrogen mediated retinal angiogenesis (Grigsby et al. 2011).

Much is yet to be learned about the role sex hormones play in the development and progression of diabetic retinopathy. It appears that any treatment of diabetic retinopathy using sex hormones, or their blockers, may not be a "one size fits all" treatment, but may vary according to the life stage, level of retinopathy and the gender of an individual. Nonetheless, it is apparent that sex hormones do play a role at several different stages of retinopathy and that sex hormone stimulation or modulation, as appropriate, can offer promise to control diabetic retinopathy.

9. Abbreviations

ACE, angiotension converting enzyme; AGE, advanced glycation end-products; AR, androgen receptor; Akt, serine/threonine protein kinase; CNV, choroidal neovascularization; COX, cyclooxygenase; CVD, cardiovascular disease; DHEA, dehydroepiandrosterone; DHT, dihydrotestosterone; DIEP, Diabetes in Early Pregnancy Study; E, estrogens; E2, 17β-estradiol; EDRF, endothelium-derived relaxing factor; ETDRS, Early Treatment of Diabetic Retinopathy Study; eNOS, endothelial nitric oxide synthase; ER, estrogen receptor; ERα, estrogen receptor alpha; ERβ, estrogen receptor beta; ERE, estrogen-response element; ERK, extracellular signal-regulated kinases; FGF, fibroblast growth factor; HAM, hypoandrogen metabolic syndrome; HDL, high-density lipoprotein; HLA, human leukocyte antigen; HRT, hormone replacement therapy; HSP, heat-shock protein; HUVEC, human umbilical endothelial cells; IDDM, insulin-dependent diabetes mellitus, type 1; ICAM, inter-cellular adhesion molecule; LDL, low-density lipoprotein; LH, luteinizing hormone; MAPK, mitogen-activated protein kinase; MCP-1, monocyte chemotactic protein-1; MPA, medroxyprogesterone; NFκ-β, nuclear factor κβ; NO, nitric oxide; NSAID, non-steroidal anti-inflammatory drugs; OAT, organic anion transporter; PAI, plasminogen activator inhibitor; PEDF, pigment epithelium-derived factor; PG, progesterones; PI3K, phosphoinositide 3 kinase; POS, polycystic ovary syndrome; PRA, progesterone receptor A; PRB, progesterone receptor B; RAGE, advanced glycation end-product receptor; RPE, retinal pigment epithelium; SERM, selective estrogen receptor modulator; tPA, tissue plasminogen activator; uPA urokinases plasminogen activator; VCAM, vascular cell adhesion molecule; VEC, vascular endothelial cells; VEGF, vascular endothelial growth factor, VEGFR, vascular endothelial growth factor receptor; VSM, vascular smooth muscle; WESDR, Wisconsin Epidemiological Study of Diabetic Retinopathy; WT, wild-type.

10. Acknowledgements

We thank NIH/NCRR/RCMI and SALSI for financial support and also Pamela Forbes and Suzanne Ferimer for their research assistance.

11. References

Aiello, L. P., R. L. Avery, P. G. Arrigg, B. A. Keyt, H. D. Jampel, S. T. Shah, et al. (1994). "Vascular endothelial growth factor in ocular fluid of patients with diabetic retinopathy and other retinal disorders." *N Engl J Med* 331(22): 1480-1487.

Albuquerque, M. L., S. K. Akiyama and H. W. Schnaper (1998). "Basic fibroblast growth factor release by human coronary artery endothelial cells is enhanced by matrix proteins, 17beta-estradiol, and a PKC signaling pathway." *Experimental cell research* 245(1): 163-169.

Ansar Ahmed, S., W. J. Penhale and N. Talal (1985). "Sex hormones, immune responses, and autoimmune diseases. Mechanisms of sex hormone action." *Am J Pathol* 121(3): 531-551.

Aragno, M., G. Meineri, I. Vercellinatto, P. Bardini, S. Raimondo, P. G. Peiretti, G. Boccuzzi (2009). "Cardiac impairment in rabbits fed a high-fat diet is counteracted by dehydroepiandrosterone supplementation." *Life sciences* 85(1-2): 77-84.

Beatson, G. T. (1896). "On the treatment of inoperable cases of carcinoma of the mamma: suggestions for a new method of treatment with illustrative cases." *Lancet*(2): 104-107.

Bell, D. S. H. (1995). "Lack of Long-Term Diabetic Complications in Spite of Poor Glycemic Control in Twins With Pure Gonadal Dysgenesis." *Diabetes Care* 18: 1286-1287.

Berg, J. M., J. L. Tymoczko and L. Stryer (2007). *Biochemistry*. New York, New York, W.H. Freeman and Company.

Berry, M., D. Metzger and P. Chambon (1990). "Role of the two activating domains of the oestrogen receptor in the cell-type and promoter-context dependent agonistic activity of the anti-oestrogen 4-hydroxytamoxifen." *EMBO J* 9(9): 2811-2818.

Brignardello, E., E. Beltramo, P. A. Molinatti, M. Aragno, V. Gatto, E. Tamagno, G. Boccuzzi (1998). "Dehydroepiandrosterone protects bovine retinal capillary pericytes against glucose toxicity." *The Journal of endocrinology* 158(1): 21-26.

Brown, G. C., M. Ridley, D. Haas, A. C. Lucier and L. K. Sarin (1984). "Lipemic diabetic retinopathy." *Ophthalmology* 91(12): 1490-1495.

Brownlee, M. (2001). "Biochemistry and molecular cell biology of diabetic complications." *Nature* 414(6865): 813-820.

Carani, C., K. Qin, M. Simoni, M. Faustini-Fustini, S. Serpente, J. Boyd, E. R. Simpson (1997). "Effect of testosterone and estradiol in a man with aromatase deficiency." *The New England journal of medicine* 337(2): 91-95.

Chen, H. C., R. S. Newsom, V. Patel, J. Cassar, H. Mather and E. M. Kohner (1994). "Retinal blood flow changes during pregnancy in women with diabetes." *Investigative ophthalmology & visual science* 35(8): 3199-3208.

Cheung, L. W., S. C. Au, A. N. Cheung, H. Y. Ngan, J. Tombran-Tink, N. Auersperg and A. S. Wong (2006). "Pigment epithelium-derived factor is estrogen sensitive and inhibits the growth of human ovarian cancer and ovarian surface epithelial cells." *Endocrinology* 147(9): 4179-4191.

Chew, E. Y., M. L. Klein, F. L. Ferris, 3rd, N. A. Remaley, R. P. Murphy, K. Chantry, D. Miller (1996). "Association of elevated serum lipid levels with retinal hard exudate in diabetic retinopathy. Early Treatment Diabetic Retinopathy Study (ETDRS) Report 22." *Arch Ophthalmol* 114(9): 1079-1084.

Chowdhury, T. A., D. Hopkins, P. M. Dodson and G. C. Vafidis (2002). "The role of serum lipids in exudative diabetic maculopathy: is there a place for lipid lowering therapy?" *Eye (Lond)* 16(6): 689-693.

Cid, M. C., H. K. Kleinman, D. S. Grant, H. W. Schnaper, A. S. Fauci and G. S. Hoffman (1994). "Estradiol enhances leukocyte binding to tumor necrosis factor (TNF)-stimulated endothelial cells via an increase in TNF-induced adhesion molecules E-selectin, intercellular adhesion molecule type 1, and vascular cell adhesion molecule type 1." *The Journal of clinical investigation* 93(1): 17-25.

Constable, I. J., M. W. Knuiman, T. A. Welborn, R. L. Cooper, K. M. Stanton, V. J. McCann and G. C. Grose (1984). "Assessing the risk of diabetic retinopathy." *American journal of ophthalmology* 97(1): 53-61.

Cowley, S. M., S. Hoare, S. Mosselman and M. G. Parker (1997). "Estrogen receptors alpha and beta form heterodimers on DNA." *J Biol Chem* 272(32): 19858-19862.

Cunha-Vaz, J. (2011). *Diabetic Retinopathy*. Hackensack, N.J., World Scientific Publishing Co. Pte. Ltd.

Cuzick, J., J. Forbes, R. Edwards, M. Baum, S. Cawthorn, A. Coates, T. Powles (2002). "First results from the International Breast Cancer Intervention Study (IBIS-I): a randomised prevention trial." *Lancet* 360(9336): 817-824.

Davis, M. D., M. R. Fisher, R. E. Gangnon, F. Barton, L. M. Aiello, E. Y. Chew, G. L. Knatterud (1998). "Risk factors for high-risk proliferative diabetic retinopathy and severe visual loss: Early Treatment Diabetic Retinopathy Study Report #18." *Invest Ophthalmol Vis Sci* 39(2): 233-252.

Dawson, D. W., O. V. Volpert, P. Gillis, S. E. Crawford, H. Xu, W. Benedict and N. P. Bouck (1999). "Pigment epithelium-derived factor: a potent inhibitor of angiogenesis." *Science* 285(5425): 245-248.

Death, A. K., K. C. McGrath, M. A. Sader, S. Nakhla, W. Jessup, D. J. Handelsman and D. S. Celermajer (2004). "Dihydrotestosterone promotes vascular cell adhesion molecule-1 expression in male human endothelial cells via a nuclear factor-kappaB-dependent pathway." *Endocrinology* 145(4): 1889-1897.

Dodson, P. M. and J. M. Gibson (1991). "Long-term follow-up of and underlying medical conditions in patients with diabetic exudative maculopathy." *Eye (Lond)* 5 (Pt 6): 699-703.

Dorchy, H., C. Claes and C. Verougstraete (2002). "Risk factors of developing proliferative retinopathy in type 1 diabetic patients : role of BMI." *Diabetes Care* 25(4): 798-799.

Du, X. L., D. Edelstein, L. Rossetti, I. G. Fantus, H. Goldberg, F. Ziyadeh, M. Brownlee (2000). "Hyperglycemia-induced mitochondrial superoxide overproduction activates the hexosamine pathway and induces plasminogen activator inhibitor-1 expression by increasing Sp1 glycosylation." *Proceedings of the National Academy of Sciences of the United States of America* 97(22): 12222-12226.

Dubey, R. K., S. Oparil, B. Imthurn and E. K. Jackson (2002). "Sex hormones and hypertension." *Cardiovascular research* 53(3): 688-708.

Duh, E., Ed. (2009). *Diabetic Retinopathy*. Contemporary Diabetes. Totowa, New Jersey, Humana.

Elamin, M. B., M. Z. Garcia, M. H. Murad, P. J. Erwin and V. M. Montori (2010). "Effect of sex steroid use on cardiovascular risk in transsexual individuals: a systematic review and meta-analyses." *Clinical endocrinology* 72(1): 1-10.

Enmark, E. and J. A. Gustafsson (1999). "Oestrogen receptors - an overview." *J Intern Med* 246(2): 133-138.

Epidemiology of Diabetes Interventions and Complications (DCCT/EDIC) Study Research Group (2005). "Intensive diabetes treatment and cardiovascular disease in patients with type 1 diabetes." *N Engl J Med* 353(25): 2643-2653.

Ernest, J. T., T. K. Goldstick and R. L. Engerman (1983). "Hyperglycemia impairs retinal oxygen autoregulation in normal and diabetic dogs." *Investigative ophthalmology & visual science* 24(7): 985-989.

Espinosa-Heidmann, D. G., M. E. Marin-Castano, S. Pereira-Simon, E. P. Hernandez, S. Elliot and S. W. Cousins (2005). "Gender and estrogen supplementation increases severity of experimental choroidal neovascularization." *Exp Eye Res* 80(3): 413-423.

Folkman, J. (1971). "Tumor angiogenesis: therapeutic implications." *N Engl J Med* 285(21): 1182-1186.

Folkman, J. (1995). "Angiogenesis in cancer, vascular, rheumatoid and other disease." *Nature medicine* 1(1): 27-31.

Fonseca, V. A., Ed. (2009). *Cardiovascular Endocrinology*. Contemporary Endocrinology. Totowa, NJ, Humana Press.

Forest, M. G. (1975). "Differentiation and development of the male." *Clinics in endocrinology and metabolism* 4(3): 569-596.

Gao, G., Y. Li, D. Zhang, S. Gee, C. Crosson and J. Ma (2001). "Unbalanced expression of VEGF and PEDF in ischemia-induced retinal neovascularization." *FEBS Lett* 489(2-3): 270-276.

Giddabasappa, A., M. Bauler, M. Yepuru, E. Chaum, J. T. Dalton and J. Eswaraka (2010). "17-beta estradiol protects ARPE-19 cells from oxidative stress through estrogen receptor-beta." *Invest Ophthalmol Vis Sci* 51(10): 5278-5287.

Grigsby, J. G., K. Parvathaneni, M. A. Almanza, A. M. Botello, A. A. Mondragon, D. M. Allen and A. T. Tsin (2011). "Effects of tamoxifen versus raloxifene on retinal capillary endothelial cell proliferation." *Journal of ocular pharmacology and therapeutics : the official journal of the Association for Ocular Pharmacology and Therapeutics* 27(3): 225-233.

Grunwald, J. E., C. E. Riva, A. J. Brucker, S. H. Sinclair and B. L. Petrig (1984). "Altered retinal vascular response to 100% oxygen breathing in diabetes mellitus." *Ophthalmology* 91(12): 1447-1452.

Grunwald, J. E., C. E. Riva, B. L. Petrig, A. J. Brucker, S. S. Schwartz, S. N. Braunstein, S. Grunwald (1995). "Strict control of glycaemia: effects on blood flow in the large retinal vessels and in the macular microcirculation." *The British journal of ophthalmology* 79(8): 735-741.

Gupta, P. D., K. Johar, Sr., K. Nagpal and A. R. Vasavada (2005). "Sex hormone receptors in the human eye." *Surv Ophthalmol* 50(3): 274-284.

Haffner, S. M., D. Fong, M. P. Stern, J. A. Pugh, H. P. Hazuda, J. K. Patterson, R. Klein (1988). "Diabetic retinopathy in Mexican Americans and non-Hispanic whites." *Diabetes* 37(7): 878-884.

Hak, A. E., J. C. Witteman, F. H. de Jong, M. I. Geerlings, A. Hofman and H. A. Pols (2002). "Low levels of endogenous androgens increase the risk of atherosclerosis in elderly men: the Rotterdam study." *The Journal of clinical endocrinology and metabolism* 87(8): 3632-3639.

Hall, A. P. (2006). "Review of the pericyte during angiogenesis and its role in cancer and diabetic retinopathy." *Toxicologic pathology* 34(6): 763-775.

Hammes, H. P. (2005). "Pericytes and the pathogenesis of diabetic retinopathy." *Hormone and metabolic research = Hormon- und Stoffwechselforschung = Hormones et metabolisme* 37 Suppl 1: 39-43.

Hammes, H. P. and M. Porta (2010). Experimental Approaches to Diabetic Retinopathy. Basal, Switzerland, Karger.

Hulley, S., D. Grady, T. Bush, C. Furberg, D. Herrington, B. Riggs and E. Vittinghoff (1998). "Randomized trial of estrogen plus progestin for secondary prevention of coronary heart disease in postmenopausal women. Heart and Estrogen/progestin Replacement Study (HERS) Research Group." *JAMA : the journal of the American Medical Association* 280(7): 605-613.

Imperato-McGinley, J. and W. J. Canovatchel (1992). "Complete androgen insensitivity Pathophysiology, diagnosis, and management." *Trends in endocrinology and metabolism: TEM* 3(3): 75-81.

Janfaza, M., T. I. Sherman, K. A. Larmore, J. Brown-Dawson and K. O. Klein (2006). "Estradiol levels and secretory dynamics in normal girls and boys as determined by an ultrasensitive bioassay: a 10 year experience." *Journal of pediatric endocrinology & metabolism : JPEM* 19(7): 901-909.

Janka, H. U., J. H. Warram, L. I. Rand and A. S. Krolewski (1989). "Risk factors for progression of background retinopathy in long-standing IDDM." *Diabetes* 38(4): 460-464.

Jensen, E. V. (1962). "On the mechanism of estrogen action." *Perspect Biol Med* 6: 47-59.

Jovanovic-Peterson, L. and C. M. Peterson (1991). "Diabetic retinopathy." *Clinical obstetrics and gynecology* 34(3): 516-525.

Kaushik, M., S. P. Sontineni and C. Hunter (2010). "Cardiovascular disease and androgens: a review." *International journal of cardiology* 142(1): 8-14.

Kazi, A. A., K. H. Molitoris and R. D. Koos (2009). "Estrogen rapidly activates the PI3K/AKT pathway and hypoxia-inducible factor 1 and induces vascular endothelial growth factor A expression in luminal epithelial cells of the rat uterus." *Biology of reproduction* 81(2): 378-387.

Kernell, A., I. Dedorsson, B. Johansson, C. P. Wickstrom, J. Ludvigsson, T. Tuvemo, G. Dahlquist (1997). "Prevalence of diabetic retinopathy in children and adolescents with IDDM. A population-based multicentre study." *Diabetologia* 40(3): 307-310.

Klein, B. E., S. E. Moss and R. Klein (1990). "Effect of pregnancy on progression of diabetic retinopathy." *Diabetes Care* 13(1): 34-40.

Klein, B. E., S. E. Moss and R. Klein (1990). "Oral contraceptives in women with diabetes." *Diabetes Care* 13(8): 895-898.

Klein, B. E., S. E. Moss, R. Klein and T. S. Surawicz (1991). "The Wisconsin Epidemiologic Study of Diabetic Retinopathy. XIII. Relationship of serum cholesterol to retinopathy and hard exudate." *Ophthalmology* 98(8): 1261-1265.

Klein, R., B. E. Klein, S. E. Moss and K. J. Cruickshanks (1994). "The Wisconsin Epidemiologic Study of diabetic retinopathy. XIV. Ten-year incidence and progression of diabetic retinopathy." *Arch Ophthalmol* 112(9): 1217-1228.

Klein, R., M. D. Knudtson, K. E. Lee, R. Gangnon and B. E. Klein (2008). "The Wisconsin Epidemiologic Study of Diabetic Retinopathy: XXII the twenty-five-year progression of retinopathy in persons with type 1 diabetes." *Ophthalmology* 115(11): 1859-1868.

Klein, R., K. E. Lee, R. E. Gangnon and B. E. Klein (2010). "The 25-year incidence of visual impairment in type 1 diabetes mellitus the wisconsin epidemiologic study of diabetic retinopathy." *Ophthalmology* 117(1): 63-70.

Knuiman, M. W., T. A. Welborn, V. J. McCann, K. G. Stanton and I. J. Constable (1986). "Prevalence of diabetic complications in relation to risk factors." *Diabetes* 35(12): 1332-1339.

Kobayashi, K., H. Kobayashi, M. Ueda and Y. Honda (1997). "Expression of 17 beta-hydroxysteroid dehydrogenase type IV in chick retinal pigment epithelium." *Experimental eye research* 64(5): 719-726.

Kostraba, J. N., J. S. Dorman, T. J. Orchard, D. J. Becker, Y. Ohki, D. Ellis, A. L. Drash (1989). "Contribution of diabetes duration before puberty to development of microvascular complications in IDDM subjects." *Diabetes Care* 12(10): 686-693.

Krolewski, A. S., J. H. Warram, L. I. Rand, A. R. Christlieb, E. J. Busick and C. R. Kahn (1986). "Risk of Proliferative Diabetic Retinopathy in Juvenile-Onset Type 1 Diabetes: A 40-yr. Follow-up Study." *Diabetes Care* 9(5): 443-452.

Lacassagne, A. (1936). "Hormonal pathogenesis of adenocarcinoma of the breast." *American Journal of Cancer* 27: 217-225.

Larinkari, J., L. Laatikainen, T. Ranta, P. Moronen, K. Pesonen and T. Laatikainen (1982). "Metabolic control and serum hormone levels in relation to retinopathy in diabetic pregnancy." *Diabetologia* 22(5): 327-332.

Lee, J. S., B. Ettinger, F. Z. Stanczyk, E. Vittinghoff, V. Hanes, J. A. Cauley, S. R. Cummings (2006). "Comparison of methods to measure low serum estradiol levels in postmenopausal women." *The Journal of clinical endocrinology and metabolism* 91(10): 3791-3797.

Levin, E. R. and S. R. Hammes, Eds. (2011). *Estrogens and Progestins*. The Pharmacological Basis of Therapeutics. New York, McGraw-Hill.

Liu, J., S. Wu, H. Wei, K. Zhou, Y. Ruan and W. Lai (2002). "Effects of sex hormones and their balance on the proliferation of rat vascular endothelial cells." *Hormone research* 58(1): 16-20.

Lloyd, C. E., R. Klein, R. E. Maser, L. H. Kuller, D. J. Becker and T. J. Orchard (1995). "The progression of retinopathy over 2 years: the Pittsburgh Epidemiology of Diabetes Complications (EDC) Study." *Journal of diabetes and its complications* 9(3): 140-148.

Love, R. R. and J. Philips (2002). "Oophorectomy for breast cancer: history revisited." *J Natl Cancer Inst* 94(19): 1433-1434.

Manni, A. and M. Verderame, Eds. (2002). *Selective Estrogen Receptor Modulators: Research and Clinical Applications*. Totowa, New Jersey, Humana Press.

Marin-Castano, M. E., S. J. Elliot, M. Potier, M. Karl, L. J. Striker, G. E. Striker, S. W. Cousins (2003). "Regulation of estrogen receptors and MMP-2 expression by estrogens in human retinal pigment epithelium." *Investigative ophthalmology & visual science* 44(1): 50-59.

Marquez, D. C. and R. J. Pietras (2001). "Membrane-associated binding sites for estrogen contribute to growth regulation of human breast cancer cells." *Oncogene* 20(39): 5420-5430.

McCrohon, J. A., W. Jessup, D. J. Handelsman and D. S. Celermajer (1999). "Androgen exposure increases human monocyte adhesion to vascular endothelium and endothelial cell expression of vascular cell adhesion molecule-1." *Circulation* 99(17): 2317-2322.

Mendelsohn, M. E. (2002). "Genomic and nongenomic effects of estrogen in the vasculature." *The American journal of cardiology* 90(1A): 3F-6F.

Mendelsohn, M. E. and R. H. Karas (2005). "Molecular and cellular basis of cardiovascular gender differences." *Science* 308(5728): 1583-1587.

Merimee, T. J. (1990). "Diabetic retinopathy. A synthesis of perspectives." *N Engl J Med* 322(14): 978-983.

Miyamoto, K., S. Khosrof, S. E. Bursell, R. Rohan, T. Murata, A. C. Clermont, A. P. Adamis (1999). "Prevention of leukostasis and vascular leakage in streptozotocin-induced diabetic retinopathy via intercellular adhesion molecule-1 inhibition." *Proceedings of the National Academy of Sciences of the United States of America* 96(19): 10836-10841.

Moloney, J. B. and M. I. Drury (1982). "The effect of pregnancy on the natural course of diabetic retinopathy." *American journal of ophthalmology* 93(6): 745-756.

Mueller, M. D., J. L. Vigne, A. Minchenko, D. I. Lebovic, D. C. Leitman and R. N. Taylor (2000). "Regulation of vascular endothelial growth factor (VEGF) gene transcription by estrogen receptors alpha and beta." *Proc Natl Acad Sci U S A* 97(20): 10972-10977.

Mukherjee, T. K., H. Dinh, G. Chaudhuri and L. Nathan (2002). "Testosterone attenuates expression of vascular cell adhesion molecule-1 by conversion to estradiol by aromatase in endothelial cells: implications in atherosclerosis." *Proceedings of the National Academy of Sciences of the United States of America* 99(6): 4055-4060.

Mumford, S. L., S. Dasharathy, A. Z. Pollack and E. Schisterman, F. (2011). "Variations in lipid levels according to menstrual cycle phase: clinical implications." *Clinical Lipidology* April: 225-235.

Murphy, R. P., M. Nanda, L. Plotnick, C. Enger, S. Vitale and A. Patz (1990). "The Relationship of Puberty to Diabetic Retinopathy." *Archives of Ophthalmology* 108(2): 215-218.

Namperumalsamy, P., R. Kim, T. P. Vignesh, N. Nithya, J. Royes, T. Gijo, V. Vijayakumar (2009). "Prevalence and risk factors for diabetic retinopathy: a population-based assessment from Theni District, south India." *The British journal of ophthalmology* 93(4): 429-434.

Nanda, S., N. Gupta, H. C. Mehta and K. Sangwan (2003). "Effect of oestrogen replacement therapy on serum lipid profile." *The Australian & New Zealand journal of obstetrics & gynaecology* 43(3): 213-216.

Nelson, R. G., J. A. Wolfe, M. B. Horton, D. J. Pettitt, P. H. Bennett and W. C. Knowler (1989). "Proliferative retinopathy in NIDDM. Incidence and risk factors in Pima Indians." *Diabetes* 38(4): 435-440.

Nishikawa, T., D. Edelstein, X. L. Du, S. Yamagishi, T. Matsumura, Y. Kaneda, M. Brownlee (2000). "Normalizing mitochondrial superoxide production blocks three pathways of hyperglycaemic damage." *Nature* 404(6779): 787-790.

Ogueta, S. B., S. D. Schwartz, C. K. Yamashita and D. B. Farber (1999). "Estrogen receptor in the human eye: influence of gender and age on gene expression." *Invest Ophthalmol Vis Sci* 40(9): 1906-1911.

Ohtsuki, S., M. Tomi, T. Hata, Y. Nagai, S. Hori, S. Mori, T. Terasaki (2005). "Dominant expression of androgen receptors and their functional regulation of organic anion transporter 3 in rat brain capillary endothelial cells; comparison of gene expression between the blood-brain and -retinal barriers." *Journal of cellular physiology* 204(3): 896-900.

Olsen, B. S., A. K. Sjolie, P. Hougaard, J. Johannesen, K. Marinelli, B. B. Jacobsen and H. B. Mortensen (2004). "The significance of the prepubertal diabetes duration for the development of retinopathy and nephropathy in patients with type 1 diabetes." *J Diabetes Complications* 18(3): 160-164.

Orshal, J. M. and R. A. Khalil (2004). "Gender, sex hormones, and vascular tone." *American journal of physiology. Regulatory, integrative and comparative physiology* 286(2): R233-249.

Osborne, C. K., H. Zhao and S. A. Fuqua (2000). "Selective estrogen receptor modulators: structure, function, and clinical use." *J Clin Oncol* 18(17): 3172-3186.

Pettersson, K., K. Grandien, G. G. Kuiper and J. A. Gustafsson (1997). "Mouse estrogen receptor beta forms estrogen response element-binding heterodimers with estrogen receptor alpha." *Mol Endocrinol* 11(10): 1486-1496.

Pieber, D., V. C. Allport, F. Hills, M. Johnson and P. R. Bennett (2001). "Interactions between progesterone receptor isoforms in myometrial cells in human labour." *Molecular human reproduction* 7(9): 875-879.

Porta, M., P. Dalmasso, G. Grassi, S. Marena, M. Maurino, P. Passera and M. Trento (2004). "Pre-pubertal onset of type 1 diabetes and appearance of retinopathy." *Diabetes Metab* 30(3): 229-233.

Porta, M., A. K. Sjoelie, N. Chaturvedi, L. Stevens, R. Rottiers, M. Veglio and J. H. Fuller (2001). "Risk factors for progression to proliferative diabetic retinopathy in the EURODIAB Prospective Complications Study." *Diabetologia* 44(12): 2203-2209.

Prabhu, A., Q. Xu, M. B. Manigrasso, M. Biswas, E. Flynn, R. Iliescu, C. Maric (2010). "Expression of aromatase, androgen and estrogen receptors in peripheral target tissues in diabetes." *Steroids* 75(11): 779-787.

Qi, Z., C. M. Hao, R. I. Langenbach, R. M. Breyer, R. Redha, J. D. Morrow and M. D. Breyer (2002). "Opposite effects of cyclooxygenase-1 and -2 activity on the pressor response to angiotensin II." *The Journal of clinical investigation* 110(1): 61-69.

Raman, R., K. Vaitheeswaran, K. Vinita and T. Sharma (2011). "Is prevalence of retinopathy related to the age of onset of diabetes? Sankara Nethralaya Diabetic Retinopathy

Epidemiology and Molecular Genetic Report No. 5." *Ophthalmic research* 45(1): 36-41.

Rand, L. I., A. S. Krolewski, L. M. Aiello, J. H. Warram, R. S. Baker and T. Maki (1985). "Multiple factors in the prediction of risk of proliferative diabetic retinopathy." *The New England journal of medicine* 313(23): 1433-1438.

Rassam, S. M., V. Patel and E. M. Kohner (1995). "The effect of experimental hypertension on retinal vascular autoregulation in humans: a mechanism for the progression of diabetic retinopathy." *Experimental physiology* 80(1): 53-68.

Rocha, E. M., L. A. Wickham, L. A. da Silveira, K. L. Krenzer, F. S. Yu, I. Toda, D. A. Sullivan (2000). "Identification of androgen receptor protein and 5alpha-reductase mRNA in human ocular tissues." *The British journal of ophthalmology* 84(1): 76-84.

Rosenn, B., M. Miodovnik, G. Kranias, J. Khoury, C. A. Combs, F. Mimouni, M. J. Lipman (1992). "Progression of diabetic retinopathy in pregnancy: association with hypertension in pregnancy." *American journal of obstetrics and gynecology* 166(4): 1214-1218.

Rossouw, J. E., G. L. Anderson, R. L. Prentice, A. Z. LaCroix, C. Kooperberg, M. L. Stefanick, J. Ockene (2002). "Risks and benefits of estrogen plus progestin in healthy postmenopausal women: principal results From the Women's Health Initiative randomized controlled trial." *JAMA : the journal of the American Medical Association* 288(3): 321-333.

Rubanyi, G. M. and R. Kauffman, Eds. (1998). *Estrogen and the Vessel Wall*. The Endothelial Cell Research Series. Amsterdam, Harwood Academic Publishers.

Salyer, D. L., T. D. Lund, D. E. Fleming, E. D. Lephart and T. L. Horvath (2001). "Sexual dimorphism and aromatase in the rat retina." *Brain research. Developmental brain research* 126(1): 131-136.

Schocket, L. S., J. E. Grunwald, A. F. Tsang and J. DuPont (1999). "The effect of pregnancy on retinal hemodynamics in diabetic versus nondiabetic mothers." *American journal of ophthalmology* 128(4): 477-484.

Shibata, H., T. E. Spencer, S. A. Onate, G. Jenster, S. Y. Tsai, M. J. Tsai and B. W. O'Malley (1997). "Role of co-activators and co-repressors in the mechanism of steroid/thyroid receptor action." *Recent Prog Horm Res* 52: 141-164; discussion 164-145.

Simoncini, T., R. De Caterina and A. R. Genazzani (1999). "Selective estrogen receptor modulators: different actions on vascular cell adhesion molecule-1 (VCAM-1) expression in human endothelial cells." *The Journal of clinical endocrinology and metabolism* 84(2): 815-818.

Simoncini, T., A. Hafezi-Moghadam, D. P. Brazil, K. Ley, W. W. Chin and J. K. Liao (2000). "Interaction of oestrogen receptor with the regulatory subunit of phosphatidylinositol-3-OH kinase." *Nature* 407(6803): 538-541.

Smith, C. L. and B. W. O'Malley (2004). "Coregulator function: a key to understanding tissue specificity of selective receptor modulators." *Endocr Rev* 25(1): 45-71.

Smith, T. S., J. Szetu and R. R. Bourne (2007). "The prevalence and severity of diabetic retinopathy, associated risk factors and vision loss in patients registered with type 2 diabetes in Luganville, Vanuatu." *The British journal of ophthalmology* 91(4): 415-419.

Sone, H., Y. Okuda, Y. Kawakami, S. Kondo, M. Hanatani, K. Matsuo, K. Yamashita (1996). "Progesterone induces vascular endothelial growth factor on retinal pigment epithelial cells in culture." *Life Sci* 59(1): 21-25.

Suzuma, I., M. Mandai, H. Takagi, K. Suzuma, A. Otani, H. Oh, Y. Honda (1999). "17 Beta-estradiol increases VEGF receptor-2 and promotes DNA synthesis in retinal microvascular endothelial cells." *Invest Ophthalmol Vis Sci* 40(9): 2122-2129.

Svensson, M., J. W. Eriksson and G. Dahlquist (2004). "Early glycemic control, age at onset, and development of microvascular complications in childhood-onset type 1 diabetes: a population-based study in northern Sweden." *Diabetes Care* 27(4): 955-962.

Szabo, A. J., A. G. Stewart and G. E. Joron (1967). "Factors associated with increased prevalence of diabetic retinopathy: a clinical survey." *Canadian Medical Association journal* 97(6): 286-292.

Takenaka, K., S. Yamagishi, Y. Jinnouchi, K. Nakamura, T. Matsui and T. Imaizumi (2005). "Pigment epithelium-derived factor (PEDF)-induced apoptosis and inhibition of vascular endothelial growth factor (VEGF) expression in MG63 human osteosarcoma cells." *Life Sci* 77(25): 3231-3241.

Tamoxifen. (2007). "Drugs @ FDA: U.S. Food and Drug Administration Web site." Retrieved 2010, from http://www.accessdata.fda.gov/scripts/cder/drugsatfda/index.cfm?fuseaction=Search.Label_ApprovalHistory#apphist.

Tanaka, N., H. Yonekura, S. Yamagishi, H. Fujimori, Y. Yamamoto and H. Yamamoto (2000). "The receptor for advanced glycation end products is induced by the glycation products themselves and tumor necrosis factor-alpha through nuclear factor-kappa B, and by 17beta-estradiol through Sp-1 in human vascular endothelial cells." *The Journal of biological chemistry* 275(33): 25781-25790.

Tanemura, M., N. Miyamoto, M. Mandai, H. Kamizuru, S. Ooto, T. Yasukawa, Y. Honda (2004). "The role of estrogen and estrogen receptor beta in choroidal neovascularization." *Mol Vis* 10: 923-932.

Tapp, R. J., P. Z. Zimmet, C. A. Harper, D. J. McCarty, P. Chitson, A. M. Tonkin, J. E. Shaw (2006). "Six year incidence and progression of diabetic retinopathy: results from the Mauritius diabetes complication study." *Diabetes Res Clin Pract* 73(3): 298-303.

The Diabetes Control and Complications Trial Group (1993). "The Diabetes Control and Complications Trial." *N Engl J Med* 329(14): 977-986.

Thompson, J. and R. A. Khalil (2003). "Gender differences in the regulation of vascular tone." *Clinical and experimental pharmacology & physiology* 30(1-2): 1-15.

Thorneycroft, I. H., D. R. Mishell, Jr., S. C. Stone, K. M. Kharma and R. M. Nakamura (1971). "The relation of serum 17-hydroxyprogesterone and estradiol-17-beta levels during the human menstrual cycle." *American journal of obstetrics and gynecology* 111(7): 947-951.

Tombran-Tink, J., G. G. Chader and L. V. Johnson (1991). "PEDF: a pigment epithelium-derived factor with potent neuronal differentiative activity." *Exp Eye Res* 53(3): 411-414.

Tombran-Tink, J. and L. V. Johnson (1989). "Neuronal differentiation of retinoblastoma cells induced by medium conditioned by human RPE cells." *Invest Ophthalmol Vis Sci* 30(8): 1700-1707.

UK Prospective Diabetes Study Group (1998). "Tight blood pressure control and risk of macrovascular and microvascular complications in type 2 diabetes: UKPDS 38. UK Prospective Diabetes Study Group." *BMJ* 317(7160): 703-713.

Vargas, R., J. T. Repke and S. H. Ural (2010). "Type 1 diabetes mellitus and pregnancy." *Reviews in obstetrics and gynecology* 3(3): 92-100.

Varma, R., G. L. Macias, M. Torres, R. Klein, F. Y. Pena and S. P. Azen (2007). "Biologic risk factors associated with diabetic retinopathy: the Los Angeles Latino Eye Study." *Ophthalmology* 114(7): 1332-1340.

Vazquez, F., J. C. Rodriguez-Manzaneque, J. P. Lydon, D. P. Edwards, B. W. O'Malley and M. L. Iruela-Arispe (1999). "Progesterone regulates proliferation of endothelial cells." *The Journal of biological chemistry* 274(4): 2185-2192.

Vidro, E. K., S. Gee, R. Unda, J. X. Ma and A. Tsin (2008). "Glucose and TGFbeta2 modulate the viability of cultured human retinal pericytes and their VEGF release." *Current eye research* 33(11): 984-993.

Villablanca, A. C., M. Jayachandran and C. Banka (2010). "Atherosclerosis and sex hormones: current concepts." *Clinical science* 119(12): 493-513.

Vitale, C., M. Fini, G. Speziale and S. Chierchia (2010). "Gender differences in the cardiovascular effects of sex hormones." *Fundamental & clinical pharmacology* 24(6): 675-685.

Wang, F. H., Y. B. Liang, F. Zhang, J. J. Wang, W. B. Wei, Q. S. Tao, T. Y. Wong (2009). "Prevalence of diabetic retinopathy in rural China: the Handan Eye Study." *Ophthalmology* 116(3): 461-467.

Webb, C. M. and P. Collins (2010). "Testosterone and coronary artery disease in men." *Maturitas* 67(1): 15-19.

Webb, P., P. Nguyen, J. Shinsako, C. Anderson, W. Feng, M. P. Nguyen, P. J. Kushner (1998). "Estrogen receptor activation function 1 works by binding p160 coactivator proteins." *Mol Endocrinol* 12(10): 1605-1618.

Wickham, L. A., J. Gao, I. Toda, E. M. Rocha, M. Ono and D. A. Sullivan (2000). "Identification of androgen, estrogen and progesterone receptor mRNAs in the eye." *Acta ophthalmologica Scandinavica* 78(2): 146-153.

Wilson, J. D., D. W. Foster, H. M. Kronenberg and P. R. Larsen, Eds. (1998). *Williams Textbook of Endocrinology*. Toronto, Ontario Canada, W.B. Saunders.

Wong, T. Y., N. Cheung, W. T. Tay, J. J. Wang, T. Aung, S. M. Saw, P. Mitchell (2008). "Prevalence and risk factors for diabetic retinopathy: the Singapore Malay Eye Study." *Ophthalmology* 115(11): 1869-1875.

Wong, T. Y., R. Klein, F. M. Islam, M. F. Cotch, A. R. Folsom, B. E. Klein, S. Shea (2006). "Diabetic retinopathy in a multi-ethnic cohort in the United States." *American journal of ophthalmology* 141(3): 446-455.

Wu, F. C. and A. von Eckardstein (2003). "Androgens and coronary artery disease." *Endocrine reviews* 24(2): 183-217.

Wu, M. V., D. S. Manoli, E. J. Fraser, J. K. Coats, J. Tollkuhn, S. Honda, N. M. Shah (2009). "Estrogen masculinizes neural pathways and sex-specific behaviors." *Cell* 139(1): 61-72.

Wynne, F. L. and R. A. Khalil (2003). "Testosterone and coronary vascular tone: implications in coronary artery disease." *Journal of endocrinological investigation* 26(2): 181-186.

Zhang, J. J., T. J. Jacob, M. A. Valverde, S. P. Hardy, G. M. Mintenig, F. V. Sepulveda, C. F. Higgins (1994). "Tamoxifen blocks chloride channels. A possible mechanism for cataract formation." *J Clin Invest* 94(4): 1690-1697.

Permissions

The contributors of this book come from diverse backgrounds, making this book a truly international effort. This book will bring forth new frontiers with its revolutionizing research information and detailed analysis of the nascent developments around the world.

We would like to thank Mohammad Shamsul Ola, for lending his expertise to make the book truly unique. He has played a crucial role in the development of this book. Without his invaluable contribution this book wouldn't have been possible. He has made vital efforts to compile up to date information on the varied aspects of this subject to make this book a valuable addition to the collection of many professionals and students.

This book was conceptualized with the vision of imparting up-to-date information and advanced data in this field. To ensure the same, a matchless editorial board was set up. Every individual on the board went through rigorous rounds of assessment to prove their worth. After which they invested a large part of their time researching and compiling the most relevant data for our readers. Conferences and sessions were held from time to time between the editorial board and the contributing authors to present the data in the most comprehensible form. The editorial team has worked tirelessly to provide valuable and valid information to help people across the globe.

Every chapter published in this book has been scrutinized by our experts. Their significance has been extensively debated. The topics covered herein carry significant findings which will fuel the growth of the discipline. They may even be implemented as practical applications or may be referred to as a beginning point for another development. Chapters in this book were first published by InTech; hereby published with permission under the Creative Commons Attribution License or equivalent.

The editorial board has been involved in producing this book since its inception. They have spent rigorous hours researching and exploring the diverse topics which have resulted in the successful publishing of this book. They have passed on their knowledge of decades through this book. To expedite this challenging task, the publisher supported the team at every step. A small team of assistant editors was also appointed to further simplify the editing procedure and attain best results for the readers.

Our editorial team has been hand-picked from every corner of the world. Their multi-ethnicity adds dynamic inputs to the discussions which result in innovative outcomes. These outcomes are then further discussed with the researchers and contributors who give their valuable feedback and opinion regarding the same. The feedback is then collaborated with the researches and they are edited in a comprehensive manner to aid the understanding of the subject.

Apart from the editorial board, the designing team has also invested a significant amount of their time in understanding the subject and creating the most relevant covers. They scrutinized every image to scout for the most suitable representation of the subject and create an appropriate cover for the book.

The publishing team has been involved in this book since its early stages. They were actively engaged in every process, be it collecting the data, connecting with the contributors or procuring relevant information. The team has been an ardent support to the editorial, designing and production team. Their endless efforts to recruit the best for this project, has resulted in the accomplishment of this book. They are a veteran in the field of academics and their pool of knowledge is as vast as their experience in printing. Their expertise and guidance has proved useful at every step. Their uncompromising quality standards have made this book an exceptional effort. Their encouragement from time to time has been an inspiration for everyone.

The publisher and the editorial board hope that this book will prove to be a valuable piece of knowledge for researchers, students, practitioners and scholars across the globe.

List of Contributors

Carlos César Lopes De Jesus
Federal University of Sao Paulo, Sao Paulo, Brazil

Mohd Wajid Ali Khan
I3-IRG, Department of Immunity, Infection and Biochemistry, Medical School of Cardiff, Cardiff University, Cardiff, United Kingdom

Kamalpreet Banga
School of Public Health, University of Saskatchewan, Health Sciences Building, Saskatoon, Canada

Wahid Ali Khan
Department of Clinical Biochemistry, College of Medicine and Medical Science, King Khalid University, Abha, Kingdom of Saudi Arabia

Mohammad Shamsul Ola and Mohd Imtiaz Nawaz
Department of Ophthalmology, College of Medicine, King Saud University, Riyadh, KSA

Yoshiyuki Kubo and Ken-ichi Hosoya
University of Toyama, Japan

Byung Joo Lee and Jeong Hun Kim
Fight against Angiogenesis-Related Blindness (FARB) Laboratory, Seoul Artificial Eye Center Clinical Research Institute, Seoul National University Hospital, Republic of Korea
Department of Ophthalmology, College of Medicine, Seoul National University, Republic of Korea

Shigeo Yoshida, Keijiro Ishikawa, Mitsuru Arima, Ryo Asato, Yukio Sassa and Tatsuro Ishibashi
Department of Ophthalmology, Kyushu University Graduate School of Medical Sciences, Fukuoka, Japan

Katarzyna Zorena, Dorota Raczyńska and Krystyna Raczyńska
Medical University of Gdańsk, Poland

Hongbin Lü
Department of Ophthalmology, Affiliated Hospital of Luzhou Medical College, Sichuan Province, China

Ying Yang, Ying Zhang and Yiping Li
Department of Endocrinology and Metabolism, Yunnan Province 2nd Hospital, Kunming, PR China

Christina Antonopoulos and Manju Subramanian
Boston University School of Medicine, USA

Desislava Koleva-Georgieva
University Eye Clinic, University Hospital"St. George", Plovdiv, Bulgaria

Zvia Burgansky-Eliash
Department of Ophthalmology, The Edith Wolfson Medical Center, Holon, Sackler Faculty of Medicine, Tel-Aviv University, Israel

C. Mariño, J. Novo, N. Barreira and M.G. Penedo
University of A Coruña, Spain

Akihiro Kakehashi
Department of Ophthalmology, Jichi Medical University, Saitama Medical Center, Saitama, Japan

Ayumi Ota, Fumihiko Toyoda, Nozomi Kinoshita, Hiroko Yamagami and Hiroto Obata
Department of Ophthalmology, Jichi Medical University, Saitama Medical Center, Japan

Takafumi Matsumoto and Junichi Tsuji
Pharmacology Research Laboratories, Dainippon Sumitomo Pharma Co. Ltd., Japan

Yoh Dobashi, Wilfred Y. Fujimoto, Masanobu Kawakami and Yasunori Kanazawa
Department of Integrated Medicine I, Jichi Medical University, Saitama Medical Center, Japan

Wilfred Y. Fujimoto
Division of Metabolism, Endocrinology and Nutrition, University of Washington School of Medicine, Seattle, WA, USA

Yeon Sung Moon and Na Rae Kim
Inha University School of Medicine, Korea

Oldřich Farsa
Faculty of Pharmacy, University of Veterinary and Pharmaceutical Sciences Brno, Czech Republic

Jeffery G. Grigsby, Kalpana Parvathaneni, Brandi S. Betts and Andrew T.C. Tsin
Department of Biology, University of Texas at San Antonio, San Antonio, Texas, United States of America

Donald M. Allen
Department of Biology, University of Texas of the Permian Basin, Odessa, Texas, United States of America

Richard B. Culbert
Department of Surgery, Texas Tech School of Medicine, Midland, Texas, United States of America

Richard B. Culbert and Gerardo Escobedo
Premier Retina Specialists, Midland, Texas, United States of America